FAMILY MEDICINE CERTIFICATION REVIEW

Second Edition

FAMILY MEDICINE CERTIFICATION REVIEW

Second Edition

Editors

Martin S. Lipsky, MD
Regional Dean
University of Illinois College of Medicine at
Rockford
Rockford, Illinois

Mitchell S. King, MD
Associate Professor of Family Medicine
Associate Dean for Academic Affairs
University of Illinois College of Medicine at
Rockford
Rockford, Illinois

Jeffrey L. Susman, MD
Editor-in-Chief, Journal of Family Practice
Medical Editor, AAFP Home Study Monographs
Fred Lazarus Jr. Professor and Chairman
Department of Family Medicine
University of Cincinnati
Cincinnati, Ohio

Robert W. Bales, MD, MPH
Assistant Clinical Professor
University Primary Care Clinic
Mt. Morris, Illinois

Matthew L. Hunsaker, MD
Director, Rural Medical Education Program (RMED)
National Center for Rural Health Professions
Assistant Professor of Family Medicine
University of Illinois College of Medicine at Rockford
Rockford, Illinois

 Wolters Kluwer | Lippincott Williams & Wilkins
Health
Philadelphia • Baltimore • New York • London
Buenos Aires • Hong Kong • Sydney • Tokyo

Acquisitions Editor: Sonya Seigafuse
Developmental Editor: Rebecca Barroso
Managing Editor: Nancy Winter
Manufacturing Coordinator: Kathleen Brown
Marketing Manager: Kimberly Schonberger
Creative Director: Doug Smock
Production Services: GGS Book Services
Printer: Data Reproductions Corporation

© 2007 by Martin S. Lipsky

530 Walnut Street
Philadelphia, PA 19106 USA
LWW.com

First edition, © 2005 Lippincott Williams & Wilkins

The publisher is not responsible (as a matter of product liability, negligence, or otherwise) for any injury resulting from any material contained herein. This publication contains information relating to general principles of medical care that should not be construed as specific instructions for individual patients. Manufacturers' product information and package inserts should be reviewed for current information, including contradictions, dosages, and precautions.

Printed in the USA

Library of Congress Cataloging-in-Publication Data
Family medicine certification review / editors, Martin S. Lipsky . . .
[et al.]. — 2nd ed.
    p. ; cm.
  Includes index.
  ISBN 13: 978-1-4051-0505-7
  ISBN 10: 1-4051-0505-4
  1. Family medicine--Examinations, questions, etc. I. Lipsky, Martin S.
  [DNLM: 1. Family Practice—Examination Questions.   2. Physicians,
Family—Examination Questions. WB 18.2 F1976 2007]
  RC58.F335 2007
  610.76--dc22

                        2007003321

Care has been taken to confirm the accuracy of the information presented and to describe generally accepted practices. However, the authors, editors, and publisher are not responsible for errors or omissions or for any consequences from application of the information in this book and make no warranty, expressed or implied, with respect to the currency, completeness, or accuracy of the contents of the publication. Application of this information in a particular situation remains the professional responsibility of the practitioner.

The authors, editors, and publisher have exerted every effort to ensure that drug selection and dosage set forth in this text are in accordance with current recommendations and practice at the time of publication. However, in view of ongoing research, changes in government regulations, and the constant flow of information relating to drug therapy and drug reactions, the reader is urged to check the package insert for each drug for any change in indications and dosage and for added warnings and precautions. This is particularly important when the recommended agent is a new or infrequently employed drug.

Some drugs and medical devices presented in this publication have Food and Drug Administration (FDA) clearance for limited use in restricted research settings. It is the responsibility of the health care provider to ascertain the FDA status of each drug or device planned for use in their clinical practice.

To purchase additional copies of this book, call our customer service department at (800) 638-3030 or fax orders to (301) 223-2320. International customers should call (301) 223-2300.

Visit Lippincott Williams & Wilkins on the Internet: at LWW.com. Lippincott Williams & Wilkins customer service representatives are available from 8:30 am to 6:00 pm, EST.

10 9 8 7 6 5 4 3 2 1

Preface

There are many reasons why the editors of this book are proud to be family physicians. Among these reasons is that family medicine was the first discipline to require recertification to maintain specialty certification. Although subsequently many other disciplines have fallen in step and require recertification, we are pleased that family medicine developed this standard.

Despite our enthusiasm for recertification and its role in maintaining current competency, no one of us looks forward to having his or her own re-examination packet arrive in the mail. All of the editors have faced this chilling moment and the feeling of not knowing where to start reviewing for a test that covers the breadth of material that defines family medicine. The goal of this book is to help candidates meet the challenge of successfully passing boards by providing a broad spectrum of questions and answers. The answer for each question is accompanied by an explanation that contains additional facts to augment an individual's review. The questions can also identify areas of weakness that can help direct further review. The second edition includes several new tables and charts to provide relevant information in a convenient and compact manner. We believe this book also provides a useful tool for students preparing for the USMLE Step III and for those individuals seeking a broad-based review book. The clinical set problems can also help students assess their clinical management skills and to learn more about the evaluation and management of several commonly encountered conditions.

The second edition of this book builds on the first edition. All the questions have been reviewed to make sure they are consistent with the latest information. For example, questions related to hypertension and lipids draw upon JNC-VII and ATP-III guidelines.

The questions are structured to match the content, complexity, and type of questions seen on the American Board of Family Medicine certifying examination and are divided into sections that match the subject categories on the exam. The allotment of questions to each category approximates the American Board of Family Medicine's published distribution of questions for each subject. In addition, 50 clinical set problems, which constitute a major portion of the exam, are provided.

As readers use this text, the editors welcome their thoughts and opinions. Please feel free to contact any of us either directly or through Lippincott Williams & Wilkins. We hope that you find this book useful in mastering the material required to pass the American Board of Family Medicine certifying exam.

Martin S. Lipsky, MD
Mitchell S. King, MD
Jeffrey L. Susman, MD
Robert W. Bales, MD
Matthew Hunsaker, MD

Editors/Contributors

EDITORS

Martin S. Lipsky, MD
Regional Dean
Professor of Family Medicine
University of Illinois College of Medicine at Rockford
Professor of Family Medicine
Rockford, Illinois

Mitchell S. King, MD
Associate Dean, Academic Affairs
Associate Professor
Department of Family Medicine
University of Illinois College of Medicine at Rockford
Rockford, Illinois

Jeffrey L. Susman, MD
Professor and Director (Chair)
Department of Family Medicine
University of Cincinnati
Cincinnati, Ohio

Robert W. Bales, MD, MPH
Assistant Professor of Family and Community Medicine
University of Illinois College of Medicine at Rockford
Rockford, Illinois

Matthew L. Hunsaker, MD, FAAFP
Director, Rural Medical Education Program, National Center for Rural Health Professions
Assistant Professor, Department of Family and Community Medicine
University of Illinois College of Medicine at Rockford
Rockford, Illinois

CONTRIBUTORS

Darice L. Zabak, MD
Assistant Professor Family Medicine
University of Illinois College of Medicine at Rockford
Staff Physician
Rockford Health Systems
Rockford, Illinois

Surgery

Joseph A. Greco, MD, FAAFP
Associate Director, Bryn Mawr Family Practice Residency Program
Bryn Mawr, Pennsylvania

Steve Growney, MD
Private practice, family medicine
Bryn Mawr, Pennsylvania

Stefana M. Pecher, MD
Bryn Mawr Family Medicine
Bryn Mawr, Pennsylvania

Obstetrics

Arpana Broor, MD
Visiting Clinical Assistant Professor
University of Illinois College of Medicine at Rockford
Department of Family and Community Medicine
Rockford, Illinois

Gynecology

Yachna Ahuja
Case Western Reserve University School of Medicine
Cleveland, Ohio

Justin C. Bohrer
Cleveland Clinic Lerner College of Medicine of
Case Western Reserve University
Cleveland, Ohio

Lynda G. Montgomery, MD, MEd
Assistant Professor of Family Medicine and
Director, Predoctoral Education
Division
Department of Family Medicine
Case Western Reserve University School of
Medicine
Cleveland, Ohio

Evelyn Morley Hemmingsen
Case Western Reserve University School of
Medicine
Cleveland, Ohio

Douglas A. Pepple
Case Western Reserve University School of
Medicine
Cleveland, Ohio

Jonah Stulberg
Case Western Reserve University School of
Medicine
Cleveland, Ohio

Christopher Tangen, DO
House Officer, Department of Family Medicine
Case Western Reserve University
Cleveland, Ohio

We thank the following individuals who contributed
questions and helped review the first edition of this
text:

John Affinito, MD
Clinical Instructor
Department of Family Medicine
Northwestern University Feinberg School of
Medicine
Chicago, Illinois
McGaw Family Practice Residency Program
Residency Faculty
Highland Park Hospital
Highland Park, Illinois

Siri Akal, MD
Assistant Professor/Assistant Residency
Director
University of Miami

Attending Physician
Jackson Memorial Hospital
Miami, Florida

Frederick Mitsu Anderson, MD
Resident
Department of Family Medicine
University of Miami
Miami, Florida

Albert J. Arias, MD
Resident Physician
Department of Psychiatry
University of Connecticut Health Center
Farmington, Connecticut

Orson J. Austin, MD
Associate Professor and Clinical Faculty
Department of Family Medicine
University of Cincinnati
Cincinnati, Ohio

Elizabeth Anne Baker, MD
Clinical Instructor
Advocate Health Care
Chicago, Illinois

Steve Bartz, MD, RPh
Assistant Professor of Family Medicine
University of Cincinnati
Cincinnati, Ohio

Shari J. Baum, MD
Private Practice
Mountain Island Urgent Care
Charlotte, North Carolina

Adam Bennett, MD
Fellow, Department of Family Medicine
Northwestern University Feinberg School of
Medicine
Chicago, Illinois

Kavitha Bhat Schelbert, MD
Clinical Assistant Professor
Department of Family Medicine
University of Iowa Hospitals and Clinics
Iowa City, Iowa

Linda Bigi, DO
Clinical Instructor
Department of Family Medicine

Northwestern University Feinberg School of
Medicine
Chicago, Illinois
Residency Faculty, McGaw Family Practice
Residency Program
Glenbrook Hospital
Glenview, Illinois

Thomas E. Bournias, MD
Assistant Professor of Clinical Ophthalmology
Department of Ophthalmology
Northwestern University Feinberg School of
Medicine;
Attending Physician
Northwestern Memorial Hospital
Chicago, Illinois

Saria Carter, MD
Resident
Department of Family Medicine
University of Miami School of Medicine
Miami, Florida

Laure DeMattia, DO
Chief Resident
Department of Family Medicine
McGaw Family Practice Residency Program of
Northwestern University
Glenview, Illinois

Kathleen Ann Downey, MD
Associate Professor of Family Medicine
University of Cincinnati
Cincinnati, Ohio

Patricia Evans, MD
Assistant Professor of Family Medicine
Georgetown University
Washington, DC

Brian Finley, MD
Associate Professor of Family Practice
University of Nebraska Medical Center
Omaha, Nebraska

Daniel S. Frank, MD
Resident
Department of Family Medicine
University of Miami School of Medicine
Miami, Florida

Janet F. Gick, MD
Assistant Professor

Clinton Memorial Hospital Family Practice
Residency
Wilmington, Ohio

Pepi Granat, MD
Clinical Professor
Department of Family Medicine
University of Miami School of Medicine
Miami, Florida

Amy E. Harrison, MD
Director of Women's Health Fellowship
MacNeal Family Practice Residency Program
Berwyn, Illinois

Julie Hobart, MD
Assistant Professor of Clinical Family Medicine
University of Cincinnati College of Medicine
Attending Family Physician
Mercy Hospital–Mt. Airy Campus
Cincinnati, Ohio

Keith B. Holten, MD
Associate Professor of Family Medicine
University of Cincinnati
Cincinnati, Ohio
Residency Director, Family Practice Residency
Program
CMH Regional Health System
Wilmington, Ohio

Julie Johnson Covin, MD
Resident
Department of Family Medicine
University of Miami School of Medicine
Miami, Florida

Mary Virginia Krueger, DO
Women's Health Coordinator
Department of Family Medicine
Madigan Army Medical Center
Fort Lewis, Washington

Kurt Kurowski, MD
Associate Professor, Department of Family
Medicine
Finch University of Health Sciences/The Chicago
Medical School
North Chicago, Illinois
Associate Director, Family Practice Residency
Swedish Covenant Hospital
Chicago, Illinois

Leslie Ann B. Mendoza, MD
Chief Resident
Department of Family Medicine
McGaw Medical Center Residency Program of
Northwestern University
Glenview, Illinois

Jory A. Natkin, DO, FAAFP
Clinical Instructor
Department of Family Medicine
Northwestern University Feinberg School of
Medicine
Chicago, Illinois
Residency Faculty–McGaw Medical Center
Glenbrook Hospital
Glenview, Illinois

Edward Onusko, MD
Associate Clinical Professor
Department of Family Medicine
University of Cincinnati
Cincinnati, Ohio

Maureen O'Hara Padden, MD, MPH, FAAFP
LCDR, MC, USN(FS)
Director of Residency Training
Family Medicine
Naval Hospital Camp Lejeune
Jacksonville, North Carolina

Layne A. Prest, PhD, IMFT
Associate Professor
Director of Behavioral Medicine
Department of Family Medicine
University of Nebraska Medical Center
Omaha, Nebraska

Rick Ricer, MD
Professor
Department of Family Medicine
University of Cincinnati
Cincinnati, Ohio

W. David Robinson, PhD, IMFT
Assistant Professor
Department of Family Medicine
University of Nebraska Medical Center
Omaha, Nebraska

Douglas R. Smucker, MD, MPH
Associate Professor
Department of Family Medicine

University of Cincinnati
Cincinnati, Ohio

Sanjaya Sooriarachchi, MD
Resident, Department of Family Medicine
McGaw Family Practice Residency Program
Glenbrook Hospital
Glenview, Illinois

Penny Tenzer, MD
Vice Chair, Department of Family Medicine
University of Miami School of Medicine
Director, Family Medicine Residency Program
Jackson Memorial Medical Center
Miami, Florida

Barbara B. Tobias, MD
Associate Professor of Clinical Family
Medicine
Department of Family Medicine
University of Cincinnati College of Medicine
Cincinnati, Ohio

Charles T. Webster, MD
Assistant Professor of Clinical Medicine
Department of Family Medicine
University of Cincinnati
Attending Physician
University of Cincinnati Medical Center
Cincinnati, Ohio

Rebecca Williams, MD
Clinical Assistant Professor of Family Medicine
University of Illinois, Chicago
Chicago, Illinois
Attending Physician
MacNeal Family Practice Residency
Berwyn, Illinois

Julie K. Wood, MD
Department of Family Medicine
Samaritan Hospital
Macon, Missouri

Darice L. Zabak, MD
Assistant Professor Family Medicine
University of Illinois College of Medicine at
Rockford
Attending Physician
Rockford Health Systems
Rockford, Illinois

Reviewers

Liz Baker, MD
3rd year resident
Rose Family Residency
Denver, Colorado

Wayne Brown, MD
2nd year resident
Utah Valley Family Practice Residency
Provo, Utah

Lucy Chen, MD
3rd year resident of family medicine
University of Washington
Seattle, Washington

Michael Gale, MD
3rd year resident
Utah Valley Family Practice
Residency
Provo, Utah

Uri Goldberg, DO
2nd year resident
Rose Family Residency
Denver, Colorado

Tracey Haas, MD
2nd year resident
Maine Medical Center Residency
Program
Portland, Maine

Jayanthi Jambulingam, MD
2nd year resident
Wayne State University
Family Practice Residency Program
Detroit, Michigan

Martin Lebl, MD
3rd year resident

Rose Family Residency
Denver, Colorado

Su-May Lee, MD
UCSF Family Practice Residency
University of California, San Francisco
San Francisco, California

Jane Li, MD
3rd year resident
University of Massachusetts Family Practice
Program
Hahnemann Family Health Center
Worcester, Massachusetts

Ana Sofia Lopes, MD
2nd year resident
University of Miami
Miami, Florida

Mamata Majmundar, MD
3rd year resident
University of Kentucky
Lexington, Kentucky

Michele Mohr, MD
2nd year chief resident
Community Health Center at the
University of Wyoming Family Practice
Residency Program
Casper, Wyoming

Brian F. Morris, MD
PGY-2
Ball Memorial Family Practice Residency
Muncie, Indiana

Rajasree J. Nair, MD
3rd year resident
Family Practice Residency at the UT

Southwestern Medical Center
Dallas, Texas

Nancy Pandhi, MD
2nd year resident
Shenandoah Valley Family Practice Residency
Virginia Commonwealth University
Front Royal, Virginia

Maggie Pasek, MD
3rd year resident
University of Colorado
Denver, Colorado

Laura Pickler, MD, MPH
3rd year resident
Rose Family Residency
Denver, Colorado

George Qiao, MD
1st year resident
University of New Mexico Family Practice Program
Albuquerque, New Mexico

Molly Roberts, MD, MS
Co-Director of Synchronicity Center for Mind/Body/Spirit
Tucson, Arizona

Sarah Sciascia, MD
4th year resident
Tufts Family Residency Program
Family Health Center
Malden, Massachusetts

Jennifer Setterdahl, MD
3rd year resident in family practice
University of Missouri
Columbia, Missouri

Saima Siddiqui, MD
3rd year resident
Wayne State University
Detroit, Michigan

Michael Stadnicki, MD
3rd year resident
Maine Medical Center Residency Program
Portland, Maine

John B. Waits, MD
3rd year resident
In His Image Family Practice Residency
Tulsa, Oklahoma

Brian West, MD
2nd year resident
Shenandoah Valley Family Practice Residency
Virginia Commonwealth University
Front Royal, Virginia

Julie Yeh, MD
3rd year resident
Thomas Jefferson University
Hospital Family Practice Residency
Philadelphia, Pennsylvania

Jane Yu, MD
2nd year resident
Tufts University Family Practice Residency
Malden, Massachusetts

Darice L. Zabak, MD
Assistant Professor Family Medicine
University of Illinois College of Medicine at Rockford
Attending Physician
Rockford Health Systems
Rockford, Illinois

Acknowledgments

This book represents the efforts of many talented individuals. First and foremost, we acknowledge the numerous contributors to the first edition of the book. Their contributions form the backbone of the second edition. We thank our fellow editors whose efforts to produce a good product made us each proud to be part of this project.

We thank Sonya Seigafuse and Lippincott Williams & Wilkins for their confidence in this book and their support for publishing the second edition. Both Nancy Winter, the managing editor for this project, and Rebecca Barroso, the development editor, deserve our thanks for all their help.

We also thank our families for their endless support and patience during the time we spent working on this project. Finally, a special thanks to one of our contributors, Darice Zabak, for her invaluable help with this project. She provided a separate independent review of the questions from the perspective of a busy practitioner who was preparing to recertify. Her insightful comments and critique were invaluable for ensuring accuracy and improving the quality.

Table of Contents

Chapter 1

Internal Medicine Questions

1. Diagnostic criteria for the metabolic syndrome include which of the following:
A. Peripheral obesity
B. High HDL-C
C. Hypomagnasemia
D. Hypertriglyceridemia
E. Hyperphosphatemia

2. A 65-year-old white female presents to your office with a chronic productive cough. She produces over 2 tablespoons of sputum each day, and her current cough has been present for 3 months. History reveals that she had a similar episode of chronic, productive cough that lasted more than 3 months each of the past 2 years, but at different seasons of the year. The most appropriate diagnosis of this patient would be:
A. Seasonal allergies
B. Emphysema
C. Chronic bronchitis
D. Asthma
E. Tuberculosis

3. Thiazolidinediones act to control hyperglycemia in type 2 diabetes primarily by:
A. Decreasing insulin resistance in muscle, fat, and liver
B. Stimulating pancreatic beta cells to increase insulin output
C. Decreasing glucose production by the liver
D. Inhibiting intestinal enzymes that break down carbohydrates, delaying carbohydrate absorption
E. Increasing plasma insulin levels

4. Which of the following statements is true concerning the ECG stress test?
A. Males are more likely than females to have a false-positive ECG stress test.
B. Baseline ST-T wave abnormalities are not associated with a false-positive test.
C. Severe hypertension may predispose to a false-positive test.
D. Left ventricular hypertrophy with strain makes the ECG stress test more sensitive.
E. Thin individuals are more likely than obese patients to have a false-positive result.

5. A 28-year-old female has severe menstrual cramps and very heavy menstrual periods. This problem has existed over the past year, and recently she has begun to have fatigue and shortness of breath with prolonged walking. She has no ankle swelling and no

other problems. Physical examination would most likely reveal which of the following?
A. Icteric sclerae
B. Pale conjunctiva
C. Hepatomegaly
D. Splenomegaly
E. Clubbing

6. The first step in treating a 60-year-old patient with weight loss, epigastric pain, and mild anemia should be:
A. *Helicobacter pylori* antibody test
B. Endoscopy
C. 6-week trial of H2 blockers
D. 90-day trial of proton pump inhibitor
E. Over-the-counter PPI for 30 days

7. An adolescent girl presents with a rash that is made up of very small, bright red, nonblanching macules. The child had nonspecific viral symptoms last week. She appears to be in excellent health except for the rash. She is not on any medications. What is the most common cause of this condition?
A. Penicillin
B. Hemolysis
C. Human immunodeficiency virus (HIV)
D. Lupus
E. Idiopathic thrombocytopenic purpura

8. A 38-year-old presents with fever, low back pain, and perineal discomfort. Which of the following statements is true?
A. Chronic prostatitis, alone, would be likely to explain this patient's symptoms.
B. The presentation of this patient is consistent with the definition of asymptomatic inflammatory prostatitis.
C. If the prostate examination is normal, acute bacterial prostatitis is unlikely.
D. If acute bacterial prostatitis is diagnosed, treatment with penicillin VK is recommended.
E. If this patient has acute bacterial prostatitis, it is unlikely that he has chronic prostatitis/chronic pelvic pain syndrome.

9. A 35-year-old presents with an enlarging neck mass just anterior to the sternocleidomastoid muscle. Which of the following statements is true?
A. The presence of cholesterol crystals makes the diagnosis of a branchial cyst unlikely.
B. The location suggests a thyroglossal duct cyst.

C. Treatment might initially begin with a course of antibiotics.

D. Excision is almost never needed for permanent treatment.

E. Epidermoid cysts are characterized by keratin and mesodermal skin elements.

10. For a child with a history of anaphylaxis, which of the following preventive measures would be inappropriate:

A. Allergen desensitization with insect venom for those sensitive to stinging insects

B. Avoidance measures

C. Patient education on the use of epinephrine

D. Pretreatment with diphenhydramine before administration of antibiotics causing anaphylaxis

E. Education of close family members concerning treatment of anaphylaxis

11. Which of the following is a first-line drug for rate control in the longer term management of stable but symptomatic atrial fibrillation:

A. Verapamil

B. Quinidine

C. Digoxin

D. Procainamide

E. Amiodarone

12. A 37-year-old female with a history of chronic corticosteroid therapy comes in with complaints of easy bruising, muscle weakness, depressive symptoms, and amenorrhea. On exam you find evidence of hirsutism, truncal obesity, striae, elevated blood pressure, and hyperglycemia. If you wanted to make the diagnosis of Cushing's syndrome, what would be the single best test to do so?

A. Overnight dexamethasone suppression test

B. Plasma cortisol

C. Renal profile

D. Plasma ACTH level

E. Abdominal CT scan

13. What should be initial therapy for a 67-year-old woman with newly diagnosed Parkinson's disease?

A. Levodopa/carbidopa combination

B. Dopamine agonist

C. Levodopa/carbidopa plus a COMT inhibitor

D. MAO-B inhibitor

E. Any of the above choices

14. A 65-year-old man comes to the office complaining of having to get up three times every night to go to the bathroom. You evaluate him for benign prostatic hypertrophy by using the American Urologic Association's symptom index. You find that his index score is 18. What is an appropriate treatment?

A. No treatment

B. Transurethral resection

C. Tolterodine

D. Tamsulosin

E. Spironolactone

15. Of the following tests, which one by itself can confirm the diagnosis of peripheral vascular disease?

A. Digital subtraction angiogram

B. Auscultation of bruits

C. Ankle-brachial index of less than 0.90

D. Systolic pressure index of less than 0.90

E. Ankle-brachial index of greater than 1.1

16. Which of the following statements is true regarding chronic obstructive pulmonary disease (COPD) treatment?

A. Oxygen therapy is responsible for more than 50% of the cost of treating COPD in the United States.

B. Long-term oxygen therapy reduces mortality and improves quality of life in patients with mild COPD.

C. Long-term oxygen therapy should be considered in patients with a partial pressure of arterial oxygen of less than 55 mmHg (PaO_2).

D. Theophylline should be used for most patients with severe COPD.

E. Immunization with the influenza vaccine is contraindicated in patients with severe COPD.

17. The most common cause of aortic stenosis is:

A. Rheumatic fever

B. Syphilis

C. Intravenous drug abuse

D. Idiopathic

E. Postinfectious

18. Which of the following conditions would disqualify an athlete from participation in noncontact sports?

A. HIV

B. Diabetes mellitus type 1

C. Unilateral kidney

D. Carditis

E. Atlantoaxial instability

19. What is the most common cause of sudden death, besides trauma, in an athlete less than 35 years of age?

A. Coronary artery disease

B. Hypertrophic cardiomyopathy

C. Status asthmaticus

D. Hyperthermia

E. Electrocution from lightning

20. A 38-year-old female presents complaining of urgency, frequency, and dysuria. She is found to have a temperature of 38°C, no flank pain, and a urinalysis positive for nitrites and leukocyte esterase. Which of the following is the most appropriate treatment regimen?

A. Trimethoprim-sulfamethoxazole DS bid for 3 days

B. Norfloxacin 400 mg PO bid for 7 to 14 days

C. Ciprofloxacin 250 mg PO bid for 5 days

D. Trimethoprim 300 mg PO every day for 3 to 5 days

E. Amoxicillin 500 mg PO bid for 10 days

21. Which of the following is a true statement concerning the treatment of obesity?

A. Orlistat is a selective reuptake inhibitor of serotonin and norepinephrine.

B. Sibutramine acts centrally to reduce energy intake by inducing a feeling of satiety.

C. According to the National Institutes of Health (NIH), surgical therapy of morbid obesity is ineffective.

D. Gastric bypass surgery achieves significant sustained weight loss in less than 10% of individuals.

E. Sibutramine decreases fat absorption in the intestine.

22. A 44-year-old male presents to the emergency room with an acutely swollen left knee. He has been in good health, and he has no chronic health conditions and no history of trauma. The most important evaluation should be:

A. MRI of the knee

B. Erythrocyte sedimentation rate

C. Diagnostic arthrocentesis of the knee

D. Complete blood count

E. Rheumatoid factor

23. The patient in the preceding question has appropriate laboratory evaluations drawn. In the meantime, the decision is made to perform an arthrocentesis. Which of the following is a true statement concerning this examination?

A. A synovial fluid WBC count of less than 2,000 cells/mm³ suggests an inflammatory process.

B. The presence of needle-shaped crystals is a normal finding.

C. The presence of crystals excludes the possibility of an infection.

D. Cloudy synovial fluid would be consistent with an inflammatory process.

E. The finding of fat droplets is to be expected.

24. A 27-year-old presents with the worst headache of his life. Which of the following is least likely to be helpful?

A. Careful history eliciting recent trauma or head injury

B. Evaluation of cranial nerves including the retina

C. Strong consideration of CT or MRI of the head

D. Plain film of the skull

E. History of previous headache problems and treatments

25. Elevated blood pressure in the setting of acute ischemic stroke needs to be judiciously treated because:

A. High blood pressure needs to be treated aggressively in order to decrease the incidence of intracranial bleeding.

B. Acute elevations in blood pressure usually do not spontaneously decline.

C. Blood pressures above 160 mmHg systolic or 100 mmHg diastolic are immediately life-threatening.

D. Areas of ischemic brain lose autoregulation and may be dependent on elevated mean arterial pressure to maintain perfusion.

E. Aggressive lowering of blood pressure with acute ischemic stroke improves outcome.

26. You are treating a patient with INH after "converting" with a positive PPD skin test. The patient presents with constitutional symptoms, fever, arthritis, and serositis. A true statement concerning this patient is:

A. This patient likely has developed disseminated tuberculosis and needs to be hospitalized.

B. It would be likely to find renal and central nervous system disease.

C. A positive ANA would be likely.

D. Antibodies to double-stranded DNA are invariably present.

E. It would be important to know if the patient was also taking penicillin.

27. A 25-year-old male patient presents with a history of a painless swelling of the right testicle. He thinks it is actually enlarging on a daily basis. His last sexual encounter was 6 months ago. He has no urinary tract symptoms. Physical examination reveals a large, non-tender testicle that does not transluminate. The epididymis appears normal. There is no tenderness. Which of the following is the most appropriate next step?

A. Refer for transscrotal open or percutaneous biopsy

B. Refer for ultrasound and a surgical opinion

C. Advise the patient to ejaculate multiple times over the next several days

D. Treat with 2 weeks of an appropriate antibiotic

E. Recheck in 6 months

28. Which of the following drug classes is least likely to cause a delirium?

A. Benzodiazepines

B. Cephalosporins

C. Opioids

D. Antihistamines

E. Cardiac glycosides (digoxin)

29. Which of the following tests should be performed in the routine evaluation of a demented patient?

A. APOE genotyping

B. Depression screening

C. Noncontrast head CT

D. SPECT scan

E. Carotid ultrasound

30. Which of the following statements is false?

A. Inappropriate or confusing responses to questions on registration forms or during the interview might suggest low literacy.

B. Low literacy is associated with higher levels of physical illness.

C. Approximately 22% of the adult U.S. population is at the lowest level of literacy and is unable to read even basic written messages.

D. Computerized formulas are able to effectively assess the quality of patient education materials aimed at lower literacy audiences.

E. A widely used instrument to assess literacy is the Rapid Estimate of Adult Literacy in Medicine (REALM).

31. A true statement about the diagnosis of urinary tract infection (UTI) includes:

A. More than 85% with pyelonephritis have fever.

B. In a patient with symptoms suggestive of UTI, the presence of a vaginal discharge does not significantly reduce the likelihood of UTI.

C. Having a positive nitrite dipstick is a very sensitive test for UTI.

D. Back pain is a specific symptom associated with upper tract infection.

E. Approximately 1 in 7 women who have a UTI will have a falsely negative leukocyte esterase test.

32. A true statement concerning the diagnosis of deep venous thrombosis (DVT) and pulmonary embolism is which of the following?

A. Ultrasound techniques are able to reliably distinguish between recurrent and chronic DVT.

B. Pulmonary embolism can reliably be diagnosed by the history and physical examination.

C. The alveolar-arterial difference on blood gas determination is invariably elevated greater than 20 mmHg with a pulmonary embolism.

D. False-positive ultrasound tests are possible in the presence of a pelvic mass.

E. Repeat ultrasound testing seldom demonstrates progression of DVT.

33. A true statement about syphilis includes:

A. The primary lesion of syphilis is a painful ulcer associated with painless regional lympadenopathy.

B. Clinical symptoms of secondary syphilis occur after 2 to 5 years following primary syphilis.

C. A maculopapular rash affecting the palms and soles rarely occurs.

D. Without treatment, clinical symptoms of secondary syphilis persist.

E. Tertiary syphilis occurs after 5 years.

34. A true statement concerning domestic violence is:

A. The lifetime prevalence of violence between spouses is 5%.

B. Victims of violence can be readily identified on the basis of demographic variables.

C. There are no valid screening tools for domestic violence.

D. Victims of violence often experience insomnia, fatigue, and chronic pain.

E. Abused women have lower health care costs than nonabused women.

35. A 45-year-old is diagnosed with colon cancer after an episode of rectal bleeding and colonoscopy. In reviewing her past family history, she also has a brother who had colon cancer and a father who died of colon cancer at age 51. They allegedly were diagnosed with a colon full of polyps. She is wondering if there may be a genetic test you could do on her 20-year-old son to determine if he is at risk. What would you tell her?

A. Most likely all of these cases are spontaneous and not related. No testing is needed.

B. It would be appropriate to test for the APC tumor suppressor gene now, which would indicate an increased risk of familial adenomatous polyposis.

C. He does not need screening until age 35, 10 years before she was diagnosed.

D. Recommend prophylactic colectomy.

E. She need not worry her son because this problem skips generations.

36. Which of the following is not a risk factor for developing knee osteoarthritis?

A. Moderate amount of routine physical activity

B. Previous history of joint trauma

C. Age

D. Obesity

E. Female gender

37. Hyperphosphatemia is most often caused by:

A. Hypoparathyroidism

B. Rhabdomyolysis

C. Renal failure

D. Tumor lysis syndrome

E. Hyperthyroidism

38. You are following up closely with a young adolescent who presented last week with chest pain. You have chosen to follow this patient closely because he had Kawasaki disease as a child. Which of the following statements is true?

A. Kawasaki disease is associated with a parvovirus infection and results in pulmonary intersitial fibrosis.

B. Kawasaki disease is associated with asthma.

C. Coronary artery abnormalities can occur in up to 25% of untreated children.

D. Kawasaki disease is associated with valvular heart disease.

E. Acute phase reactants such as the erythrocyte sedimentation rate (ESR) and C-reactive protein (CRP) are usually normal.

39. The most appropriate therapy for renal cell carcinoma that is confined to the kidney is:

A. Radical nephrectomy of the involved kidney

B. Bilateral nephrectomy, because of the high incidence of occult malignancy in the contralateral kidney

C. Chemotherapy, because the incidence of metastases at the time of diagnosis of renal cell carcinoma is 90%

D. Radiation therapy, because of the highly sensitive nature of renal cell carcinoma to radiation

40. A 55-year-old female comes to you for a facial rash (Figure 1-1). She has fixed rubor and telangiectasias across her nose and on both cheeks. She has tried multiple topical agents and several different oral antibiotics. She has been told that there are no other treatment

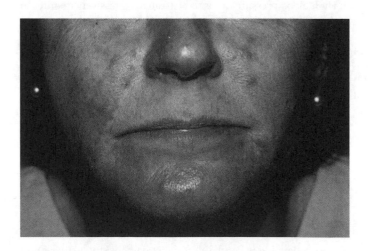

Figure 1-1. As seen here, the patient has inflammatory papules and pustules and telangiectasias located on the central third of the face. From Goodheart HP. Goodheart's Photoguide of Common Skin Disorders. *2nd ed. Philadelphia: Lippincott Williams & Wilkins; 2003.*

options. You explain that you have had a lot of success with which of the following treatments:

A. Regular sun exposure
B. Nizoril cream
C. Hydrocortisone 1% cream
D. Benadryl oral daily
E. Metronidazole topical

41. Which of the following statements is false about the BRCA 1 or 2 gene?

A. It is a gene for breast cancer.
B. Five percent of patients with breast cancer will have the BRCA 1 or 2 gene.
C. A positive test may affect future insurance policies for the patient.
D. The test is expensive.
E. All types of familial breast cancer can be detected by these two genes.

42. Which of the following statements is true concerning chronic bronchitis?

A. Associated with a productive cough
B. Fever daily for 3 months
C. Improvement with exercise
D. Seasonal symptoms
E. Jaundice

43. The leading infectious cause of death worldwide is:

A. HIV
B. Tuberculosis
C. Pneumococcal pneumonia
D. Influenza A
E. Avian influenza (bird flu)

44. Which of the following is not a risk factor for osteoporosis?

A. Long-term corticosteroid therapy
B. Asian race
C. Cigarette smoking
D. Excessive alcohol use
E. Long-term thyroid replacement therapy

45. Empiric outpatient treatment of community-acquired pneumonia (CAP) should *not* consist of:

A. A macrolide (including erythomycin, clarithromycin, or azithromycin)
B. Doxycycline or tetracycline (if patient is younger than 8 years old)
C. An antipneumococcal beta-lactam (including cefuroxime axetil, high-dose amoxicillin, amoxicillin-clavulanate)
D. A quinolone (including lomefloxacin, ciprofloxacin, ofloxacin)
E. Sulfamethoxazole

46. Which of the following anemias would classically show microcytic hypochromic indices on a complete blood count?

A. Vitamin B12 deficiency
B. Sideroblastic anemia
C. Chronic alcoholism
D. Folate deficiency
E. Anemia of chronic disease

47. Hormonal (endocrine) therapy is the best choice for what stage of prostate cancer?

A. Stage A
B. Stage B
C. Stage D
D. Hormonal therapy is seldom indicated.
E. Hormonal therapy is indicated as part of every prostate cancer treatment program.

48. A 29-year-old patient with known rheumatoid arthritis presents with a 2-day history of fever and a painful, red, and swollen right knee. Physical exam reveals a knee that is painful to move and is noticeably warm. Laboratory studies indicate a moderate leukocytosis. Which statement is correct in evaluating this condition?

A. An aspiration should not be performed to avoid contaminating the joint.
B. If infected, likely organisms include *N. gonorrhea* and *S. aureus*.
C. IV antibiotics should be instituted after cultures are positive.
D. A bone scan will be helpful in providing an early diagnosis.
E. A plain x-ray of the knee is likely to be diagnostic.

49. Lung cancer is:

A. The leading cause of cancer deaths in both men and women
B. The leading cause of cancer deaths in men, and the third leading cause of cancer deaths in women
C. The leading cause of cancer deaths in women, and the second leading cause of cancer deaths in men
D. Less likely to occur in female smokers than in male smokers
E. An important disease for which the U.S. Preventive Services Task Force recommends regular screening

50. Which of the following group of findings would be most consistent with the syndrome of inappropriate ADH (SIADH)?

A. Hypernatremia, euvolemia, urine osmolality greater than 100 mosm/kg
B. Hyponatremia, euvolemia, urine osmolality greater than 100 mosm/kg
C. Hypernatremia, hypovolemia, urine osmolality greater than 100 mosm/kg
D. Hypernatremia, hypovolemia, urine osmolality less than 100 mosm/kg
E. Hyponatremia, euvolemia, urine osmolality less than 100 mosm/kg

51. A 28-year-old male presents with urethral discharge. He states that he has been with the same sexual partner for 6 months and is having no other symptoms. He denies any prior history of STDs. Which of the following tests is least helpful?

A. HIV
B. Chlamydia and GC PCR probes
C. Urinalysis
D. KOH and wet mounts
E. Urine culture

52. All of the following are treatment options for hyperkalemia *except*:

A. Calcium gluconate
B. Insulin
C. Sodium bicarbonate

D. Beta-blockers
E. Kayexalate

53. A 29-year-old farmer presents with a 2-day history of low back pain and tingling of the right great toe. He has recently been using a small tractor to till a field and recalls no injury or fall. He is in good health, takes no medication, and denies illicit drug use. He has had several episodes of back pain in the past and self-medicated with acetaminophen. His wife urged him to come to the physician because she heard that tingling in the toe signifies a "slipped disk" that requires surgery.

On physical examination, the patient is alert, cooperative, and in no acute distress. He is afebrile. There is poorly localized pain on palpation of the lower sacral area. A straight leg-raising test on the right is positive at 30 degrees and negative on the left.

There is minimal sensory loss in right great toe and the motor examination and reflexes are normal.

Management of this patient should include:
A. Immediate neurosurgical referral for evaluation
B. Magnetic resonance imaging of the lumbo-sacral spine
C. Plain lumbo-sacral spine films
D. Strict bed rest for the next week
E. Watchful waiting over the next month unless symptoms are progressive or unrelenting

54. In a patient with severe persistent asthma, which of the following is true?
A. They have intermittent symptoms.
B. Controller agents should be used sparingly.
C. Oral steroids may be required frequently or on a long-term basis.
D. The peak flow is typically 60% to 80% of predicted.
E. Their physical activity is typically normal.

55. A 44-year-old is being treated for fibromyalgia. She complains that she limits her activity because of pain. After doing a thorough physical and confirming your diagnosis, you suggest:
A. Try to remain active despite the pain.
B. Begin a period of strict bed rest to reduce her discomfort.
C. Begin oxycodone 10 mg daily and increase until pain is eliminated.
D. Try chiropractic manipulation of the cervical spine for the next year.
E. Initiate a trial of St. John's Wort.

56. A 59-year-old patient returns from the urologist with the diagnosis of prostate cancer. The note from the urologist indicates that he has stage B and a Gleason score of 6. He has no other medical problems. The patient wants your opinion of what he should do.
A. Do nothing and observe it for now
B. External beam radiation
C. Interstitial seeds
D. Lumpectomy
E. Radical prostatectomy

57. During a physical exam you hear a blowing diastolic murmur that is best heard at the left sternal border and that gets louder when you have the patient squat down. The patient denies any cardiac symptoms, has never been told he has a murmur, and has no significant past medical history. What is the most likely cause of the murmur?
A. Aortic stenosis
B. Aortic regurgitation
C. Mitral stenosis
D. Mitral regurgitation
E. Mitral valve prolapse

58. Which of the following signs is unlikely in a patient with allergic rhinitis?
A. Nasal obstruction
B. Pale, bluish turbinates
C. Allergic shiners
D. Mouth breathing
E. Cervical adenopathy

59. A 46-year-old experiences a sensation of fullness in his ear, tinnitus, sensorineural hearing loss, and vertigo. A true statement is:
A. If this patient has a hearing loss early in the course of his disease, it is likely to be at lower frequencies.
B. Hearing loss could be predicted to be confined to the higher frequencies.
C. Diuretics would be contraindicated in this person.
D. Tinnitus would be unlikely to fluctuate and is solely associated with dizzy spells.
E. Unsteadiness would be unlikely to persist for more than 1 hour.

60. A 50-year-old symptomatic man with three negative hemocult cards had a routine screening sigmoidoscopy. On exam, a 0.5-cm tubular adenoma was found and completely removed. You recommend:
A. Repeat sigmoidoscopy in 90 days
B. Repeat sigmoidoscopy in 1 year
C. Repeat sigmoidoscopy in 5 years
D. Colonoscopy as soon as possible
E. CT with contrast of abdomen to evaluate the extent of colon cancer, surgical, and oncologic consultations

61. Which characteristic would be least likely to be found in a patient with migraine?
A. Unilateral
B. Photophobia
C. Disabling
D. Nasal congestion, rhinorrhea, and lacrimation
E. Nausea

62. A 68-year-old woman comes in for her annual exam and has no complaints. She needs a refill of her hormone replacement medication and wants some screening labs done. She has no significant past medical or family history. On physical examination, nothing remarkable is found. You get her labs back and find that the only thing outside of the normal range is her calcium, which is 11.9 mg/dL. Which of the following would not be a possible cause of this?
A. Parathyroid adenoma
B. Metastatic cancer
C. Sarcoidosis

D. Paget's disease
E. Vitamin E intoxication

63. True statements regarding risk factors for colorectal cancer include:
A. Hereditary nonpolyposis colorectal cancers are an autosomal recessive condition.
B. Females are more likely than males to have colorectal cancer.
C. Inflammatory bowel disease substantially reduces the risk of colorectal cancer.
D. Increased fat intake protects against the development of colorectal cancer.
E. Gardner's syndrome is characterized by hereditary polyposis and is associated with the development of colorectal cancer.

64. Which of the following interventions is considered a standard treatment for COPD but is not considered a standard treatment for asthma?
A. Selective beta-2 agonist inhaler
B. Long-acting selective beta-2 agonist inhaler
C. Ipratroprium inhaler
D. Corticosteroids
E. Patient education

65. A true statement about gout is:
A. Gout is predominately a disease of younger women.
B. The duration and magnitude of hyperuricemia is associated with the occurrence of gout and age of onset of gouty symptoms.
C. Pain gradually evolves in gout over a period of weeks to months.
D. Systemic symptoms such as fever and malaise infrequently occur in gout.
E. It is associated with chunky, box-like, positively birefringent crystals.

66. A 37-year-old presents with unilateral headache associated with stuffed-up nose, red eyes, and excruciating pain. Your management would include which of the following:
A. Emergency MRI
B. Verapamil for acute headache
C. Sumatriptan for chronic suppression
D. Oxycodone for chronic suppression
E. 100% oxygen inhalation acutely

67. A 70-year-old female with a history of osteoarthritis comes to you complaining of right knee pain that she describes as 5 out of 10 on a pain scale. What would be the initial choice for medication therapy?
A. Acetaminophen 1 g tid
B. Ibuprofen 600 mg tid
C. Celecoxib 200 mg qid
D. Codeine 30 mg/acetaminophen 325 mg 1 or 2 tablets qid prn
E. Hydrocodone 5 mg/acetaminophen 500 mg tid to qid

68. A 17-year-old presents with a 2-day history of sore throat, fever, and tender cervical adenopathy. She has no upper respiratory symptoms and your examination discloses a red pharynx with tonsillar exudate, no rhinorrhea, and tender anterior adenopathy. Which management strategy would be the least likely to be successful?
A. An IM shot of penicillin G benzathine (900,000 U) and penicillin G procaine (300,000 U)
B. Watchful waiting since the likelihood of streptococcal (strep) infection is so low
C. Pen VK 500 mg PO bid for 10 days
D. If the patient is allergic to penicillin, treatment with erythromycin
E. Counseling that early treatment of strep throat will reduce the risk of rheumatic fever

69. A 32-year-old G2P1001 female at 13 weeks comes to your office with complaints of palpitations, anxiety, and heat intolerance. An ECG shows sinus tachycardia with a rate of 110 beats/minute and a TSH is less than 0.1. How would you treat this patient during her pregnancy?
A. Radioactive iodine
B. Follow her clinically and treat after delivery
C. Partial thyroidectomy
D. Propothiouracil
E. Iodine

70. A previously healthy 54-year-old presents with fatigue. He denies other symptoms. Which is the least likely to be helpful in his evaluation?
A. History of recent travel, particularly internationally
B. History of risky behaviors for HIV
C. Previous history of cancer
D. Family history of coronary artery disease
E. History of hepatitis

71. Which of the following medications is the first-line drug of choice in treating partial seizures?
A. Carbamazepine
B. Phenobarbital
C. Valproic acid
D. Gabapentin
E. Topiramate

72. A true statement concerning health care of lesbians includes which of the following:
A. Cervical cancer is of no concern; therefore, pap smears are unnecessary.
B. Routine mammography screening recommendations should be followed.
C. PAP smears should be performed every 5 years because of the decreased risk of cervical cancer.
D. There is no need to assess HIV risk factors in lesbians.
E. Discussions of parenting are unwarranted with lesbian couples.

73. Which of the following statements is false?
A. Live vaccines are easier to store secondary to better vaccine stability.
B. There is a risk of transmission of the clinical illness to household contacts of vaccine recipients if live virus is used.
C. The live virus may increase the antigenic stimulus by replicating in the host.

D. Live virus vaccines have a similar side effect profile compared to other vaccine types.

E. Examples of live virus vaccines include varicella and oral polio virus.

74. A 22-year-old patient says that he has a family history of polycystic kidney disease. You explain to him:

A. Men are affected 5:1 compared to women.

B. The disease is associated with intracranial aneurysms.

C. It is inherited in an autosomal recessive fashion.

D. It is usually symptomatic by the patient's early 20s.

E. Fortunately, other than renal disease, polycystic kidney disease is not associated with any other problems.

75. A 45-year-old male with alcoholism presents with a history of chronic epigastric pain, steatorrhea, and weight loss. You suspect chronic pancreatitis. A true statement includes:

A. Invariably the serum amylase and lipase are elevated.

B. Impaired glucose tolerance is seen in up to 50% of patients.

C. Malabsorption is seldom associated with B12 deficiency.

D. There is no increased risk of pancreatic carcinoma.

76. You are seeing a patient with hemophilia A. Which of the following statements about hemophilia A is true?

A. Is a sex-linked recessive disorder

B. Is associated with low factor VIII-related antigen (von Willebrand's factor)

C. Has an abnormal PT

D. Is associated with factor IX deficiency

E. May be treated with vitamin K

77. A patient presents with polyuria. You are suspicious of diabetes insipidus. A true statement is:

A. Central diabetes insipidus is associated with a greater than 9% increase in urinary osmolality after dehydration and vasopressin administration.

B. In nephrogenic diabetes insipidus there is a large increase in urine osmolality after vasopressin administration.

C. Urine volume is almost always less than 5 L/day.

D. Sarcoidosis, metastatic tumors, and recent head trauma are unlikely causes of diabetes insipidus.

78. Which one of the following statements is true regarding the immunization of adolescents?

A. A 2- or 3-dose hepatitis B series should be initiated if not previously given.

B. A hepatitis B booster should be given if the initial 3 doses were given in infancy.

C. A varicella booster should be given if the adolescent develops a case of the shingles (herpes zoster).

D. Give a repeat MMR if the second dose of MMR was given prior to age 2 years.

79. Which statement is true regarding a patient with mild cognitive impairment?

A. The diagnosis is best made by clinical history.

B. The mini-mental status exam (MMSE) is typically abnormal.

C. Most patients will not eventually develop a dementia.

D. Vitamin E can be preventative.

E. Typical studies to test cognitive status are abnormal.

80. The Seventh Report of the Joint National Committee on Prevention, Detection, Evaluation and Treatment of High Blood Pressure (JNC VII-1997) suggests the following class of drugs for the initial treatment of hypertension in the absence of other comorbid conditions:

A. Alpha-adrenergic blockers

B. Beta-blocker

C. Calcium channel blockers

D. ACE inhibitors

E. Thiazide diuretic

81. Which of the following statements about control of heart rate with digoxin in atrial fibrillation is true?

A. It is especially effective during exercise.

B. It is vagally mediated.

C. Its onset of action is quicker than intravenous diltiazem or beta-blockers.

D. Digoxin has a broad therapeutic index.

E. Digoxin should always be given in conjunction with quinidine.

82. Current rates of vaccination for persons 65 years and older in the United States for influenza and pneumococcal vaccine are approximately:

A. Influenza 65%, pneumococcal 66%

B. Influenza 95%, pneumococcal 66%

C. Influenza 65%, pneumococcal 30%

D. Influenza 95%, pneumococcal 10%

E. Influenza 30%, pneumococcal 95%

83. Patients with COPD should receive supplemental oxygen to correct hypoxemia when their partial pressure of oxygen (PaO_2) is less than:

A. 85 mmHg

B. 75 mmHg

C. 65 mmHg

D. 55 mmHg

E. 45 mmHg

84. Alpha-glucosidase inhibitors (e.g., acarbose and miglitol) act to control hyperglycemia in type 2 diabetes mostly by:

A. Decreasing insulin resistance in muscle, fat, and liver

B. Stimulating pancreatic beta cells to increase insulin output

C. Decreasing glucose production by the liver

D. Inhibiting intestinal enzymes that break down carbohydrates, delaying carbohydrate absorption

E. Increasing plasma counter-regulatory hormones

85. Which of the following treatments would be least likely to help a patient with an acute exacerbation of asthma?

A. Methylprednisolone

B. Theophylline

C. Albuterol inhalation treatments

D. Atrovent (ipratropium) inhalation treatments

E. Oxygen

86. Pharmacologic stress testing with adenosine or Persantine is contraindicated in patients with:

A. Morbid obesity

B. Valvular cardiac disease

C. Hypertension

D. Active bronchospasm

E. Type 2 diabetes mellitus

87. Which of the following is an effective antibiotic for group A beta-hemolytic streptococcal pharyngitis:

A. Clindamycin

B. Gentamycin

C. Trimethoprim-sulfa

D. Tetracycline

E. Sulfamethoxazole

88. An acute cerebrovascular accident (CVA) characterized by right-sided hemiparesis and expressive aphasia is most consistent with occlusion of which one of the following:

A. Left middle cerebral artery

B. Right middle cerebral artery

C. Left anterior cerebral artery

D. Right anterior cerebral artery

E. Brain stem

89. External beam radiation for prostate cancer is associated with all of the following *except*:

A. Erectile dysfunction

B. Proctitis

C. Memory loss

D. Cystitis

E. Enteritis

90. Which of the following statements about scleroderma is true?

A. It is always associated with diffuse, systemic disease.

B. The CREST syndrome is a form of diffuse scleroderma associated with carditis, renal disease, endocrinopathy, sclerodactyly, and tumors.

C. Diffuse cutaneous scleroderma is associated with antinucleolar antibodies and the absence of anticentromere antibody.

D. It is uncommonly associated with Raynaud's phenomena.

E. Diffuse cutaneous scleroderma is almost never associated with dysphagia, cardiac disease, or renal disease.

91. For both acute otitis media (AOM) and bacterial sinusitis, the most common cause is:

A. *Streptococcus pneumoniae*

B. *Hemophilis influenza*

C. *Moraxella catarrhalis*

D. *Neisseria meningitis*

E. *Staph aureus*

92. Which of the following is most consistent with a diagnosis of rheumatoid arthritis (RA)?

A. Malaise, fatigue, and a positive rheumatoid factor

B. Acute monoarthritis lasting less than 6 weeks

C. Symmetric polyarthritis of the wrists, hands, and feet

D. Asymmetric polyarthritis associated with low back and sacroiliac pain

E. Fever and chills associated with limited range of motion of the hip in a 5 year old

93. A patient presents to your office with a 3-month history of itching. This is causing the patient to have multiple skin lesions in various stages (linear erosions, scabs, and scars that are both hypopigmented and hyperpigmented). The patient states he cannot keep himself from scratching and has tried multiple over-the-counter remedies. The medical causes of neurotic excoriations include all of the following *except*:

A. Hepatic disease

B. Congestive heart failure

C. Urticaria

D. Pregnancy

E. Malignancy

94. An antibiotic that usually does *not* have adverse drug–drug interactions caused by its effect on the cytochrome P-450 system is:

A. Azithromycin (Zithromax)

B. Clarithromycin (Biaxin)

C. Erythromycin base

D. Erythromycin estolate

E. Rifampin

95. Which of the following is *not* true regarding Reiter's syndrome?

A. It is one of the most common causes of acute inflammatory arthritis in young men.

B. There is an increased incidence in patients who are HLA-B27 antigen positive.

C. The classic triad of arthritis, conjunctivitis, and urethritis is seen in only one-third of affected patients.

D. Post-dysenteric Reiter's syndrome has a male:female ratio of 5:1.

E. Mucocutaneous lesions are a feature of the disease.

96. Which of the following historical or physical findings determines if a man is at high risk for prostate cancer?

A. Tobacco use

B. Alcohol

C. Family history of cancers

D. Benign prostatic hypertrophy

E. African American heritage

97. A patient undergoes a contrast-enhanced computed tomography (CT) scan of the kidneys for evaluation of hematuria. Which of the following statements is false?

A. If the mass has cystic components, it is not cancer.

B. If a solitary mass is detected that enhances with intravenous contrast, the likelihood of renal cell carcinoma (RCC) is high.

C. Multiple masses suggest metastatic disease.

D. A renal CT scan is superior to an ultrasound as an initial imaging study in detecting RCC.

E. Multiple masses may represent lymphoma.

98. Pica, especially of ice, is found most commonly with which of the following processes?

A. Iron deficiency anemia

B. Bipolar disorder

C. Post-traumatic stress disorder

D. Vitamin B12 deficiency

E. Social anxiety disorder

99. According to the recommendations of the third report of the Expert Panel on Detection, Evaluation and Treatment of High Blood Cholesterol in Adults, which of the following risk factors is *not* an indication for setting a goal low-density lipoprotein (LDL) cholesterol level lower than 100 mg/dL?
A. Hypertension in a 45-year-old male with no other risk factors
B. Diabetes mellitus
C. Known coronary heart disease
D. Peripheral arterial disease
E. 65-year-old male with history of hypertension who smokes

100. Antiviral treatment for chronic hepatitis C virus infection is recommended by the NIH for patients whose disease is most likely to progress. Risk factors for progressive disease include which of the following?
A. Very mild histologic disease by biopsy
B. Persistently abnormal alanine aminotransferase levels
C. Undetectable circulating hepatitis C virus RNA
D. Mild hepatitis and fibrosis on biopsy
E. Female gender

101. A true statement concerning obstructive sleep apnea (OSA) is:
A. OSA is often associated with daytime fatigue and sleepiness.
B. OSA is often improved by intake of alcohol or sedatives, which improve the duration and quality of sleep.
C. The most effective intervention is recommendation of a weight loss regimen.
D. Nasal administration of continuous positive airway pressure (CPAP) is usually not effective because most people sleep with their mouth open.
E. Physical signs of OSA include a small neck size.

102. Which of the following is not a contraindication to Metformin use?
A. History of lactic acidosis
B. Concurrent use of thiazolidinediones
C. Type 2 diabetics with severe congestive heart failure
D. Type 2 diabetics with renal insufficiency
E. Diabetic ketoacidosis

103. During epidemics of influenza, the highest rates of infection are among:
A. Children
B. Adults older than 65 years
C. Adults with diabetes
D. Adults with chronic respiratory illnesses
E. Well adults

104. Which of the following statements about cervical cancer is true?
A. A woman's lifetime risk of cervical cancer is 5%.
B. Greater than 40% of women dying of cervical cancer are 65 years of age or older.
C. Stage 1 cervical cancer is associated with a 5-year survival rate of 50%.
D. Women who smoke are not at higher risk of cervical cancer.
E. Colposcopy with biopsy and endocervical curettage can be performed in a pregnant female.

105. Several clinical trials have demonstrated that the treatment of an individual for hypertension has the greatest beneficial effect on the individual's relative risk of which one of the following?
A. Stroke
B. Myocardial infarction
C. Renal failure
D. Congestive heart failure
E. All-cause cardiovascular mortality

106. A 27-year-old male comes into your office with a history of exercise-induced asthma. He has been training for a marathon and wondered if there might be a medication besides albuterol he could use. What could you recommend?
A. Nedocromil inhaler
B. Theophylline
C. Oral steroid therapy
D. Atrovent (Ipratropium) inhaler
E. No change in therapy, Albuterol is the best option.

107. The most clinically useful marker for the presence of acute or chronic hepatitis B infection is:
A. Antibody to hepatitis B surface antigen
B. Hepatitis B surface antigen
C. Hepatitis B core antigen
D. Hepatitis E antigen
E. Alkaline phosphatase

108. Sulfonylureas act to control hyperglycemia in type 2 diabetes mostly by:
A. Decreasing insulin resistance in muscle, fat, and liver
B. Stimulating pancreatic beta cells to increase insulin output
C. Decreasing glucose production by the liver
D. Inhibiting intestinal enzymes that break down carbohydrates, delaying carbohydrate absorption
E. Decreasing the plasma breakdown of insulin

109. What is the key diagnostic test in making the diagnosis of congestive heart failure?
A. Chest x-ray
B. Electrocardiogram
C. Cardiac catheterization
D. Echocardiogram
E. Shortness of breath

110. In assessing a patient with shortness of breath, what finding on spirometry would be the most consistent with asthma?
A. An increase in the forced expiratory volume per second (FEV1)
B. An increased FEV1/FVC ratio
C. A decrease in the FEV1
D. A normal FEV1/FVC ratio
E. A restrictive pattern

111. Agents that should *not* be initiated in patients who present with an acute myocardial infarction (MI) and persistent chest discomfort are:
A. Beta-blockers
B. Dihydropyridine calcium channel blockers (e.g., nifedipine)
C. Nitrates

D. Heparin

E. Aspirin

112. Which is the preferred antipsychotic agent for patients with Parkinson's disease who develop hallucinations?

A. Haloperidol (Haldol)

B. Olanzapine (Zyprexa)

C. Quetiapine (Seroquel)

D. Clozapine (Clozaril)

E. Chlordiazepoxide

113. When using oxygen supplementation for patients with COPD, patients should limit the minimum rate of the oxygen to that necessary to achieve what percent oxygen saturation?

A. Greater than 90%

B. 80% to 85%

C. 70% to 75%

D. 60% to 65%

E. Titer to render patient asymptomatic

114. Which of the following statements concerning nonsteroidal anti-inflammatory drug (NSAID) treatment is true?

A. Refecoxib (Vioxx) is associated with a cardioprotective effect.

B. Celecoxcib (Celebrex) is associated with a renoprotective effect.

C. Naproxen has similar efficacy for rheumatoid arthritis.

D. Celecoxib plus low-dose aspirin confer no greater risk of GI bleeding.

E. Higher doses of celecoxib have a cardioprotective effect.

115. The best choice among the following antibiotics for treatment of urinary tract infection in the third trimester of pregnancy is:

A. Trimethoprim-sulfa

B. A fluoroquinolone

C. Erythromycin

D. Cephalexin

E. Penicillin VK

116. In a patient with hypocalcemia that is symptomatic, all of the following treatments would be appropriate *except*:

A. Increasing the dosage of digoxin in a patient using this medication since hypocalcemia can decrease the effectiveness of digoxin

B. Administration of calcium gluconate

C. Correction of hypomagnesemia

D. Oral calcium carbonate supplementation

E. Correction of underlying causes

117. A 35-year-old male accountant presents with a 3-day history of pain just distal to the elbow on the radial side. The pain is exacerbated when he raises the pencil from his paperwork. Further history reveals that last weekend he was building a deck for his house and used a hammer all weekend. The pain began the following morning. The most likely diagnosis is:

A. Brachioradialis tendonitis

B. Medial epicondylitis (Golfer's elbow)

C. Lateral epicondylitis (Tennis elbow)

D. Olecranon bursitis

E. Carpal tunnel syndrome

118. An antibiotic that often does not provide adequate coverage of *Haemophilus influenzae* is:

A. Azithromycin

B. Clarithromycin

C. Erythromycin

D. Cefuroxime axetil (Ceftin)

E. Amoxicillin-clavulanate

119. A 40-year-old male comes to the office with weakness, abdominal pain, and arthralgias. Initial blood tests show a mild elevation in SGOT/SGPT (AST/ALT). In reviewing the family history, the patient's father had hemochromatosis. What additional blood test would be most specific in screening for hemochromatosis?

A. Renal profile

B. Transferrin saturation

C. Glucose

D. Complete blood count

E. Amylase

120. A patient presents with palpitations. You obtain an ECG that demonstrates delta waves at the beginning of the QRS complex. A true statement concerning this patient is which of the following?

A. Calcium channel blockers are the treatment of choice.

B. Adenosine is contraindicated.

C. Radiofrequency catheter ablation is definitive therapy.

D. Beta blockers are contraindicated.

E. The PR interval is long.

121. Which of the following is true regarding testicular cancer?

A. Testicular cancer usually presents with gross hematuria or bloody ejaculate.

B. Fifty percent of patients will present with metastases.

C. Testicular cancer presents with a tender and firm testicular mass.

D. A CT with contrast of the testes is the mainstay for initial diagnosis.

E. Twenty percent of patients will present with gynecomastia.

122. Which of the following statements is true regarding Graves' disease?

A. Graves' disease is the most common autoimmune disorder in the United States.

B. There is a higher incidence of Graves' disease among blacks compared to Caucasians and Asians.

C. Males have a higher prevalence of Graves' disease than females.

D. Among patients with hyperthyroidism, 10% have Graves' disease.

E. Mutation to the TSH receptor is responsible for Grave's disease.

123. Which would be the least likely complication of prolonged steroid use in a patient with severe persistent asthma?

A. Hypothyroidism

B. Osteoporosis

C. Adrenal suppression

D. Hyperglycemia

E. Psychosis

124. Which of the following statements is not true regarding the diagnosis and treatment of multiple sclerosis?

A. It is more common in women than in men.

B. MRI is useful in making the diagnosis.

C. The diagnosis requires exclusion of all alternative processes.

D. Treatment is most efficacious early in the disease.

E. Viral infections can cause sudden deteriorations of the symptoms.

125. True statements about screening for colorectal cancer in an average risk population include:

A. Colonoscopy every 20 years is acceptable.

B. Hydrating the fecal occult blood test increases the specificity of this screen.

C. Suggest patients use vitamin C at least 1 week prior to screening.

D. Carcinoembryonic antigen screening (CEA) is recommended as a routine measure.

E. Most authorities recommend initiating screening between ages 40 and 50.

126. An 18-year-old presents with fever up to 102°F and ear pain. You find that she has a left acute otitis media and treat her with amoxicillin. You schedule a follow-up in 3 weeks. When you see her at that time, the physical exam shows fluid behind the tympanic membrane (TM). The TM moves a little with insufflation and is not erythematous. What type of medication has been shown to be helpful in this situation?

A. Antibiotics

B. Antihistamines

C. Corticosteroids

D. Decongestants

E. Watchful waiting

127. A patient presents with dizziness that started 3 months ago and has been continuous and worsening. The patient denies any other symptoms and has no significant past history. She denies any head trauma or recent colds or infections. On physical exam you find only some vertical nystagmus. Which one of the following tests should be done immediately?

A. MRI

B. Electroencephalography (EEG)

C. Audiogram

D. Lumbar puncture

E. Blood cultures

128. In patients with endoscopy-proven duodenal ulcers, *H. pylori* eradication treatment alone:

A. Increases the proportion of ulcers healed after 6 weeks

B. Is not associated with reduction of 1-year recurrence of ulcers

C. Showed an increased risk of re-bleeding over controls in the subsequent year

D. Typically must be repeated due to the high rates of re-infection

E. May be associated with *H. pylori* resistance

129. The most sensitive sign of a deep venous thrombosis is:

A. The presence of Homan's sign

B. Erythema

C. Local tenderness

D. Calf pain

E. Edema

130. Which of the following is the leading cause of COPD?

A. Allergies

B. Air pollutants

C. Cigarette smoking

D. Occupational exposure (coal mining, farming)

E. Exposure to toxic antigens

131. Which of the following would be a red flag, and warrant further evaluation, in a patient with presumed irritable bowel syndrome?

A. Painful constipation

B. Diarrhea stools

C. Crampy abdominal pain

D. Blood in stool

E. Bloating

132. Which of the following is the best indicator of disease activity in rheumatoid arthritis?

A. Rheumatoid factor elevation

B. Number of joints involved

C. Response to NSAIDs

D. Duration of morning stiffness

E. Extra-articular manifestations

133. Which of the following statements about breast cancer is true?

A. Only 20% of women who have breast cancer have a significant family history.

B. One in 20 women will develop breast cancer in their lifetime.

C. The accuracy of diagnosing breast cancer with mammography in women both before and after menopause is approximately 50%.

D. Ultrasound can accurately diagnose breast cancer.

E. Diagnosis of breast cancer by needle biopsy is often misleading.

134. One of the tests listed below has been identified as useful in confirming the diagnosis of congestive heart failure. Which one is it?

A. CBC

B. TSH

C. Comprehensive metabolic panel

D. Liver function tests

E. Brain natriuretic peptide

135. Pregnant women with inflammatory bowel disease should:

A. Not use methotrexate as long-term studies are lacking

B. Be advised not to get pregnant because it may exacerbate the disease

C. Undergo monthly flexible sigmoidoscopy to assess disease progression

D. Avoid medical treatment of their disease due to the risk of teratogenicity

E. Be counseled that severe inflammatory bowel disease may be associated with post-maturity

136. Which of the following groups is not considered at increased risk for complications of influenza?

A. Individuals older than age 65

B. Residents of nursing homes

C. Patients of any age with significant chronic disease

D. Health care workers

E. Pregnant women

137. Which of the following is true concerning the health care of prisoners?

A. The tuberculosis (TB) infection rate in prison is lower than the general population.

B. All employees of correctional facilities should be screened for TB.

C. Schizophrenia is the most common mental health condition in adolescent prisoners.

D. Hepatitis C usually presents with dramatic and acute symptoms in prisoners.

E. Excessive drinking and drug use reduce the risk of suicide in prisoners by providing an "escape."

138. Which of the following is a true statement concerning celiac sprue?

A. Testing is recommended in all patients with constipation.

B. Abdominal CT scan is sensitive for the diagnosis of celiac disease.

C. IGA anti-gliadin antibody testing is highly specific for celiac disease.

D. A single small intestine biopsy is highly sensitive.

E. IGA endomysial antibody testing is highly specific for celiac disease.

139. A 63-year-old male presents to the emergency room with complaints of abdominal pain, paresthesias, fatigue, and irritability. He has a history of amyloidosis, and you find his calcium level to be low at 7.2 mg/dL. Which would be the least likely to be found?

A. Chvostek's sign

B. Trousseau's sign

C. Seizures

D. Tetany

E. Shortened QT interval

140. A 65-year-old male patient presents with maroon-colored stools and dizziness. The NG tube aspirate is negative for blood. Which would be the least helpful?

A. Tagged RBC scan

B. EGD

C. Helical CT scan

D. IV proton pump inhibitor

E. Typing and screening for potential transfusion

141. A true statement about chronic urticaria is:

A. You can usually find the cause of chronic urticaria.

B. Antihistamines are ineffective.

C. Selective serotonin reuptake inhibitors (SSRIs) are a treatment option.

D. Only 5% of patients will resolve in 1 year.

E. H1 and H2 blockers are seldom helpful.

142. Which of the following symptoms or signs is not one of the major diagnostic criteria in making the clinical diagnosis of heart failure?

A. Paroxysmal nocturnal dyspnea

B. S-3 gallop

C. Rales

D. Pulmonary edema

E. Hepatomegaly

143. Incidental finding of gallstones on x-ray in an otherwise asymptomatic patient with no additional risk factors warrants:

A. Urgent referral to surgery

B. Follow-up RUQ ultrasound

C. Helical CT scan

D. Observation

E. Restricted-fat diet

144. A 36-year-old male presents with a 4-month history of sinus congestion, pressure, and greenish nasal discharge. He has been treated with broad-spectrum antibiotics three different times and is seeing you for a second opinion. Which of the following has been shown to treat this condition?

A. Decongestants

B. Antihistamines

C. Corticosteroids

D. Antibiotics

E. Watchful waiting

145. In patients with erosive GERD, compared with H2 blockers, proton pump inhibitors have been shown to be more effective in:

A. Decreasing relapse rates

B. Achieving more rapid relief of symptoms

C. Treatment of Barrett's esophagus

D. Improving lung function in patients with asthma

E. Reducing development of esophageal cancer

146. A long-term smoker asks you about the pulmonary complications of smoking. You tell him that:

A. He has a 90% chance of developing COPD.

B. A minority of patients with COPD are smokers.

C. Any pulmonary symptoms are probably related to COPD.

D. He has a 10% to 15% chance of developing clinical evidence of COPD.

E. If he quits, his loss of lung function will not improve.

147. A true statement concerning soft tissue sarcoma is:

A. Most involve the upper extremity.

B. They typically metastasize hematogenously.

C. MRI is used to make a definitive diagnosis.

D. The 5-year survival rate is over 90%.

E. Recurrent disease is most commonly metastatic to the liver.

148. A female patient is sent to you by her dentist to get subacute aterial endocarditis (SBE) prophylaxis prior to getting her extensive dental work done. On questioning the patient, she tells you that her previous cardiologist told her that she had a murmur on physical exam consistent with mitral valve prolapse (MVP) and would need SBE prophylaxis for the rest of her life. She states that she has never had an echocardiogram. What should you do?

A. Tell her that the rules have all changed and MVP always requires prophylaxis.

B. Give her a script for amoxicillin-clavulonate.

C. Order an echocardiogram.

D. Send her to a stress test.

E. Do a 24-hour Holter monitor.

149. A 62-year-old man is found to have a mass on digital rectal prostate examination at a routine health maintenance check. A true statement concerning this gentleman is:

A. There is no need to do a PSA test since he has a prostate mass.

B. He probably has stage A disease since the mass was found incidentally.

C. Biopsy is positive for cancer in greater than 90% of men with nodules.

D. Exposure to cadmium oxide is a risk factor for prostate cancer.

E. If the patient is found to have prostate cancer confined to one lobe of his prostate, the chance of pelvic lymph node involvement is greater than 50%.

150. Which of the following statements is true concerning cancer screening?

A. All women older than age 50 should have yearly pelvic ultrasound to screen for ovarian cancer.

B. PSA testing is universally recommended for prostate cancer screening in men older than age 65.

C. CT scan or chest x-ray is recommended for lung cancer screening in all smokers.

D. Mammography is recommended for women age 50 to 65.

E. Pap smears should be continued indefinitely after age 70 even if the patient has been routinely screened for cervical cancer during the past 20 years.

151. Which of the following statements is true concerning the diagnosis of acute HIV infection?

A. The CD4 count will usually be significantly abnormal.

B. Western blot testing is a sensitive screen for acute HIV infection.

C. Acute HIV infection is usually totally asymptomatic.

D. The viral load will be high.

E. Enzyme-linked immunosorbent assay (ELISA) testing will invariably be positive.

152. A 30-year-old female presents to your office with complaints of weakness and paresthesias of her left leg and right arm. She previously had been healthy and was not taking any medications. She has no past surgical history. She does not drink or smoke. She was adopted (so she does not know her family history). She has noticed these symptoms for the past 3 to 6 months and they seem to come and go with no reason or pattern.

Her physical exam shows a very mild but definite weakness in the left leg and right arm. Which one of the following tests is not helpful in making the diagnosis of multiple sclerosis?

A. MRI

B. Oligoclonal banding

C. Ig index

D. CT scan

E. Lumbar puncture

153. Which treatment modality has been FDA approved for the treatment of osteoarthritis?

A. Intra-articular hyaluronic acid (Hylan)

B. Intra-articular glucocorticoids

C. Tramadol (Ultram)

D. Glucosamine

E. Feverfew

154. The most common cause of jaundice in pregnancy is:

A. Cholecystitis

B. Acute viral hepatitis

C. Sclerosing cholangitis

D. Gilbert's disease

E. Metastatic hepatic cancer

155. Which of the following is true concerning maternal–fetal transmission of HIV infection?

A. Infection cannot occur in utero.

B. The probability of maternal–fetal HIV transmission is approximately 90%.

C. C-section does not lower the risk of maternal–fetal transmission of HIV infection.

D. Universal screening of pregnant women is recommended.

E. Transmission is not reduced by postpartum treatment.

156. Which of the following statements concerning giardia lambia is *false*?

A. It is the most common parasitic enteritis in the United States.

B. The preferred method of diagnosis in the United States hinges on the collection and microscopic examination of three fresh stool specimens.

C. Transmission is via the fecal–oral route.

D. Infectious cysts may be shed for months after symptomatic disease.

E. Common symptoms are diarrhea, abdominal pain, and bloating.

157. A patient with a history suggestive of skin psoriasis now complains of swollen, painful fingers. Which of the following is true?

A. Unlike rheumatoid arthritis, psoriatic arthritis is usually asymmetrical.

B. Unlike ankylosing spondylitis, psoriatic arthritis does not cause back complaints.

C. Psoriatic arthritis may respond well to NSAID therapy; disease-modifying antirheumatic drugs (DMARDs) are used for nonresponders.

D. Unlike a reactive arthritis (i.e., from inflammatory bowel disease), psoriatic arthritis is seropositive for rheumatoid factor.

E. Psoriatric arthritis is never associated with nail changes.

158. Which of the following is *incorrect* regarding testicular cancer?

A. Forty percent of males with testicular cancer have a history of an undescended testicle.

B. Testicular cancer is associated with no clear etiology or genetic factors.

C. Except for seminomas, testicular cancer has a rapid doubling rate, with doubling times of 10 to 30 days.

D. The amount of tumor burden is proportional to the degree of elevation of AFP or HCG.

E. Navaho Indians living in Arizona do not have an increased risk of developing testicular cancer.

159. A 24-year-old intravenous drug abuser presents with fever. Which of the following is true?

A. The absence of a heart murmur would make endocarditis unlikely.

B. If endocarditis is considered likely, a normal transthoracic echocardiogram essentially rules out this infection.

C. Initial treatment of possible endocarditis should be based on the results of culture.

D. Injection drug users are at most risk for having bacterial endocarditis of the right side of the heart (tricuspid and pulmonic valves).

E. A single negative blood culture during the time of a temperature greater than 101°F is sufficient to rule out endocarditis.

160. The patient in question 159 is found to have enterococcal endocarditis. A true statement concerning his treatment is which of the following?

A. Penicillin, as a single drug, is the treatment of choice.

B. Aminoglycoside resistance is rare.

C. Cephalosporins are recommended for treatment.

D. Vancomycin is currently recommended as a substitute for penicillin in patients who are penicillin allergic.

E. Vancomycin resistance is unknown.

161. You are called concerning a 72-year-old nursing home patient who has developed increasing anorexia, weakness, and mental status changes. The nurse has recorded a respiratory rate of 36. A true statement concerning this patient is which of the following?

A. Pneumonia is unlikely in the absence of cough.

B. The elevated respiratory rate is probably a nonspecific finding.

C. Mental status changes are present in two-thirds of elders with community-acquired pneumonia.

D. Fever is invariably present in an elder with pneumonia.

E. An arterial PO_2 is of little value in managing this patient.

162. A true statement concerning the treatment of influenza is:

A. Oseltamivir and zanamivir are effective in the treatment of only influenza A.

B. Rimantadine and amantadine interfere with viral replication and are effective for both influenza A and B.

C. Amantadine is metabolized predominately by the kidneys.

D. Rimantadine is metabolized predominately by the kidneys.

E. Vaccination confers immediate protection.

163. A 69-year-old active male elder presents to your office and a urinalysis discloses white cells. A true statement about this patient is:

A. If the patient is asymptomatic, but the colony count is greater than 10^5, treatment is needed.

B. A small number of white cells in the urine is uncommon in elders and usually indicates the presence of disease.

C. If the patient has symptoms suggestive of a UTI, treatment should be avoided since most patients are cured spontaneously.

D. The nitrate test on the urine may be negative in the face of a UTI caused by staphylococcus.

E. If diagnosed with a UTI, the patient's age and gender make it less likely he would have a complicated or severe infection.

164. Which of the following statements concerning dental disease is true?

A. As patients age, the gingiva proliferates.

B. Diabetes is associated with a high risk of periodontal disease, and periodontal disease is associated with poorer glycemic control.

C. Xerostomia is improved by the use of diuretics.

D. Patients with dentures no longer need routine dental care.

E. Ten percent of poor elders have lost all of their natural teeth.

165. A 59-year-old woman with mild congestive heart failure controlled with furosemide and enalapril presents with hearing loss and vestibular symptoms. She takes two extra-strength aspirin four times a day for her osteoarthritis. Which of the following is true?

A. Furosemide is unlikely to be associated with hearing loss.

B. Enalapril is likely to be associated with hearing loss.

C. Aspirin is seldom associated with ototoxicity.

D. Recent treatment with cisplantin might explain her symptoms.

E. The time course of symptoms is unlikely to change evaluation.

166. Your patient has COPD. On physical examination, you note that he is a very thin individual who breathes through pursed lips. Which of the following is used to describe this type of physical appearance of someone with COPD?

A. Pink puffer

B. Blue bloater

C. Pickwickian

D. Pectus excavatum

E. Marfanoid

167. All of the following are criteria for the metabolic syndrome, *except*:

A. Body weight greater than 120% of ideal body weight

B. HDL: less than 40 in men, less than 50 in women

C. Blood pressure greater than 130/85 or the use of blood pressure medication

D. Triglycerides greater than 150

E. Fasting glucose greater than 110

168. A 15-year-old boy is brought to your office with a lesion on his lower lip that his mom has noticed for the past 2 days. The lesion has a honey colored crust on an erythematous base and surrounding it are several small blisters. His mom thinks it started as a bug bite. What is the best way to treat this?

A. Penicillin orally

B. Amoxicillin-clavulanate orally (Augmentin)

C. Nafcillin IV

D. Mupirocin (Bactroban) topically

E. Bacitracin topically

169. Thirty minutes after receiving a yellow fever shot, the patient returns to the office with the complaint of itching, nausea, abdominal cramps, and shortness of breath. Proper treatment of this condition begins with:

A. Starting an IV

B. Hydroxyzine 50 mg PO

C. Subcutaneous epinephrine

D. Cimetidine 30 mg IV

E. Steroids 60 mg PO

170. A 25-year-old woman complains of pain and swelling of both her hands and feet lasting several hours every morning for almost 4 months. One month ago, her physician started NSAIDs with partial relief of her symptoms. However, during the past week she has noticed morning stiffness of both knees, which improves after a hot shower. Physical examination shows warmth and swelling of the MCP joints of both hands as well as symmetric fusiform swelling of the PIPs. Both wrists are swollen and tender. There is mild swelling of the ankles and knees and pain with compression of the MTP joints of both feet. One month ago, a sedimentation rate was 54 and a rheumatoid factor (RF) was negative. Which option is most appropriate for this patient?

A. Change to a different NSAID.

B. Obtain baseline laboratory studies and start a DMARD.

C. Begin low-dose prednisone.

D. Repeat the RF in 2 months.

E. Reassure the patient that her prognosis is good and there is time to observe the course of her illness without additional medications.

171. A 14-year-old female presents with acne. She wants to know what things she must avoid. You educate her on the four factors that interact to cause acne lesions. Which one of the following has not been shown to cause acne?

A. Fast foods and chocolate

B. *Propionibacterium acnes*

C. Follicular plugging from abnormal desquamation

D. Hypersensitivity to *P. acnes*

E. Androgen-induced sebum production

172. Risk factors for complications from cholelithiasis include patients with which of the following?

A. Scandinavian descent

B. Older than age 40

C. Sickle cell disease

D. Sickle cell trait

E. Female gender

173. Which of the following statements is true about colorectal cancer staging?

A. Dukes' stage C cancer extends to distant lymph nodes.

B. In the NIH TNM staging system, M stands for mobile, as in a mobile lymph gland.

C. The higher the stage, the better the prognosis.

D. In TMN stage 1, there are distant metastases.

E. Staging of colorectal cancer provides important prognostic information and has treatment implications.

174. Which of the following is least likely to be associated with supraclavicular adenopathy?

A. Lymphoma

B. Tuberculosis

C. Cat scratch disease

D. Histoplasmosis

E. Coccidiomycosis

175. An 18-year-old male comes into the STD clinic with the complaint of a 3-day history of dysuria and staining on the underwear. On your exam, you find a thin yellowish-green discharge. His UA shows 5 to 10 WBCs and is positive for leukocyte esterase. On Gram stain, you find gram-negative, intracellular diplococci. What should he be treated with?

A. Ceftriaxone 125 mg IM

B. Ciprofloxin 500 mg PO

C. Levofloxin 250 mg PO

D. Spectinomycin 2 g IM

E. Any of the above plus azithromycin 1 g PO

176. Which of the following is not associated with temporal arteritis?

A. Jaw claudication and headache

B. Thoracic aortic aneurysm

C. Polymyalgia rhematica

D. Continuous inflammation on temporal artery biopsy

E. An elevated C-reactive protein

177. Which of the following would be unlikely to be an effective treatment for genital or anal warts?

A. Imiquimod

B. Podophyllin

C. Laser

D. Cryotherapy

E. Systemic interferon

178. Which of the following nonpharmacological treatment modalities is beneficial in osteoarthritis?

A. Patient education

B. Knee bracing

C. Corrective footwear

D. Strengthening exercises

E. All of the above

179. A 47-year-old patient presents with substernal chest pain and dyspnea, and an electrocardiogram demonstrates 4-mm elevation of leads II, III, and AVF. A true statement regarding this patient is which of the following?

A. If 2 hours have elapsed, it is too late to administer a thrombolytic.

B. Streptokinase is a superior thrombolytic for young patients.

C. Aspirin is contraindicated if a thrombolytic is going to be used.

D. Thrombolytic administration after acute MI is associated with improved survival.

180. Which of the following statements is true concerning low-molecular-weight heparin (LMWH) compared to heparin in the treatment of DVT:

A. Laboratory monitoring remains important.

B. Dosing is based on gender and body mass index.

C. LMWH is given subcutaneously.

D. Major bleeding is more likely.

E. It obviates the need for oral anticoagulation.

181. A patient presents with a rash (Figure 1-2) and you make the diagnosis of which of the following?

A. Rocky Mountain spotted fever

B. Lyme disease

C. Steven Johnson's syndrome

D. Tinia corporus

E. Cat scratch disease

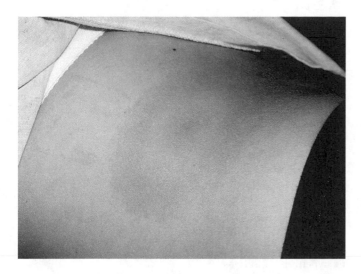

Figure 1-2. From Goodheart HP. Goodheart's Photoguide of Common Skin Disorders. *2nd ed. Philadelphia: Lippincott Williams & Wilkins; 2003.*

182. A true statement concerning IgE-mediated anaphylaxis includes which of the following?
A. It is seldom caused by immunotherapy.
B. Penicillin is uncommonly associated with anaphylaxis.
C. Yellow jackets do not cause anaphylaxis.
D. Peanut allergy may be caused by peanut oil in processed foods.
E. Latex allergy rarely affects health care workers.

183. The peak incidence of testicular malignancies occurs in which age group?
A. Infants
B. Children younger than 10 years
C. Teenagers
D. Young adults, age 20 to 40 years
E. Adults older than 60 years

184. A patient with hyperparathyroidism is least likely to present with the following?
A. Hypercalcemia
B. Elevated parathyroid hormone levels
C. Elevated serum chloride levels
D. Elevated serum phosphate levels
E. Metabolic acidosis

185. Which of the following is true concerning rheumatoid arthritis?
A. Laboratory, histologic, and radiographic findings confirm the diagnosis of rheumatoid arthritis.
B. Documentation of an inflammatory synovitis is essential for diagnosis.
C. Rheumatoid factor is found in 100% of patients with rheumatoid arthritis.
D. The rheumatoid factor titer is of great prognostic value.
E. Elevated synovial fluid white cell count is inconsistent with the diagnosis.

186. The most common cause of anemia across all age groups is which of the following?
A. Iron-deficiency anemia
B. Anemia of chronic illness
C. Sickle cell anemia
D. Vitamin B12 deficiency
E. Thalassemia

187. Which of the following statements is true regarding lymphadenopathy?
A. The differential diagnosis of lymphadenopathy is limited.
B. Adenopathy is more common in adults compared to children.
C. Supraclavicular nodes are common in children.
D. A common cause of axillary adenopathy is cat scratch disease.
E. Diaper dermatitis is not associated with inguinal adenopathy.

188. The combination drug amoxicillin-clavulanate (Augmentin) is at times more effective than amoxicillin alone because:
A. The combination drug is effective against methicillin-resistant *Staph. aureus* (MRSA).
B. The combination drug improves coverage of atypical organisms such as chlamydia and mycoplasma.
C. The combination drug provides improved coverage of organisms that produce beta-lactamases, such as *Haemophilus influenzae*.
D. The combination drug is better absorbed than amoxicillin alone.
E. It is less expensive, therefore enhancing adherence.

189. Your patient is a 45-year-old female whose hobby is needlepoint. During the past week, she has had pain on the radial side of her wrist and thumb, especially when she uses her thumb. Her pain is reproduced when you have her grasp her thumb with the adjacent digits, and ulnarly deviate and palmar flex the wrist. This is a classic presentation of which of the following?
A. Stress fracture of the scaphoid bone
B. Trigger finger
C. Ganglion cyst
D. DeQuervain's tenosynovitis
E. Carpal tunnel

190. Which of the following statements about colon cancer screening is not true?
A. Spinach, prunes, and plums do not cause falsely positive hemocult stool card results.
B. Testing of stool for occult blood obtained by digital rectal exam is of unproven value due to the high rate of false-positive tests.
C. Patients who have a single second-degree relative diagnosed after the age of 60 with colon cancer can be considered of average risk of getting colon cancer, and recommendations for screening are the same as those for other average risk patients.
D. Colonoscopy screening should be started at puberty in patients with a family history of hereditary nonpolyposis colorectal cancer.
E. Colonoscopy screening every 1 or 2 years should be offered to patients with ulcerative colitis, 7 or 8 years after they have been diagnosed with pan-colitis.

191. A true statement concerning treatment of rhinitis is:
A. Use nasal decongestant drops for at least 2 weeks to desensitize the mucous membranes.
B. Diphenhydramine (Benadryl) is a first choice for treating symptoms in elders.

C. Physicians can reliably predict which of the second-generation antihistamines (including azelastine, cetirizine, fexofenadine, and loratadine) will be most effective in a given patient based on these drugs' onset of action and half-life.

D. Intranasal steroids should be avoided in elders.

E. Immunotherapy is effective at improving quality of life.

192. Which is not correct regarding seminomatous testicular cancer?

A. Seminomas are slow growing, and at presentation 75% are confined to the testis.

B. Overall survival from seminomas is 99%.

C. Seminomas are very radiosensitive.

D. An elevated alpha-fetal protein (AFP) excludes the diagnosis of pure seminoma.

E. Greater than 95% of patients receive a radical inguinal orchiectomy for diagnosis and local control of their cancer.

193. A 55-year-old is noted to have an irregular pulse on examination. You are concerned the patient has developed atrial fibrillation (AF). A true statement is:

A. If rheumatic heart disease is present, the risk of stroke is reduced substantially.

B. Warfarin is contraindicated in a patient with a remote history of a nonhemorrhagic stroke.

C. In general, patients with AF should have warfarin therapy to achieve an INR of 3 to 4.

D. Paradoxically, alcohol abuse reduces the risk of AF.

E. Rate control with chronic anticoagulation, rather than rhythm control, is recommended for the majority of patients.

194. When INH is given for prophylaxis of TB:

A. Pyridoxine hydrochloride supplementation should be given to patients at risk for drug-induced hepatitis.

B. Pyridoxine hydrochloride supplementation should be given to patients at risk for the development of neuropathy.

C. Pyridoxine hydrochloride supplementation should routinely be given to all patients on INH.

D. Pyridoxine hydrochloride supplementation has not been demonstrated to be effective in preventing complications of INH therapy.

E. Young adults are at greatest risk of INH-induced neuropathy.

195. A 47-year-old with a history of known coronary artery disease seeks your advice about goals for hyperlipidemia treatment. He was just diagnosed with hyperlipidemia and has an LDL of 166. You suggest which of the following based on the National Cholesterol Education Program?

A. An LDL of less than 160

B. An LDL of less than 130

C. An LDL of less than 70

D. Begin immediate drug therapy—therapeutic lifestyle changes are unnecessary

E. Current LDL is fine

196. Which of the following statements concerning *Entamoeba* infection is true?

A. It is transmitted by the respiratory route.

B. There are two genetically identical but morphologically distinct species, *E. histolytica* and *E. dispar*.

C. Diarrhea is caused by coinfection with *Shigella*.

D. Bloody diarrhea (dysentery) is rarely seen with *Entamoeba* infection.

E. Differentiation of *E. histolytica* and *E. dispar* can be reliably performed via microscopic examination of the stool.

197. A 40-year-old male with a history of asthma comes in to the emergency room with an acute exacerbation. He is in severe respiratory distress and is intubated soon after arriving. What would you expect to find on his first arterial blood gas?

A. Chronic respiratory alkalosis

B. Acute respiratory acidosis

C. Chronic respiratory acidosis

D. Acute respiratory alkalosis

E. Normal arterial blood gas

198. A true statement concerning the treatment of benign prostatic hypertrophy (BPH) is:

A. Saw palmetto has been shown to improve urologic symptoms and flow measures.

B. Finasteride (Proscar) is an alpha blocker associated with orthostatic hypotension.

C. Tamsulosin (Flomax) is a 5-alpha reductase inhibitor associated with impotence.

D. Medications are just as effective as surgery at relieving symptoms.

E. There is no reliable way to monitor symptoms associated with BPH.

199. Which of the following signs or symptoms is not normally associated with patients that have COPD?

A. Chronic cough

B. Restlessness

C. Panic-like attacks

D. Mania

E. Pulsus paradoxus

200. A 59-year-old presents with a 3-month history of hoarseness. Which of the following statements is false?

A. Hoarseness for longer than 2 to 4 weeks suggests the possibility for a more serious problem.

B. If the patient had a history of heavy alcohol or tobacco use, the risk of cancer would be increased.

C. If unilateral vocal cord paralysis is demonstrated, imaging along the course of the recurrent laryngeal nerve is indicated if the cause of paralysis remains occult.

D. Direct visualization of the larynx is necessary.

E. Squamous cell carcinomas would be an uncommon form of malignancy if cancer is found.

201. During your history with the patient in the previous question, you uncover that he is a professional singer. A true statement is:

A. Direct visualization of the larynx is now unnecessary.

B. If vocal cord polyps are found, voice rest alone is usually curative.

C. If vocal cord granulomas were found, GERD should be suspected.

D. The finding of papillomas should prompt voice rest, which is usually curative.

E. A smoking and alcohol history is superfluous in this case.

202. Which of the following is most useful in diagnosing an upper GI bleed?
A. BUN:creatinine ratio of 100
B. Supine sinus tachycardia (pulse greater than 100 bpm)
C. Palmar crease pallor
D. Facial pallor
E. Abnormal liver function test

203. A true statement concerning rhinitis in pregnancy is which of the following?
A. Rhinitis is uncommon in pregnancy.
B. Increased estrogen diminishes capillary engorgement during pregnancy.
C. Pregnancy-related vasomotor rhinitis usually resolves promptly during the postpartum period.
D. Nasal steroids are contraindicated in pregnancy.
E. Pregnancy is associated with a decreased sensitivity to smoke, chemical fumes, and environmental irritants.

204. A 42-year-old male comes in with concern about a lump he has felt in his neck for about 2 weeks. On exam, you find a nodule in the right lobe of the thyroid about 1 cm in size that is mobile and soft with no associated lymphadenopathy. What is the most appropriate next step in evaluating this patient?
A. Ultrasound of the thyroid
B. Bloodwork including TSH and free T4
C. Reevaluation in 2 months to determine if the nodule has resolved
D. Referral to surgeon for total excision
E. Needle aspiration biopsy

205. If the man in the previous question was found to have a malignant nodule, what would be the most likely form of thyroid malignancy you would find?
A. Follicular carcinoma
B. Medullary carcinoma
C. Anaplastic carcinoma
D. Papillary carcinoma
E. Lymphoma

206. A 17-year-old presents to your office because of a 2-day history of severe headache, very high temperature up to 105°F orally, lethargy, and a new rash. The patient returned from summer camp 2 days ago but had no illness during his week in a wooded area at summer camp. He has no ill contacts. Physical examination reveals a very ill-appearing child with a rash most prominent at the ankles and wrists. The rash does not blanch with pressure (Figure 1-3). The most likely diagnosis is:
A. Poison ivy
B. Lyme disease
C. Rocky Mountain spotted fever
D. Henoch–Schonlein purpura
E. Dermatomyositis

207. Which of the following statements concerning dust mites is true?
A. They may be killed by washing bedding and nightclothes in water hotter than 130°F.
B. They will never return once they are eradicated.

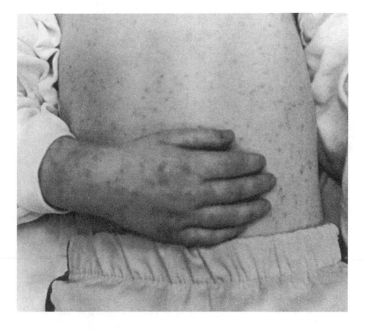

Figure 1-3. From Fleisher GR, Ludwig W, Baskin MN. *Atlas of Pediatric Emergency Medicine. Philadelphia: Lippincott Williams & Wilkins; 2004.*

C. They can be reduced by raising the household humidity over 50%.
D. High-efficiency particulate air (HEPA) filters have conclusively been shown to remove dust.
E. Leaving mattresses bare minimizes colonization by mites.

208. Which of the following statements concerning the health care of prisoners is false?
A. More than 6 million people were in jail, or prison, or on parole in 1999.
B. Most inmates are young, undereducated, and poor.
C. Mental health problems affect greater than 15% of prisoners.
D. Prisoners with self-identified mental illness are more likely to commit violent crimes and have a higher rate of having sustained sexual and physical abuse.
E. The rate of suicide in the incarcerated population is 10 times less than that of the general population.

209. A 42-year-old presents with a 6-month history of fatigue and weight loss. He has been diagnosed with asthma and irritable bowel syndrome by another physician. Your record documents a 20-pound unintentional weight loss. Your response might include which of the following:
A. Suggestion for psyllium daily
B. Supplementing diet with Ensure daily
C. Treatment trial with fluoxetine (Prozac)
D. Treatment trial with dicyclomine
E. Initiating an evaluation of the lower GI tract

210. Which one of the following statements is false concerning the impact of religious commitment on health?
A. There appears to be lower mortality.
B. Functional ability is increased for elders.

C. There are fewer health-compromising behaviors.

D. Substance abuse rates are higher.

E. Coping skills may be improved.

211. Which of the following statements is true concerning the management of spasticity?

A. A goal is to increase functional ability.

B. Local muscle blocks are unable to control localized spasticity.

C. Botulinum toxin type A (Botox) has a duration of action of approximately 2 years.

D. Baclofen (Lioresal) is contraindicated for treating spasticity associated with spinal cord injury.

E. Spasticity is characterized by hypoactive reflexes, weakness, and rapid initiation of movement.

212. A true statement concerning tension headache is:

A. Associated with fatigue and difficulty concentrating

B. Exacerbated by certain foods

C. Disabling functionally—unable to continue current activities

D. Unilateral

E. Repeated, severe attacks, which occur over a period of days to weeks

213. To detect early hepatocellular carcinoma in patients with cirrhosis, the two best screening techniques are:

A. Liver biopsy and AFP level

B. Liver ultrasound and AFP level

C. Liver ultrasound and biopsy

D. CEA and AFP levels

E. Rely on patient symptoms

214. Which of the following statements is true concerning occupational transmission of HIV?

A. The risk of transmission of HIV is 30% when an accidental needle stick occurs with an instrument contaminated with HIV.

B. There has never been a case of HIV transmission documented via the mucous membranes.

C. There has never been a case of HIV transmission documented via intact skin.

D. Health care workers have little to worry about since mass screenings for HIV have been initiated.

E. There are no effective post-exposure prophylactic strategies.

215. Long-term use of minocycline antibiotics in the treatment of acne should be avoided because of the risk of causing what drug-induced condition?

A. Anaphylaxis

B. Anaphylactoid reaction

C. Keloid formation

D. Lupus-like syndrome

E. Hemolysis

216. The most common indication for liver transplantation is:

A. Hepatitis B

B. Primary sclerosing cholangitis

C. Alcohol-related cirrhosis

D. Hepatitis C

E. Hepatitis A

217. Fifteen minutes after receiving an intramuscular penicillin injection, a patient becomes flushed and short of breath. Which is the least important intervention?

A. A blood pressure should be recorded.

B. An auscultory examination of the chest should be performed.

C. An arterial blood gas should be ordered.

D. An oral examination should be performed.

E. A skin examination should be performed.

218. On examination, the patient in the previous question has wheezing, lip edema, a pulse rate of 106, and a blood pressure of 120/80. The appropriate initial treatment is:

A. Observation

B. IV bolus of normal saline 500 cc

C. Diphenhydramine 50 mg IV over 2 minutes

D. Epineprine 1:1,000 0.5 cc subcutaneously

E. Methylprednisolone 250 mg IV over several minutes

219. Your patient is a 32-year-old white female who presents with signs and symptoms of COPD. She has hypoxia, a prolonged expiratory phase of respiration, and a poor FEV1. She has never smoked but does have a family history of early emphysema. This person should be evaluated for which of the following problems?

A. Farmer's lung

B. Coal miner silicosis

C. Alpha-1-antitrypsin deficiency

D. Histoplasmosis

E. Hemochromatosis

220. Which of the following statements regarding allergen immunotherapy ("allergy shots") is false?

A. Repeated doses of small doses of allergen are effective in reducing symptoms of allergic rhinitis.

B. Immunotherapy should be avoided during an asthma exacerbation.

C. Patients with life-threatening reactions to bee and wasp stings must have immunotherapy.

D. Immunotherapy does not need to be directed at specific allergens but causes a generalized "blanket" desensitization.

E. Immunotherapy improves asthma symptoms and decreases need for medications.

221. Which of the following patients could watchful waiting be safely employed?

A. Palpable anterior cervical nodes in a school-age child

B. An enlarged node with erythema, tenderness, warmth, or fluctuance

C. An adult with a 2-cm inguinal node

D. Multiple firm, nontender groups of nodes

E. Multiple firm, supraclavicular nodes in a child with no medical problem

222. A previously healthy 13-year-old has 2 days of fatigue, fever, and limping. He now refuses to bear weight. His mother denies a history of trauma. Examination reveals an apprehensive adolescent

with a temperature of 101.8°F. His right hip is flexed, abducted, and externally rotated. He winces when the physician attempts to internally rotate and extend the hip. Remaining examination reveals no source of infection. Serum white blood count is 17,000/mm³ and the sedimentation rate is 39. Which of the following is now the most important test for this adolescent?
A. Ultrasound of the hip
B. Aspiration of the hip joint
C. MRI of the hip
D. STAT blood cultures
E. Plain films of the hip

223. All of the following are typical characteristics of COPD *except*:
A. Onset in middle age
B. Long history of cigarette smoking
C. Rapidly progressive symptoms
D. Exertional dyspnea
E. Mostly irreversible airflow limitation

224. Which one of the following is not associated with classic aortic stenosis?
A. Angina
B. Palpitations
C. Exertional syncope
D. Dyspnea
E. A long asymptomatic period

225. A 64-year-old presents with tenderness in the proximal muscles of the arms and legs. She tells you that another physician had diagnosed her with fibromyalgia. She has to struggle to get up from the armchair in your office. Your appropriate action should include:
A. Reassurance that undoubtedly her previous physician was correct and suggest regular daily exercise
B. Initiation of high-dose steroids for the next 3 months
C. Drawing labs, including an ESR and muscle enzymes
D. Performing a biopsy of the patient's temporal artery
E. Performing a muscle biopsy

226. Which of the following is a true statement concerning patients with mitral valve regurgitation (MVR)?
A. The ejection fraction in patients with MVR should never be above the normal range.
B. Valve replacement should be contemplated when the ejection fraction falls below 60%.
C. Valve replacement should be contemplated when the end systolic dimension of the left ventricle is more than 25 mm.
D. Early on in patients with MVR, volume overloading and left ventricular hypertrophy almost never occur.
E. Fatigue is seldom a presenting complaint.

227. The most common cause of preventable peripheral vascular disease is:
A. Hyperlipidemia
B. Congestive heart failure
C. Hypertension
D. Rheumatic fever
E. Diabetes

228. Diet and lifestyle modifications including which of the following can alleviate the symptoms of irritable bowel syndrome:
A. Large meals spaced 4 hours apart
B. Increased dietary fiber until stools are bulky
C. Daily laxatives
D. Increased milk products
E. Sedentary lifestyle

229. A 59-year-old man presents with a left-sided neck mass. Upon examination, you find a solitary thyroid nodule in the left lobe of the thyroid. It is not tender, moves easily, and is not causing any symptoms. Which of the following is considered the most useful diagnostic test in this setting?
A. Thyroid ultrasound
B. MRI
C. Thyroid isotope scan
D. Fine-needle biopsy
E. CT scan

230. A red flag for a serious underlying condition as the cause of headache is:
A. Scotoma
B. Functionally incapacitating
C. Chronic headaches
D. Nausea
E. History of motor vehicle accident and head trauma

231. Of the following four modalities, which is the most sensitive for evaluation of osteoporosis?
A. Ultrasound
B. CT scan
C. Plain x-rays
D. DEXA scan
E. Serum calcium

232. Vaccination with BCG (Bacille Calmette-Guérin) for prevention of TB:
A. Is contraindicated for use in the United States by the Centers for Disease Control and Prevention (CDC)
B. Confers lifetime immunity in about 50% of recipients
C. Employs a live vaccine and therefore may occasionally cause disseminated, fatal disease
D. Is a contraindication to PPD skin testing
E. Is recommended for routine use by the CDC

233. When considering the prognosis in a 75-year-old woman who just suffered a hip fracture, which of the following statements is true?
A. Patients with hip fractures have an average 1-year mortality rate of approximately 20% to 25%.
B. Twenty percent of patients are still unable to walk unassisted.
C. Fifty percent of patients enter a nursing home 1 year after a hip fracture.
D. A majority of patients are able to maintain their previous lifestyle after hip replacement.
E. Patients with hip fracture almost never recover.

234. A 32-year-old male patient with chronic diarrhea, constipation, and joint pain presents with a recent hip fracture. The most likely diagnosis is:
A. Irritable bowel syndrome
B. Crohn's disease
C. Ulcerative colitis
D. Gastroenteritis
E. Celiac disease

235. A 44-year-old patient is brought into the emergency room by ambulance for severe dizziness. You find the patient lying absolutely still and refusing to move. She states that if she moves her head she becomes very dizzy and throws up. She describes the room as spinning when this occurs. This problem started this morning, has never happened before, and the patient has no relevant past medical history. She denies difficulty or changes in hearing. The Hall–Pike maneuver demonstrates rapidly extinguishable, brief, horizontal nystagmus. The rest of the cranial nerve and neurologic exam is normal. Which of the following is the most likely diagnosis?
A. Acoustic neuroma
B. Viral syndrome
C. Arrythmia
D. Infarct of the middle meningeal artery
E. Infarct of the posterior circulation

236. Which of the following is not associated with *H. pylori*?
A. Gastric B lymphoma
B. Duodenal ulcers
C. Gastric ulcers
D. Pancreatic cancer
E. Gastric carcinoma

237. An advantage of oral ampicillin over amoxicillin is:
A. Improved oral absorption
B. A wider antimicrobial spectrum
C. Better coverage of susceptible enteric pathogens
D. Less frequent dosing interval required
E. Associated with higher serum concentration

238. Which of the following is least likely to be seen in the patient with COPD?
A. Fully reversible airflow limitation
B. Destruction of lung parenchyma
C. Loss of lung elasticity
D. Closure of small airways
E. Bullae

239. Which of the following is true about patients with gallstones?
A. Rapid weight loss is a factor implicated in the development of gallstones.
B. Ninety percent of patients with asymptomatic gallstones will ultimately become symptomatic.
C. When monitored, patients with asymptomatic gallstones ultimately present with complications of gallstone disease rather than biliary colic.
D. Prophylactic cholecystectomy is recommended for most patients with asymptomatic gallstones.
E. Biliary colic is characterized by constant pain over 2 or 3 days.

240. In which situation would consultation or referral to a rheumatologist be unnecessary for a patient with rheumatoid arthritis?
A. Evidence of progressive synovitis unresponsive to NSAIDs, low-dose prednisone, and a DMARD.
B. Extra-articular manifestations of the disease, including systemic vasculitis, Sjogren's syndrome, or pericardial involvement
C. Lack of knowledge or experience in treating rheumatoid arthritis on the part of the primary care physician
D. Extremely high rheumatoid factor titer in a patient with debilitating disease
E. Initiation of a DMARD

241. When evaluating a patient with lung cancer, it is important to differentiate between small cell versus non-small cell tumors because:
A. Small cell (also called oat cell) lung cancer has usually metastasized at the time of diagnosis; therefore, surgical cure is not likely to be achieved.
B. Small cell lung cancer is more commonly found in nonsmokers than in smokers.
C. Small cell cancer makes up over 75% of all lung cancers.
D. Prognosis is better overall in small cell versus non-small cell lung cancer.
E. There is no important reason to distinguish the two.

242. The most appropriate next step in younger patients with new-onset symptoms of heartburn, especially after meals or while recumbent with or without regurgitation, is:
A. Perform EGD to rule out esophagitis.
B. Withhold treatment until evaluation for *H. pylori* is complete.
C. Empirically treat with H2 blockers or PPI.
D. Perform 24-hour gastric pH study.
E. Obtain a gastric biopsy.

243. Which of the following signs and symptoms must be present to make the diagnosis of acute otitis media?
A. Erythema
B. Fever
C. Irritability
D. Fluid under pressure in the middle ear
E. Anorexia or vomiting

244. Which of the following Pap smear results could be managed without referral for colposcopy?
A. Atypical glandular cells of undetermined significance
B. Low-grade squamous intraepithelial lesion
C. High-grade squamous intraepithelial lesion
D. ASCUS of undetermined significance
E. ASCUS high grade

245. Which area of the country has the highest prevalence of Rocky Mountain spotted fever?
A. The Rocky Mountain states
B. The Pacific Northwest
C. New England
D. Mid-Atlantic states
E. South Florida

246. Which of the following is false regarding the recommendations of the third report of the National Cholesterol Education Program (NCEP 3-2001)?
A. Elevated LDL cholesterol is identified as the primary target of cholesterol-lowering therapy.
B. In all adults aged 20 years or older, a fasting lipid profile is to be obtained at least once every 5 years.
C. Patients admitted to the hospital for an acute coronary event should not have lipid profiles performed because of the high rate of false-positive results secondary to stress.
D. African Americans should be carefully screened for lipid abnormalities because of their high risk for coronary heart disease.
E. Abdominal aortic aneurysm is a coronary heart disease equivalent.

247. A 27-year-old patient is brought to the emergency room for an overdose of an unknown substance. She has a history of recurrent depression and is being treated with citaprolam (Celexa). On laboratory exam, she is noted to have an anion gap of 18 and metabolic acidosis. Which of the following substances would most likely cause this finding?
A. Tylenol (acetaminophen)
B. Aspirin
C. Morphine
D. Citalopram
E. Cocaine

248. In a 15-year-old with diabetes mellitus type 1, which of the following findings is inconsistent with diabetic ketoacidosis?
A. Hypokalemia
B. Hyperglycemia
C. Hypophosphatemia
D. pH of 7.2
E. Hypermagnesemia

249. Which *one* of these antimicrobial agents provides the most effective coverage of *Streptococcus pneumoniae*?
A. The third-generation cephalosporin cefixime (Suprax)
B. The third-generation cephalosporin ceftibuten (Cedax)
C. The second-generation fluoroquinolone ciprofloxacin (Cipro)
D. The third-generation fluoroquinolone levofloxacin (Levaquin)
E. Doxycycline

250. Central pontine myelinolysis can occur when a deficiency of this electrolyte is corrected too rapidly:
A. Calcium
B. Potassium
C. Sodium
D. Phosphorus
E. Magnesium

251. A 32-year-old man presents with a myocardial infarction. In reviewing his past history, you find that his father, uncle, and grandfather all had myocardial infarctions in their 30s or 40s. Which of the following is not likely to be a cause of this family's coronary disease?
A. Familial hyperlipidemia
B. Hypertrophic cardiomyopathy
C. Marfan syndrome
D. Anomalous origin of the left coronary artery
E. Wolf–Parkinson–White syndrome

252. In acute infectious mononucleosis, symptoms (headaches, sore throat, malaise, and fever), monospot test, atypical lymphocytosis, and IgM antibody against Epstein–Barr virus capsid antigen all tend to *peak* at:
A. Two days after initial exposure
B. Four weeks after initial exposure to the virus
C. Ten to 14 days after initial exposure to the virus
D. Eight weeks after initial exposure to the virus
E. Twelve weeks after initial exposure to the virus

253. A 55-year-old postmenopausal woman comes to your office with concern about osteoporosis. You order a DEXA scan and it is consistent with osteoporosis. What would you tell her about estrogen replacement therapy based on the Women's Health Initiative (WHI) study?
A. The trial showed a reduction in invasive breast cancer in those on combined hormone therapy.
B. The WHI showed a substantial reduction in the incidence of dementia and improved mini-mental status scores significantly.
C. The risk of hip, wrist, and vertebral fractures was reduced in the WHI.
D. The rate of coronary events was significantly reduced in those on combined hormone therapy.
E. The risk of stroke was reduced by 31%.

254. If the patient in the previous question decided on an alternative to hormone replacement therapy, what might be the next best option for her?
A. Calcitonin
B. Calcium
C. Raloxifene
D. Alendronate
E. Vitamin D

255. A 45-year-old woman comes in with a lump in her breast. She describes it as painful and not changing in size during the last couple of weeks. She has no family history of breast cancer. You tell her:
A. The risk of breast cancer is 5% or less.
B. If the mass changes around the menstrual cycle, it is more likely to be cancer.
C. Do not worry about the mass, and follow up in a year.
D. Urgent referral to a surgical oncologist is warranted.
E. Do BRCA1 and BRCA2 gene testing.

256. Complications of celiac sprue include:
A. Cancer
B. Rectal fissures
C. Diverticulosis
D. Cholelithiasis
E. Liver cysts

257. Which of the following is the least important to include in the workup of a 56-year-old after the diagnosis of breast cancer?
A. Testing for estrogen and progesterone receptors on the cancer tissue
B. Complete blood count and liver function tests
C. Chest radiograph
D. Bone scan
E. Sedimentation rate

258. Which of the following is a risk factor for cervical cancer?
A. One lifetime sexual partner
B. Chlamydia infection
C. Later onset of first intercourse
D. Smoking
E. Nulliparity

259. A 39-year-old comes into the hospital with complaints of muscle weakness and fatigue. His history is significant for a history of hypertension, and he is currently on Lisinopril (Zestril) 40 mg a day. He occasionally takes NSAIDs for headaches. On laboratory exam, what would you most likely find?
A. Hypokalemia
B. Hyperkalemia
C. Hyponatremia
D. Hypernatremia
E. Hypercalcemia

260. In the patient in the previous question, you discover his potassium level is 7.0. Which of the following findings on ECG would be inconsistent with hyperkalemia?
A. Peaked T waves
B. Widening of the QRS complex
C. Shortened PR interval
D. Sine wave pattern
E. Loss of p waves

261. Infectious mononucleosis (an Epstein–Barr virus infection) is usually transmitted by:
A. Direct contact of saliva from an infected person with the oropharyngeal epithelium of a nonimmune individual
B. The blood-borne route
C. Expired respiratory droplet particles
D. Expectorated mucous particles
E. Fomite-borne infection

262. Which of the following is true regarding COPD?
A. COPD is the leading cause of death in the United States.
B. While mortality from COPD is increasing in developing nations, industrialized nations, such as the United States, are experiencing decreases in mortality from this disease.
C. Environmental pollutants are rarely important causes of COPD in developing nations.
D. High birth weight is a risk factor for COPD.
E. Occupational exposure to environmental dust and organic antigens may predispose to COPD.

263. A 26-year-old patient comes in with the complaint of irregular periods during the past 6 months. She is approximately 260 pounds, has a family history of diabetes, and denies any history of thyroid problems. On exam, she is noted to be obese, mildly hypertensive, and has evidence of hirsutism. Assuming the rest of her exam is normal, what finding on laboratory exam is inconsistent with polycystic ovarian disease?
A. Hyperglycemia
B. Elevated prolactin level
C. Decreased LH/FSH ratio
D. Elevated fasting insulin level
E. Elevated plasma testosterone level

264. A 72-year-old male has a solitary complaint of a 2-month history of fecal incontinence. He has never had abdominal or rectal surgery. A colonoscopy 4 years ago showed diverticulosis. Physical exam reveals a moderately decreased anal sphincter tone without stool in the rectal vault. A moderate-sized hemorrhoid is present but no rectal prolapse is present. Neurologic exam is normal. What would be the next step in the evaluation and management of this patient?
A. Empiric treatment with an antidiarrheal agent
B. Ultrasonography of the rectal vault
C. Sigmoidoscopy to visualize the rectal area
D. Anorectal manometry to measure rectal pressures
E. Surgical referral

265. A 49-year-old male with an unremarkable medical history has a first episode of loss of consciousness. Which would most likely provide new information as to the cause of syncope?
A. Tilt table testing
B. Head CT
C. EEG
D. ECG
E. Signal averaged ECG

266. A 71-year-old male complains of a 2-month history of neck and bilateral shoulder pain and stiffness, which tends to be worse in the morning. Pain is worsened by movement but is not palpable on examination. There is no noticeable joint redness or swelling. His ESR is 63. Which diagnosis is likely?
A. Fibromyalgia
B. Polymyositis
C. Polymyalgia rheumatica
D. Rheumatoid arthritis
E. Scleroderma

267. Which of the following is a true statement concerning menopause?
A. Menopause occurs between the age of 40 and 50 in 95% of women.
B. Estrogen is ineffective at relieving symptoms of emotional lability.
C. Hormone replacement therapy is absolutely contraindicated for women with menopausal symptoms.
D. The risk of endometrial hyperplasia and cancer may be significantly reduced with cyclic estrogen therapy.
E. The combination of continuous estrogen therapy and low-dose progesterone is associated with amenorrhea in almost two-thirds of women.

268. Laboratory evaluation of the adult patient requiring hospitalization for community-acquired pneumonia (CAP) should routinely include:
A. A blood culture
B. ESR
C. CRP
D. Bronchoscopy
E. Serum calcium

269. A 37-year-old patient complains of a 4-month history of a painful left shoulder. Physical exam reveals marked reduction in range of motion and significant pain to passive and active manipulation. Which statement is true about adhesive capsulitis (frozen shoulder)?

A. The primary etiology is intracapsular glenohumeral joint synovial adhesions.

B. Trauma is usually the inciting event.

C. Diabetes mellitus, hyperthyroidism, and hypertriglyceridemia are frequent associated conditions.

D. The primary loss of shoulder movement is extension and internal rotation.

E. Corticosteroid injections are proven to reduce pain and inflammation.

270. Which of the following descriptions is typical of the onset of a delirium?

A. Insidious onset, fluctuating time course, clear sensorium, poor attention

B. Acute onset, progressive time course, clouded sensorium, poor attention

C. Insidious onset, progressive time course, clear sensorium, intact attention

D. Acute onset, fluctuating time course, clouded sensorium, poor attention

E. Insidious onset, fluctuating time course, clouded sensorium, poor attention

271. Which of the following statements is true concerning osteoarthritis?

A. Osteoarthritis is primarily a disease of bone.

B. Marginal erosions are often seen on radiograph.

C. Acetaminophen is the drug of choice.

D. A hot erythematous and markedly swollen joint is a typical presentation.

E. Prolonged morning stiffness longer than 30 minutes is common.

272. Which HPV types cause most external genital warts in immunocompetent patients?

A. 6 and 11

B. 16 and 18

C. 31 and 33

D. 35 and 38

E. 42 and 43

273. A patient with breast cancer requires increasing doses of oral morphine (MS Contin) to control her pain from metastatic disease. She complains of increasing constipation and abdominal discomfort. What is the appropriate daily recommendation?

A. Encourage more fiber in her diet.

B. Use a fiber pellet since she is unlikely to drink a psyllium slurry.

C. Start docusate sodium to soften her stool.

D. Add senna granules to stimulate peristalsis.

E. Start nightly mineral oil to promote evacuation.

274. Which statement regarding *Clostridium difficile* infection is true?

A. *Clostridium difficile* infection accounts for most cases of antibiotic-associated diarrhea.

B. Oral metronidazole and vancomycin have similar cure rates.

C. Relapsing infections should be treated for 2 or 3 weeks versus the usual 10 days.

D. Confirmatory assays for cure should be performed after a treatment course.

E. It is never asymptomatic.

275. A 42-year-old presents with sore throat, rhinorrhea, and cough. On examination, he is afebrile, his throat is red, but there is no exudate or adenopathy. He requests azithromycin for his strep infection. What would be the least appropriate response?

A. The most common age for streptococcal (strep) infection is childhood to adolescence.

B. You recommend penicillin treatment rather than azithromycin.

C. The presence of rhinorrhea and cough make it less likely a strep infection is present.

D. You suggest a rapid strep screen, which may help bolster your suspicion that strep is absent.

E. The likelihood of strep infection is less than 10%.

276. Which of the following statements is false regarding the treatment of COPD?

A. Most patients with stable COPD get improvement with oral corticosteroids.

B. Pulmonary rehabilitation has been shown to increase quality of life in patients with severe COPD.

C. Smoking cessation slows the progression of COPD.

D. Long-term oxygen therapy has been shown to increase quality of life and reduce mortality in hypoxemic patients with COPD.

E. Long-term oxygen therapy has been shown to increase quality of life and reduce mortality in patients with COPD with normal oxygenation.

277. Which statement about Parkinson's disease is true?

A. Selegiline has been shown to provide neuroprotective benefit.

B. Tremor must be present to make the clinical diagnosis.

C. Deep brain stimulation is primarily effective for disabling tremors.

D. A vertical gaze palsy is a common finding.

E. Essential tremor is a risk factor for Parkinson's disease.

278. Which of the following drug's action is not affected by the coadministration of a proton pump inhibitor?

A. Theophylline

B. Griseofulvin

C. Vitamin B12

D. Ketoconazole

E. Amoxicillin

279. Your patient is a 35-year-old male who was involved in an auto accident 4 years ago. He had blunt abdominal trauma and had to have the distal end of his small intestine and the proximal end of the large intestine removed surgically. He did well postoperatively and other than chronic diarrhea has continued to do well. During the past 6 months, he has developed fatigue and shortness of breath. He takes no medications. A complete blood count reveals a macrocytic anemia. Which of the following would best explain his signs and symptoms?

A. Folate deficiency

B. Chronic depression

C. B12 deficiency

D. Post-traumatic stress disorder

E. Malingering

280. Which of the following statements is true concerning seronegative spondyloarthropathies?

A. It is associated with the HLA-B17 gene.

B. Reiter's syndrome or reactive arthritis is almost never associated with extra-articular symptoms.

C. Ankylosing spondylitis is a disease of older women associated with asymmetric monoarthritis.

D. Arthritis may be the first manifestation of inflammatory bowel disease, especially Crohn's disease.

E. Inflammation at bony sites of tendon, ligament, and fascial attachment (enthesitis) is rarely seen with reactive arthritis.

281. The most common cause of congestive heart failure is:

A. Hypertension

B. Coronary artery disease

C. Diabetes mellitus

D. Valvular heart disease

E. Cardiomyopathy

282. Which of the following statements regarding COPD is correct?

A. Chronic bronchitis is characterized by a productive cough occurring for more than 6 months duration for greater than 5 successive years.

B. Emphysema often results in reduction of air spaces and proliferation of lung parenchyma.

C. Alpha-1-antitrypsin deficiency is present in approximately 10% of COPD patients.

D. Cigarette smoking accounts for the majority of cases of COPD in the United States.

E. Advanced COPD is unlikely to cause significant disability and morbidity.

283. A true statement concerning strongyloidiasis is which of the following?

A. It is not endemic to any portion of the continental United States.

B. Larvae cannot penetrate human skin.

C. It produces only an acute disease.

D. Transmission is via the respiratory route.

E. It can produce hyperinfection characterized by filariform larvae migrating through the bowel to many organs throughout the body.

284. Biguanides (e.g., metformin) act to control hyperglycemia in type 2 diabetes mostly by:

A. Decreasing insulin resistance in muscle, fat, and liver

B. Stimulating pancreatic beta cells to increase insulin output

C. Decreasing glucose production by the liver

D. Inhibiting intestinal enzymes that break down carbohydrates, delaying carbohydrate absorption

E. Decrease degradation of circulating plasma insulin

285. Which of the following is a true statement concerning chronic abdominal pain and irritable bowel syndrome in adolescents?

A. Rare in adolescents

B. There is no gender predilection

C. Unlikely to be associated with depression

D. Is seldom severe enough to restrict activity

E. Associated with cerebral aneurysms

286. Which of the following medications has been shown to be the mainstay in treating any patient who has been diagnosed with congestive heart failure?

A. Angiotensin-converting enzyme inhibitors

B. Digoxin

C. Amiodarone

D. Calcium channel blockers

E. Aldosterone antagonist

287. Which one of the following statements is true concerning administration of cephalosporins to patients with a history of penicillin allergy?

A. Allergy can be accurately predicted on the basis of penicillin skin testing.

B. Cephalosporins are contraindicated in patients who have developed a rash following the administration of penicillin.

C. Cephalosporins are contraindicated in patients who have a family history of penicillin allergy.

D. Penicillins in general produce fewer immediate and delayed hypersensitivity reactions than cephalosporins.

E. Cefprozil and ceftriaxone confer little risk of allergic cross-reaction.

288. Which of the following is true concerning the seronegative spondyloarthropathies?

A. Associated with arthritis of the spine

B. Strong association with HLA-B17 antigen

C. Onset before age 40

D. Associated with retinitis

E. Never seen in association with skin lesions

289. A patient is admitted to the hospital with a 3-day history of symptoms and physical exam findings consistent with pneumonia. A laboratory finding that would suggest *Legionella* pneumonia is:

A. Hypernatremia

B. Detection of *Legionella* antigen in the urine

C. Many gram-negative bacteria seen on Gram stain of the sputum

D. Absence of leukocytosis

E. Hypocalcemia

290. Which of the following is unlikely to be associated with increased mortality from COPD?

A. Older age

B. Cigarette smoking

C. Malnutrition

D. FEV1 less than 1 L

E. Bradycardia

291. Which of the following therapies has not been shown to be useful in the treatment of peripheral vascular disease?

A. Angioplasty

B. Antiplatelet therapy

C. Amputation

D. Vascular bypass surgery

E. Exercise

292. An 80-year-old patient asks you about prostate cancer. You reply:

A. The risk of dying due to prostate cancer is more than 20%.

B. Although the majority of men of your age have at least microscopic evidence of prostate cancer, the chance of dying from prostate cancer is less than 5%.

C. The U.S. Preventive Services Task Force recommends a screening PSA test for all men age 65 and older.

D. There is good evidence that early detection of prostate cancer saves lives.

E. With a projected life expectancy of 20 years, PSA testing is recommended.

293. Drugs that should *not* be initiated for long-term secondary prevention in survivors of myocardial infarction are:

A. Beta-blockers

B. Lipid-lowering agents

C. Hormone replacement therapy in postmenopausal women

D. Angiotensin-converting enzyme inhibitors

E. Aspirin

294. Which of the following is the most common in men?

A. Acrochodon

B. Verrucae

C. Benign prostatic hypertrophy

D. Condyloma accuminata

E. Carcinoma of the prostate

295. Which of the following statements is *incorrect* regarding acute exacerbations of COPD?

A. COPD exacerbations are most often bacterial.

B. Environmental causes of COPD are relatively common.

C. COPD inflammation occurs primarily in the lung parenchyma and bronchioles.

D. COPD often has nonpulmonary (systemic) effects.

E. Smoking cessation can help forestall the progression of COPD.

296. Which of the following is least likely to be a complication of having a radical prostatectomy?

A. Erectile dysfunction

B. Proctitis

C. Urinary incontinence

D. Myocardial infarction

E. Local infection

297. Which of the following statements is true concerning HIV disease?

A. Heterosexual transmission is uncommon worldwide.

B. Heterosexual transmission of HIV is decreasing each year in the United States.

C. Transmission of HIV through heterosexual intercourse is less likely from an infected male to uninfected female, rather than an infected female to uninfected male.

D. Receptive oral sex may transmit HIV.

E. The risk of HIV infection via blood transfusion in the United States is approximately 1 in 15,000 donations.

298. A 37-year-old female presents with multiple tender points in her upper back, chest, and arms. She is fatigued and complains of pain. You have seen her for 2 years with these complaints. She denies joint swelling or stiffness. Your history and physical examination is otherwise unremarkable. You should undertake the following:

A. Rheumatoid factor and antinuclear antibody to assess for rheumatoid arthritis and systemic lupus erythematosis

B. An EMG

C. An MRI of the spine

D. Counseling the patient about the benefits of regular exercise

E. Suggesting a trial of a benzodiazepine as a muscle relaxer

299. Ulcerative colitis is least associated with which of the following?

A. Increased risk of colon cancer

B. Bloody diarrhea

C. Decreased risk of occurrence with smoking

D. Anal fissures

E. Isolated proctitis

300. A 65-year-old male presents to the clinic for his annual exam. He has no complaints. He has no significant medical history and his physical is normal except you notice a moderately enlarged, boggy prostate that is not tender. He denies any significant symptoms suggestive of BPH. When you get his labs back, the only thing that is positive is the urinalysis, which shows WBCs and bacteria. However, a culture is reported as no growth. What is an appropriate treatment?

A. Ciprofloxin 500 mg PO bid for 14 days

B. Oflxacin 200 mg PO bid for 21 days

C. Trimethoprim/sulfamethoxazole DS tab PO bid for 28 days

D. Carbenicillin 382 mg PO qid for 90 days

E. Tamsulosin 0.4 mg daily

301. A 33-year-old female comes in with symptoms of fatigue, constipation, cold intolerance, and somnolence. What would be the single best test to order to evaluate her thyroid?

A. Free T4

B. T3

C. TSH

D. Free thyroxine index

E. Thyroxine-binding globulin

302. Which of the following is the most common type of primary testicular malignancy?

A. Nongerminal tumor

B. Seminoma

C. Nonseminoma

D. Choriocarcinoma

E. Lymphoma

303. Which of the following is *true* regarding the nonpharmacologic treatment of COPD?

A. There is little evidence that pulmonary rehabilitation improves quality of life in COPD patients.

B. Smoking cessation improves quality of life but does not slow COPD progression.

C. Lung volume-reduction surgery is not considered a viable option in the treatment of COPD.

D. Noninvasive positive-pressure ventilation may decrease the need for mechanical ventilation in hospitalized COPD patients.

E. Oxygen therapy is ineffective in improving survival in patients who are hypoxemic.

304. Which of the following is the least likely to predispose to renal cell carcinoma?

A. A history of tobacco smoking

B. Obesity

C. Chronic dialysis use

D. Alcohol overuse

E. Tuberous sclerosis

305. A 24-year-old homosexual male presents with fatigue. Your initial evaluation should include which of the following?

A. HIV testing

B. CD4 counts and viral load studies

C. A careful history

D. Initiation of antiretroviral therapy

E. A chest x-ray

306. You are evaluating a 46-year-old patient for new onset of seizures. Which of the following imaging methods is the preferred study of the brain structure?

A. CT scan

B. Ultrasound

C. MRI

D. PET scan

E. Angiogram

307. A patient comes into the office complaining of several bouts of dizziness and ringing noise in his ears. The individual denies any recent infection, head trauma, or past history of these symptoms. He has no significant past medical or surgical history. He is not taking any medications at the present time. The episodes can last from several days to several months. During the episodes, the patient feels unsteadier and has a difficult time hearing his wife, but he is not incapacitated. On physical exam, you find horizontal nystagmus, decreased hearing in the right ear, and an abnormal Weber's test (noise heard in the left ear). Which of the following diagnoses is most likely?

A. Benign positional vertigo

B. Meniere's disease

C. Viral labyrinthitis

D. Vestibular neuronitis

E. Tumor

308. A 23-year-old female comes in to establish as a new patient and tells you she has a history of asthma. In reviewing her history, you find she is currently using an albuterol inhaler approximately 4 times a week and wakes up once a week with symptoms. How would you classify her asthma?

A. Mild intermittent

B. Mild persistent

C. Moderate persistent

D. Severe persistent

E. Exercise-induced

309. Is the asthma of the patient in the previous question controlled or not? What recommendations might you give her regarding her therapy?

A. Controlled, do not change her therapy

B. Controlled, educate regarding triggers

C. Not controlled, give a short burst of oral prednisone

D. Not controlled, add a long-acting bronchodilator such as salmeterol

E. Not controlled, add a low-dose inhaled corticosteroid or leukotriene antagonist

310. The same 23-year-old patient comes in to your office 2 months later after having a kitchen fire at home and is complaining of shortness of breath. What factor on your history and physical might make you consider admitting her to the hospital?

A. Wheezing on lung exam

B. Pulse oximetry less than 93%

C. Respiratory rate of 30 breaths per minute

D. No response to one treatment with an albuterol nebulizer

E. $PaCO_2$ of 25

311. A 56-year-old asymptomatic male with no family history of colon cancer has returned his hemocult cards. One of the three cards is positive for blood. A colonoscopy is performed and reveals a 0.5-cm hyperplastic polyp in the descending colon. It is removed in total. Follow-up recommendations should be:

A. Referral to a surgeon for a partial colectomy

B. Repeat colonoscopy in 1 year

C. Setting up a referral to a colostomy nurse prior to the referral to the general surgeon

D. CT scan with contrast of the abdomen to stage the extent of the colon cancer

E. Colonoscopy in 10 years

312. In the treatment of diabetic ketoacidosis, insulin therapy should be initiated:

A. Immediately upon significant clinical suspicion of the condition since delay in therapy can be life-threatening

B. Only after the serum potassium level is determined to be normal or elevated

C. Only after the serum potassium level is determined to be low

D. Only after the serum or venous pH is determined to be above 7.0

E. When the ECG suggests hypokalemia

313. Which of the following is true concerning HIV?

A. Transmitted by respiratory-droplet mode

B. Is a DNA virus

C. Is unknown among native African populations who have developed immunity to this virus

D. Is widely distributed throughout the world

E. Primary mode of transmission in Africa is by mosquito

314. You see the following patient in your office (Figure 1-4). A true statement concerning treatment is:

A. Patients with extensive disease may respond to moisturizers and ultraviolet B light.

B. Topical steroids are contraindicated.

C. Patients treated with PUVA have a reduced incidence of skin cancer.

D. Capsaicin cream may help with pruritis.

E. Anthralin ointment may worsen this disease.

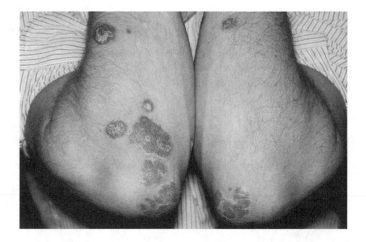

Figure 1-4. *From Goodheart HP. Goodheart's Photoguide of Common Skin Disorders. 2nd ed. Philadelphia: Lippincott Williams & Wilkins; 2003.*

315. Which of the following statements is false?

A. Side effects of zafirlukast (Accolate) include headache and diarrhea.

B. Zileuton (Zyflo) requires liver function testing for the first few months because of potential liver toxicity.

C. Both Zyflo and accolate are contraindicated in breast-feeding.

D. Montelukast (Singulair) has once-a-day dosing.

E. The leukotriene inhibitors can be a useful addition during acute asthma exacerbations.

316. A 22-year-old male presents with low back pain for the past 2 weeks. There is no radiculopathy. He is a baggage handler at a local airline. Which of the following statements concerning his management is true?

A. Plain films of the lumbosacral spine are an important aspect of evaluation.

B. He should be advised to wear a back belt to help reduce the risk of recurrent back strain.

C. His job satisfaction best predicts recovery.

D. A trial of traction is indicated.

E. Acupuncture is an acceptable option.

317. Please select the correct statement regarding COPD prognostic indicators.

A. The long-term prognosis for patients with chronic bronchitis is generally good.

B. Older age and a decreased FEV1 are the strongest predictors of mortality.

C. Older age is the major risk factor responsible for accelerated reductions in FEV1.

D. Although malnutrition and weight loss can be associated with COPD, these factors do not impact survival.

E. Right-sided heart failure is not associated with morbidity.

318. An antiviral agent that is effective for prophylaxis against influenza B virus is:

A. Amantadine (Symmetrel)

B. Rimantadine (Flumadine)

C. Oseltamivir (Tamiflu)

D. Etanercept (Enbrel)

E. Ribavirin

319. A patient with bronchogenic carcinoma located at the apex of the lung at the superior pulmonary sulcus (thoracic inlet) is *most* likely to present with:

A. Nocturnal cough

B. Weight loss

C. Hemoptysis

D. Shoulder pain

E. Headache

320. A patient has heard about hemochromatosis in the news. He asks your opinion about testing. You suggest which of the following?

A. Hemachromatosis occurs in less than 1 in 10,000 individuals, and screening is not recommended.

B. There is no screening test for hemochromatosis.

C. Hemachromatosis occurs in approximately 1 in 200 individuals.

D. A skin biopsy is diagnostic with hemochromatosis.

E. Only females are affected.

321. Which of the following is a recommended management strategy for recurrent abdominal pain in adolescents?

A. Emphasizing that the pain is "in their head"

B. Emphasizing a bland, restricted diet

C. Empiric treatment for *Helicobacter* infection

D. Psychologic evaluation

E. A trial of olanzapine (Zyprexa)

322. All of the following items in the history and physical would prompt you to screen for Marfan's syndrome *except*:

A. Kyphoscoliosis

B. Cardiac murmur

C. Arm span greater than height

D. Family history of Marfan's syndrome

E. Extreme obesity

323. A 30-year-old African American male presents to your office with fatigue, weight loss, fevers, and shortness of breath. On his chest x-ray you see bilateral hilar lymphadenopathy and decide to evaluate for sarcoidosis. What test would be the most definitive in making your diagnosis?

A. Pulmonary function tests

B. Bronchoscopy with biopsy

C. Serum angiotensin-converting enzyme levels

D. Bronchoalveolar lavage with measurement of CD4/CD8 cell ratio

E. Stress thallium

324. If the patient in the previous question was diagnosed as having stage II sarcoid, hilar lymphadenopathy with infiltrates, what could you tell him his chances for remission would be?

A. 5%

B. 25%

C. 50%

D. 90%

E. This disease never remits.

325. Which of the following is not a recommended way to diagnose diabetes mellitus?

A. Elevated fasting glucose (confirmed on a separate occasion)

B. Elevated hemoglobin A1c (confirmed on a separate occasion)

C. Abnormal response to glucose challenge (confirmed on a separate occasion)

D. Presentation in acute diabetic ketoacidosis

E. FBS greater than 200 with symptoms

326. The leading cause of mortality in U.S. travelers is:

A. Infectious

B. Injury

C. Cancer

D. Cardiovascular

E. Suicide or homicide

327. A 54-year-old woman presents with sore throat. She denies difficulty swallowing and has no upper respiratory symptoms. She noted neck tenderness when her 1-year-old grandson was hugging her earlier that day. A true statement concerning evaluation and management includes:

A. Presumptive treatment for strep is indicated.

B. A referral to a dentist is appropriate.

C. If a tender submandibular gland is found, steroids are indicated.

D. Thyroid abnormalities would be unusual.

E. Tenderness of the thyroid could cause ear pain as well.

328. A 76-year-old patient with diabetes has an IVP for suspected renal stones. True statements concerning acute tubular necrosis (ATN) include all of the following *except*:

A. Oliguria usually lasts 10 to 14 days.

B. A low urinary sodium may be found.

C. Hyperkalemia may ensue.

D. RBC casts and heavy proteinuria are expected.

E. The patient's age and diabetes are risk factors for ATN.

329. Which of the following nondrug treatments for psoriasis has been shown to be better than placebo?

A. Sun beds

B. Fish oil supplements

C. Oral vitamin D

D. Antistreptococcal treatments

E. Acupuncture

330. A patient visiting North Carolina returns with fever, rash, headache, and myalgias. Which of the following would be least likely if the patient has Rocky Mountain spotted fever?

A. History of mosquito exposure

B. Rash on the palms and soles

C. Hemorrhagic areas over the bony prominences

D. Azotemia

E. Normal CSF

331. What is a treatment of choice for the patient in the last question?

A. Doxycycline

B. Penicillin

C. Lincomycin

D. Rifampin

E. Gentamycin

332. A patient presents with blurred vision. Which of the following findings would *not* be supportive of the diagnosis of multiple sclerosis?

A. An MRI demonstrating white matter lesions greater than 3 mm in diameter

B. A previous episode of visual loss lasting for 3 days, 2 years ago

C. Onset of symptoms at age 32

D. Normal CSF

E. Impaired somatosensory evoked response test

333. Which of the following statements is true concerning thrombolytic agents in myocardial infarction?

A. Benefits from treatment are unrelated to time of administration.

B. The American College of Cardiology recommends thrombolytic therapy for acute ST elevation myocardial infarction within 24 hours of the onset of symptoms.

C. Recombinant tissue-type plasminogen activator is less efficacious than streptokinase.

D. Independent risk factors for intracranial hemorrhage include male gender, white, and age older than 60 years.

E. An absolute contraindication to thrombolytic therapy is ischemic stroke within 3 months.

Chapter 1

Answer Key

1.	D	43.	B	85.	B	127.	A	169.	C	211.	A	253.	C	295.	A
2.	C	44.	B	86.	D	128.	A	170.	B	212.	A	254.	D	296.	B
3.	A	45.	E	87.	A	129.	E	171.	A	213.	B	255.	A	297.	D
4.	C	46.	B	88.	A	130.	C	172.	C	214.	C	256.	A	298.	D
5.	B	47.	C	89.	C	131.	D	173.	E	215.	D	257.	E	299.	D
6.	B	48.	B	90.	C	132.	D	174.	C	216.	D	258.	D	300.	D
7.	E	49.	A	91.	A	133.	A	175.	E	217.	C	259.	B	301.	C
8.	C	50.	B	92.	C	134.	E	176.	D	218.	D	260.	C	302.	B
9.	B	51.	E	93.	B	135.	A	177.	E	219.	C	261.	A	303.	D
10.	D	52.	D	94.	A	136.	D	178.	E	220.	D	262.	E	304.	D
11.	A	53.	E	95.	D	137.	B	179.	D	221.	A	263.	C	305.	C
12.	A	54.	C	96.	E	138.	E	180.	C	222.	B	264.	A	306.	C
13.	E	55.	A	97.	A	139.	E	181.	B	223.	C	265.	D	307.	B
14.	D	56.	E	98.	A	140.	C	182.	D	224.	B	266.	C	308.	B
15.	C	57.	B	99.	A	141.	C	183.	D	225.	C	267.	E	309.	E
16.	C	58.	E	100.	B	142.	E	184.	D	226.	B	268.	A	310.	C
17.	D	59.	A	101.	A	143.	D	185.	B	227.	E	269.	C	311.	E
18.	D	60.	D	102.	B	144.	C	186.	A	228.	B	270.	D	312.	B
19.	B	61.	D	103.	A	145.	B	187.	D	229.	D	271.	C	313.	D
20.	B	62.	E	104.	B	146.	D	188.	C	230.	E	272.	A	314.	D
21.	B	63.	E	105.	A	147.	B	189.	D	231.	D	273.	D	315.	E
22.	C	64.	C	106.	A	148.	C	190.	D	232.	C	274.	B	316.	C
23.	D	65.	B	107.	B	149.	D	191.	E	233.	A	275.	B	317.	B
24.	D	66.	E	108.	B	150.	D	192.	B	234.	B	276.	A	318.	C
25.	D	67.	A	109.	D	151.	D	193.	E	235.	B	277.	C	319.	D
26.	C	68.	B	110.	C	152.	D	194.	B	236.	D	278.	E	320.	C
27.	B	69.	D	111.	B	153.	A	195.	C	237.	C	279.	C	321.	D
28.	B	70.	D	112.	D	154.	B	196.	B	238.	A	280.	D	322.	E
29.	B	71.	A	113.	A	155.	D	197.	B	239.	D	281.	B	323.	B
30.	D	72.	B	114.	C	156.	B	198.	A	240.	E	282.	D	324.	C
31.	E	73.	A	115.	D	157.	C	199.	D	241.	A	283.	E	325.	B
32.	D	74.	B	116.	A	158.	A	200.	E	242.	C	284.	C	326.	D
33.	A	75.	B	117.	A	159.	D	201.	C	243.	D	285.	B	327.	E
34.	D	76.	A	118.	C	160.	D	202.	A	244.	D	286.	A	328.	D
35.	B	77.	A	119.	B	161.	C	203.	C	245.	D	287.	E	329.	A
36.	A	78.	A	120.	C	162.	C	204.	E	246.	C	288.	C	330.	A
37.	C	79.	A	121.	B	163.	D	205.	D	247.	B	289.	B	331.	A
38.	C	80.	E	122.	A	164.	B	206.	C	248.	E	290.	E	332.	D
39.	A	81.	B	123.	A	165.	D	207.	A	249.	D	291.	B	333.	E
40.	E	82.	C	124.	C	166.	A	208.	E	250.	C	292.	B		
41.	E	83.	D	125.	E	167.	A	209.	E	251.	D	293.	C		
42.	A	84.	D	126.	E	168.	D	210.	D	252.	B	294.	C		

Internal Medicine Answers

1. D

The metabolic syndrome is a constellation of abnormalities that include abdominal (central) obesity, low HDL-C, impaired glucose tolerance, hypertension, and hypertriglyceridemia. Changes in magnesium and phospate metabolism are not part of this syndrome. The metabolic syndrome is associated with an increased risk of heart disease, diabetes mellitus, and morbidities associated with obesity. Lifestyle changes including weight loss and exercise, metformin, and other oral medications may reverse the progression to diabetes. Although the unique contribution of the metabolic syndrome to morbidity and mortality is debated, these abnormalities are frequently seen together and offer the clinician leverage for behavioral changes.

2. C

The definition of chronic bronchitis is a productive cough that has been present for 3 months in each of 2 successive years. Seasonal allergies can produce a chronic and productive cough during the time when the allergen is prevalent. This patient is not symptomatic during the same season each year, which would argue against a seasonal allergy. If she had chronic perennial allergies, she might present with symptoms all year long. Emphysema is the permanent enlargement of the air spaces distant to the terminal bronchioles. Emphysema usually presents with shortness of breath, wheezing, or a limitation in activity. Emphysematous changes may be present on x-ray, particularly with advanced disease. Asthma can present with a cough. Many times it is a nocturnal cough and is rarely productive. This patient does not report any wheezing.

3. A

Thiazolidinediones bind to peroxisome proliferator-activated receptor-gamma in muscle, fat, and liver to decrease insulin resistance. Because they do not raise insulin levels, they do not induce hypoglycemia when used alone. To a lesser degree, they also decrease hepatic gluconeogenesis. They may cause fluid retention and hepatic toxicity and therefore should be avoided in patients with congestive heart failure or liver disease. Monitoring of liver enzymes is also required.

4. C

Women are more likely to have false-positive treadmill ECG testing results than men and may be better candidates for pharmacologic or echocardiographic stress tests. Pretest ECG abnormalities caused by left ventricular hypertrophy with strain, severe hypertension, or baseline ST-T wave changes increase the likelihood of false-positive test results, as does obesity.

5. B

This presentation is suggestive of iron deficiency anemia caused by increased blood loss through very heavy menstrual periods. Once her hemoglobin has dropped below 10, physical examination may reveal pale conjunctiva, nail beds, and palms. She should not show jaundice unless she is actively lysing red blood cells in the intravascular spaces, which is not suggested by her history. There is no reason for her to have splenomegaly unless she would have spherocytosis, which is rare. She should not have hepatomegaly unless she has congestive heart failure, which is unlikely at her age without other physical findings. Clubbing is not associated with iron deficiency anemia. Common causes of clubbing include pulmonary disease, endocarditis, chronic renal disease, and ulcerative colitis.

6. B

Endoscopy is the procedure of choice in patients with "red flag" symptoms—dysphagia, weight loss, jaundice, anemia, epigastric mass, or older than 55 years with new onset or continuous epigastric pain—because these symptoms are associated with an upper GI malignancy.

7. E

Thrombocytopenia can be caused by decreased platelet production, increased platelet destruction, dilutional phenomena, platelet sequestration, or pseudothrombocytopenia. Common causes of platelet descruction include DIC, the anti-phospholipid antibody syndrome, drugs such as heparin, infections such as HIV and infectious mononucleosis, and ITP. ITP is characterized by isolated, idiopathic thrombocytopenia. Purpura, bruising, and bleeding are encountered. Other symptoms are usually absent—hepatosplenomegaly, lymphadenopathy, fever, or bone or joint pain. Medications can cause thrombocytopenia and purpura, but we have no history of any medication use. Medications that can cause ITP include penicillin, valproic acid, quinidine, sulfonamides, cimetidine, and heparin. HIV and lupus are less common causes of ITP; viral illnesses will often be associated with ITP in children. Eighty to ninety percent of younger individuals recover in a few weeks, but ITP can be more recalcitrant in adults. See Figure 1-5.

8. C

Prostatitis is a heterogeneous disease of men age 18 to 50. Acute bacterial prostatitis is characterized by constitutional symptoms, low back or perianal pain, a tender swollen prostate, and signs of infection such as white cells or bacteruria on urinalysis. Chronic bacterial prostatitis is associated with recurrent bacterial urinary tract infections with the same organism where the prostate is the nidus of infection. As many as 90% of patients with acute prostatitis have chronic prostatitis or chronic pelvic pain syndrome. Asymptomatic inflammatory prostatitis is usually an incidental finding associated with inflammatory cells identified in the prostate gland or secretions. By definition, such patients are asymptomatic.

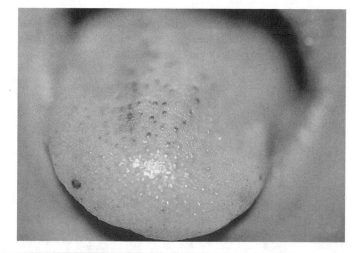

Figure 1-5. *Hemorrhagic bullae of the lips (A) and petechiae on the tongue (B) mark the presentation of this child with idiopathic thrombocytopenic purpura. From Fleisher GR, Ludwig W, Baskin MN.* Atlas of Pediatric Emergency Medicine. *Philadelphia: Lippincott Williams & Wilkins; 2004.*

Table 1.1 Neck masses

Lesion	Location	Embryology	Treatment
Thyroglossal duct cyst	Midline, near thyroid	Epithelial remnant of thyroglossal tract	Follow, or surgical removal if symptomatic
Branchial cyst	Anterior to sternocleido-mastoid, in lower portion of neck	First and second branchial arches; may include lymphoid tissue	Antibiotic therapy and removal
Dermoid cyst	Anterior fontanelle, lateral forehead, upper eyelid	Along fusion lines of neuronal axis or face, with lining of epidermis and keratin and mesodermal elements	Potential for sinus development; surgical excision recommended
Epidermal cyst	Any place	Proliferation of epidermal cells within dermis that does not communicate with skin surface; an acquired lesion	Watchful waiting or excision

9. B

Thyroglossal duct cysts are embryologic remnants of the thyroid gland and located at the midline over thyroid cartilage. Branchial cysts are located anterior to the sternocleidomastoid. Branchial cysts will often contain cholesterol crystals. Antibiotic therapy and then removal are recommended. Dermoid cysts gradually enlarge with sebum and can become infected. Simple excision is recommended. Dermoid cysts are characterized by focal keratinization and mesodermal elements; these features distinguish them from epidermoid cysts. Anterior cervical lymph nodes are found in found in front of the sternocleidomastoid and posterior cervical nodes run the groove behind the sternocleidomastoid and in front of the trapezius. See Table 1.1.

10. D

Patients with the history of antibiotic-induced anaphylaxis should not receive the drug again, unless proper desensitization has been carried out recently. The desensitization is temporary. Patient education regarding avoidance, use of epinephrine, and consideration of allergen desensitization are very important.

11. A

The long-term goal of management for stable but symptomatic atrial fibrillation is rate control in most patients. Although a wide variaty of agents are used, beta-blockers and calcium channel blockers such as diltiazem are preferred. Because of digoxin's side effect profile, and lower efficacy, most experts now recommend digoxin as second-line therapy for atrial fibrillation. Procainamide does not control ventricular response rate. Quinidine is not indicated for rate control. Amiodarone may be useful in select patients, but side effects limit its tolerability. Anticoagulation is another important consideration. In low-risk patients without risk factors, aspirin alone might be sufficient. For most medium- or high-risk patients, anticoagulation with warfarin to achieve a target INR of 2.5 is recommended.

12. A

The overnight dexamethasone suppression test is a very sensitive test as well as a 24-hour urine cortisol measurement. Cushing's syndrome, which is a result of excess glucocorticoid hormone, is most often iatrogenic. Other causes include an ACTH-producing pituitary tumor, ectopic ACTH production by a small cell carcinoma of the lung, adrenal adenomas, and adrenal carcinomas.

13. E

Historically, Parkinson's disease has been treated with levodopa or carbidopa as a first-line agent. Levodopa is very effective and almost all patients will respond to treatment. Carbidopa, a decarboxylase inhibitor, reduces nausea and vomiting by preventing peripheral conversion of levodopa to dopamine and allowing more levodopa to act centrally. Evidence suggests that individuals initially started on levodopa tend to develop dyskinesias earlier than those started on dopamine agonists. Many clinicians have now started using dopamine agonists as first-line treatment. However, this is not universally followed. Factors such as age, coexisting cognitive impairment, need for rapid response, and cost all can influence agent choice. Younger patients are at higher risk of developing lifetime motor complications, so a dopamine agonist is preferable; however, older individuals are less likely to develop levodopa-related complications. Since dopamine agonists tend to cause more psychiatric complications, levodopa is preferred in cognitively impaired patients. Levodopa is also preferred when rapidity of onset is desired and when cost is a factor. Adding a COMT inhibitor to levodopa may reduce motor complications and is another early treatment strategy; however, this approach raises costs significantly. MAO-B inhibitors, such as selegiline, may be useful for mild disease.

14. D

The AUA index asks the patient how often he has experienced the following symptoms: bladder not feeling empty after voiding, urinating less than 2 hours after going, the urinary stream starting and stopping while voiding, finding it difficult to postpone urinating, having a weak stream (dribble on your shoes), having to strain to get the stream started, and having to get up to go many times per night. Each question is scored from 0 to 5. Those with mild symptoms (a score of less than 11) require no treatment. Those with a moderate to severe symptom index can benefit greatly from therapy. Treatment options include doxazosin (Cardura), tamsulosin (Flomax), terazosin (Hytrin), finasteride (Proscar—only proven to help in men with prostates that measure more than 40 mL in volume), saw palmetto (conflicting evidence), and surgery (TURP).

15. C

The ankle-brachial index is the best test for confirming the diagnosis of peripheral vascular disease in the lower extremity. The rest of the tests are helpful but are neither sensitive nor specific enough to confirm the diagnosis. A normal ankle-brachial index is .9 to 1.3. An ankle-brachial index of 0.9 or less is very sensitive in dectecting angiographic evidence of peripheral vascular disease, whereas an index of less than 0.4 suggests advanced disease.

16. C

Because liquid oxygen is expensive, in-home oxygen therapy accounts for a significant amount of the COPD treatment cost in the United States (more than 30%). Whereas long-term O_2 therapy has been shown to decrease mortality and improve quality of life in severe COPD, an improved survival benefit has not been demonstrated in patients with less severe disease. Thus, oxygen therapy should be considered for long-term use in patients with a PaO_2 of less than 55. Routine use of methylxanthines (e.g., theophylline) in COPD is not warranted. There may be a small role for these agents in COPD patients who do not respond to common bronchodilators.

17. D

The most common cause of aortic stenosis (AS) is idiopathic. Individuals born with a bicuspid valve are at most risk for developing AS. The classic murmur of AS is a systolic ejection murmur that radiates to the neck and is made quieter by having the patient perform the Valsalva maneuver. Patients with AS do well until they begin to develop symptoms, and they have a 75% mortality rate in the next 3 years if they do not undergo valve replacement. See Figure 1-6.

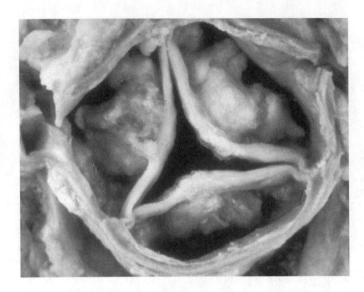

Figure 1-6. Calcific aortic stenosis. Large deposits of calcium salts are evident in the cusps and the free margins of the thickened aortic valve, as viewed from above. From Rubin E, Farber JL. Pathology. *3rd ed. Philadelphia: Lippincott Williams & Wilkins; 1999.*

18. D

Atlantoaxial instability would disqualify athletes from participation in contact sports, but noncontact sports other than diving are acceptable. Carditis is a disqualifying condition from all sports. Most authorities recommend disqualifying individuals with a solitary kidney from contact sports. Although insulin regimens may need to be adjusted for athletes, type 1 diabetes is not a contraindication to competing in sports. Other contraindications to participation in contact sports include recent seizure, solitary functioning eye, loss of conciousness with recent concussion, active coagulopathy, eye disease such as congenital glaucoma or retinal detachment, and a variety of other cardiovascular conditions.

19. B

Hypertrophic cardiomyopathy is the cause in approximately 50% of cases of sudden death in athletes. Coronary artery disease is the number one cause in patients older than age 35. The classic murmur of hypertrophic cardiomyopathy is a harsh, crescendo–decrescendo murmer radiating to the base, but not the neck. The intensity of this murmur will increase when outflow obstruction is increased, for example, with the Valsalva maneuver or standing from a supine position. See Figure 1-7.

20. B

The first thing to realize is that this does not meet the requirements for an uncomplicated cystitis (UTI). The patient has a fever of 102°F and thus by definition needs to be treated as an uncomplicated pyelonephritis. Due to the high rates of resistance to amoxicillin, it is no longer a recommended treatment. There is also increasing resistance to sulfonamides and trimethoprim sulfamethoxazole. The recommended initial oral agent for uncomplicated pyelonephritis (prior to knowing the resistance pattern) is a fluoroquinalone (usually ciprofloxacin, levofloxacin). For the uncomplicated UTI you can choose between a short course therapy of 3 days and the longer therapy of 7 days. Older patients and women with recurrent history of UTIs need the

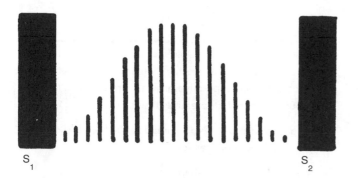

Figure 1-7. Hypertrophic cardiomyopathy. From Bickley LS, Szilagyi P. Bates' Guide to Physical Examination and History Taking. 8th ed. Philadelphia: Lippincott Williams & Wilkins; 2003.

longer regimen. Although the duration of treatment for a complicated UTI is controversial, most experts would favor a course of at least 7 to 14 days.

21. B

Orlistat is an inhibitor of pancreatic lipase and decreases fat absorption in the intestine. Sibutramine acts centrally to induce a feeling of satiety by reuptake inhibition of serotonin and norepinephrine. According to an NIH consensus panel, surgical therapy for severe obesity is effective and provides the most sustained weight loss. Gastric bypass surgery is the most commonly performed operation and results in sustained weight loss in up to 90% of patients. Surgery is typically indicated as an option for individuals with a BMI greater than 35 with comorbidities. The high incidence of morbidity and even mortality for surgery needs to be considered.

22. C

Although all of these tests might ultimately be useful, the most immediate concern is to rule out an infection, which could cause permanent disability, even mortality. Arthrocentesis is critical for almost every patient with monoarticular joint disease.

23. D

Synovial fluid analysis is an important diagnostic procedure in the patient with monoarticular arthritis. Normal synovial fluid should be clear, whereas cloudy fluid suggests an inflammatory arthritis. The presence of needle-shaped crystals suggests monosodium urate crystals. The presence of crystals does not exclude the possibility of infection. Fat droplets suggest a fracture. See Table 1.2.

24. D

Patients with the "worst headache of their life" must be considered to have a potentially catastrophic process such as a ruptured or leaking aneurism or intracranial bleed. A thorough history of past headaches (e.g., migraine), recent trauma or head injury, and associated symptoms such as fever is important. The physician should perform a careful neurologic examination. The physician should strongly consider a CT or MRI of the head in such situations. A plain film of the skull will provide little useful information and is insensitive to the conditions of most concern. Imaging prior to a lumbar puncture is usually performed to rule out a mass lesion that could predispose to brain herniation. A negative CT scan will not rule out a subarachnoid bleed, particularly a small (sentinel) bleed days later in the course.

25. D

In an acute ischemic stroke, some neurons die within a few minutes of complete loss of their blood supply. Other surrounding areas have relative ischemia and are at risk for cell death if blood flow is not maintained or improved. These areas may be dependent on a short-term elevation of the mean arterial pressure in order to maintain adequate perfusion for survival. In general, unless systolic blood pressure remains above 220 mmHg or diastolic pressure remains above 120 mmHg, elevated blood pressure should not be treated within the first 48 to 72 hours after an acute ischemic stroke. Multiple trials have shown that more aggressive management of blood pressure in the setting of acute ischemic stroke is associated with worse outcomes.

26. C

This patient presents with symptoms and signs suggesting drug-induced lupus. Drug-induced lupus is definitely associated with isoniazid, chlorpromazine, methyldopa, hydralizine, and procainamide. There is no clear association with penicillin or other antibiotics. The patient would be likely to have a positive ANA and antihistone antibodies but not antibodies to double-stranded DNA. Renal disease and central nervous system (CNS) involvement are rare.

Table 1.2 Synovial fluid analysis

Characteristic	Normal	Noninflammatory	Septic	Inflammatory
Lucency	Transparent	Transparent	Opaque	Cloudy/opaque
Viscosity	High	High	Variable	Low
WBC (mm³)	<200	200–2000	>100,000	2,000–10,000
PMNs (%)	<25	<25	<75	>50
Protein (g/dL)	1–2	1–3	3–5	3–5
LDH (compared to serum)	Very low	Very low	Variable	High
Glucose (compared to serum)	Equal	Equal	Variable	High

In patients with HIV, recent contact with indivuals known to have TB, fibrotic changes on chest x-ray consistent with TB, or immunosupression, a tuberculin test with ≥5 mm of induration should be considered positive. A reaction of ≥10 mm of induration is positive in those with an increased probability of TB not previously specified. Otherwise, a reaction of 15 mm or greater is considered positive in those of low risk.

27. B

This case is a classic presentation of testicular cancer. Antibiotics would be the appropriate treatment if epididymitis was suspected, but the history and physical do not support this diagnosis. Testicular congestion, secondary to decreased sexual activity, can give tenderness and swelling in the testicles; however, a painless rapidly growing testicle is cancer until proven otherwise. A transscrotal approach to biopsy is contraindicated because of the risk of spreading the cancer to another lymph node system. The skin of the scrotum and the testicles have different lymph drainage systems. Embryologically, the testicle originally was in the abdomen and migrated through the inguinal canal down into the scrotum followed by its vascular system, lymphatic drainage system, and nerves. Watchful waiting would be inappropriate for this patient.

28. B

Although antibiotics in general can cause delirium, cephalosporins seldom are associated with this problem. Other antibiotics such as fluroquinones and trimethoprim or sulfamethoxasole are more likely to cause delirium. Many classes of drugs are well documented for causing CNS side effects. These include opioids, benzodiazepines, cardiac glycosides, steroids, and any medication with significant anticholinergic effects (antihistamines, muscle relaxants, and antispasmotics).

29. B

Screening for depression is essential in the workup of a possible dementia since a depressed mood can cause memory disturbance. Also included in the routine evaluation is a TSH and vitamin B12 level since they can cause reversible memory impairment. An RPR formerly was routinely recommended but is now suggested for individuals living in a high-risk environment area. Clinicians frequently obtain a noncontrast head CT or brain MRI; however, if a patient demonstrates the typical mental status decline of Alzheimer's and if there are no physical exam findings suggestive of an alternative diagnosis, the costly imaging offers little to the overall evaluation.

A common, easily completed oral screener for geriatric depression is the short version of the geriatric depression scale (Table 1.3).

Besides a depression inventory, the mini-mental status exam (Folstein exam) and the clock-drawing test are neurologic exams frequently used by primary care physicians. More extensive tests (Weschler, Blessed Dementia Rating Scale) are occasionally used if the diagnosis is in question.

APOE genotyping is not specific enough to be clinically useful since many individuals with the 4 allele will not develop the disease and some without the allele will still develop Alzheimer's. Likewise, a SPECT scan is too nonspecific and too costly to be considered in the routine evaluation. CSF analysis can be helpful in atypical cases including a rapidly progressive dementia, reactive syphilis serology, suspected CNS infection, or for early onset dementia (less than age 55). It cannot be recommended for routine

Table 1.3 Geriatric depression scale

Undertake the test orally. Obtain a clear yes or no answer. If necessary, repeat the question. Cross off either yes or no for each question (depressive answers are bold/italic). Count up 1 for each depressive answer.

Scoring intervals: 0–4, No depression; 5–10, Mild depression; 11+, Severe depression

1. Are you basically satisfied with your life? Yes **No**

2. Have you dropped many of your activities and interests? **Yes** No

3. Do you feel happy most of the time? Yes **No**

4. Do you prefer to stay at home rather than going out and doing new things? **Yes** No

If none of the above responses suggests depression, STOP HERE. If any of the above responses suggests depression, ask questions 5–15.

5. Do you feel that life is empty? **Yes** No

6. Do you often get bored? **Yes** No

7. Are you in good spirits most of the time? Yes **No**

8. Are you afraid that something bad is going to happen to you? **Yes** No

9. Do you feel helpless? **Yes** No

10. Do you feel that you have more problems with memory than most? **Yes** No

11. Do you think it is wonderful to be alive? Yes **No**

12. Do you feel pretty worthless the way you are now? **Yes** No

13. Do you feel full of energy? Yes **No**

14. Do you feel that your situation is hopeless? **Yes** No

15. Do you think that most people are better off than you are? **Yes** No

evaluation. CSF Tau protein, although elevated in Alzheimer's, can also be elevated in other disorders. A carotid ultrasound is not indicated in the routine evaluation of the patient with dementia.

30. D

Low literacy is a hidden epidemic associated with poor adherence, lower health status, and less than ideal communication. More than one-fifth of the adult U.S. population is unable to comprehend even basic written materials. Easily administered tools, such as the REALM, can help screen for literacy. Sole reliance on computerized assessments of patient education materials will often overestimate the understandability of the handouts.

31. E

There is no single ideal test for UTI. For example, approximately 1 in 7 women who have a UTI will have a falsely negative leukocyte esterase test. The nitrite dipstick has a sensitivity of approximately 50%. If vaginal discharge is present, the patient more likely has vaginitis than UTI. A pelvic exam is important in this situation. Back pain is a nonspecific symptom suggestive of many conditions. Only approximately one-half of women with pyelonephritis have fever.

32. D

The diagnosis of DVT and pulmonary embolism (PE) is fraught with challenges. The history and physical examination alone are unable to accurately make these diagnoses. Common tests, such as Doppler ultrasound, also have important limitations for the diagnosis of DVT. False-positive tests are possible with pelvic tumors. False-negative results are common and serial or alternative testing is often needed in patients who remain symptomatic. Unless impedence plethysmography or ultrasound tests have returned to normal, it is impossible to know if an abnormal test is associated with a recurrent or chronic DVT. Although hypoxemia and an elevated alveolar–arterial gradient are often seen in PE, it is insufficiently sensitive to obviate further testing. A normal d-dimer test in most populations makes the likelihood of DVT or PE very low; however, in very high-risk patients, such as those with known malignancy, the negative predictive value of the d-dimer is not as helpful. An elevated d-dimer is nonspecific and only suggests the need for further testing.

33. A

Syphilis presents with the chancre, a painless solitary ulcer associated with painless adenopathy. Although classically on the genitalia, a chancre can occur on the lip. A maculopapular rash involving the palms and soles is often seen (see Figure 1-8). Secondary syphilis occurs after 4 to 10 weeks following primary infection and abates within 3 to 12 weeks. Tertiary syphilis occurs 10 to 30 years later.

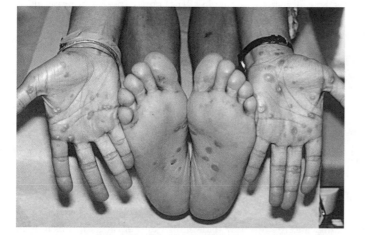

Figure 1-8. Secondary syphilis. Characteristic copper or "ham" colored, palmoplantar papulosquamous lesions seen on the patient's palms and soles. From Goodheart HP. Goodheart's Photoguide of Common Skin Disorders. *2nd ed. Philadelphia: Lippincott Williams & Wilkins; 2003.*

34. D

Domestic violence is very common. The lifetime prevalence of domestic violence has been found to be up to 40%. There is no way to identify victims of violence on the basis of demographic variables alone. Fortunately, brief, valid screening tools exist. Abused women often seek care in the medical system and their health care costs are more than double those of nonabused women.

35. B

Genetic testing for the APC tumor suppressor gene would be helpful for this patient's son. Patients with familial adenomatous polyposis (FAP) start developing tumors in childhood and teenage years, and there is a 100% incidence of colon cancer in affected patients by age 50. FAP is an autosomal dominant diseae but also can arise from spontaneous mutation. There is a risk for extracolonic cancers including gastric cancer, hepatoblastoma and medulloblastoma in children, and duodenal cancer.

36. A

Prolonged heavy physical activity including participation in long-term intense sports activity is a major risk factor for subsequently developing large joint osteoarthritis. Engaging in a moderate level of physical activity does not increase the risk of developing disease. Conversely, regular moderate activity can reduce morbidity and improve symptoms primarily by strengthening muscles that support the joint. Increasing age, obesity, and a previous history of joint trauma are all associated with potentially developing osteoarthritis. Other risk factors include quadriceps muscle weakness, inactivity, reduced proprioception, and female gender.

37. C

The most common cause of hyperphosphatemia is renal failure. Other causes include adrenal insufficiency, acidosis, and sickle cell anemia, in addition to those listed.

38. C

Kawasaki disease is associated with high fever, mucocutaneous changes including bilateral conjunctivitis and mucosal erythema, lymphadenopathy, and a high risk of coronary artery abnormalities in untreated patients. Aspirin is the drug of choice for treatment. Corticosteroids are contraindicated and associated with a greater risk of coronary artery complications. Aspirin and gamma globulin are common treatment options. The cause of Kawasaki disease remains unknown. See Figure 1-9.

39. A

Renal cell carcinoma is the tenth most common cancer in Western countries, constituting approximately 2% of all malignancies. It is usually resistant to chemotherapy, radiation, and immunotherapy. At the time of diagnosis, 25% to 30% of patients have metastatic disease. Radical nephrectomy with removal of the ipsilateral adrenal gland and the regional lymph nodes is the standard therapy for disease localized to the kidney. Prophylactic bilateral nephrectomy is not routinely recommended since bilateral renal cell carcinomas occur in only 2% of sporadic cases.

40. E

Benzoyl peroxide and topical antibiotics such as metronidozole gel are first-line agents and will usually treat and maintain remission of rosacea. Azelaic acid, tretinoin, and oral antibiotics

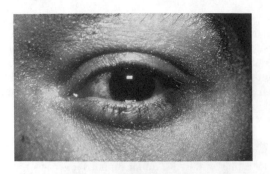

Figure 1-9. Kawasaki's syndrome. Ocular involvement. From Goodheart HP. Goodheart's Photoguide of Common Skin Disorders. 2nd ed. Philadelphia: Lippincott Williams & Wilkins; 2003.

are also effective. Isotretinoin is the most effective treatment for severe or resistant rosacea, but it has strict prescribing requirements.

41. E

Only approximately one-third of all familial breast cancers are associated with the BRCA 1 and 2 genes. A patient with the BRCA 1 gene has a lifetime risk of approximately 50% to 80% for breast cancer and 16% to 60% for ovarian cancer. Patients with BRCA 1 and 2 comprise only 5% of patients with breast cancer.

42. A

Chronic bronchitis is defined as a productive cough for 3 months in at least 2 successive years. Chronic bronchitis is associated with rhonchi secondary to mucus or debris in the bronchi, but classically does not cause rales, since chronic bronchitis is a disease process of the larger airways. A seasonality to symptoms suggests allergies or environmental exposures. Jaundice and ongoing fever are not seen with chronic bronchitits.

43. B

Tuberculosis may be caused by three closely related organisms: *Mycobacterium tuberculosis, Mycobacterium bovis,* and *Mycobacterium africanum.* TB is the leading cause of death from an identified infectious organism worldwide, with 8 million new infections and 3 million deaths per year. In some Asian and sub-Sahara African nations, nearly 50% of the HIV-infected population is coinfected with *M. tuberculosis.* In the United States, where the rate of TB infection is relatively low, populations at risk for the disease include immigrants, homeless persons, intravenous drug users, HIV-infected patients, prison inmates, residents of nursing homes and mental health institutions, and health care workers.

44. B

Individuals who are white are at increased risk for osteoporosis, not those who are Asian, who appear to have reduced risk. African Americans also appear to have a lower risk of hip fracture than white females. Other risk factors include some anticonvulsant therapies, estrogen deficiency, increased age, family history of osteoporosis, and a low body mass index.

45. E

Although there are multiple options for empiric (when culture results are pending) antibiotic treatment of CAP, effective coverage of *Streptococcus pneumoniae* should be provided because it is the most

common bacterial cause of CAP. The Infectious Disease Society of America and the American Thoracic Society have published guidelines on the treatment of CAP that stratify the patient by illness severity, recent antibiotic therapy, underlying diseases, and local pathogen resistance. Macrolides, doxycycline, tetracycline, and antipneumococcal beta-lactams all provide good efficacy against *Strep. pneumoniae* and are appropriate choices for CAP. High-dose amoxiciallin is still favored by some experts. The quinolones as a class have variable coverage of *Strep. pneumoniae.* Lomefloxacin, ciprofloxacin, and ofloxacin provide poor or variable coverage of *Strep. pneumoniae*—levofloxacin, sparfloxacin, gatifloxacin, moxifloxacin, and gemifloxacin have acceptable coverage. Sulfonamides, alone, would be a poorer choice of coverage.

46. B

Chronic alcoholism classically presents with macrocytic indices. Theoretically, an alcoholic could develop gastritis and develop an iron deficiency anemia from blood loss, but a high MCV is typical. B12 and folate deficiency classically show a macrocytic, hyperchromic laboratory evaluation. The anemia of chronic disease is classically a normochromic, normocytic anemia. Sideroblastic anemia is in the differential of microcytic hypochromic anemia, which also includes iron deficiency anemia, sickle cell anemia, thalassemia, the anemia of chronic illness, lead intoxication, and spherocytosis. Figure 1-10 outlines an approach for evaluating an anemia.

47. C

Hormonal or endocrine therapy is used for treating more advanced prostate cancer (stages C and D). Orchiectomy, lutenizing hormone-releasing factor analogues such as leuprolide, estrogens, and other hormonally active treatments are commonly used.

48. B

The differential diagnosis of this patient should include infection, acute rheumatoid arthritis, acute osteoarthritis, crystal-induced arthritis, ischemic arthritis, and a foreign body in the joint.

The likely diagnosis, with the presence of fever and a significant leukocytosis, is septic arthritis. A variety of organisms can cause an infectious process, but young adults are at particular risk for *Neisseria gonorrhea* and patients with rhematoid arthritis are at increased risk for *Staphylococcus aureus* due to compromised joints and glucocorticoid treatment. This age group is also at higher risk for IV drug abuse, again making *S. aureus* more likely.

Immediate knee aspiration is essential in the initial workup. Intravenous antibiotics should be started after the aspiration is performed. Choice of antibiotics should be based on the initial Gram stain of the joint fluid and adjusted based on the culture results. Withholding antibiotics until after a culture is positive could have disastrous consequences.

Obtaining a bone scan initially will be of limited value. Except for a joint effusion, an x-ray of the involved joint may not show any radiographic changes. The diagnosis should be made on clinical criteria and guided by microbiological studies.

49. A

Lung cancer is currently the leading cause of cancer deaths in both men and women. Women appear to be more sensitive than men to the carcinogens in tobacco smoke, both for active and passive (secondhand) exposure. The incidence of lung cancer also increases with exposure to asbestos or radon. The U.S. Preventive Services Task Force concluded that the evidence is insufficient to recommend for or against screening asymptomatic persons for lung cancer.

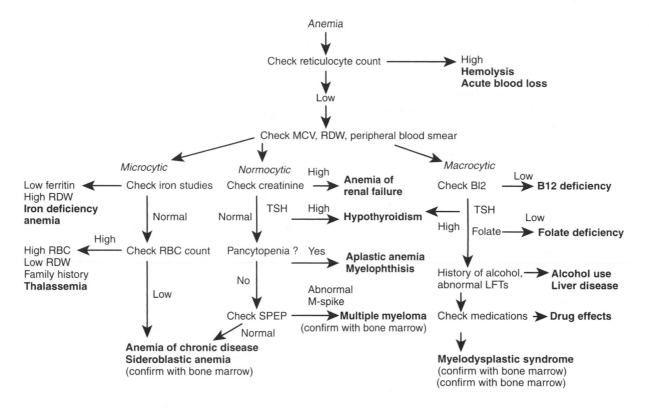

Figure 1-10. An approach to the evaluation of anemia. From Young V, Kormos W, Goroll A. Blueprints in Medicine. *2nd ed. Malden, MA: Blackwell Science; 2001:260.*

50. B

Hyponatremia, euvolemia, and urine osmolality >100 mosm/kg are consistent with SIADH. When considering the cause of hyponatremia, the first step is to evaluate the patient's volume status. SIADH is the most common cause of normovolemic hyponatremia and is characterized by low plasma osmolality coupled with an inappropriately elevated urine osmolality. The urine Na is usually above 40 meq/L and there is a normal plasma Cr and acid–base balance. The causes of SIADH include malignant tumors, pulmonary diseases, and drugs such as carbamazepine, opioids, clofibrate, vincristine, and chlorpropramide.

51. E

The above presentation is classic for urethritis and all of the above tests may be indicated depending on your location and the test reliability. However, the urine culture has a very low probability of helping you make a diagnosis and does not need to be obtained.

52. D

The above treatments could all be helpful, with the exception of beta-blockers, which might cause additional harm. Beta-2 adrenergic agonists can be helpful as well as thiazide and loop diuretics in patients with stable renal function. Patients with renal failure might be best treated with dialysis.

53. E

The patient has a history and physical examination consistent with a herniated disc, but most patients will recover uneventfully without surgery. Although a neurosurgical referral would be in order if the patient demonstrated signs of cauda equina syndrome (suggested by bowel or bladder complaints associated with other neurologic

symptoms and signs), the patient does not manifest these symptoms. Likewise, MRI, CT, plain films, and imaging studies are not indicated. Such studies would be beneficial if the patient was a candidate for surgery, but a 4- to 6-week trial of conservative therapy is indicated in the absence of more serious problems. Even relatively short bed rest has been associated with prolonging, not shortening, recovery.

54. C

Severe persistent asthma is characterized by continuous symptoms, functional limitation, and a peak flow usually less than 60% of predicted. Peak flows of 60% to 80% of predicted are typical of moderate persistent asthma. Treatment of severe persistant asthma includes a long-acting beta agonist, a controller medication such as inhaled steroids, and oral steroids when needed. See Table 1.4.

55. A

Fibromyalgia can be very challenging for patients, families, and their physicians. Despite discomfort, patients should be counseled to engage in regular exercise. Bed rest should be avoided. Opioid analgesics are inappropriate for this chronic condition. There are no good data demonstrating the effectiveness of manipulation for fibromyalgia. Although many patients with fibromyalgia will have disordered sleep and depression, more conventional antidepressants would be a better choice if such disorders were suspected.

56. E

Prostate cancer is defined by its stage and its Gleason score. Staging is categorized by the following: A, confined to the prostate and not palpable; B, confined to the prostate and palpable; C, extends into the seminal vesicles; and D, has already metastasized (most commonly to bone). The pathologist performs the Gleason

Table 1.4 Classification of asthma

Class	Symptoms	PFTs
Mild intermittent	Symptoms less than three times per week Asymptomatic between exacerbations Uncommon nocturnal symptoms	Peak expiratory flow relatively constant and FEV1 ≥80% predicted
Mild persistent	Symptoms more than twice per week but less than once a day; nocturnal symptoms more than twice a month	PEF varies 20%–30% FEV1 ≥80% predicted
Moderate persistent	Daily symptoms with functional limitation and regular nocturnal symptoms	PEF variability >30% FEV1 >60 but <80
Severe persistent	Continual symptoms with marked functional limitation and regular exacerbations	PEF variability >30% FEV1 ≤60% predicted

scoring by determining how aggressive the cancer looks in two different tissue specimens (scale is from 1 to 5 in each specimen and the two scores are added together). A score of 2 to 4 represents a nonaggressive tumor (well-differentiated) and a score of 8 to 10 represents a very aggressive tumor (poorly differentiated). A score of 5 to 7 is of moderate aggressiveness. The two treatment options are radical surgery and radiation. In general, surgery is best for the younger, healthy patient, and radiation is better for the older man or one with other significant health problems. This patient is healthy and younger than 65 years old and has the greatest probability of cure with aggressive treatment—radical prostatectomy.

57. B
Aortic regurgitation (AR) is caused by any disease that affects the aortic root or leaflets. The common causes include endocarditis, rheumatic fever, collagen vascular disease, and syphilis. With AR, the main problem is an increase in stroke volume, which causes high pulse pressures and increased afterload. These problems lead to progressive left ventricular dysfunction. AR presents with symptoms of left-sided failure, including fatigue, dyspnea, and orthopnea. Studies show that the only way to prevent permanent damage to the heart is to have surgery before left ventricular dysfunction becomes bad. Deterioration may occur even before symptoms develop, so physicians must do serial echocardiograms on such patients. Medications that reduce afterload, such as nifedipine, can help postpone surgery.

58. E
Nasal obstruction, pale, bluish turbinates, allergic shiners, and mouth breathing are all common signs of allergic rhinitis. Other less common associated findings include tearing, scleral injection, decreased hearing, a crease across the lower part of the nose, and atopic dermatitis. Findings such as cervical adenopathy or fever suggest the presence of underlying infection.

59. A
The patient has the classic triad of Meniere's disease: episodic vertigo, sensorineural hearing loss, and tinnitus. Other symptoms such as a sense of fullness in the ear or pressure are also common. Hearing loss, early in the course of this disease, is confined to lower frequencies. As Meniere's disease progresses, all frequencies are affected. Tinnitus often fluctuates and may be present between episodes of vertigo; unsteadiness and dizziness may persist for days. Diuretics and a low-salt diet are initial treatment.

60. D
A tubular adenoma is a precancerous colon lesion. The larger the lesion, the increased likelihood for malignant degeneration and colonic invasion with cancerous cells. A colonoscopy should be strongly considered because almost one-third of such patients have neoplastic lesions in the proximal colon. Patients found to have tubular adenoma should have repeat colonoscopy at least every 3 years.

61. D
The diagnostic criteria for migraines includes the following features: unilateral, pulsating, aggravated by activity, associated with nausea and vomiting, photophobia, phonophobia, and functionally incapacitating. Nasal congestion, rhinorrhea, lacrimation, facial sweating, miosis, and ptosis are associated with cluster headache.

62. E
Vitamins A and D can cause an elevated calcium level but not vitamin E. Endocrine disorders and cancer cause the vast majority of hypercalcemia. Hyperparathyroidism is two to four times more likely in women than men, and approximately 65% of all cases occur in postmenopausal women.

63. E
Many conditions increase the risk of colorectal cancer, including male gender, increasing age, inflammatory bowel disease, especially ulcerative colitis, and high-fat intake. Hereditary nonpolyposis and Gardner's syndrome are autosomal dominant conditions that predispose to colorectal cancer.

64. C
Short- and long-acting selective beta agonists are standard therapy in both COPD and asthma. In asthma, a short-acting beta agonist is utilized in all steps of treatment; a long-acting agonist is used in step 2 or 3. Treatment of COPD can also be performed in stepwise fashion. For the treatment of bronchospasm, a short-acting beta agonist is recommended for step 1, and a long-acting beta agonist can be added at step 2. Inhaled corticosteroids are utilized as step 2 treatment in asthma and can be an alternative to oral corticosteroids in step 3 therapy of COPD. Ipratropium is a standard treatment in COPD, beginning at step 2, but has not been shown to be effective therapy for asthma. Patient education is appropriate in both conditions.

65. B
Gout is associated with rapid onset of symptoms, reaching a peak in 12 hours. It more commonly occurs in middle-aged men, but it can also affect older adults of either gender. The duration and magnitude of hyperuricemia is associated with the age of onset of symptoms. Systemic symptoms are common. Synovial fluid analysis will disclose needle-like, negatively birefringent crystals. Chunky, box-like, positively birefringent crystals are consistent with calcium pyrophosphate dehydrate crystals. See Figure 1-11.

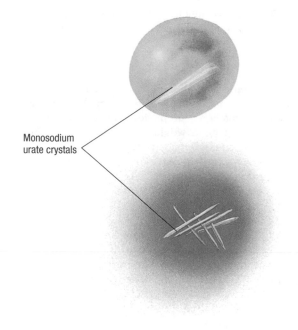

Monosodium
urate crystals

Figure 1-11. Gouty arthritis of the knee. Monosodium urate crystals. Provided by Anatomical Chart Co.

66. E

This patient has cluster headache—a chronic, disabling headache associated with lacrimation, rhinorrhea, red eyes, restlessness, and severe unilateral pain. Oral medications are of limited use in acute cluster headache. One hundred percent oxygen inhalation, triptans, and ergots may be effective. For chronic suppression, steroids (for duration of expected cluster), calcium channel blockers, lithium, and valproic acid may be effective. Opioid analgesics would be a last resort because of the chronic and recurrent nature of cluster headache. An emergency MRI is not indicated.

67. A

Initial treatment for mild to moderate osteoarthritic knee pain should begin with plain acetaminophen because of its proven safety, efficacy, and low cost. Studies have shown that for mild to moderate pain relief, acetaminophen is comparable to traditional NSAIDs. Acetaminophen should be used with caution or avoided in persons with preexisting liver disease and in alcohol abusers because of increased risk for hepatic toxicity. The other treatment options listed can be tried if acetaminophen treatment fails or if a patient presents with severe pain.

68. B

This patient has a high likelihood of strep, and at a minimum a rapid strep test or culture should be pursued. Twice daily penicillin is effective and enhances compliance. For penicillin-allergic patients, a macrolide such as erythromycin or a second-generation cephalosporin are acceptable alternatives. Early treatment of strep infections does reduce the risk of rheumatic fever but not the risk of nephropathy.

69. D

This patient is symptomatic and should be treated with PTU or methimazole. A low-dose beta-blocker could also be used to control symptoms until the PTU is effective. Radioactive iodine is not

safe in pregnancy and is contraindicated. Iodine may cause goiter in the neonate.

70. D

The evaluation of the adult with fatigue can be challenging. Consideration of infection, inflammatory illness, neoplastic, psychiatric, and other common conditions should be entertained. Although a careful history and physical examination is important, a family history of coronary artery disease is unlikely to be helpful.

71. A

The current recommendations for the treatment of partial seizures are the use of either carbamazepine (Tegretol) or phenytoin (Dilantin). Phenobarbital has a much higher incidence of side effects and so is not recommended as first-line. Gabapentin and topiramate can be effective in helping to control partial seizures but are used in combination with either tegretol or dilantin. Lamotrigine and tiagabine may have an important role in select patients with partial siezures.

72. B

There are many misconceptions concerning health care of lesbians. In general, routine health care screening recommendations should be followed. Many lesbians will have had heterosexual intercourse and, regardless, should undergo routine PAP smears. Likewise, HIV risk factors, such as risky sexual behaviors and intravenous drug use, should be assessed. Other developmental issues, such as parenting, should remain an important part of health care for lesbians.

73. A

Live vaccines (e.g., varicella vaccine, oral polio, and MMR) often have more restrictive handling requirements than non-live vaccines. Some live vaccines may cause clinical disease in contacts of recipients (e.g., oral polio virus). The ability of the live virus to replicate in the recipient improves its efficacy. The side effect profile of live virus vaccines is similar to that of other vaccines.

74. B

Polycystic kidney disease affects men and women equally and is inherited in an autosomal dominant fashion. Symptoms of flank pain, urinary tract infections, hematuria, and nocturia begin in the third or fourth decade. Hepatic cysts and intracranial aneurysms are seen. Diagnosis is via ultrasound or other imaging modality.

75. B

Chronic pancreatitis is often associated with normal pancreatic enzyme levels. Steatorrhea occurs late in the course of the illness and malabsorption of B12 is seen in up to 40% of patients. Impaired glucose tolerance is found in one-half. There is an increased risk of pancreatic carcinoma. Common causes of chronic pancreatitis include alcohol abuse, genetic etiologies, obstruction, and immune disorders such as SLE.

76. A

Hemophilia A is a sex-linked recessive disorder of factor VIII coagulant activity with normal factor VIII-related antigen (von Willebrand's factor). The PT is normal and the PTT is elevated. Treatment is with factor VIII replacement. See Table 1.5.

77. A

Diabetes insipidus (DI) is associated with inappropriate release of (central) or response to ADH (nephrogenic—tubular insensitivity).

Table 1.5 Conditions associated with an abnormal PT and PTT

Condition	PT	PTT
Factor VII deficiency	Prolonged	Normal
Liver disease	Prolonged	Normal or prolonged
Vitamin K deficiency or warfarin administration	Prolonged	Normal
Heparin administration	Normal	Prolonged
Factor VIII, IX, or XI deficiency or von Willebrand disease	Normal	Prolonged
Prothrombin, fibrinogen, or factor V or X deficiency	Prolonged	Prolonged

Urine volume can be more than 15 L/day. DI is associated with intracranial or neoplastic processes of the hypothalamus, hypothalamic surgery, head injury, aneurysms, and idiopathic causes. With central DI, there is a greater than 9% increase in urine osmolality after dehydration and vasopressin administration. With nephrogenic DI, there is little or no rise in urine osmolality following this test.

78. A

Physicians should ascertain whether adolescents have had the recommended hepatitis B series. A recent study demonstrated that a two-dose hepatitis B vaccine regimen was as effective as a three-dose regimen for adolescents 11 to 19 years of age. Recombivax HB [Hepatitis B Vaccine (Recombinant)] is now approved as a two-dose regimen for ages 11 to 15 years. Booster doses after the initial two- or three-dose series are not routinely required. Varicella vaccine is not recommended in individuals with previous or current varicella infection (neither chicken pox nor herpes zoster). The MMR series is complete if two doses are given at least 4 weeks apart after the first birthday.

79. A

As with Alzheimer's disease, mild cognitive impairment (MCI) is best diagnosed by a detailed clinical history. Patients with MCI will have cognitive deficits only in the area of memory. Orientation, calculation, recognition skills, constructual ability, and language skills are all in the normal range. Typical diagnostic studies, used to evaluate for a dementia, are negative. These include memory questionnaires such as the MMSE or clock-drawing test. In fact, most patients will achieve a normal score on basic screening questionnaires.

Studies indicate that approximately 10% to 15% of patients who have MCI will develop a formal dementia, such as Alzheimer's disease, annually. Since these patients are at much higher risk than the general population, they should be screened periodically for a dementing illness.

Vitamin E has not been shown to be protective for the development of MCI. Studies in Alzheimer's disease patients suggest a benefit in doses between 1,600 and 2,000 IUs daily.

Acetyl-cholinesterase inhibitors, shown to be useful in Alzheimer's disease and in vascular dementia, may also prove to be beneficial for MCI.

80. E

JNC VII recommended diuretics as the first choices for initial treatment of hypertension unless other comorbid conditions were present that would be a contraindication to use of these or in situations in which patients would benefit from the use of another class of antihypertensive (e.g., using a beta-blocker in a patient requiring migraine prophylaxis). An ACE, ARB, calcium channel blocker, or beta-blocker can be substituted or added if diuretic therapy fails to provide adequate control.

81. B

One of the disadvantages of chronic heart rate control with digoxin in atrial fibrillation is that it is vagally mediated. This results in a resting bradycardia but little protection against exercise-induced tachycardia. The onset of action of intravenous digoxin is relatively slow and the drug is relatively toxic, with a narrow therapeutic index. Perferred drugs include beta- and calcium channel blockers.

82. C

Influenza vaccination rates are more than twice that of pneumococcal vaccination rates, even though the recommended populations in adults are almost identical. Indications for influenza and pneumococcal vaccination include older than 65 years of age; adult with chronic cardiovascular, pulmonary, or liver disease; diabetes; and patients with HIV infection.

83. D

The American Thoracic Society suggests that long-term oxygen therapy be used for patients whose PaO_2 is 55 mmHg or less, 59 mmHg with cor pulmonale, or 60 mmHg with specific conditions such as sleep apnea. The use of supplemental oxygen to correct hypoxemia is associated with increased survival and increased quality of life.

84. D

Alpha-glucosidase inhibitors work by delaying carbohydrate absorption in the gut through their inhibition of intestinal enzymes. They need to be taken with a meal containing carbohydrates in order to be effective. They may be useful in the individual with postprandial hyperglycemia, but in general they are less effective than the other available oral diabetic agents. They have the advantage of not directly causing hypoglycemia. Because these agents cause undigested sugars to pass into the distal small bowel, their major side effects are diarrhea, flatulence, bloating, and cramps.

85. B

In general, methylxanthines or theophylline are not indicated in an acute attack of asthma. They would be more appropriate as an adjuvant therapy in the patient with persistent asthma.

86. D

The administration of adenosine or persantine (dipyridamole) causes dilation and increased blood flow in normal coronary arteries. Studies with radioisotopes such as thallium can demonstrate this response. Diseased, stenotic coronary arteries do not respond with increased blood blow and therefore do not show an increase in perfusion following the administration of these drugs. This type of pharmacologic stress test is useful in patients who cannot tolerate physical stress, such as individuals with severe emphysema or morbid obesity. These agents may precipitate acute bronchospasm, however, and are contraindicated in patients with asthma or other bronchospastic pulmonary diseases. They cannot be given to patients taking theophylline or caffeine products.

87. A

The treatment of choice for group A beta-hemolytic streptococcal pharyngitis is penicillin. Alternative antibiotics include a macrolide (erythromycin, clarithromycin, and azithromycin), clindamycin, or a second-generation oral cephalosporin. The combination antibiotic preparation trimethoprim-sulfa or sulfa alone, gentamycin, and tetracycline do not provide reliable coverage for group A beta-hemolytic streptococcal pharyngitis.

88. A

Acute CVAs usually present as clinical syndromes based on the anatomical areas of the brain involved in the ischemic insult. An acute stroke in the left middle cerebral artery distribution will present with symptoms of right-sided hemiparesis and expressive aphasia. These patients often manifest symptoms of depression in the postacute phase of the stroke. A stroke in the right middle cerebral distribution would cause left-sided hemiparesis but not expressive aphasia. Injury in the area of the brain supplied by the right or left anterior cerebral artery results in weakness and sensory loss in the opposite-side lower extremity more than upper extremity without aphasia.

89. C

External beam radiation for prostate cancer is associated with ED, proctitis, cystitis, and enteritis. It does not cause memory loss.

90. C

Scleroderma is a chronic autoimmune disease associated with vasculopathy and fibrosis. It is classified into either systemic or limited cutaneous disease. The CREST syndrome is a form of limited cutaneous sclerodermas and is associated with calcinosis, Raynaud's phenomena, esophageal dysmotility, sclerodactyly, and telangectasia. This form of scleroderma carries a relatively good prognosis and is associated with anticentromere antibody. In contrast, diffuse cutaneous scleroderma is associated with approximately 50% 10-year survival and harbors the risk of life-threatening visceral disease. Diffuse cutaneous scleroderma is associated with antinucleolar antibodies and the absence of anticentromere antibody.

Other common autoantibodies and their associated illnesses include:

Rheumatoid factor—80% of patients with rheumatoid arthritis, but also in SLE, Sjogrens, and mixed connective tissue disorder.
Antinuclear antibody—SLE, but also scleroderma, Sjogrens, mixed connective tissue disease, polymyositis/dermatomyositis, and rheumatoid arthritis.
Anti-ds DNA—SLE in 60%.
Anti-histone—Drug-induced SLE, 90%; SLE, 50%.
Anti-centromere—Scleroderma, 30%.
c-ANCA—Wegener's granulomatosis.

91. A

Both acute otitis media (AOM) and bacterial sinusitis are almost always preceded by a viral URI; strep pneumonia is the most common bacterial isolate. In sinusitis, symptoms of 5 days' duration or less suggest a viral etiology, whereas symptoms lasting longer than 7 to 10 days usually warrant antibiotic treatment. For AOM, a waiting period of 72 hours before antibiotics is warranted unless the child is toxic appearing or immunocompromised. By using a watchful waiting approach, antibiotic usage is reduced substantially. Treatment failure is defined as fever, malaise, or ear pain that persists for more than 72 hours after antibiotic initiation. The choice of antibiotics may be determined by your local area resistance pattern, but in general you should start with one of the "older," narrower spectrum antibiotics.

92. C

Fatigue and malaise are frequent symptoms of RA, but they are not specific enough to be diagnostic criteria. A positive rheumatoid factor (RF) alone is never conclusive evidence of RA. Approximately 80% of patients with RA are RF positive. However, many conditions are associated with a positive test, including infections, other inflammatory diseases, and normal aging. Monoarthritis is an unusual presentation for RA. Failure to progress to polyarthritis and symptoms less than 6 weeks are both inconsistent with RA. Patients with self-limited polyarthritis frequently have another diagnosis, such as reactive arthritis or polymyalgia rheumatica. RA's usual insidious onset may at first be asymmetric, but with time symmetric involvement of the wrists, MCPs, and PIPs follows. The feet are commonly affected and frequently there is parallel disease activity in the hands. Knees, ankles, shoulders, and elbows are often affected. Synovitis of C1 and C2 can lead to atlantoaxial instability, but the lumbosacral spine and sacroiliac joints are not involved in RA.

The American Rheumatologic Association criteria for rheumatoid arthritis is made when patients have at least four of the following seven criteria:

1. Morning stiffness
2. Arthritis of three or more joint areas
3. Arthritis of hand joints
4. Symmetric arthritis
5. Rheumatoid nodules
6. RF positive
7. Radiographic changes

93. B

All of the above, except heart failure can cause pruritus. Recent studies have shown that the selective serotonin reuptake inhibitors produce the strongest antipuritic effect. Other medications that may be helpful are antihistamine (H1 and H2 blockers) and tricyclic antidepressants.

94. A

Azithromycin, although usually grouped with erythromycin and clarithromycin in the macrolide family of antiobiotics, is more properly termed an azalide antibiotic. This drug is not metabolized in the P-450 system and therefore has less potential than the macrolides for adverse interactions with drugs such as cimetadine (Tagamet) and theophylline. Rifampin also interacts extensively with the CYP-450 system.

95. D

Reiter's syndrome (RS) or reactive arthritis is an inflammatory disease that follows, within 1 to 4 weeks, an infection of the genital tract with chlamydia or ureaplasma, or of the gastrointestinal tract with salmonella, shigella, campylobacter, or yersinia. The incidence ratio of male to female is 1:1 in post-dysenteric RS. However, post-venereal RS is seen mostly in men, with a ratio of 9:1. Urethritis (cervicitis and vaginitis in women) occurs in both forms of the disease and, when present, is usually the initial symptom. Conjuctivitis may develop concurrently or after urethritis has resolved. Arthritis typically appears last. These classic symptoms may develop sequentially and are seen in only one-third of patients. Since genital infections can be asymptomatic, this component of the diagnostic triad may be missed. HLA-B27 is positive in 80% of patients with spondylitis. Low back and buttock pain occurs in one-half of patients and may be from sacroiliitis or spondylitis. However, only 20% of patients show radiographic changes of the spine or sacroiliac joints. Peripheral arthritis is common and usually presents as an asymmetric oligoarthritis of the joints in the lower extremities. Enthesitis is also frequently seen, particularly in the heel. Circinate balanitis consists of painless ulcers of the shaft or glans of the penis and keratoderma blennorrhagicum, a vesiculating eruption that becomes scaly and hyperkeratotic, and appears commonly on the soles. Painless oral ulcers and nonpitting nail changes also occur. See Figure 1-12.

96. E

The only factors identified as making a man high risk for the development of prostate cancer are having a first-degree relative with prostate cancer and being of African American heritage. African American men have a fourfold greater mortality from prostate cancer. Tobacco and alcohol place men at high risk for other cancers (lung, bladder, liver, and stomach). BPH has not been shown in itself to increase the risk of prostate cancer; however, it can make screening more difficult. The old myth that men who had a vasectomy were at higher risk for prostate cancer has been found to be just that: a myth. Studies have found no relationship between having a vasectomy and developing prostate cancer.

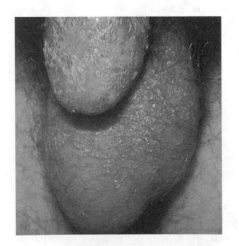

Figure 1-12. Reiter's syndrome. In circinate balanitis, psoriasiform lesions occur on the glans penis and the scrotum. From Goodheart HP. Goodheart's Photoguide of Common Skin Disorders. 2nd ed. Philadelphia: Lippincott Williams & Wilkins; 2003.

97. A

Renal masses may be detected by abdominal CT scans done to evaluate hematuria, flank pain, or a flank mass. Not uncommonly, however, renal tumors may also be discovered incidentally during imaging for other indications. A solid, contrast-enhancing, solitary renal mass has a high likelihood of being renal cell carcinoma (RCC). Multiple masses would suggest metastases or lymphoma, particularly with a history of a primary malignancy. The more highly cystic a renal mass is, the less likely it is to be cancer, although RCC may have cystic components.

98. A

Pica, or the desire to consume nonfood items, is peculiar to pregnancy and iron deficiency anemia. The craving to eat dirt and paint has been reported, but intense craving to eat ice should lead one to consider iron deficiency anemia. This craving has not been reported in other anemias, and it has not been reported in bipolar disorder or post-traumatic stress disorder.

The differential of microcytic anemia includes not only iron deficiency anema but also common hemoglobinopathies including sickle cell and thalasemia and blood loss. See Figure 1-13.

99. A

ATP-3 suggests a goal LDL cholesterol of less than 100 for patients with a greater than 20% risk of a major coronary event during the next 10 years. This risk group includes patients with known coronary heart disease, other clinical forms of cardiovascular disease, diabetes, or multiple risk factors that confer a 10-year risk for coronary heart disease (CHD) greater than 20%.

100. B

The NIH identifies very mild histologic disease by biopsy, undetectable levels of hepatitis C virus in the blood, and normal liver function tests as indicators that the disease is less likely to progress and that the patient is not likely to sufficiently benefit from antiviral therapy.

101. A

Sleep apnea occurs when there is either disruption of the central drive to breath (e.g., as in advanced COPD and head trauma) or blockage of nasal–oral airflow (obstructive sleep apnea). Patients with OSA have frequent nighttime arousals and therefore may experience daytime fatigue and sleepiness. Alcohol or sedatives may worsen obstruction by decreasing pharyngeal muscle tone. Weight loss can be a successful treatment for OSA, but unfortunately only a small fraction of people can permanently lose weight, so recommending it is usually ineffective. Most people sleep with their mouth closed, so nasal CPAP is usually effective. A chinstrap can be used if needed to keep the mouth closed. A larger neck size, especially greater than 17 inches in males, is associated with OSA.

102. B

Combination therapy of metformin with any of the classes of drugs used to treat type 2 diabetes, including insulin, is reasonable. Patients with CHF or renal insufficiency are at increased risk for the development of lactic acidosis and should not be given metformin. Any form of significant acidosis would be a contraindication to metformin.

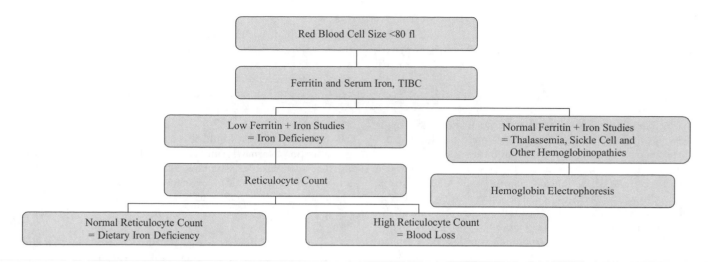

Figure 1-13. *Differential diagnosis of microcytic anemia.*

103. A

Epidemics of influenza viruses (A and B) are typically seen during the winter months. Although influenza viruses can cause disease among all age groups, the rates of infection are highest among children. Rates of serious illness and death, however, are highest among persons older than 65 years of age and persons of any age with chronic illnesses (e.g., diabetes or asthma), which increase risk for complications of influenza.

104. B

A significant proportion of women with cervical cancer are older than 65 years, which is important to remember when screening. A woman's lifetime risk of cervical cancer is approximately 1%, and stage 1 cervical cancer has a 5-year survival rate of approximately 80%. Women who smoke are at increased risk. Colposcopy with biopsy can be performed in high-grade lesions, but an endocervical curettage should not be performed in pregnancy.

105. A

Effective treatment of hypertension has a much greater reduction of relative risk of stroke than of myocardial infarction, renal failure, congestive heart failure, or cardiovascular mortality.

106. A

Both nedocromil and cromolyn sodium are mast cell stabilizers that can be used for exercise-induced asthma. In some studies, nedocromil has been shown to be more effective in inhibiting bronchospasm associated with exercise and cold air exposure. These medications can also be used in children and pregnant women with mild persistent asthma.

107. B

Antibody to hepatitis B surface antigen indicates the development of an immune response to the virus, via either immunization or natural infection. Hepatitis core antigen is not detectable in the serum. Hepatitis E antigen occurs during periods of high viral replication and may not be present in the chronic carrier state. High titers of E antigen correlate with infectivity. The most clinically useful marker for hepatitis B infection is the hepatitis B surface antigen.

108. B

Insulin secretagogues (sulfonylureas and repaglinide) stimulate the pancreas to release more insulin. They may become less effective as the disease process progresses and the pancreas loses its capacity to increase insulin output.

109. D

All of the tests can be useful in the patient with suspected heart failure; however, the test that is best at confirming the diagnosis of congestive heart failure is the echocardiogram. The most widely accepted definition of heart failure is a patient with an ejection fraction of less than 40%. This is, of course, only for left ventricular systolic dysfunction. Although many agree that diastolic dysfunction is a common cause of heart failure, there is controversy about its diagnosis and treatment.

110. C

A decrease in the FEV1 and decrease in the FEV1/FVC ratio are most consistent with asthma.

111. B

The initiation of treatment with dihydropyridine calcium channel blockers is generally contraindicated in routine treatment of acute MI because of reflex sympathetic activation (tachycardia), and hypotension associated with their use. Of course, beta-blockers must be used cautiously in the face of congestive heart failure.

112. D

All antipsychotic agents have the potential to cause, or worsen, extrapyramidal symptoms. Clozapine has been shown in several trials to treat hallucinations without significantly worsening motor symptoms. Clozapine can cause agranulocytosis, necessitating frequent CBC monitoring. Haloperidol, along with other traditional antipsychotics, can cause significant motor dysfunction especially at higher doses. In one trial, olanzipine was shown to worsen symptoms. Quetiapine is reported to have more favorable effects, but this has not yet been proven in clinical trials. Chlordiazepoxide, a benzodiazepine, may worsen psychosis, increase the likelihood of falls, and would be relatively contraindicated.

113. A

Oxygen supplementation should be limited to the minimum flow rate necessary to achieve a PaO_2 greater than 60 mmHg or an oxygen saturation greater than 90%. Higher flow rates can produce CO_2 narcosis or retention.

114. C

The Cox-2 inhibitor class of NSAIDs has been shown to provide effective pain relief with less risk of gastrointestinal bleeding, but there has been increasing concern about the association with cardiovascular disease. Indeed, refecoxib (Vioxx) was withdrawn from the market when the association with MI and stroke was found. There appears to be a dose-related risk of cardiovascular events with celecoxib, with higher doses associated with cardiovascular events and death. Cox-2 inhibitors have significant risk of GI bleeding when combined with low-dose aspirin. Valdecoxib (Bextra) and naproxen have similar efficacy for rheumatoid arthritis. The Cox-2 inhibitor class, however, still has identical renal effects as traditional NSAIDs and should be used with caution in those at particular risk, such as elderly patients with preexisting kidney disease or those on diuretics and ACE inhibitors.

115. D

Trimethoprim-sulfa may increase hyperbilirubinemia in the newborn period and therefore should be avoided late in pregnancy. Fluoroquinolones are contraindicated in pregnancy because of defects in cartilage formation found at high doses in animal studies. Erythromycin is safe in pregnancy but does not provide good coverage of the gram-negative organisms that usually cause UTI. Cephalexin is considered safe and well tolerated in pregnancy and has reasonable efficacy against common urinary pathogens. Although penicillin is safe, it would be unlikely to provide appropriate antibiotic coverage.

116. A

Hypocalcemia can potentiate digitalis toxicity, so the ECG should be monitored. The goal of replacement should be to maintain the level of calcium between 8 and 9 mg/dL. Because calcium is approximately 40% bound to albumin, an important first step is measuring this protein. The calcium level will fall approximately 0.8 mg/dL for each gram/dL decrease in serum albumin. Common causes of hypocalcemia include: extravascular deposition (e.g., hyperphosphatemia), acute pancreatitis, hypoparathyroidism, vitamin D deficiency, sepsis, and surgery.

117. A

This is a classic presentation of a brachioradialis tendonitis. A brachioradialis inserts just medially and distally to the lateral epicondyle and flexes the wrist radially, as opposed to the dorsoflexor tendons, which flex the wrist dorsally. This would be the classic motion of someone using a hammer or a pencil. This would most likely be confused with the lateral epicondylitis or tennis elbow; however, this condition results from inflammation of the extensor muscles of the forearm, particularly the extensor carpi radialis brevis. Pain in tennis elbow would be directly over the lateral epicondyle. Pain with brachioradialis tendonitis is distal to the epicondyle in the forearm. Golfer's elbow is similar to tennis elbow, but it involves the medial epicondyle. This is not where the patient hurts. Olecranon bursitis is a painful swelling over the posterior aspect of the elbow over the olecranon. This is not where the patient hurts.

118. C

In the macrolide-azalide family, azithromycin and clarithromycin provide broader coverage than erythromycin; for example, they are effective against *Haemophilus influenzae*. Second-generation cephalosporins such as cefuroxime axetil (with the exception of cefaclor [Ceclor]) provide good coverage of *H. influenzae*.

119. B

The best screening test would be a serum ferritin level or transferrin saturation. Normal serum ferritin levels for men are up to 300 mg/mL, and those for women are up to 200 mg/mL. Anything above those levels would necessitate additional testing for hemochromatosis, such as genetic testing or a liver biopsy.

120. C

This patient has Wolff–Parkinson–White syndrome. Calcium blockers will enhance conduction via the accessory pathway and are contraindicated. Rate control is achieved acutely with adenosine or beta-blockers. Radiofrequency catheter ablation therapy is the definitive treatment. The PR interval would be short reflecting rapid AV conduction via accessory pathways.

121. B

Testicular cancers usually present with a nontender, firm testicular mass and perhaps a heavy sensation in the abdomen. It usually does not cause hematuria. Fifty percent of patients have metastases at the time of presentation, but only 10% are symptomatic. Testicular ultrasound with color-flow Doppler is the initial imaging tool for detecting testicular cancer. CTs of the abdomen and chest are most effective for evaluating metastastic lesions. Five percent of patients will have gynecomastia. Testicular cancer is the most common type of cancer in men age 15 to 35 years. Germ cell tumors such as seminomas and nonseminomatous germ cell tumors comprise more than 95% of these cancers.

122. A

Grave's disease is the most common cause of autoimmune disease in the United States and accounts for more than one-half of those with hyperthyroidism. The prevalence of Graves' disease is actually lower in blacks than in Caucasians or Asians. Graves' disease will usually have a diffusely increased iodine uptake on thyroid scan. Antithyroid antibodies (e.g., antimicrosomal antibodies) are usually present. Autoantibodies to the thyrotropin receptor, not a mutation of the TSH receptor, cause Grave's disease.

123. A

Hypothyroidism is not associated with steroid use. Abrupt withdrawal of steroids or illness can cause adrenal crisis and should be treated promptly. Long-term use of steroids is associated with osteoporosis. Calcium supplementation, vitamin D, use of antiresorptive agents, and calcitonin are usual strategies for forestalling glucocorticoid-induced osteoporosis. Regular bone density evaluation is recommended.

124. C

MS is more common in women than men (threefold) and is more common in those of northern European descent. The exact cause of MS is still unknown, but we do know that both genetics and early environmental factors influence the incidence of MS. It is known that a family history is significant. The farther away from the equator one lives, the higher the prevalence. Historical data indicate that there have been sudden outbreaks of MS in isolated populations; this suggests the possibility of exposure to a transmissible agent that leads to disease expression. Antibodies to several viruses have been found in patients with MS, but no virus has been consistently associated with the condition. Treatment options depend on the pattern of disease activity. Common agents include avonex, steroids, copaxone, interferon, and immune modifiers such as cyclophosphamide.

125. E
The U.S. Preventive Task Force, American Cancer Society, and American Academy of Family Physicians agree on many broad points of screening for colorectal cancer. Colonoscopy is emerging as an acceptable and preferable mode of screening on an every-10-year basis. Although very sensitive and specific, patient acceptance and availability of this procedure temper this recommendation. Fecal occult blood testing remains acceptable when combined with flexible sigmoidoscopy. Hydrating specimens increases the sensitivity but lessens the specificity of this test. Avoiding aspirin and NSAID use, not eating red meat, parsnips, beets, and horseradish, and refraining from the use of vitamin C will help limit false results. CEA is not recommended for screening. All authorities recommend initiation of screening between ages 40 and 50 years.

126. E
This patient has serous otitis media or otitis media with effusion. Many patients will still have effusion 1 month after treatment for acute otitis media, and no intervention has been proven effective. A common approach is to monitor the effusion over the next 3 months and then check and determine if it is affecting the hearing. Pressure equalization tubes may be helpful in this situation. Most effusions resolve spontaneously without intervention.

127. A
Always assume that the vertical nystagmus is caused by a condition of the central nervous system and needs urgent (probably inpatient) evaluation. You may need to get an LP, but a CT or MR should be done first to rule out a mass lesion. An audiogram may be helpful to assess for unilateral hearing loss, but it is not urgently needed. Blood cultures are unlikely to be helpful unless signs of systemic infection are present.

128. A
Treatment of *Helicobacter pylori* reduces 1-year recurrence rates and increases the proportion of healed ulcers. Adult reinfection rates are less than 1% per year. Treatment for initial *H. pylori* infection typically involves a triple approach with a proton pump inhibitor (PPI; e.g., omeprazole) and several antibiotics (e.g., amoxicillin and clarithromycin). Dual drug regimens have a greater recurrence rate than triple therapies. Bismuth, metronidazole, and tetracycline is an alternative first-line therapy.

129. E
Edema is approximately 97% sensitive for a deep venous thrombosis, calf pain is 86% sensitive, and local tenderness is 76% sensitive. The Homan sign is only 56% sensitive, whereas erythema is 24% sensitive. The most specific signs include erythema (62%), Homan sign (39%), and edema (33%). Although clinical prediction rules have been developed, there is no combination of signs and symptoms that can rule out or rule in DVT, particularly in a high-risk patient. Use of the modified Well's criteria may help stratify the risk of DVT. See Table 1.6.

130. C
Cigarette smoking is the leading cause of COPD, with active smoking accounting for 80% to 90% of all cases. Other risk factors include Caucasian race, male gender, low social economic status, exposure to air pollutants, the presence of allergies, and a family history of COPD. More than 90% of patients with COPD either previously smoked or currently smoke cigarettes. Alpha-1-antitrypsin deficiency should be considered in patients younger than age 45 with a family history of respiratory disease who present with features of COPD, particularly in the absence of smoking. Up to 10% of these patients will have serious liver disease and may have findings consistent with hepatitis or cirrhosis.

131. D
Irritable bowel syndrome may be characterized by diarrhea, constipation, abdominal pain, bloating, and mucus in stools. Weight loss, hematochezia, and melena should be evaluated for other causes. Effective treatments for IBS include antispasmodics and serotonin-3 and serotonin-4 antagonists. Many other approaches, such as the use of antidepressant medications such as tricyclics and psychosocial interventions, are less well supported.

132. D
Morning stiffness is more prolonged when there is greater synovitis and joint swelling. Rather than the exact number of involved joints, it is the severity of joint inflammation that helps determine disease activity. Rheumatoid factor does not parallel fluctuations in disease activity, although patients with high titers may have a worse prognosis. Erythrocyte sedimentation rate and C-reactive protein are good objective measures of active disease. NSAIDs are beneficial for symptom relief in RA; however, they do not decrease joint damage. Therefore, caution should be used in assessing disease progression based on the patient's response to an NSAID. Swelling in more than 20 joints and extra-articular involvement

Table 1.6 Well's criteria

Score 1 for each of the following:
Active cancer
Pitting edema greatest in affected limb
Non-varicose collateral superficial veins
Paralysis or immobilization of lower extremity
Noncalized tenderness along distribution of deep vein
Whole leg swollen
Subtract 2 if an alternative diagnosis is more likely
Low probability is 0 or less
Moderate: 1 or 2
High: 3 or greater

such as vasculitis, Felty's syndrome, or interstitial lung disease are also associated with a poorer prognosis.

133. A

Only 20% of women with breast cancer have a positive family history. One in eight women will develop breast cancer during their lifetime, and mammography is sensitive before and after menopause. Nonetheless, there is a high false-positive rate. Approximately 2,000 screens need to be performed to prevent one death over a 10-year period in a woman in her 40s. Although ultrasound can distinguish between solid and cystic masses, it is not as reliable in the diagnosis of breast cancer. A tissue biopsy, including needle biopsy, is the most reliable method to diagnose breast cancer.

134. E

Both atrial and brain natriuretic peptides (BNP) have been found to be elevated in patients with heart failure. Initial studies indicate they are useful in diagnosing heart failure and may be useful in predicting the prognosis and in monitoring patients with heart failure. Levels of BNP greater than 100 pg/mL were approximately 90% sensitive and 80% specific for heart failure in one study comparing BNP and clinical judgment. Atrial fibrillation will signficantly increase the level of BNP. All of the other tests are standard lab tests that may indicate the presence of an underlying cause of the heart failure.

135. A

In general, immunosuppressant drugs should not be used in pregnancy; however, azathioprine and mecaptopurine do not show an increased incidence of congenital malformations. Corticosteroids, 5-ASA compounds, and sulfasalazine have been used safely during pregnancy. Long-term studies with methotrexate, however, are lacking. Whereas severe, active disease is associated with a higher risk of miscarriage, premature delivery and low-birth-weight infants, those with quiescent disease, can be managed successfully medically. Flexible sigmoidoscopy is associated with preterm labor.

136. D

Prophylaxis with an oral antiviral drug may be useful for patients at high risk for influenza-related complications if an outbreak of influenza occurs before or less than 2 weeks after influenza vaccination. High-risk individuals include those older than age 65, residents of nursing homes, and patients with significant chronic disease. All of the above groups should be targeted to receive vaccination starting in September. Health care workers should be vaccinated to prevent illness in the high-risk individuals with whom they may come into close contact.

137. B

Tuberculosis infection is common in prisoners, and all new prisoners and employees should be screened. Hepatitis C is often asymptomatic or presents only at the time of end-stage liver disease. Depression, not schizophrenia, is the most common adolescent mental health problem. Risk factors for suicide among prisoners include drinking and drug use, recent bad news, and depression.

138. E

Testing for celiac disease is recommended for patients with chronic diarrhea, not constipation. Although a wide range of immunologic tests (IgA anti-endomysial antibodies, IgA and IgG anti-gliadin antibodies, and anti-reticulin antibodies) are useful in the diagnosis of celiac sprue (gluten sensitive enteropathy), IGA antigliadin is associated with a large percentage of false positives. The IGA endomysial antibody testing is highly specific. A single small intestine biopsy may be falsely negative. Imaging has little value in the diagnosis unless used to exclude a mass lesion. Barium contrast studies often show increased transit time, obliteration of mucosal folds, and bowel dilation.

139. E

A prolonged QT interval on ECG is consistent with hypocalcemia. Chvostek's sign is facial twitching when the facial nerve is tapped anterior to the ear. Trousseau's sign is carpal spasm after inflating a blood pressure cuff above the systolic pressure for 2 or 3 minutes. Severe symptoms are usually only seen with moderate to severely depressed calcium levels.

140. C

Helical CT is not indicated. Tagged RBC scan can be helpful in determining the site of bleeding, especially in the small bowel. EGD can be useful in diagnosing and determining the risk of future bleed. Proton pump inhibitors have been shown to reduce rebleeding and the need for emergency surgery. Patients with active GI bleeding should always be managed conservatively with the placement of several large-bore IVs and type and screening for potential transfusion.

141. C

Despite extensive workup, only 10% to 20% of the cases of chronic urticaria will be linked to a specific etiology. Fifty percent of patients with chronic urticaria spontaneously resolve within 1 year, 20% more take up to 3 years, and 20% more take up to 5 years. Treatment options include antihistamines (second generation better than first generation), H1 and H2 blockers, tricyclic antidepressants, oral B-agonists, and the selective serotonin reuptake inhibitors.

142. E

All of the above symptoms and signs are designated as major diagnostic criteria by the American Heart Association except hepatomegaly. Jugular venous distension (JVD) is one of the major criteria. It suggests venous congestion and can be shown by pushing on the liver. True hepatomegaly would be a very late sign of end-stage heart failure and is not useful in making the clinical diagnosis of heart failure. The S3 is associated with atrial filling and should be considered a sign of CHF until proven otherwise. The S4 is associated with filling of a noncompliant ventricle as with hypertension, aortic stenosis, IHSS, and coronary artery disease.

143. D

Less than one-half of all patients with gallstones will become symptomatic. Patients may be instructed about the symptoms of gallstones and instructed to follow up with their primary care physician if symptoms develop. Further testing is not indicated.

144. C

Inhaled corticosteroids are the treatment of choice for chronic sinusitis. More invasive treatments can be useful as well but should be reserved for those who fail to respond to the corticosteroids. Antibiotics are appropriate only for acute flare-ups of chronic sinusitis. The other medications can be used for symptomatic relief but have not been shown to help resolve this condition.

145. B

Compared with H2 blockers in patients with erosive GERD, PPIs did achieve relief of symptoms more rapidly. However, there was no difference in relapse rates, treatment of Barretts esophagus, or improvement in lung function in those patients also suffering from asthma.

146. D

Approximately 10% to 15% of all smokers develop clinical evidence of COPD. Even though cigarette smoking is the leading cause of COPD, the majority of smokers will not develop clinical evidence of COPD. COPD is defined as either emphysema or chronic bronchitis. The majority of smokers may develop respiratory symptoms, but only 10% to 15% actually develop the clinical criteria for emphysema or chronic bronchitis. After smoking cessation, the loss of lung function improves back toward baseline.

147. B

Soft tissue sarcomas most commonly involve the lower extremities and are definitively diagnosed by biopsy. The 5-year survival rate is approximately 50%. They may present painlessly or impinge on nerves or surrounding tissues causing pain. Soft tissue sarcomas metastasize hematogenously, and recurrent disease is most commonly metastatic to the lung. MRI may be useful for determining the etiology of a soft tissue mass.

148. C

Mitral valve prolapse (MVP) is suspected with a midsystolic click followed by a late systolic murmur that becomes louder when the patient stands. Mitral valve prolapse has been blamed for many symptoms and long-term health problems. However, recent studies have shown that there is no increased risk of cardiac consequences unless mitral regurgitation is present. Also, with more advanced echocardiography equipment and more precise criteria, the prevalence of MVP has dropped from 15% to only 2.4%. Patients with MVP do not need SBE prophylaxis unless they have MVP with mitral regurgitation. Amoxicillin–clavulonate would not be a preferred choice for prophylaxis.

Antibiotic prophylaxis is also recommended for patients with prosthetic heart valves, previous SBE, many congenital cardiac malformations, most acquired valve problems, and hypertrophic cardiomyopathy. Prophylaxis is not indicated in patients with an isolated ASD, CABG, physiologic murmurs, previous Kawasaki disease without valve dysfunction, and in those with pacemakers or defibrillators.

The standard oral regiment for dental, respiratory, and esophageal procedures includes amoxicillin or ampicillin or, if penicillin allergic, clindamycin, cephalexin, cefadroxil, cefazolin or azithromycin, or clarithromycin.

Gastrointestinal and GU procedures will usually require pre-treatment with gentamicin and postprocedure prophylaxis.

149. D

Risk factors for prostate cancer include African American race, family history of prostate cancer, working in the rubber industry, and exposure to cadmium oxide. By definition, stage A disease is nonpalpable and only discovered at surgery. Biopsy of a prostate nodule yields cancer in approximately 50% of cases. Stage B prostate cancer (palpable disease confined to one lobe of the prostate) is metastatic to the pelvic lymph nodes in less than 20% of cases.

150. D

There are no widely accepted measures for screening for lung and ovarian cancer. PSA testing is an option for prostate cancer detection, but its effectiveness in older men remains controversial. Despite recent debate, mammography is still recommended for women age 50 to 65 years. Because of the low incidence of new cervical cancer in elders who have been regularly screened in the past, most authorities recommend discontinuing or offering this test as an option in such older women.

151. D

Patients with the acute HIV syndrome often have fever, constitutional symptoms, lymphadenopathy, and headache. A high index of suspicion is required to intervene promptly. The best test for acute HIV infection is a measure of viral load, which will usually be elevated significantly. ELISA and Western blot tests, which reflect antibody production, will usually be negative acutely. CD4 counts will also often be normal.

152. D

The diagnosis of MS is established only when the physiologically consistent signs and symptoms and laboratory tests converge to suggest involvement of myelinated tracts in multiple areas of the central nervous system. No single laboratory test result is pathognomonic for MS. The MRI can be helpful in confirming the clinical diagnosis; however, several diseases can mimic the changes seen on an MRI with MS. They include Lyme disease, sarcoidosis, viral encephalomyelitis, moyamoya disease, subcortical infarcts, and multiple small emboli. Oligoclonal bands and an elevated Ig index are sensitive indicators for MS but are not highly specific. Most MS patients have cerebrospinal fluid white cell counts of less than 40 cells/mL and protein levels less than 100 mg/dL. CT is not recommeded for the diagnosis of MS.

153. A

Hyaluronic acid has been FDA approved for knee osteoarthritis, although its efficacy remains controversial. Although the other treatments listed are not officially approved, they are often used prior to hyaluronic acid because of the high cost and multiple injections needed for treatment. Tramadol, a centrally acting opioid agonist, is an effective pain reliever indicated for moderate to severe general pain. Glucosamine sulfate has been shown in some trials to provide effective pain relief in patients with osteoarthritis, but other trials have been less convincing. Since it is a relatively inexpensive medication with few side effects, a treatment trial early in the disease process is reasonable. Intra-articular glucocorticoids can be a useful adjunct since they are also inexpensive and well tolerated. They have been proven to decrease pain.

154. B

Acute hepatitis is the most common cause of jaundice in pregnancy. Pregnancy does increase the risk of cholecystitis because cholelithiasis affects approximately 6% of pregnancies. Sclerosing cholangitis, metastatic hepatic cancer, and Gilbert's disease are relatively rare.

155. D

The risk of HIV transmission in utero is approximately 15% to 35%, and probably reflects differences in prenatal care, health status, and levels of viremia. Infection can occur in utero as early as the first trimester, although the majority of transmission occurs during delivery and in the perinatal period. C-section decreases the transmission of HIV significantly. Universal screening of all pregnant women is recommended. Transmission may be substantially reduced by as little as a single dose of zidovudine or lamivudine, even when administered in the immediate postpartum period. Breast-feeding can also increase the risk of maternal–infant HIV transmission.

156. B

Giardia is the most common parasitic infection in the United States and a common problem worldwide. Transmission is via the fecal–oral route, and infectious cysts may be shed for months following infection. Common symptoms are diarrhea, pain, and bloating. Dehydration may ensue. Diagnosis in the United States now hinges on enzyme immunoassay (ELA) of a single stool specimen, not the microscopic examination of three specimens. The ELA is more sensitive. Risk factors for giardia include travel to Third World countries, attending daycare, and attending camps.

157. C

Psoriatic arthritis does not have any diagnostic or classification criteria to establish the diagnosis. The diagnosis is usually made when a patient with psoriasis presents with an inflammatory arthritis. The disease shares many characteristics of other inflammatory arthropathies, including red, swollen, painful joints. Psoriatic arthritis can be monoarticular but is more commonly oligoarticular and symmetric. Like rheumatoid arthritis, it usually involves the small joints of the hands and feet but can involve the ankles, knees, and elbows. As with other forms of seronegative arthritis, rheumatoid factor is negative. Nail changes may be seen (Figure 1-14).

Spondylitis is a frequent finding but is less severe and tends to occur in an older age group (more than 30 years) than in ankylosing spondylitis. Sacroiliitis occurs in 30% of patients but the spondylitis can affect any portion of the back in random fashion.

NSAIDs are a primary treatment. Disease-modifying-antirheumatic drugs (DMARDs) should be initiated in nonresponders and if the disease becomes progressive, erosive, and polyarticular. Dosages and monitoring are similar as in rheumatoid arthritis.

158. A

Ten percent of patients with testicular cancer have a prior history of an undescended testis; 50% of these were intra-abdominal. It is true that although cure rates are very high for testicular cancer, the cause is unknown and genetic factors have not been found. Testicular cancer doubles in size every 10 to 30 days. Many germ cell tumors produce oncofetal protein markers, such as AFP or HCG. They can be detected in the patient's serum. The amount of tumor burden is proportional to the degree of maker elevation. Navaho Indians do not have an increased risk of testicular cancer.

159. D

The diagnosis of endocarditis requires a high index of suspicion. Nonspecific symptoms, low-grade fever, and malaise may be present, whereas other patients will present with stroke, CHF, or pneumonia. The patient may present with immunologically mediated epiphenomena such as Osler's nodes, Roth spots, and glomerulonephritis. Although physical findings such as a new onset murmur, heart failure, petechiae, and splenomegaly may be

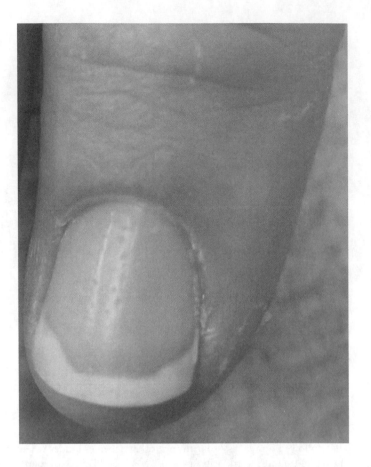

Figure 1-14. Psoriasis—nail pitting. Image provided by Stedman's.

present, the examination may be completely normal. The recommended approach to diagnosis is two blood cultures at least 12 hours apart. Although most cardiac lesions are visualized on transthoracic echocardiography, transesophageal imaging should be pursued in persons with a negative transthoracic test who are strongly suspected of having endocarditis. Right heart involvement is most common in injection drug users. Treatment should be initiated empirically while waiting for culture results.

160. D

Treatment of enterococcal endocarditis is challenging. Enterococci are resistant to low-dose penicillin G, and penicillin is not recommended as a single agent for treatment. Moreover, resistance to aminoglycosides is increasingly common. For patients with organisms sensitive to the aminoglycosides, a regimen of high-dose penicillin and gentamicin for 4 to 6 weeks is recommended. Streptomycin may be substituted for gentamicin on the basis of antibiotic susceptibility. Cephalosporins are ineffective, and vancomycin may replace penicillin for penicillin-allergic patients. Unfortunately, vancomycin resistance is emerging.

161. C

Pneumonia in elders may present very subtly. Anorexia, functional decline, weakness, and mental status changes are common symptoms. Approximately two-thirds of elders with community-acquired pneumonia will have acute mental status changes. Such changes are associated with an increased risk of mortality. Tachycardia and tachypnea greater than 28 respirations/minute suggest pneumonia. An elevated temperature over baseline is often absent. It is important to assess the patient's baseline temperature (which might be lower than "normal"). An arterial PO$_2$ or blood gas can help identify patients with more severe illness who would benefit from hospitalization.

162. C

Oseltamivir (Tamiflu) and zanamivir (Relenza) inhibit viral replication for both influenza A and B. Rimantadine (Flumadine) and amantadine (Symmetrel) interfere with viral replication and are effective against influenza A, not B. Amantadine is metabolized by the kidneys and rimantadine by the liver. Vaccination does not confer immediate protection. Two weeks of adjunctive therapy after vaccination during an outbreak is recommended.

163. D

Asymptomatic bacteriuria is common in elders and does not require treatment unless the patient is scheduled for a genitourinary procedure, has had recent obstructive uropathy, or has a history of recurrent symptomatic infections. However, the symptoms of infection may be subtle, such as anorexia, functional decline, or mental status changes. Small numbers of white cells are frequently found in the urine of elders and have limited prognostic value. The nitrate test, which depends on the conversion of nitrates to nitrite by bacteria in the urine, will be negative with pseudomonas, staphylococcus, and enterococcus, which do not metabolize nitrate. Risk factors for complicated or severe UTI include age older than 60 years, male gender, history of obstruction or stones, recent hospitalization, and concurrent diabetes or immunosuppression.

164. B

Wearers of dentures still need routine dental and oral health examinations. Dentures need to be regularly refitted. As many as 30% of denture wearers have oral lesions that may be inflammatory, infectious, or fibrous in nature. Chewing and nutrition may be compromised by poorly fitting dentures. As patients age, the gingiva recede, making root cavities more common. Xerostomia is associated with medications including diuretics, antihistamines, and anticholingergics. More than one-half of poor elders have lost their teeth.

165. D

Common ototoxic and vestibulotoxic medications include aminoglycosides, furosemide, aspirin, vancomycin, and cisplatin. It is important to evaluate the time course of symptoms and other potential causes of vestibular and hearing loss.

166. A

A pink puffer refers to thin individuals with COPD who breathe through pursed lips. A blue bloater refers to obese individuals with a bluish hue resulting from hypoxia. Pickwickian also refers to very obese individuals who have a tendency to fall asleep easily. Pectus excavatum is a physical deformity of the chest that has nothing to do with COPD. Patients with Marfan's syndrome may be thin, but again, this is irrelevant to the diagnosis of COPD.

167. A

Whereas a high BMI or weight may be suggestive of the metabolic syndrome, waist size (abdominal obesity) is used to determine inclusion criteria: men with waist size greater than 40 inches and women with waist size greater than 35 inches. In the presence of

glucose intolerance, three of these criteria must be met to qualify for the diagnosis of metabolic syndrome.

168. D

For localized impetigo, it is best managed with topical mupirocin. *Staph. aureus* and *Strept. pyogenes* most commonly cause it. Penicillin will probably not work due to bacterial resistance. Augmentin and Nafcillin should be reserved for severe infections. Bacitracin ointment is a less effective treatment. Remember, if impetigo recurs, consider colonization of the nares or intertriginous areas.

169. C

All of the above treatments are appropriate for acute anaphylaxis. However, due to widespread systemic symptoms, you should start with the subcutaneous epinephrine, oxygen, and an aerosolized B-agonist. Then consider further treatments as outlined above. Unfortunately, even today, epinephrine is underutilized in the treatment of anaphylaxis.

170. B

This patient has rheumatoid arthritis with active synovitis. The American College of Rheumatology in February 2002 recommended that DMARD therapy be started within 3 months of a confirmed diagnosis in patients who show evidence of active disease despite adequate dosing of NSAIDs. Joint damage can occur as early as 1 or 2 years after onset of the disease, and in some cases as soon as 6 months. Since DMARDs have been shown to reduce joint destruction and preserve function, early use of DMARDs is appropriate for all patients with active rheumatoid arthritis.

171. A

Studies have shown that there is no relationship to diet and acne. Hormones (cyclic for females), stress, and an important date or test always seem to bring out that noticeable pimple.

172. C

"Female, fat, forty, and fertile" define an at-risk profile for the *development* of gallstones, not the complications. In addition to "female," "fair" is another "F" that refers to people of northern European descent. Of note is that Hispanic and Native American patients are also at risk for the formation of gallstones. Patients with diabetes, sickle cell disease, and cirrhosis are all at risk for complications from gallstones, including cholecystitis, choledocholithiasis, and cholangitis.

173. E

The Dukes' and TNM staging systems are used to stage colorectal cancer. Staging has important prognostic and treatment implications, with lower stage tumors having a better prognosis. The Dukes' classification includes stage A, invasion of the mucosa and submucosa; stage B, erosion into the muscularis or serosa; stage C, involvement of regional lymph nodes; and stage D, characterized by distant metastases. The TNM staging system refers to T, level of invasion of the tumor; N, the presence or absence of nodes; and M, the presence or absence of distant metastases.

174. C

Cat scratch disease commonly presents with axillary adenopathy. Supraclavicular adenopathy more commonly is associated with serious illness, such as lymphoma, tuberculosis, histoplasmosis, and coccidiomycosis.

175. E

The 2006 CDC guidelines for the treatment of gonococcal urethritis are any of the above antibiotics (including cefixime) plus either azithromycin 1 g or doxycycline 100 mg PO bid for 7 days. STD clinics now use the most cost-effective one-time treatment, thereby ensuring compliance. If a rapid nucleic acid amplification test (MAAT) is negative for chlamydia, treatment for GC alone can be initiated.

176. D

Headache (67%), jaw claudication (50%), and low-grade fever are common clinical symptoms with temporal arteritis (giant cell arteritis). The most serious symptom is a partial or complete vision loss that can occur in up to 20% of patients and is often irreversible. When one eye is affected—and if left untreated—within 1 or 2 weeks the other eye likely will become involved. Amaurosis fugax is a frequent precursor to permanent visual loss.

Once diagnosed with temporal arteritis (TA), a patient should have a yearly chest x-ray to check for a widened mediastinum. Thoracic aortic aneurysm is 17 times more likely than in the general population. The complication typically occurs years after initial diagnosis and after other symptoms have resolved.

TA, like polymyalgia rheumatica, is an inflammatory condition, which can be generalized. Up to one-third of patients with PMR can develop TA and one-half of patients with TA develop symptoms of PMR. Increased inflammatory markers such as C-reactive protein and erythrocyte sedimentation rate characterize both. An abnormal CRP is found in 99% of cases.

TA is characterized by skip lesions of vasculitis on temporal artery biopsy. A sufficient segment of artery, 3 to 5 cm, should be obtained to confirm the diagnosis. If the pathology is negative but clinical suspicion is high, a contralateral artery biopsy should also be obtained. Steroid treatment should not wait until results of the biopsy are known due to the serious consequences of a delayed diagnosis.

177. E

Systemic interferon has not been shown to be any more effective than placebo. Both intralesional and topical interferon were found to clear warts better than placebo. All the other treatment options have been shown to be effective. However, there are no studies that show one treatment is superior to another.

178. E

Although not universally proven in randomized, controlled trials, all of the above interventions have demonstrated benefit for the treatment of osteoarthritis. Patient education discussing the natural history, treatment, and self-management of the disease process should be offered. Education has been shown to produce improvements in physical functioning and pain.

Bracing and corrective footwear provide symptom relief in knee osteoarthritis. Bracing controls lateral instability, whereas shock-absorbing footwear reduces impact-loading forces and heel wedging reduces lateral thrust on the knee joint.

Physical therapy to strengthen joint muscles is beneficial for symptom improvement of the knee and hip. Deconditioned muscles lead to inadequate motion, periarticular stiffness, and increased pain levels. An active lifestyle promoted by exercise also has psychological benefits on overall wellness and the perception of pain.

179. D

Early administration of a thrombolytic is associated with improved outcomes, including survival, of acute MI. Administration is typically suggested within 6 hours of pain onset. Aspirin is warranted as an immediate intervention and has been shown to substantially reduce mortality. There is no decisive data that one thrombolytic is better than another. Contraindications to thrombolytic therapy include active gastrointestinal bleeding, recent transthoracic or abdominal surgery (within 1 month), head trauma, recent stroke, and pancreatitis. PCTA and stent placement is another alternative for select patients.

180. C

Low–molecular-weight heparin has dramatically changed the treatment of deep venous thrombosis. Many patients can be managed as outpatients using this drug subcutaneously. Drug dosing is fixed and most individuals will not need laboratory monitoring. Major bleeding is less likely. Oral anticoagulation remains important for longer term prophylaxis.

181. B

Erythema chronicum migrans is the classic rash of Lyme disease. This usually begins as a red macule or papule at the site of the tick bite and spreads slowly peripherally as it clears centrally. It is usually erythematous. The rash appears to expand over time (migrans) and it lasts for a prolonged period of time (chronicum). Rocky Mountain spotted fever classically has a petechial rash at the ankles and wrists especially. Tinea corporus is a fungal infection of the skin. It also clears centrally as it enlarges peripherally, but it usually has a red, scaly border. A KOH prep shows fungal elements. The rash associated with Stevens–Johnson syndrome is erythema multiforme, or target (bulls-eye) lesions.

182. D

All of these are potential causes of anaphylaxis. Allergy injections are a common trigger for anaphylaxis, but life-threatening reactions are rare. Risk factors for severe anaphylaxis are poorly controlled asthma, concurrent use of beta-blockers, high allergen dose, errors in administration, and lack of sufficient observation after allergy injection administration. Penicillin is the most common drug associated with anaphylaxis, whereas bees, yellowjackets, hornets, wasps, and fire ants are the most common insects associated with IgE-mediated reactions. Peanuts, shellfish, and eggs are common food triggers and may cause anaphylaxis when consumed in small quantities in processed foods.

183. D

Testicular cancer is a young man's disease. Peak incidence is between ages 20 and 40 years, with smaller peaks in children younger than 10 years of age and adults older than 60 years of age.

184. D

Hypophosphatemia is typical in hyperparathyroidism. Common complaints include "bones, stones, moans, and groans," a reminder of the symptoms of abdominal pain, kidney stones, bone pain, and mental complaints such as fatigue, depression, or anxiety.

185. B

The diagnosis of rheumatoid arthritis is made on the basis of a set of symptoms over time. Inflammatory synovitis must be present. Rheumatoid factor is present in approximately 85% of patients but once positive, it holds little prognostic value. An elevated synovial fluid white cell count is consistent with the diagnosis.

186. A

Iron deficiency is the most common cause of anemia in the United States. It affects 7% to 10% of the adult population, 10% to 20% of infants and toddlers, and 15% to 45% of pregnant patients.

187. D

The differential diagnosis of lymphadenopathy is broad and is more commonly seen in children. It most commonly involves the cervical, inguinal, and axillary nodes. Cat scratch disease is a common cause of axillary adenopathy. Inguinal adenopathy can be due to local infection, diaper dermatitis, insect bites, syphilis, and lymphogranuloma venereum. Supraclavicular adenopathy is highly concerning for lymphoma and should never be ignored.

188. C

Beta-lactamase inhibitors (clavulanate, sulbactam, and tazobactam) have only weak intrinsic antibacterial activity but enhance the efficacy of antibiotics susceptible to breakdown from beta-lactamases. MRSA is usually resistant to these combination agents. Furthermore, the combination is unlikely to enhance coverage of resistant pneumococcus. When amoxicillin is chosen, high-dose therapy can usually overcome pneumococcal resistance. Clavulanic acid is associated with an increased incidence of diarrhea.

189. D

The physical examination maneuver described above is the Finkelstein's test. This test differentiates tendonitis from underlying arthritis and is the physical examination documentation of DeQuervain's tenosynovitis. The first dorsal compartment contains the abductor pollicis longus and the extensor pollicis brevis. This is located just proximal and radial to the anatomic snuffbox. Inflammation in this area is common in persons who do excessive repetitive handwork. The scaphoid or navicular bone, when fractured, classically gives pain on palpation of the anatomic snuffbox. However, there is no history of trauma, and this bone would be a very unusual location for a stress fracture. A trigger finger is a tenosynovitis that involves the flexor tendons of the digit or thumb at the level of metacarpophalangeal joint just proximal to the first pulley of the flexor tendon sheath, on the palmar surface of the hand. A ganglion cyst is a herniation of the synovium of the wrist and can occur in the wrist. This should appear as a nodule and should not give a positive Finkelstein test.

190. D

Patients given hemocult cards should be advised to avoid rare or lightly cooked red meat, turnips, broccoli, horseradish, cantaloupe, parsnips, radishes, vitamin C in excess of 250 mg/day, iron supplements, aspirin, and NSAIDs. However, spinach, prunes, and plums do not affect testing adversely. A digital rectal exam is traumatic to the rectal mucosal surface and causes 20% to 25% positive hemocult testing. Statement C is correct. If a patient has a first-degree relative who has had colon cancer at a young age, he is at increased risk of colon cancer. Colon cancer screening for familial adenomatous polyposis should start at puberty. Hereditary nonpolyposis colorectal cancer screening should begin at age 21. Ulcerative colitis does increase colon cancer risk. If a patient has had left-sided colitis only, the physician may delay

colon cancer screening 12 to 15 years after the diagnosis of colitis has been made.

191. E

Decongestant drops are effective in the short term, but if used for more than 3 to 5 days they can cause rebound congestion. Diphenhydramine is sedating and has anticholinergic properties. There are better treatment choices for elders; intranasal steroids, for example, are usually effective and well tolerated. The best choice of a second-generation antihistamine cannot be predicted in any given patient. Immunotherapy has been associated with improved quality of life and is an appropriate option for allergic rhinitis therapy. Conservative, environmental measures should be implemented for every patient.

192. B

In fact, seminomas are slow-growing and very radiosensitive. The overall survival is 85%, but it is greater than 90% if confined to the testis. If alpha-fetoprotein (AFP) is present, then the cancer is a mixed tumor because seminomas do not produce AFP. Treatment for seminoma is radical inguinal orchiectomy and radiation unless there is a high volume of tumor or distant metastases; then, chemotherapy may be recommended.

193. E

Atrial fibrillation is associated with valvular heart disease, diabetes, hypertension, pulmonary disease, thyrotoxicosis, and alcohol abuse. The risk of stroke is markedly increased in patients with rheumatic heart disease. Warfarin is the mainstay of therapy, and the INR is adjusted between a target of 2 and 3. A remote history of stroke is not a contraindication to warfarin therapy. Indeed, patients with previous remote stroke have even more striking benefit from warfarin therapy. Rate control and anticoagulation is recommended for the majority of patients.

194. B

Pyridoxine hydrochloride (vitamin B6) is effective in preventing the development of peripheral neuropathy secondary to treatment with INH. Use of pyridoxine supplementation is recommended for patients at risk for the development of neuropathy (patients with diabetes, uremia, seizure disorders, HIV, alcoholism, malnutrition, or pregnancy). INH-induced neuropathy is more likely in the very young and elderly, pregnant women, alcoholics, diabetes, those with HIV infection, and individuals with renal disease. Risk factors for INH-induced hepatitis include persons over age 35 years, alcoholics, individuals with chronic liver disease, and pregnant women.

195. C

In the patient with existing CHD, an LDL goal of less than 70 is recommended. Risk equivalents include diabetes, other atherosclerotic disease, and multiple risk factors that confer a more than 20% 10-year risk of CHF. Therapeutic lifestyle changes are recommended for 3 months prior to initiating drug therapy.

196. B

Entamoeba histolytica has been recently reclassified into two genetically identical but morphologically distinct species, *E. histolytica* and *E. dispar*. *Entamoeba histolytica* is responsible for amebic colitis, liver abcess, and intestinal invasion. *Entamoeba dispar* causes infection in asymptomatic carriers as well as in men engaging in risky sexual behaviors with men. Infection is transmitted via the fecal–oral route. Diarrhea, including dysentery, is the hallmark of *E. histolytica* infection. Differentiation of *E. histolytica* and *E. dispar* cannot be reliably performed via microscopic examination of the stool (Figure 1-15). Polymerase chain reaction assays are the most rapid, specific, and reliable means to differentiate these two species.

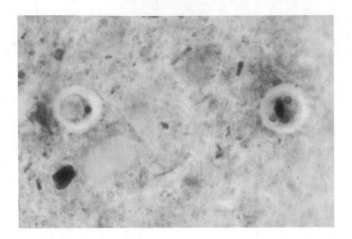

Figure 1-15. (Right) A cyst of E. histolytica with three nuclei and a cigar-shaped chromatoidal body. (Left) A precyst of the same species with a large vacuole and a thin rim of cytoplasm with a condensed nucleus. Trichrome, ×300. From Kean BH, Sun T, Ellsworth RM. Opthalmic Parasitology. *New York: Igaku-Shoin; 1991:36.*

197. B

Acute respiratory acidosis is most consistent with ventilatory failure due to asthma. The cause is the rise in PCO_2 secondary to decreased alveolar ventilation.

198. A

Symptoms associated with BPH can be assessed and monitored reliably with tools such as the American Urologic Association Symptom Checklist. Watchful waiting is often appropriate for patients with low symptom scores. Patients with more moderate or severe symptoms should be carefully counseled about treatment options. Although surgery is more effective at relieving symptoms than medications, many patients will prefer drug therapy. Finasteride (Proscar) is a 5-alpha reductase inhibitor and is associated with impotence. Tamsulosin (Flomax) is an alpha-blocker associated with orthostatic hypotension.

199. D

Patients with COPD initially present with a chronic cough and breathlessness. They may complain of a chest cold early on in the disease, but the history usually reveals that the cough has been present for several months. The cough may be productive of a clear white or even purulent sputum. As COPD progresses, patients complain of dyspnea on exertion, wheezing, and panic-like attacks when they become hypoxic. They frequently find that they are limited in their activity and they feel trapped by their disease. They may complain of feelings of isolation and depression, but mania is not a typical symptom of this disease process. Pulsus paradoxus—inspiratory decrease in systolic blood pressure of

more than 20 mmHg—is seen with cardiac tamponade, COPD, asthma, and other cardiorespiratory disorders.

200. E

Prolonged hoarseness suggests the possibility of a more serious problem and warrants direct visualization of the larynx. Other red flags include such symptoms as shortness of breath, dysphagia, aspiration, the presence of a neck mass, and a history of heavy alcohol or tobacco use. Imaging of the recurrent laryngeal nerve is imperative if the cause of unilateral vocal cord paralysis remains elusive. Squamous cell carcinoma is the most common form of cancer in this situation.

201. C

It is important to remain alert for more serious causes of laryngeal symptoms such as hoarseness. Direct visualization of the larynx remains important and may uncover other correctable lesions. Vocal cord polyps must usually be surgically removed. Papillomas respond to laser ablation. Laryngitis may respond to voice rest and proper voice technique. Granulomas are frequently associated with GERD. A thorough history, especially of alcohol and smoking, remains important.

202. A

A urea:creatinine ratio of 100 or more is indicative of an upper GI bleed. The greater the ratio, the greater the volume of blood loss. Supine tachycardia, palmar crease pallor, and facial pallor are all far less sensitive indicators.

203. C

Rhinitis is common in pregnancy and is probably related, at least in part, to capillary vasocongestion associated with higher circulating levels of estrogen. Such side effects can also be seen with birth control pills. Pregnancy is often associated with an increased sensitivity to environmental irritants. Vasomotor symptoms associated with pregnancy usually resolve promptly within a week of delivery. Hypothyroidism can also cause nasal congestion. Nasal steroids are considered first-line treatment.

204. E

Thyroid nodules in general should all be evaluated with needle aspiration biopsy to rule out the small percentage that are malignant. Findings that might increase suspicion for malignancy include a hard fixed nodule, lymphadenopathy, hoarseness, and a family history of medullary carcinoma.

An ultrasound might show if it was more likely to be a cyst but could not effectively rule out malignancy. Thyroid function tests will most likely be normal.

205. D

The most common form of thyroid malignancy is papillary, which is found in 60% to 70% of thyroid tumors. Thirty percent had metastasized at the time of diagnosis, and they can be associated with radiation exposure. The next most common is follicular carcinoma, which accounts for 10% to 20% of thyroid malignancies.

206. C

The history suggests that he could have been exposed to poison ivy. However, poison ivy does not give a petechial lesion and would not give such a severe illness. He has been exposed to tick areas, so Lyme disease is a possibility. However, this is not the classic rash of Lyme disease, and Lyme disease does not classically give such a severe illness. The rash of Lyme disease is erythema chronicum migrans. This description is classic for Rocky Mountain spotted fever with petechial rash especially at the ankles and wrists, with severe headache, severe illness, and very high fever. This is a medical emergency, and this patient will need hospitalization. Henoch–Schonlein purpura is an acute vasculitis affecting children. It does give purpuric lesions, mostly in the dependent area of the body. It is most common in the spring and autumn. Children and adolescents with this condition are rarely this ill.

207. A

Dust mites are killed by washing bedding and nightclothes in water hotter than 130°F but will return quickly as they feed on shed human epithelial cells. Steps to reduce mite antigen levels include removing rugs, carpets, and upholstered furniture; encasing mattresses in plastic; keeping humidity below 50%; and eliminating furred pets from the household. Although HEPA filters are often recommended, a placebo-controlled trial did not support this contention.

When faced with the patient with allergy symptoms, it is useful to classify symptoms as seasonal or perennial. Seasonal symptoms will suggest particular etiology such as ragweed in the late summer to frost. Perennial symptoms would suggest allergy to dust mites, animal dander, and molds.

208. E

Prisoners are a large, underserved, and at-risk population of more than 6 million individuals. Mental health problems, including suicide, are quite common. Patients with mental health problems are more likely to commit violent crimes and to have suffered sexual or physical abuse.

209. E

The patient's history of unintentional weight loss is concerning and calls into question the diagnosis of irritable bowel syndrome. Cancer, malabsorption syndromes (e.g., celiac sprue), and inflammatory bowel disease should all be considered. Pulmonary conditions mimicking asthma must also be entertained. A careful history, physical, and diagnostic evaluation is prudent.

210. D

Attendance at religious services and religious commitment are associated with a lower mortality rate, increased functional ability for elders, better coping skills, fewer health-compromising behaviors, and lower substance abuse rates. People who attend religious services frequently are more likely to stop smoking, increase exercise, and stay married.

211. A

Spasticity is characterized by hyperactive reflexes, weakness, fatigue, and slow initiation of movement. Motor dexterity is compromised. Spasticity may be either localized or more generalized. Local muscle blocks, with such agents as botulinum toxin or phenol, can be effective for more local phenomena. The duration of effect of botox is 3 to 6 months. Baclofen is usually the drug of choice for spasticity associated with spinal cord injury because of its effect on spinal cord GABA.

212. A

Tension headaches frequently occur several times a month for several hours off and on throughout the day. They are characterized by squeezing pain involving the whole head, associated fatigue, irritability, and difficulty concentrating, and they are aggravated by stress and noise. Despite headache, most patients are able to continue their activities, using analgesics, massage, or other nonprescription remedies. Migraines are often aggravated or precipitated by certain foods. Cluster headaches and migraines are usually unilateral. Cluster headaches occur in clusters lasting for several days to weeks.

The International Headache Society criteria for tension headache suggest episodic tension-type headache is more likely with the following:

1. 10 episodes occuring more than 1 day/month
2. Headache of 30 minutes to 7 days
3. Headache that is bilateral, pressing (nonpulsating), mild or moderate in intensity, and not aggravated by routine physical activity
4. No nausea, vomiting, or photophobia or phonophobia

213. B

Although controversial, most experts recommend liver ultrasound and AFP levels should be performed on a regular basis in patients with cirrhosis. CEA and liver biopsy is not indicated routinely. Unfortunately, there are no data to show that this surveilliance increases longevity or improves morbidity or is cost-effective. Thus, options for follow-up should be presented to patients and an informed decision made.

214. C

Although the risk of HIV transmission is small, even when directly inoculated via accidental needle stick with a contaminated instrument (approximately 0.3%), the consequences are potentially devastating. Although rare, cases of transmission of HIV have been documented via the mucous membranes and abraded skin. However, there has been no documented case of transmission via intact skin. Universal precautions are recommended for all health care workers. Postexposure prophylaxis for HIV is warranted, but recommendations change regularly and usually involve two or three drug regimens. PEP is not 100% effective even when provided promptly.

215. D

Long-term usage of minocycline can induce a lupus-like syndrome. Other tetracycline derivatives are preferred for long-term therapy, particularly doxycycline.

216. D

Hepatitis C is responsible for 30% to 35% of all liver transplants and is the most frequent cause of chronic liver disease. Hep C accounts for approximately 20% of patients with acute hepatitis and up to 80% have persistently elevated liver enzymes. Most patients with chronic infection are asymptomatic and approximately 15% will develop cirrhosis. The development of hepatocellular carcinoma occurs almost exclusively in those patients with cirrhosis.

217. C

Anaphylaxis is possible based on the initial symptoms. Anaphylaxis can present with flushing, urticaria, pruritus, bronchospasm, abdominal cramping, or hypotension. It is a systemic, acute reaction caused by the release of chemical mediators by the mast cells and basophils. IgE antibodies are responsible for this chemical cascade in most cases. More than one organ system should be involved to consider the reaction anaphylaxis.

218. D

Based on initial symptoms, this patient should be aggressively treated and observation is not appropriate. The most appropriate initial management for anaphylaxis is epinephrine. It maintains the blood pressure, antagonizes the mediators, and inhibits further release of mediators from mast cells and basophils. Following epinephrine administration, fluids, diphenhydramine, and methylprednisolone may be administered.

219. C

This patient is very young for the development of farmer's lung or coal miner's lung and has no history of these exposures. These diseases can produce restrictive lung disease but usually do not produce debilitating obstructive disease, unless the patient also smokes. Histoplasmosis is a very common infectious fungal process, especially in river valleys, but does not produce severe COPD. Aspergillosis is a fungus that can worsen or mimic COPD, and often needs to be considered. Alpha-1-antitrypsin deficiency is an autosomal dominant disorder and can cause COPD in very young patients, even as young as adolescence. The alveoli are destroyed by uninhibited proteases. Some patients also develop hepatitis and cirrhosis. This patient with COPD at a young age who is a nonsmoker with a family history of early emphysema should be checked for alpha-1-antitrypsin deficiency.

220. D

Repeated small doses of allergen have been proven effective for allergic rhinitis. Immunotherapy should be avoided while a patient is having an asthma exacerbation (PEFR less than 70% patient's personal best). It is mandatory that patients with life-threatening bee or wasp sting reactions be desensitized. Immunotherapy should only be considered when specific allergens have a proven relationship to symptoms. Immunotherapy does improve asthma symptoms and decreases the need for medications.

221. A

Palpable anterior cervical nodes and occipital nodes are common in school-aged children—they can be monitored without further evaluation. An enlarged node with erythema, tenderness, warmth, or fluctuance is assumed to be lymphadenitis and should be treated. Multiple firm, nontender nodes are consistent with malignancy.

222. B

The combination of fever, refusal to bear weight, and elevated sedimentation rate and serum leukocyte count are all strong indicators of joint infection. Synovial fluid analysis for Gram stain and culture is the definitive diagnostic test for evaluation of a suspected septic joint. A synovial white blood cell count greater than 50,000/mm³ is presumptive evidence of infection. The hip position assumed by the adolescent allows maximum capsular capacity to accommodate the excessive joint fluid, thus reducing intra-articular pressure and pain. Plain films are not sensitive enough to diagnose early septic arthritis. However, ultrasound is useful to detect joint effusion and to guide needle placement during aspiration. MRI is a sensitive test to diagnose osteomyelitis and soft tissue pathology. Blood cultures should be obtained on all children with joint infections because they may be positive for the responsible microbe. *Staphylococcus aureus* is the most common organism identified. Since increased

intra-articular pressure from pus can impede blood flow and cause joint destruction, a child or adolescent with a septic hip should be referred immediately for surgical decompression.

223. C

The symptoms of COPD are usually slowly progressive. Typically, COPD is characterized by an onset in mid-life, a long smoking history, dyspnea during exercise, and largely irreversible airflow limitation. The differential diagnosis includes asthma, congestive heart failure, bronchiectasis, tuberculosis, and other pulmonary entities.

224. B

There is currently no medical management for aortic stenosis (AS). The decision to undergo valve replacement is based on at least moderately severe AS, left ventricular dysfunction, and symptoms such as angina, exertional dyspnea, or dyspnea at rest. Although palpitations may suggest arrythmia, a-fib and ventricular arrythmias are uncommon. Patients with severe AS should limit vigorous physical activity and need endocarditis prophylaxis before selected procedures.

225. C

Although the patient may have had a history of fibromyalgia, her proximal muscle weakness and tenderness suggest a myopathy. A careful history is in order to uncover potential coexisting symptoms, causes of myopathy, and other rheumatologic symptoms. Screening laboratory for a myopathy, including a measure of inflammatory activity such as an erythrocyte sedimentation rate and muscle enzymes, is in order. Although a muscle biopsy may eventually be indicated, many diagnoses, such as polymyositis, would not necessarily warrant a biopsy. A temporal artery biopsy would be appropriate in the patient with suspected temporal arteritis. The initiation of steroids, particularly at high dose, is best deferred until a firmer diagnosis is made.

226. B

Early on in patients with MVR, their ejection fraction will be above normal due to the volume overloading that occurs in the left atrium and the left ventricular hypertrophy. These two conditions can compensate for MVR for a long time. Good medical management means that as soon as the ejection fraction falls below 60% or the end systolic dimension of the left ventricle is more than 45 mm, the valve needs to be repaired or replaced. Studies show that repairing the valve is associated with a lower mortality but is a technically difficult procedure. Thus, surgical referral is prudent at the first sign of ventricular dysfunction. There are currently no medical treatments that help with MVR.

227. E

Diabetes is the most common cause of preventable peripheral vascular disease. The newest studies have shown that achieving near euglycemia, controlling blood pressure aggressively, can delay or prevent the common complications of DM. Smoking cessation, when applicable, is also quite important in the prevention of peripheral vascular disease.

228. B

Dietary fiber, although initially causing some bloating, should be increased until stools are bulkier and easier to pass. Large meals cause bowel contractions and exacerbate the symptoms of IBS. Milk products contain lactose, which may cause cramping in lactose-sensitive patients, and have a high fat content, which stimulates contractions. Daily laxative use is habit forming and should be avoided.

229. D

For a man of this age, the most likely cause of this mass is malignancy, so a biopsy would be most diagnostic. As a general rule, fine-needle biopsy has become the standard in evaluating any thyroid mass. It is simple to do, relatively safe, and can be done in the office. All of the other studies listed can be used in the workup of a thyroid nodule, but their use should be determined on a case-by-case basis and be dependent on performing a detailed medical history and physical exam that searches for risk factors for thyroid cancer.

230. E

It is important to consider serious underlying causes when a patient presents with headache. Although not diagnostic, the following "red flags" suggest a much more cautious approach to the patient: sudden onset or change in previously stable headache pattern, neurologic signs or symptoms, changes in level of consciousness, meningeal signs, new headache in patient older than 40 years, headache worsened by Valsalva maneuver, and history of recent trauma.

231. D

DEXA scanning is the most sensitive test used to screen for osteoporosis. It is also an excellent way to monitor for treatment response, and it exposes the patient to a low amount of radiation compared to CT scanning. Plain radiographs do not detect osteopenia until 20% to 40% of bone mass has already been lost.

232. C

Despite the high incidence of TB worldwide, the use of BCG vaccine is controversial. It is approximately 50% to 65% effective in conferring immunity, but the immunity wanes over time and is typically lost within 10 years. BCG is a live, attenuated strain of *Mycobacterium bovis* and may occasionally cause disseminated disease, usually occurring in immunocompromised vaccine recipients. Although BCG is widely used in other areas of the world, the CDC does not recommend its routine use in the United States. The CDC does recommend its use for infants and children with negative skin test reactivity who fit one of the following uncommon situations:

1. The child cannot be given prophylaxis and will be continuously exposed to an actively infectious person.
2. The child will be continuously exposed to multidrug-resistant TB.
3. The child belongs to a group with an annual rate of TB greater than 1% per year, for whom other interventions have not been successful.

Previous administration of BCG vaccine is not a contraindication to PPD testing.

233. A

Actually, 40% of patients are still unable to walk unassisted 1 year after fracture and approximately one-third of patients will enter a nursing home during that time.

234. B

Crohn's disease can involve all layers of the small and large intestine and is most often associated with malabsorption and vitamin deficiencies, in this case osteoporosis. Ulcerative colitis only involves the large intestine and is not typically associated with malabsorption because the pathology is generally shallow but continuous throughout the colon. Gastroenteritis and irritable bowel syndrome are not considered inflammatory bowel diseases.

The following are factors favoring Crohn's disease versus ulcerative colitis:

Pain not relieved with bowel movement
Abdominal mass in right lower quadrant
The presence of granulomas (transmural disease)
Skip lesions or discontinuous disease
Fistula development
Involvement of the small bowel
Rectal sparing
The absence of gross bleeding

235. B

The patient is suffering from acute labyrinthitis. Acute labyrinthitis is most commonly caused by a viral infection but can be caused by bacterial infection, toxicity, or barotrauma. The patient is relatively young, has no other signs of neurologic impairment (including normal hearing), and is thus unlikely to have suffered a posterior circulatory event or have an acoustic neuroma. An infarct of the middle cerebral artery would produce hemiplegia and a visual field deficit. An arrythmia would be unlikely to cause isolated true vertigo. The Hall–Pike manuever suggests a benign cause of true vertigo, such as a labrythitis or possibly benign positional vertigo.

236. D

Helicobacter pylori is believed to be causally associated with gastric B lymphoma, duodenal and gastric ulcers, and distal gastric cancer. No association has been shown with pancreatic cancer.

237. C

Antibiotics within a class may have very similar antimicrobial activity but vary in other important characteristics. Ampicillin and amoxicillin are both aminopenicillins and have almost identical antimicrobial spectra, but amoxicillin has much better oral absorption and may be dosed less frequently than ampicillin. The poorer absorption of ampicillin results in a higher concentration of the drug remaining in the gut, however, and may increase delivery of the drug to the site of infection in cases of enteric bacterial infections, such as *Salmonella* species.

238. A

COPD is characterized by progressive airflow limitation. This limitation in airflow is not fully reversible. COPD includes chronic obstructive bronchitis, which occurs with obstruction of small airways, and emphysema, which causes air space enlargement and lung parenchyma destruction along with loss of lung elasticity. Closure of small airways also occurs.

239. D

Most patients with asymptomatic cholelithiasis may be safely monitored and only 20% become symptomatic over 15 years of follow-up. Patients present with typical biliary colic, not complications of gallstones. Biliary colic is characterized by crescendo pain, typically over

3 or 4 hours. Prophylatic cholecystectomy is not recommended for average risk patients. Risk factors for complications include diabetes, sickle cell disease, and as a complication of gastric bypass surgery. Rapid weight loss is also a risk factor for gallstone development. Nonetheless, prophylatic cholecystectomy is not recommended unless done incidently as part of another abdominal procedure.

240. E

Patients with progressive disease despite adequate therapy are at risk for severe joint damage and future functional impairment. They frequently need two, and possibly three, DMARDs. Experience with RA will determine an individual physician's comfort level with prescribing these sometimes toxic and costly drugs. Those physicians who are not familiar with the indications, toxicities, and monitoring of DMARDs should seek consultation with a rheumatologist. Patients with extra-articular manifestations of RA, high RF titers, debilitating disease, and a more aggressive disease course all tend to have a worse prognosis. The physician should strongly consider consultation or referral in such patients.

241. A

Small cell lung cancer occurs in less than 25% of all lung cancers but has a poorer prognosis than non-small cell cancer. Small cell lung cancer has usually metastasized at the time of initial diagnosis, precluding surgical cure. Tobacco smoking is more closely associated with small cell rather than non-small cell lung cancer.

Survival for stage I non-small cell lung cancer (NSCLC) is approximately 60% and it is approximately 25% for stage 2, whereas 5-year survival is rare for those with metastatic disease. Tumor size, resectability, and pathologic features substantially impact survivorship. Surgery is the treatment of choice for early stage NSCLC. Radiation is an option for those unwilling or unable to undergo surgery. Adjuvant chemotherapy may offer a small survival benefit. Stage 3 NSCLC is usually treated with multimodality therapy, whereas patients with more advanced stage 3 (3B) and stage 4 are treated pailliatively.

242. C

Based on the history, treatment may begin empirically with either H2 blocker or PPI. EGD is not recommended upon initial evaluation but may be indicated if symptoms are not controlled with a therapeutic trial. Evaluation for *H. pylori* may also be included initially, but treatment does not have to be withheld. A 24-hour gastric pH study is not indicated upon initial presentation.

243. D

The diagnosis of acute otitis media requires the presence of fluid under pressure in the middle ear plus one sign of acute local or systemic illness. This includes earache, fever, cough, otorrhea, hearing loss, irritability, headache, lethargy, and anorexia or vomiting.

244. D

ASCUS pap smears can be defined as high grade or of undetermined significance. ASCUS of undetermined significance could be managed with human papiloma virus (HPV) typing. If the patient is positive for a higher risk type of HPV, referral for colposcopy would be appropriate. If the patient is negative for high-risk type, repeat the Pap smear in 1 year.

245. D

The highest prevalence of Rocky Mountain spotted fever occurs in the mid-Atlantic states, especially North Carolina. Although it is titled Rocky Mountain spotted fever, the Rocky Mountain states actually have one of the lowest prevalence rates of this disease in the entire United States.

246. C

NCEP-3 continues to identify LDL cholesterol as the primary focus of therapy. Screening is recommended starting at age 20 to assess a person's risk status. Despite the fact that during hospitalization for an acute coronary event, the LDL cholesterol may be substantially lower (not higher) than is usual for the patient, it should be measured and treatment initiated if indicated. African Americans have the highest overall coronary heart disease rate and the highest out-of-hospital coronary death rates of any ethnic group in the United States.

247. B

Salicylates would be a cause of anion gap acidosis. Other causes of metabolic acidosis include lactic and ketoacidosis, methanol, ethanol, iron, isoniazid, and cyanide ingestions, and chronic renal failure.

248. E

Hypomagnesemia is more common in diabetic ketoacidosis, along with hypokalemia and hypophosphatemia. Electrolytes need to be carefully monitored as the glucose is corrected. Hypokalemia should be presumed and K supplemented as insulin treatment can cause an intracellular shift of potassium.

249. D

Not all generations of antibiotics will have the same coverage. The second-generation fluoroquinolone ciprofloxacin (Cipro) does not provide as effective coverage of *Strep. pneumoniae* as the third-generation fluoroquinolone levofloxacin (Levaquin). Likewise, the coverage of antibiotics within the same generation may vary. Of the four oral third-generation cephalosporins available, cefdinir (Omnicef) and cefpodoxime (Vantin) provide excellent *Strep. pneumoniae* coverage, but cefixime (Suprax) and ceftibuten (Cedax) do not.

250. C

Correction of hyponatremia too quickly can cause demyelination. Other risk factors for central pontine myelinolysis include malnutrition and hypokalemia. A general guideline is to raise the sodium no more than 8 mmol/L in a 24-hour period.

Hyponatremia may be caused by disorders of elevated ADH (e.g., SIADH, adrenal insufficiency, volume depletion, and CHF), disorders in which ADH is appropriately supressed (e.g., advanced renal failure and primary polydipsia), and hyponatremia with normal or elevated plasma osmolality (e.g., hyperglycemia, pseudohyponatremia, and renal failure).

251. D

The family history of early onset of myocardial infarction suggests an inherited disorder, and familial hyperlipidemia would be most likely. Other genetic causes include hypertrophic cardiomyopathy, Wolff–Parkinson–White syndrome, or Marfan syndrome.

252. B

The incubation period for EBV infection is 10 to 14 days. At the onset of symptoms, atypical lymphocytosis and testing for heterophile antibodies (the Monospot test) may or may not be positive. Approximately 4 weeks after exposure (approximately 2 weeks after onset of symptoms), symptoms peak, as do heterophile antibodies, atypical lymphocytes, and IgM antibody against EBV. By 8 to 12 weeks, symptoms have usually resolved and the previously mentioned lab tests have normalized.

253. C

The Women's Health Initiative trial showed an increase in invasive breast cancer in those on combined hormone therapy, no improvement in mini-mental status scores or the incidence of dementia, a signficant risk of increased coronary events, and a 31% increase in stroke risk. The risk of hip, wrist, and vertebral fractures was significantly reduced. This landmark study has tempered the enthusiasm for HRT given the host of unfavorable outcomes apparent in less than 7 years of follow-up.

254. D

Alendronate would be the next best option, with clinical trials available that have shown treatment can reduce the fracture risk by up to 50% in patients with osteoporosis. Calcitonin, raloxifene, and calcium plus vitamin D also have been shown to reduce the risk of fracture but not as well as estrogen and alendrondate.

255. A

The likelihood of a painful breast mass being breast cancer is less than 5%. Fibrocystic breast disease is much more likely in this scenario, especially if the mass changes around the time of the menstrual cycle. Nonetheless, all breast masses warrant close observation and should be diagnosed definitively. The presence of a cyst versus a solid mass is reassuring; thus, aspiration can not only be diagnostic but also curative in the younger, low-risk woman. An aspiration yielding clear fluid and disappearance of the mass is suggestive of a cyst. Many experts would recommend pathologic examination of a bloody aspirate. Failure to eradicate a mass with aspiration requires further evaluation. BRCA gene testing is not recommended for patients with a history of sporadic breast cancer or with a negative family history of breast and ovarian cancer.

256. A

Celiac sprue is associated with a risk of malignancy estimated between 11% and 13%. Small bowel lymphoma is the most common type. Diverticular disease, cholelithiasis, and liver cysts are not associated with celiac sprue. Rectal fissures are associated with Crohn's disease.

257. E

The sedimentation rate could be elevated but that would be expected in a neoplasm, and it would not aid in the evaluation for metastatic disease. Estrogen and progesterone receptors would guide treatment, and the other tests would be helpful in location of metastasis.

258. D

Patients at risk for cervical cancer are those with early onset of first intercourse, those with multiple sexual partners, smokers, and those with multiparity and infection with HPV, particularly types 16 and 18.

259. B

ACE inhibitors can cause hyperkalemia because of the decrease in aldosterone production and decreased potassium excretion. NSAIDs can also increase potassium as well. ACE inhibitors are often associated with a transient increase in Cr and can cause renal failure in those with bilateral renal artery stenosis. Nontheless, many experts are now more liberal with ACE and ARB use in

patients with CHF, diabetes, and renal disease, even in the face of a worsening creatinine, because of the possible favorable effects on the natural history of medical renal disease.

260. C

With hyperkalemia, the ECG initially shows some increase in the T wave amplitude, or peaked T waves. If not corrected, this can progress to a prolonged PR interval and loss of P waves. Then widening of the QRS occurs. The QRS complex can then merge with the T wave, resulting in a sine wave pattern. Asystole and ventricular fibrillation can also occur. Cardiac toxicity is the most serious effect of hyperkalemia and must be treated aggressively. See Figure 1-16.

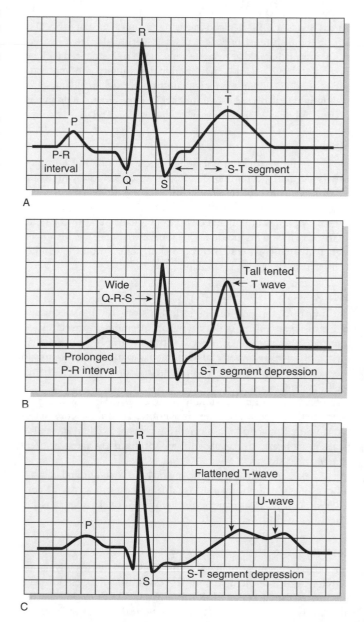

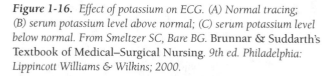

Figure 1-16. *Effect of potassium on ECG. (A) Normal tracing; (B) serum potassium level above normal; (C) serum potassium level below normal. From Smeltzer SC, Bare BG.* Brunnar & Suddarth's Textbook of Medical–Surgical Nursing. *9th ed. Philadelphia: Lippincott Williams & Wilkins; 2000.*

261. A

Survival of Epstein–Barr virus in expectorated saliva is probably brief and not a significant source of transmission. In infancy, transmission most commonly results from eating food chewed by an infected mother. In lower socioeconomic groups, most children experience primary infection in the first decade of life. Among middle and higher socioeconomic groups, infection usually occurs as a result of adolescent or postadolescent kissing (hence the nickname "kissing disease"). Previously infected individuals are immune to the development of infectious mononucleosis.

262. E

The incidence of COPD in the United States is still increasing. In fact, it is the only common cause of death that still is increasing in incidence. COPD is now the fourth leading cause of death in the United States. COPD is also increasing in prevalence and by 2020 will be the fifth most prevalent disease worldwide. Most cases of COPD are attributable to cigarette smoking in industrialized nations. In the developing world, environmental pollutants are important causes of COPD. Because poor fetal nutrition causes small lungs, low birth weight is also a risk factor for COPD. Exposure to environmental dust and organic antigens may predispose to COPD.

263. C

Typically, the luteinizing hormone:follicle-stimulating hormone ratio is elevated greater than 3:1. Recent studies are showing a correlation with insulin resistance and polycystic ovarian disease. Treatment with glucophage (metformin) is still often used to induce ovulation in patients desiring pregnancy and in the treatment of PCOS. The incidence of type 2 diabetes has also been higher in female patients with PCOS—in some studies four times as high as in the general population.

264. A

Without prior surgical or obstetrical history, the most common cause of fecal soiling is degeneration of smooth muscle in the internal anal sphincter. Rectal ultrasonography, to visualize the rectal vault, and anorectal manometry, to measure pressures in the rectal vault, are diagnostic options that are unlikely to change initial management.

Fecal impaction is common in the elderly. Many will experience fecal soiling around an impaction. Treatment consists of clearing the impaction and promoting peristalsis. If an impaction is absent, empiric treatment with an antidiarrheal agent is a reasonable next step.

A relatively recent colonoscopy makes the likelihood of a significant mass lesion unlikely. Visualizing the rectum may be considered if initial treatment is not helpful. Surgical referral is not warranted at this time.

265. D

Although frequently obtained, all the above studies usually do not provide additional insight into the cause of syncope. However, because of the high risk of death in patients with cardiac causes, an ECG is an essential initial investigation. If structural heart disease is suspected, or if syncope is associated with exercise, an echocardiogram and stress testing are also needed. If initial cardiac testing is negative, an outpatient Holter monitor or event recorder may provide additional diagnostic information.

Most episodes of syncope are neurally mediated, with vasovagal causes implicated most frequently. Situational syncope (cough, micturation, and defecation) and carotid-sinus syncope are other neurally implicated causes. A head CT only provides new diagnostic information in 4% of cases and usually there will be focal neurologic changes on physical exam. Similarly, an EEG is positive in only 2% of cases and the history is almost always suggestive of a seizure. Tilt-table testing is associated with a high degree of false-positive and false-negative tests and current guidelines downplay its usefulness.

Without heart disease or an abnormal ECG, patients who are likely to have neurally mediated syncope can be evaluated as an outpatient and do not necessarily need hospitalization.

266. C

Polymyalgia rheumatica is an inflammatory condition of unknown etiology typically characterized by aching and muscle stiffness. Pain usually involves the shoulder (70% to 90% of patients) or the neck and hips (50% to 70%) and is often bilateral. Symptoms are common in the morning, worsening with either active or passive movement. Systemic symptoms are present in 30% of cases and include fever, fatigue, and anorexia. An ESR level typically is greater than 40 mm/hour.

Fibromyalgia occurs in younger patients and is characterized by multiple localized areas of muscle pain often called trigger points. Injections of an anesthetic or even saline can alleviate localized tenderness. Depression and irritable bowel syndrome are common comorbidities. The ESR is usually normal.

Muscle weakness and an elevated CPK are more typical of polymyositis. Rheumatoid arthritis typically involves peripheral joints symmetrically. Signs of an inflammatory condition (redness and swelling) are common. An x-ray usually will indicate joint erosions and most patients are seropositive for rheumatoid factor.

267. E

Menopause occurs between the ages of 45 and 55 in 95% of women. Estrogen is effective against most of the symptoms of menopause including emotional lability. HRT is often used, particularly for short-term control of menopausal symptoms. The risk of endometrial hyperplasia and cancer is not reduced with cyclic estrogen therapy. However, the combination of estrogen and low-dose progesterone is effective and may be associated with amenorrhea in almost two-thirds of women.

268. A

The majority (80%) of patients with CAP are managed effectively with outpatient treatment. The remaining 20% will require hospitalization, secondary to either the severity of illness or comorbid conditions. A blood culture should be obtained at the time of admission in an attempt to isolate a bacterial etiology. Sputum Gram stain and culture can be useful, although it is often difficult to obtain an adequate specimen. The ESR and CRP are nonspecific markers for inflammation and not particularly useful for initial management of CAP, unless used as part of a clinical prediction rule. Bronchoscopy is reserved for cases in which more aggressive evaluation is indicated, such as with persisting infiltrates or worsening clinical status despite appropriate antibiotic therapy.

269. C

The etiology of adhesive capsulitis is unknown, but the primary process is thought to be extracapsular versus intracapsular. Significant capsular adhesions are not typical; rather, extracapsular fibrosis and collagen formation in the supporting ligaments, muscles, and bursa form contractures leading to the characteristic pain and limited range of motion. Contrary to common belief, trauma is not usually the inciting event. Many patients will have a recent history of shoulder immobility, often due to a stroke with resultant hemiplegia. Diabetes mellitus, hyperthyroidism, and hypertriglyceridemia are commonly associated with a frozen shoulder, and younger patients (younger than 40 years old) should be screened for these diseases.

On exam, patients will have the most difficulty with shoulder abduction and external rotation. Patients will complain about difficulty with associated movements such as reaching for a seat belt, hooking a brassiere strap, or grabbing a wallet. Progressive loss in shoulder range of motion ensues with difficulty in flexion, adduction, and extension (in descending order of severity).

NSAIDs and physical therapy are the mainstays of treatment. Corticosteroid injections are of unproven benefit.

270. D

A delirium is characterized by a relatively rapid onset, a variable course of symptoms often cycling between worsening and improvement within the same day, an impaired level of consciousness, and a poor attention span. Resolution of a delirium episode can be quite variable. Younger, healthy individuals quickly recover when the offending agent is removed. Individuals with impaired brain function can take several days to many weeks before clearing, and some may never fully regain prior mental functioning. A dementia is defined by answer C, a slow insidious onset over a prolonged but progressive time course, a clear sensorium until later stages, and relatively intact attention span. Depression can have a variable onset, clear sensorium, and a generally poor attention span.

271. C

Osteoarthritis is a disease of cartilage. Morning stiffness is common but usually lasts less than 30 minutes. Findings such as bony enlargement are often localized to a small number of joints, particularly the knee, hip, spine, and DIP, PIP, and CMC joints. Inflammation can be present, but a hot, erythematous, frankly swollen joint suggests another process, such as septic arthritis, gout, or pseudogout. Marginal erosions on x-ray would suggest an inflammatory arthritis such as rheumatoid arthritis.

Inflammatory arthritis is suggested by prolonged morning stiffness, pain at both rest and motion, synovitis and synovial hypertrophy, joint effusion, and erythema or warmth.

272. A

Genital warts are sexually transmitted and there are no studies showing that barrier contraceptives prevent HPV transmission. HPV 6 and 11 cause condyloma accuminata that are usually benign. HPV 16, 18, 31, 33, and 35 are the types that have been identified as the most oncogenic genotypes. HPV 16 seems to cause more squamous cell carcinomas, and HPV 18 seems to cause more adenocarcinomas.

273. D

Constipation is a well-known side effect of opioid (narcotic) medications. Frequently, as a patient's pain control improves with increasing opioid analgesic doses, a significant degree of constipation can ensue. Adding more fiber to one's diet, either through foodstuffs or as a supplement, will do little to correct significant constipation. A fiber pellet can actually cause intestinal blockage if a patient is dehydrated and does not drink sufficient fluid with the supplement.

Once opioids are used, a stimulant laxative on a routine dosing schedule is advised. Several products are available without a prescription, including senna granules, bisacodyl, and cascara.

The stimulant class has the advantage of being available in a variety of dosing forms—senna (granules for dissolution, tablet, and liquid), bisacodyl (tablets and suppository), and cascara (liquid).

Mineral oil is an old remedy that is no longer recommended for treatment. It can potentially cause a pneumonitis if accidentally aspirated. This is especially pertinent in patients on high doses of opioid analgesics. With the availability of alternate laxatives, mineral oil should be avoided.

274. B

The majority of antibiotic-associated diarrhea is not related to *Clostridium difficile* colitis. Most cases are due to the antibiotic. Ampicillin, amoxicillin-clavulanate, and cefixime account for the most cases, although fluoroquinones, macrolides, and tetracycline are also implicated. Intravenous medications have similar rates of diarrhea as orally administered drugs.

Both oral metronidazole and vancomycin have cure rates of greater than 90%. Metronidazole should be the drug of choice because it is more economical and prevents the emergence of vancomycin-resistant bacteria. Although oral treatment is preferred, intravenous metronidazole can be used at much greater expense. Intravenous vancomycin should not be used because high levels of medication in the colon do not occur.

Relapsing infections are not uncommon. Generally accepted guidelines are to treat recurrences for 4 to 6 weeks to obtain a cure. Post-treatment assays are not recommended since up to one-third of patients will have a positive test.

275. B

This gentleman has a very small chance of having a strep infection based on clinical prediction rules developed to assess the risk of strep in patients presenting with pharyngitis. Factors associated with strep infection include age 6 to 16 years, the presence of fever, posterior cervical adenopathy, tonsillar exudate, and the absence of respiratory symptoms such as cough or rhinorrhea. Given this patient's presentation, his risk of strep infection is less than 10%. A rapid strep screen may help convince the patient that a strep infection is absent. No antibiotic, however narrow in therapeutic spectrum, is appropriate for a viral infection. At a minimum, the physician should educate the patient about the low likelihood of strep and potential harms of antibiotic treatment.

276. A

The inflammation seen in COPD is not believed to be suppressed by inhaled or oral steroids. However, approximately 10% of patients with stable COPD do exhibit improvement with oral corticosteroids. It has been suggested that these patients may have coexistent asthma. There is no evidence that long-term steroid use reduces the progression of COPD.

Pulmonary rehabilitation consists of a program structured to include education, exercise, and physiotherapy. This rehabilitation has been shown to improve exercise capacity and quality of life among patients with severe COPD.

Smoking cessation is the only treatment that has been shown to slow COPD progression. At least two large trials have shown quality of life improvement and reduced mortality in severe COPD, hypoxemic patients who use long-term oxygen therapy.

277. C

Deep brain stimulation, pallidotomy, and thalamotomy are effective treatments for patients with disabling tremors refractory to treatment. The results can often be quite dramatic. Studies have shown improvement in up to 90% of patients. Selegiline has long been hypothesized to prevent as well as treat Parkinson's disease. Studies have never proved this effect, and trials have been confounded by Selegiline's improvement in treating symptoms. Although frequently thought to be a pathonomonic sign of Parkinson's, the absence of a tremor does not exclude the diagnosis. Many patients have bradykinesias as their primary symptom. Cogwheel rigidity and poor postural reflexes are the other commonly seen findings. A vertical gaze palsy is typically associated with progressive supranuclear palsy, one of the "Parkinson's plus" syndromes. These syndromes can mimic Parkinson's disease but typically do not respond to a trial of levodopa.

278. E

Proton pump inhibitors inhibit the absorption of griseofulvin, vitamin B12, and ketoconazole by decreasing gastric acidity. Lansoprazole increases the metabolism of theophylline by altering the cytochrome P 450 enzymes.

279. C

Depression and PTSD could certainly cause fatigue but would have no effect on blood indices. Folate deficiency can give a macrocytic anemia, but folate is absorbed early in the small bowel. This person has had the terminal ilium removed, which is where vitamin B12 is absorbed. Therefore, this person will develop vitamin B12 deficiency unless he receives supplemental IM vitamin B12 injections. His anemia will not develop until vitamin B12 stores are completely depleted, and this process can take 2 to 4 years.

280. D

Seronegative spondyloarthropathies are a family of multisystem inflammatory conditions. Most, but not all, are associated with the HLA-B27, more than 90% in ankylosing spondylitis. Ankylosing spondylitis is a disease of young male adults and presents with low back pain or sacroiliitis. Arthritis may be the first manifestation of inflammatory bowel disease, particularly Crohn's disease, although more subtle abdominal symptoms have often been present for some time. Enthesitis is a prominent feature of reactive arthritis, which is also associated with extra-articular problems such as keratoderma blennorrhagicum, a papulosquamous disorder; circinate balanitis, a shallow ulcer of the penis; nail changes; uveitis; and, more rarely, aortitis.

281. B

All of the above are known causes of heart failure, but by far the leading cause of heart failure is CAD. Heart failure is defined as a dysfunction of the myocardium in its pumping function. Whereas all of these conditions cause heart problems, CAD causes injury to the myocardium directly and is the most common cause of heart failure.

282. D

Progressive airflow limitation that is not fully reversible is characteristic of COPD. COPD includes a constellation of entities including chronic bronchitis. Chronic bronchitis is defined as the presence of a chronic productive cough for more than 3 months over a time period of more than 2 successive years. COPD also encompasses emphysema, a condition that results in enlargement of air spaces and destruction of lung parenchyma. Emphysema also causes loss of lung elasticity and closure of the small airways. Alpha-1-antitrysin deficiency occurs in less than 1% of patients with COPD;

it should be suspected when COPD occurs in a patient younger than 45 years of age, especially if there is no history of prior tobacco use or chronic bronchitis. Cigarette smoking accounts for the majority of cases of COPD in industrialized nations. Environmental causes are more prominent in developing nations.

283. E

Strongyloidiasis, or infection with strongyloides stercoralis, is a problem endemic to tropical regions, including areas of the southern United States. Infection occurs via the fecal–oral route or when larvae penetrate skin. Migration under the skin causes cutaneous eruptions and migratory urticarial lesions. Larvae may migrate to the lungs causing peripheral eosinophilia. These larvae may be coughed and swallowed. In the upper GI tract they mature, and adults and eggs inhabit the mucosa of the GI tract. Infection may become chronic or latent. Hyperinfection most commonly occurs in immunocompromised hosts and is characterized by penetration of the bowel wall and widespread organ involvement. Necrosis, inflammation, and peritonitis can occur.

284. C

Metformin has some effect on insulin resistance at the tissue level but works primarily by decreasing hepatic gluconeogenesis. Because it does not primarily increase the level or the action of insulin, it is not associated with weight gain in the patient with type 2 diabetes.

285. B

Recurrent abdominal pain and irritable bowel syndrome are common in adolescents. Students with IBS and recurrent abdominal pain are also more likely to report anxiety and depression than students without them. Pain and IBS are often severe enough to restrict activity. There is no significant gender association and no association with cerebral aneuryms.

286. A

Recent studies demonstrate that the ACE inhibitors are beneficial to all patients (NYHA classes I–IV) with heart failure and that they decrease mortality and improve symptoms. Digoxin has been shown to reduce morbidity, improve quality of life by reducing symptoms, and prevent rehospitalization. However, digoxin has not been shown to have any effect on mortality and has a long list of side effects. The current recommendation is to use digoxin in patients who are in atrial fibrillation and in those who are still symptomatic despite being on ACE inhibitors, diuretics, and beta-blockers. Recent work suggests that beta-blockers are useful not only for treating heart failure but also for decreasing mortality and improving symptoms. They should be used for patients who are hemodynamically stable, have no contraindications, and are currently not dyspneic at rest. Thus, beta-blockers should be used for patients with mild and moderate heart failure (NYHA class II and III). Calcium channel blockers are not useful. Spironolactone has been found to decrease mortality and hospitalization rates in those patients who have symptomatic heart failure at rest; it is currently recommended for individuals with severe (NYHA class IV) heart failure. Amiodarone is useful in select patients with recurrent or life-threatening ventricular fibrillation.

287. E

Cephalosporins have a low rate of allergic reactions in general. They are usually well tolerated in patients with a history of penicillin allergy. Unfortunately, allergy cannot be accurately predicted on the basis of penicillin skin testing. Many cephalosporins, including cefprozil and ceftriaxone—because of their side chains—confer little risk of allergy and cross-reactivity to penicillin.

288. C

The seronegative spondyloarthropathies are a group of heterogeneous diseases with clinical and laboratory features in common. These diseases include ankylosing spondylitis (AS), Reiter's syndrome (RS) or reactive arthritis, psoriatic arthritis (PsA), and arthritis associated with inflammatory bowel disease. Elevated sedimentation rates and negative autoantibodies characterize these disorders. There is a high association with HLA-B27 antigen. Ninety-five percent of patients with ankylosing spondylitis, 80% with RS with spondylitis, and 50% with colitic and psoriatic arthritis with sacroiliitis have a positive B27 antigen. Nonetheless, many patients may be HLA-B27 positive and never develop signs of arthropathy. Age of onset is typically before 40 years. Spondylitis and sacroiliitis may be seen in all the spondyloarthropathies and are the hallmark presentation of AS. Peripheral arthritis affects a minority of patients with AS, IBD, and psoriasis but is more common and acute in RS. It typically presents as an asymmetric oligoarthritis of the lower extremity joints. PsA, however, may also present as a symmetric polyarthritis similar to rheumatoid arthritis or, more classically, as arthritis of the distal interphalangeal joints of the hands. Arthritis mutilans is a very destructive form of PsA affecting the hands, feet, and spine. Iritis occurs in all the spondyloarthropathies, although conjunctivitis predominates in RS. Mucocutaneous lesions are seen in all these diseases except AS. They include oral and genital ulcers and hyperkeratotic skin and nail changes. See Figure 1-17.

289. B

Legionella antigen is detectable in the urine of 80% of infected patients on days 1 to 3 of the clinical illness. Other findings that may be present are mild leukocytosis (60% to 80%), hyponatremia, and a sputum Gram stain that demonstrates many leukocytes but a paucity of micro-organisms (sometimes small, weakly gram-negative bacilli may be seen). Serial serologic testing may take 4 to 8 weeks to demonstrate a diagnostic increase in antibody titer.

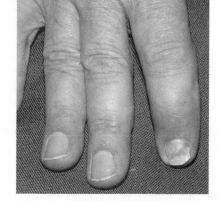

Figure 1-17. *Psoriatic arthritis. "Sausage finger deformity" of the distal interphalangeal joint. Note onycholysis. From Goodheart HP.* Goodheart's Photoguide of Common Skin Disorders. *2nd ed. Philadelphia: Lippincott Williams & Wilkins; 2003.*

290. E

Factors associated with decreasing survival in COPD include older age and a decreased forced expiratory volume per second (FEV1). An FEV1 of less than 1 liter is indicative of severe disease. Cigarette smoking is clearly the major risk factor associated with reductions in FEV1. Mortality increases with longer term and higher quantity cigarette use. Weight loss and malnutrition are potential systemic effects of COPD and are also associated with an increase in COPD mortality. Right-sided heart failure and resting tachycardia are also associated with mortality increases.

291. B

Antiplatelet therapy has not been shown to be any more effective than placebo in the treatment of peripheral vascular disease. All of the other options are proven ways to deal with the peripheral vascular disease. Antiplatelet therapy, such as aspirin, is used to reduce the risk of heart attack in patients with peripheral vascular disease.

292. B

If all men lived long enough, virtually every one would have microscopic evidence of prostate cancer. To date, there are no data to support that early detection and treatment of any stage of prostate cancer helps decrease mortality. Indeed, only 3% of men actually die directly due to their prostate cancer, as opposed to dying with their prostate cancer.

293. C

HRT with estrogen plus progestin for secondary prevention of coronary events should not be given de novo to postmenopausal women after acute MI (because of lack of efficacy and harms demonstrated in the Heart and Estrogen-Progestin Replacement Study—HERS). Postmenopausal women who were already on HRT at the time of an acute MI should be counseled concerning the risks and benefits of continuing HRT.

294. C

BPH is the most common benign "tumor" in men. Fifty percent of men have it by age 60, and by age 85, 90% of men have the condition. It is responsible for more than 1.7 million office visits annually. However, only approximately 50% of men who develop hypertrophy require treatment.

295. A

Previously, it was believed that most acute COPD exacerbations were secondary to bacterial pathogens. We now believe that many acute COPD exacerbations are due to viral and environmental causes. Upper respiratory viral infections, pollutants of various kinds, and temperature changes can cause COPD flare-ups. Histopathologic evidence indicates that COPD's inflammatory process occurs most often in the peripheral airways (bronchioles) and parenchyma of the lung. In addition to its pulmonary effects, COPD clearly has systemic effects and can cause significant weight loss.

The treatment of COPD exacerbations with antibiotics remains controversial. Some experts recommend routine treatment with a narrow spectrum agent such as amoxicillin, whereas others bide watchful waiting or treatment only with purulent secretions. Bronchodilators including inhaled beta-2 agonists, inhaled anticholinergics, and corticosteroids are all effective in clinical trials. Oxygen is administered to maintain a saturation of 90% or greater (depending on baseline).

The diagnosis of exacerbations may be made more objective and severity stratified by the presence of three criteria: increased sputum voume, increased sputum purulence, and increased dyspnea. The presence of such features as upper respiratory tract infection, increased wheezing, increased cough, fever, or increased heart rate or respiratory rate may signify a more serious episode.

296. B

The odds of erectile dysfunction after surgery are 75% versus 50% after radiation therapy. Twenty-five percent of men will have some urinary incontinence after surgery, whereas 7% to 10% will have total urinary incontinence. Some form of nerve injury is almost assured with surgery and occurs in 50% to 75% of men after radiation. One in 10 men will develop postradiation proctitis. Cardiac complications and local infection are relatively common complications.

297. D

Heterosexual transmission is the most common route of HIV infection worldwide, and it is particularly common in developing countries. Heterosexual transmission is increasing each year in the United States. Transmission of HIV is more likely from an infected male to an uninfected female rather than vice versa. There are an appreciable number of documented cases of HIV transmission from receptive oral sex. The risk of HIV infection via blood transfusion or blood products is very low in the United States—less than 1 in 500,000.

298. D

This patient sounds like she has fibromyalgia. The patient has multiple tender points, fatigue, and pain. Although it is conceivable that the patient has early rheumatoid arthritis or SLE, her physical examination and course of illness do not support these diagnoses. Likewise, there are no symptoms or signs warranting an EMG or MRI. Benzodiazepines are ineffective for fibromyalgia and associated with substantial sedation and side effects. Regular exercise is beneficial in patients with fibromyalgia.

299. D

Anal fissures are associated with Crohn's disease but not ulcerative colitis. Bloody diarrhea is associated with both Crohn's disease and ulcerative colitis. Smoking has been found to increase the risk of Crohn's disease but decreases the risk of ulcerative colitis. Some studies have also shown a decrease in the symptoms of ulcerative colitis with use of a nicotine patch. Ulcerative colitis is associated with a greater risk of colon cancer.

300. D

The most likely cause of this problem is chronic prostatitis. The patient is usually older and may not have any symptoms or just some nonspecific pressure or pain in the perineal, rectal, or low back area. The diagnosis can be made by the examination of the prostatic secretions for white blood cells and the presence of bacteriuria. Any of the above antibiotics can be used for treatment, but due to the poor penetration of antibiotics into an uninflamed prostate it usually takes at least 3 months of treatment. Tamsulosin would not be appropriate for this asymptomatic individual.

301. C

The thyroid stimulating hormone is the single best test to evaluate for hypothyroidism. If it were only moderately elevated, a low free T4 would confirm the diagnosis.

302. B

Primary testicular cancers are divided into germinal, which include 90% to 95% of all cancers, and nongerminal tumors. The germinal tumors are further divided into seminoma and nonseminomas. The nonseminoma types include embryonal, teratoma, choriocarcinoma, and yolk sac tumors. Seminoma is the most common type of testicular cancer.

303. D

Noninvasive positive pressure ventilation, using a nasal mask, may reduce the need for intubation in hospitalized patients with COPD exacerbations. However, it should be noted that controlled trial evidence is needed to confirm this finding. Pulmonary rehabilitation involves the provision of a structured program in education, exercise, and physiotherapy in COPD patients. Controlled trials have shown pulmonary rehabilitation to improve exercise capacity and quality of life in patients with severe COPD. Smoking cessation is the only intervention that has been shown to slow the progression of COPD. Lung volume-reduction surgery involves surgery to remove the part of the lung most affected by emphysema. The goal is to improve ventilatory function. Lung volume-reduction surgery has shown short-term benefits in indices such as FEV1, reduced total lung and exercise capacity, and improved respiratory muscle function. These benefits, and a resultant improvement in quality of life, last for approximately 1 year in most patients.

304. D

Risk factors for renal cell carcinoma (RCC) include a history of tobacco smoking, obesity, chronic dialysis, advanced age, and male gender. Certain genetic syndromes (familial renal cell carcinoma, von Hippel–Lindau syndrome, and tuberous sclerosis) have a relatively high incidence of RCC—of these, 25% have bilateral renal involvement. Alcohol is not known to be a risk factor for RCC.

305. C

A careful history and physical examination, not testing, should be the initial evaluation in any individual no matter their sexual orientation. Although the possibility of HIV infection should be entertained, other common causes of lassitude should also be considered. The patient's sexual history, previous HIV testing, and findings on physical examination will guide rational management.

306. C

The MRI is the preferred imaging study in evaluating a patient with epilepsy. It can help establish the precise diagnosis because of its high sensitivity and specificity for any structural abnormalities of the brain tissue and identifying lesions within the cranial cavity. Except for the rapid evaluation of the patient in whom a bleed is suspected post-trauma, MRI is usually preferred over CT scan.

307. B

Benign positional vertigo is usually associated with head movement and most commonly associated with an otolith. It is not associated with hearing loss. Viral labyrinthitis is usually associated with a viral infection of the upper respiratory tract and serous fluid is found behind the tympanic membrane. It can present with vertigo, nystagmus, and hearing loss; however, it is usually not recurrent. Vestibular neuronitis is intense vertigo that lasts hours to days but there are no other findings. These four conditions produce 80% to 85% of all cases of true vertigo (patient either spinning or the environment around the patient is spinning).

308. B

This patient has mild persistent asthma, which is defined as having asthma symptoms more than two times a week but less than one time a day. These patients also have nocturnal awakenings more than two times a month.

309. E

This patient is not well controlled since she is using her inhaler more than twice a week and experiencing symptoms so frequently. Addition of a low-dose inhaled corticosteroid or a leukotriene antagonist are appropriate options for mild persistent asthma.

310. C

A respiratory rate of greater than 28 or pulse of greater than 110 beats per minute would both indicate a severe episode. Wheezing is an unreliable indicator of the severity of attack. A pulse oximetry measurement of 90% is the goal unless the patient is pregnant or has cardiac disease. A $PaCO_2$ of 25 is expected in a patient who is hyperventilating. A $PaCO_2$ that is normal or elevated may be a sign of impending respiratory failure and such patients should be monitored closely in the intensive care unit.

311. E

A hyperplastic polyp in itself is of little concern; however, there is controversy concerning the association of hyperplastic polyps with more serious lesions. If only a sigmoidoscopy is performed, hyperplastic polyps may be a marker for more proximal disease. Since this patient's entire colon exam was normal except for the hyperplasic polyp, follow-up colonoscopy in 10 years would be reasonable. Certainly, none of the more aggressive approaches noted would be recommended.

312. B

In the rare patient who presents in diabetic ketoacidosis with a low potassium level, administration of insulin will shift extracellular potassium into the cells and may precipitate life-threatening cardiac arrhythmias. Therefore, the potassium level should be known prior to the initiation of insulin therapy in diabetic ketoacidosis.

313. D

HIV is an RNA virus that is widely distributed throughout the world and transmitted by blood and blood products. There is no evidence that the virus is spread via an insect vector or respiratory droplet transmission. The virus displays great heterogeneity, making development of an effective vaccine challenging.

314. D

This patient has the typical lesions of psoriasis. Patients with recalcitrant and extensive disease may be treated with ultraviolet A light and psoralens. Twenty-five percent of patients receiving PUVA will develop squamous cell skin cancers. Depending on how extensively the skin is involved, the progression of treatment options for localized psoriasis is a combination of moisturizers, tanning preparations, topical corticosteroids, tazarotene gel, or anthralin ointment. Ointments are preferred over creams because they moisturize the skin better. Capsaicin cream is very effective for the pruritis associated with psoriasis. Long-term maintenance therapy consists of calcipotriene or tazoratene without steroids.

315. E

Leukotrienes should not be started during an acute exacerbation of asthma. It would be more appropriate to consider adding them as an additional agent in persistent asthma.

316. C

In patients with low back pain without radiculopathy, the physician should explore "red flags" for more serious problems. Plain films are seldom helpful unless problems are suggested by the history and the physical. Job satisfaction is an important predictor of recovery. Ineffective options for acute low back pain include traction, acupuncture, and steroids. Manipulation, analgesics, and muscle relaxants are acceptable options. Back belts have not been helpful in reducing the recurrence of low back pain.

317. B

The long-term prognosis for patients with symptomatic chronic bronchitis is not good. In fact, 60-year-old chronic smokers with bronchitis have a 10-year mortality of 60%. Studies suggest that older age and a decreased FEV1 are the strongest predictors of mortality in COPD. Cigarette smoking is the major risk factor associated with accelerated declines in FEV1. Poor COPD prognostic factors associated with survival reductions include malnutrition, weight loss, hypoxemia (PaO_2 less than 55 mmHg), and right-sided heart failure.

318. C

Amantadine and rimantadine inhibit the function of the M2 protein channels of influenza A virus and prevent viral uncoating. They are indicated for both prophylaxis and therapy for influenza A. They have no effect on influenza B viruses, all of which lack the M2 protein. Oseltamivir is a neuramidase inhibitor and is effective against both influenza A and B. Neuramidase is a viral enzyme that cleaves the bonds between the emerging virus and the cell, allowing the virus to penetrate into respiratory secretions. Etanercept inhibits tumor necrosis factor and is used in treating advanced rheumatoid arthritis. Ribavirin is not used for the treatment of influenza.

319. D

Apical lung tumors extending into the superior thoracic inlet are called superior sulcus tumors or Pancoast tumors. The constellation of symptoms they cause (Pancoast's syndrome) are shoulder and arm pain, Horner's syndrome (ptosis, miosis, and anhidrosis), and weakness and atrophy of the muscles of the hand. Anatomic structures that may be involved include the eighth cervical trunk; first and second thoracic nerve trunks; the paravertebral sympathetic chain; the inferior cervical ganglion; vertebral bodies; the first, second, and third ribs; the phrenic nerve; the recurrent laryngeal nerve; and the superior vena cava. Most cases of Pancoast's syndrome are caused by non-small cell bronchogenic carcinoma.

320. C

Hemochromatosis occurs in approximately 1 in 200 people. It is the most commonly inherited genetic disorder in the United States. Case finding is done with a serum ferritin test or transferrin test searching for signs of iron overload. Genetic testing is available to screen for this disease.

321. D

Recurrent abc
with acknowledg
chiatric condition
inflammatory bowel di
out. Often, psychological
A normal diet should be c
H. pylori is not recommended
tance. A trial of an atypical antipsy

322. E

Typically, two of the above in men taller tr
taller than 5 feet 10 inches require screening w
and slit lamp exam. Other findings that should he
picion include an anterior thoracic deformity, upper
ratio more than one standard deviation below the mea
and an ectopic lens.

323. B

Bronchoscopy with biopsy showing noncaseating granulomas
would be the most specific. Even with that, however, other causes
would need to be eliminated, such as Wegener's granulomatosis and
fungal diseases such as histoplasmosis or mycobacterial infection.
Elevated ACE levels are seen in 95% of patients with sarcoidosis.
Pulmonary testing typically demonstrates a restrictive pattern.

Approximately 60% to 80% of cases are self-limited, whereas
approximately 10% to 20% of cases are severe and cause substantial
disability. Treatment options include corticosteroids, methotrexate,
and other immune modifying agents.

324. C

Stage I disease, hilar lymphadenopathy without parenchymal infiltrates on radiography, has a remission rate of 60% to 80%.

Stage II is 50% to 60%, and stage III, which consists of infiltrates
without lymphadenopathy, has a remission rate of less than 30%.

325. B

The Hemoglobin A1c is not recommended by the ADA or other
experts for diagnosis of diabetes mellitus because a diagnostic
threshold value has not yet been established. The elevated fasting
glucose remains the most commonly used diagnostic test for
diabetes.

326. D

Cardiovascular causes are present in 40% to 50% of cases. Injury
is the cause of approximately 20% of cases, and cancer is the cause
of 6%.

327. E

Although a 54-year-old could have viral or bacterial pharyngitis,
the physician should remain alert for other ENT disorders, including dental abnormalities, glandular blockage or infections, and
thyroid difficulties. Referred pain is common and may deflect the
physician from making the correct diagnosis. Treatment will be
based on the underlying cause of pain. Steroids would not be indicated in the case of siloadenitis or parotitis.

328. D

Acute tubular necrosis is associated with ischemia, nephrotoxins
including aminoglycosides and contrast dye, and myoglobinuria.

t.
The
Conflu
Azotemia

331. A

Doxycycline is a tre
Mountain spotted fever.
by *Rickettsia rickettsii* tran
that can be used include
Although tetracyclines can caus
younger than 9 years of age, the risk
apy and should be weighed against the
ness. Pencillin and lincomycin both cove
well but not *Rickettsia*. Rifampin is an antit
that can also be used as a prophylaxis for menin

332. D

The CSF is abnormal in approximately 80% of patients
Such abnormalities include oligoclonal bands, elevate
elevated myelin basic protein, and mild lymphocytic pleocyto
Abnormal findings on somatosensory evoked response testing and
of the white matter on MRI are also typical. The onset of symptoms occurs usually from age 15 to 60 years, and diagnosis relies
on objective neurologic symptoms involving two or more areas of
the CNS separated in time.

333. E.

Benefits from thrombolytic treatment of STEMI are related to
time of administration, and the American College of Cardiology
recommends thrombolytic therapy for acute ST elevation MI
within 12 hours of the onset of symptoms. Recombinant tissue-
type plasminogen activator is slightly more efficacious than streptokinase. Independent risk factors for intracranial hemmorhage
include female gender, black race, and age older than 75 years.
Absolute contraindications to thrombolytic theapy include
ischemic stroke within 3 months, previous intracerbral hemmorhage, known malignant intracranial neoplasm, and bleeding
diathesis.

Chapter 2

Pediatrics Questions

1. You are caring for a newborn infant of a mother who reports a history of syphilis but had uncertain treatment and no follow-up evaluation for her disease. Which of the following is most useful in determining whether the child has congenital syphilis?
A. Venereal Disease Research Laboratory test (VDRL)
B. Blood culture
C. Dark field microscopy of a vaginal swab specimen
D. Physical examination for abnormalities
E. Umbilical cord culture

2. Which of the following are diagnostic of urinary tract infection in a 12-month-old child?
A. A bag specimen that grows 50,000 bacterial colonies
B. Transurethral catheter specimen with 5,000 bacterial colonies
C. A suprapubic aspirate specimen with 1,000 bacterial colonies
D. A bag specimen with 10 to 15 WBCs per high-powered field
E. A bag specimen positive for nitrite and/or leukocyte esterase

3. An 8-year-old boy presents with the scalp lesion shown in Figure 2-1. Which of the following is most appropriate treatment for this lesion?
A. Topical 2% hydrocortisone
B. Topical terbinafine
C. Topical clotrimazole
D. Oral griseofulvin
E. Oral prednisone

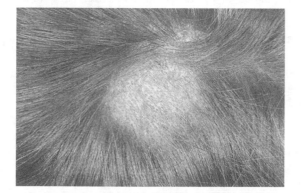

Figure 2-1. Reproduced with Permission from Rudolf M, Levence M. Paediatrics and Child Health. *Oxford: Blackwell Science Ltd, 1992:2100.*

4. A 10-month-old female presents with gastroenteritis and dehydration. She continues to have diarrhea and her urine output has decreased. On physical examination, she is tachycardic, has normal blood pressure, and her mucous membranes are dry. Her weight has decreased from 9.5 to 8.7 kg. Which of the following are the most appropriate for providing rehydration in this child?

A. Clear liquids orally
B. D5 0.45 NaCl at 50 cc/kg/day
C. Normal saline at 50 cc/kg/day
D. Normal saline 500 cc as a bolus
E. Normal saline 20 cc/kg as a bolus

5. A 6-year-old female presents with 6 days of fever. On physical examination, she has a temperature of 102°F, a heart rate of 120 beats per minute, conjunctival erythema, an indistinct maculopapular rash, digital desquamation, pharyngeal erythema, and cervical lymphadenopathy. A rapid strep screen and throat culture are negative. The next step in evaluating and treating this patient includes which of the following?
A. Await repeat throat culture to determine therapy
B. Empiric penicillin for streptococcal coverage
C. Empiric vancomycin for staphylococcal and streptococcal coverage
D. Intravenous immunoglobulin
E. Oral corticosteroids

6. A 6-year-old girl presents with her first episode of otitis media. She has been treated with antibiotics on one prior occasion for a urinary tract infection. She has no known drug allergies. Which of the following is the most appropriate antibiotic to treat this patient?
A. Cefuroxime
B. Azithromycin
C. Amoxicillin
D. Cephalexin
E. Amoxicillin/clavulanic acid

7. Which of the following is appropriate therapy for treating an adolescent with chlamydial cervicitis?
A. Azithromycin 1 g in a single dose
B. Doxycycline 100 mg twice daily for 3 days
C. Ceftriaxone 250 mg as a single IM dose
D. Metronidazole vaginal gel twice daily for 5 days
E. Penicillin 500 mg orally three times daily for 7 days

8. A 7-year-old female presents for evaluation of enuresis. She is dry during the day but has never been dry at night. Her father had enuresis as a child. Urinalysis and urine culture are normal. Which of the following is appropriate to recommend at this time?
A. Taking away her television time until her bedwetting resolves
B. Urology consultation
C. Bed alarm and behavioral modification program
D. Psychiatric referral
E. Therapy with sertraline

9. Which of the following is an indication for bone marrow biopsy in a patient with suspected idiopathic thrombocytopenic purpura?

A. Use of corticosteroid therapy for treatment

B. Use of intravenous immunoglobulin for treatment

C. Platelet count less than 50,000

D. Thrombocytopenia persisting for more than 1 month

E. Thrombocytopenia with normal hemoglobin and white blood cell counts

10. The parents of a 2-month-old male diagnosed with sickle cell disease want to know more about "pneumonia" vaccine. When discussing this vaccine with the parents, which of the following is true?

A. High-risk infants should receive the 23-valent pneumococcal vaccine.

B. Heptavalent pneumococcal vaccine alone is recommended for high-risk children older than age 2 years.

C. Children with sickle cell disease or asplenia who receive the pneumococcal vaccine still require antibiotic prophylaxis.

D. Pneumococcal vaccine is not recommended for healthy infants.

E. Pneumococcal vaccine may not be administered at the same time as MMR, varicella, or poliovirus vaccines.

11. A 2-year-old female with two previous episodes of pneumonia presents again with pneumonia. Her past medical history and family history are unremarkable. For prior office visits, she has been seen for constipation in addition to her pneumonias. Her weight has decreased over the past few visits despite what the mother reports as a hearty appetite. During current evaluation, she is diagnosed with cystic fibrosis. Which of the following is true regarding cystic fibrosis?

A. Anorexia is a common finding with cystic fibrosis.

B. Most patients with cystic fibrosis have a positive family history.

C. Decreased sweat chloride levels confirm the diagnosis.

D. Staphylococcus is a frequent organism causing pneumonia with cystic fibrosis.

E. Genetic testing is the only test available to establish the diagnosis.

12. A 10-year-old male presents with pharyngitis that proves to be group A strep by rapid testing in the office. He has no significant history except that he is allergic to penicillin. His mother has many questions about the treatment and contagiousness of this disease. Which of the following is true regarding group A streptococcal pharyngitis?

A. He may be treated with a sulfonamide antibiotic.

B. Treatment significantly shortens the course of illness.

C. All family members should be treated with antibiotics.

D. He may return to school after 24 hours of antibiotic therapy.

E. Clindamycin should not be used to treat streptococcal pharyngitis.

13. During evaluation of a 5-year-old child for sore throat, you obtain a throat culture that is positive for group A meningococcus. You call the family to check on the status of the patient and discover that she is now asymptomatic. Which of the following additional measures is appropriate in caring for this child?

A. No treatment needed

B. Oral rifampin for 7 days

C. Oral penicillin for 10 days

D. One dose of intramuscular ceftriaxone

E. Ciprofloxacin 500 mg orally for one dose

14. A 2-year-old female who is new to your practice presents for physical examination prior to entering day care. She is below the 5th percentile for weight and at the 50th percentile for height. She has had limited care during her first 2 years and she had no reported significant past history. After obtaining the rest of the history, you want to follow this child closely because you suspect failure to thrive. When considering causes for failure to thrive, which of the following is most common?

A. Milk protein intolerance

B. Psychosocial

C. Cystic fibrosis

D. Gastroesophageal reflux disease

E. Asthma/atopy

15. An 8-year-old boy with a history of asthma presents reporting wheezing and coughing once per month and no nocturnal symptoms. He is currently on no medications. Which of the following is the most appropriate treatment for this patient?

A. Short-acting B2 agonist MDI

B. Steroid MDI

C. Cromolyn sodium MDI

D. Long-acting B2 agonist MDI

E. Monteleukast orally

16. During the course of a physical examination, a 12-year-old girl states that she is concerned that most of her friends have begun having periods, but she has not begun her menstrual periods. She has no significant past medical history and is on no medications. Physical examination is normal and the patient has stage 2 breast and pubic hair development. Which of the following is the most appropriate step in managing this patient?

A. Pelvic ultrasound

B. Serum FSH and LH

C. Genetic karyotyping

D. Reassurance

E. Progesterone withdrawal testing

17. The mother of a 3-year-old male is concerned about her son's chronic congestion. The congestion has improved somewhat with over-the-counter diphenhydramine. You suspect allergies as the underlying cause and pursue further testing. Which of the following is true regarding allergy testing?

A. Radioallergosorbant testing (RAST) is more sensitive than skin testing.

B. RAST is more specific than skin testing.

C. Antihistamines do not interfere with skin testing.

D. Skin testing cannot be performed in children younger than age 4 years.

E. RAST is indicated in those with a history of severe anaphylactic reactions.

18. A 16-year-old male presents for a sports physical. He has no significant past or family history. He reports no sports-related symptoms or injuries. His physical examination is entirely within normal limits, including his blood pressure and cardiac exam. Which of the following is true regarding student athletes?

A. Cardiovascular deaths are more common in female athletes than male athletes.

B. Family history is of no screening value in athletes.

C. Hypertrophic cardiomyopathy is the most common cause of cardiovascular sports deaths.
D. Routine electrocardiography is recommended to screen athletes.
E. Echocardiography is recommended as routine screening for athletes.

19. During hospital care for a newborn, you are providing counseling to the mother regarding breast-feeding her infant. When counseling this mother, which of the following is true?
A. Breast-fed term newborns do not require vitamin supplementation.
B. Breast milk must not be frozen.
C. Breast-fed infants have a higher incidence of respiratory and gastrointestinal infections.
D. Whole milk may be introduced at 6 months of age.
E. Breast milk may be refrigerated indefinitely.

20. Which of the following is true regarding scoliosis?
A. Scoliosis cannot progress after skeletal and sexual maturity of the individual.
B. Higher degrees of curvature are associated with greater risk of progression.
C. Males have a higher risk for progression of curvature.
D. Incidence of scoliosis is greater in females than males.
E. Onset at a younger age lessens the risk for progression of curvature.

21. A 3-year-old boy is hospitalized with a acute febrile illness and is found to have a urinary tract infection. When planning the evaluation and treatment of this patient, which of the following is indicated at this time to assess an acute urinary tract infection?
A. Renal ultrasound
B. Cystoscopy
C. Voiding cystourethrography
D. Indwelling Foley catheter drainage
E. Urethral culture

22. Which of the following findings is supportive of a diagnosis of familial short stature?
A. Delayed sexual maturity
B. Height at 50th percentile at age 5
C. Bone age equal to chronologic age
D. Bone age less than chronologic age
E. Bone age greater than chronologic age

23. A child presents with an acute febrile illness of 5 days' duration along with physical findings consistent with Kawasaki syndrome. Additional supportive findings on laboratory testing include which of the following?
A. Thrombocytopenia
B. Polycythemia
C. Elevated ASO titer
D. Elevated ESR
E. Positive monospot test

24. The leading causes of death for children in the United States are:
A. Cardiovascular disease, infections, malignancy
B. Infections, malignancy, homicide
C. HIV-related disease, accidents, malignancy
D. Accidents, homicide, suicide
E. Malignancy, cardiovascular disease, pulmonary disease

25. A 2-month-old female who was born at 34 weeks of gestation presents for a well-child examination. She had an uncomplicated newborn period and did not require mechanical ventilation. Her family history is significant for a seizure disorder in a cousin. When discussing vaccination, the mother does not want to vaccinate the child, especially with the DtaP vaccine. You learn that one of the patient's siblings had a febrile reaction to the vaccine in the past. Current recommendations regarding administering DTP/ DtaP to this child are:
A. Give initial dose of DtaP at 4 months of age.
B. DTP/DtaP is contraindicated because of the family history of seizures.
C. DTP/DtaP is contraindicated because of the family history of adverse reaction to the vaccine.
D. Give DtaP at the current visit.
E. Give the initial dose of DtaP when the child weighs 8 pounds.

26. Which of the following tests is most helpful in determining the need for additional treatment or referral in a 7-year-old child with persistent bilateral middle ear effusions?
A. Audiometry
B. Tympanometry
C. Electronystagmography
D. Brain stem auditory evoked responses
E. Tympanocentesis

27. You are seeing a 10-year-old asthmatic child with moderate persistent asthma who is experiencing an exacerbation. He is currently on an inhaled bronchodilator every 4 hours as needed. You determine that he does not require hospitalization. For better control of this patient's disease, a recommended next step in trying to chronically manage his asthma should include:
A. No additional therapy
B. Antibiotic therapy
C. Inhaled corticosteroid therapy
D. Inhaled anticholinergic therapy
E. Oral antihistamine therapy

28. Which of the following is an accepted use for developmental screening tests?
A. Diagnosing mental retardation
B. Diagnosing learning disabilities
C. Identifying children requiring formal evaluation
D. Diagnosing behavioral disorders
E. Identifying genetic disorders

29. Which of the following therapies is appropriate treatment for chlamydial conjunctivitis in the newborn?
A. Topical erythromycin for 7 days
B. Topical aminoglycosides for 14 days
C. Oral erythromycin for 14 days
D. Oral erythromycin for 7 days
E. Topical sulfonamide therapy for 7 days

30. The mother of a 10-year-old boy presents because she wants her son's cholesterol checked. He had it checked 2 years ago and it was 220 mg/dL. The child's father has a history of hyperlipidemia and is currently on medication to lower his lipids. Which of the following is true regarding cholesterol and cholesterol screening in children?
A. Normal cholesterol in children is ≤240 mg/dL.
B. Childhood cholesterol levels predict adult levels.

C. Parental history of hypercholesterolemia is an indication for screening.

D. Cholesterol screening should begin at 12 months of age if there is a family history of lipid disorders.

E. Cholesterol screening should begin by age 10 years in all children.

31. The mother of a 6-month-old infant presents for routine follow-up care for her infant. This is her first child. In the course of questioning, she inquires about normal sleep patterns in infants this age. She notes that he gets up at night and cries and that she must feed him a bottle in order to get him back to sleep. She has always put him to bed after feedings when he falls asleep in her arms. Which of the following is appropriate advice for this mother?

A. Reassure her that this is normal.

B. Advise her to awaken him and feed him to avoid the crying.

C. Advise her to put him to bed sleepy but awake.

D. Advise her to ignore the crying.

E. Advise her not to hold him while feeding him the bottle.

32. Which of the following ages and stages of cognitive development (Piaget) are correctly paired?

A. Birth to age 2—concrete operational

B. Ages 2 to 6 years—sensorimotor

C. Ages 6 to 11 years—preoperational

D. Ages 11 and above—formal operations

E. Ages 2 to 6—concrete operational

33. An 8-year-old male presents for annual physical examination. He has no medical problems. In the course of the physical examination, you note that he is uncircumcised and that the foreskin is not yet retractable. Indications for circumcision in males with phimosis include which of the following?

A. Recurrent urinary tract infections

B. Recurrent tinea cruris

C. Cosmetic appearance

D. To maintain penile cleanliness

E. Prevention of penile cancer

34. A mother brings in her 2-month-old daughter for routine care and during the evaluation initiates a discussion regarding when to start feeding her daughter solid foods. The infant was 6 pounds at birth and currently weighs 10 pounds. She is taking 24 ounces of formula per day during six feedings. She is content and not colicky or fussy and sleeps 6 hours at night. She has a normal physical examination and is developmentally normal for her age. In counseling the mother, which of the following would be an appropriate recommendation?

A. She should not introduce solids until 4 to 6 months of age.

B. She should initiate feedings with meats at 3 months of age.

C. Feeding solid foods must wait until eruption of teeth.

D. She may begin feeding cereals now.

E. She should first add cereal to the formula to determine tolerance to solids.

35. A 3-year-old girl presents for a well child visit. During the course of the evaluation, the mother notes that the child only says 10 to 15 words and does not yet form sentences. Your physical examination, including neurologic examination and developmental assessment, is normal. What is the appropriate next step in assessing this child?

A. Referral for genetic karyotype

B. Referral for hearing evaluation

C. Referral for neuropsychiatric testing

D. Order CT scan of the head

E. Reassure the mother that this is normal

36. A 6-year-old male presents for a routine school physical. He has not started school yet and did not attend preschool due to limited financial resources available to the family. His last physician visit was a few years ago for a sick visit. On review of his immunization record, you note that he has not had any vaccinations since 6 months of age. In attempting to provide "catch-up" for this child's immunization requirements, which of the following is true?

A. You may not administer more than three vaccines simultaneously.

B. You may not give two live vaccines simultaneously.

C. He does not require the *Haemophilus* vaccine (Hib).

D. All of the vaccines must be given at least 2 months apart.

E. You cannot give live vaccines along with DtaP.

37. Recommendations for routine health care of children with trisomy 21 include which of the following?

A. Annual electrocardiograms

B. Annual chest x-rays

C. Annual hearing evaluation

D. Echocardiograms every 3 years

E. C-spine films every 2 years

38. Which of the following is a recommended strategy to advise parents in dealing with sibling rivalry?

A. Encourage competition between siblings.

B. Allow physical fighting to take its natural course.

C. Allow children to vent negative feelings.

D. Buy children the same presents and clothing to avoid differences.

E. Schedule all activities together as a family.

39. The mother of a 2-year-old boy presents with concerns that her child is not yet toilet trained. He has no significant past medical history and is normal on physical exam. He shows no interest in toilet training at this time, and when the mother initiates attempts to use the toilet, he becomes upset. At this time, the most appropriate recommendation is which of the following?

A. Discontinue current attempts and try again in 2 months.

B. Provide physical punishment for soiling his diapers.

C. Advise her that boys are typically toilet trained by this time and to keep trying.

D. Change his diaper less frequently so he will be uncomfortable and want to use the toilet.

E. Give him "time-outs" each time he soils his diaper.

40. You are seeing a 15-month-old male in the office for evaluation of fever. The mother notes that his temperature has been 103°F for the past 2 days. She reports that he is coughing but notes no other symptoms. He has no significant past medical history and does not attend day care. He has had no medications other than acetaminophen, which has lowered his temperature after each dose. When his temperature is 100°F or less, he is more active and takes both liquids and solid food. He has had no known sick contacts. He has been your patient since birth, has had regular medical care, and is current with regard to his immunizations. His temperature is 102°F in the office. His physical examination is otherwise unrevealing. Which of the following are appropriate in management of this patient?

A. Observation and continued acetaminophen
B. CBC, blood culture, chest x-ray, and urinalysis with culture
C. Empiric amoxicillin/clavulanic acid therapy for 10 days
D. Ceftriaxone 50 mg/kg IM and re-evaluate the patient in 1 week
E. Switch the acetaminophen to ibuprofen

41. Which of the following is an indication for use of soy-based milk?

A. Colic
B. Lactose intolerance
C. Prematurity
D. Cystic fibrosis
E. Gastroesophageal reflux disease

42. Which of the following would place a child at highest risk for lead exposure?

A. Living in a home built in 1988
B. Prior blood lead level of 5 μg/dL
C. Having a parent who works as a cashier at a gas station
D. Living in a building in which other children have had elevated blood lead levels
E. History of premature birth at 34 weeks of gestation

43. Which of the following is true regarding children and divorce of their parents?

A. The children should be asked their opinion about whether the parents should divorce.
B. The children should be asked where they want to live.
C. The children should be discouraged from sleeping with the custodial parent.
D. Disputes between the parents should be openly discussed.
E. The children should be encouraged to choose sides when differences between the parents occur.

44. A child in your practice dies in an accident and the parents call for advice regarding their other children. Which of the following is true regarding children and death in the family?

A. The children should be allowed to attend the funeral.
B. The death should be explained in inexact terms (e.g. "they're sleeping").
C. The children should not resume their usual activities for at least 2 weeks.
D. The parents need to relax on the usual house rules in order to allow for grieving.
E. All pictures and mementos of the deceased child should be removed from the house as soon as possible.

45. The mother of a 6-year-old girl presents with concerns that her daughter is staining her underwear with stool on almost a daily basis. The patient seems mildly embarrassed by this and states she is unaware when this occurs. She normally has bowel movements every 3 or 4 days and these are quite large by the mother's description. She is otherwise healthy, eats well, and is active. With regard to encopresis, which of the following is a true statement?

A. It is more common in girls.
B. It should be punished.

C. It is most commonly due to chronic constipation.
D. Thirty percent remission occurs after 6 months of treatment.
E. Agents to slow intestinal motility (e.g., loperamide) are the preferred treatment.

46. When obtaining consent for medical care, which of the following would not require parental notification and consent?

A. 14-year-old for surgical removal of a benign-appearing skin lesion
B. 15-year-old with penile discharge
C. 10-year-old with rash
D. 12-year-old for immunizations
E. 16-year-old with sore throat

47. A teenager presents for an annual physical examination and during the exam reveals that he has had oral sex with another male that resulted in orgasm. He is confused about this experience. He states that he normally dates girls and is aroused through interactions with girls. He has had no other experiences with boys and is not interested in or aroused by males, other than what happened on this one occasion. Which of the following is true?

A. He is homosexual or bisexual.
B. Up to one-third of males have a sexual experience with another male that results in orgasm.
C. This behavior is not associated with any risk for sexually transmitted diseases.
D. He needs psychotherapy.
E. Homosexual experimentation is more common in girls than in boys.

48. An 18-year-old sexually active female presents to discuss contraception. She would like to take the birth control pill but is concerned about its effects. You discuss the potential risks of hormonal contraception and then balance this with the advantages. Which of the following is a health benefit of taking the birth control pill?

A. Relief from dysmenorrhea
B. Prevention of sexually transmitted diseases
C. Lowers risk of heart disease
D. Protection from breast cancer
E. Lowers risk of venous thrombosis

49. Which of the following is true regarding eating disorders?

A. Anorexia nervosa is the most common eating disorder.
B. Bulimia nervosa is more common in males than females.
C. Psychiatric comorbidities occur rarely with eating disorders.
D. The average age of onset of bulimia is between 17 and 25 years.
E. Bulimia nervosa classically results in dramatic weight loss.

50. With regard to teenagers and suicide, which of the following is a true statement?

A. Boys attempt suicide more often than girls.
B. Girls have more successful suicide attempts than boys.
C. Suicide is the second most common cause for death in teenagers.
D. Family history of suicide confers no increase in risk for teenage suicide.
E. Psychiatric disease confers no added risk for suicide in adolescents.

51. A 6-month-old male is noted to have an undescended left testicle during the course of his well child check. The parents are very concerned. Which of the following is a true statement regarding cryptorchidism?

A. The child needs immediate surgery.

B. Hormonal therapy with human chorionic gonadotropin is 70% to 80% effective in treatment.

C. This condition is associated with decreased risk for testicular cancer.

D. Eighty percent or more of testicles will spontaneously descend by 1 year of age.

E. Surgery is indicated if descent has not occurred by age 4 years.

52. Which of the following statements about scrotal hernias and masses is correct?

A. Reducible hernias should be repaired within 2 to 4 weeks.

B. Hydroceles must be promptly repaired during infancy.

C. The most common abdominal viscera within hernias in girls is large intestine.

D. Hernia occurs more commonly in children older than 5 years of age.

E. Incarcerated hernias should be repaired within 4 to 6 weeks.

53. A 6-year-old male is noted to have asymptomatic hematuria with 15 RBCs/hpf on urinalysis. He has no significant past medical history and his physical examination is unremarkable. Initial evaluation should include which of the following?

A. Urine cytology

B. Serum PTH

C. Renal biopsy

D. Cystoscopy

E. Repeat urinalysis for RBCs and protein

54. A 5-year-old presents for routine school physical examination and is noted to have a blood pressure of 130/88. Repeat measurements confirm this finding. He is asymptomatic and has an otherwise normal physical examination. Which of the following is the most common cause for hypertension in this age group?

A. Primary hypertension

B. Renal parenchymal disease

C. Broncopulmonary dysplasia

D. Pheochromocytoma

E. Renal artery stenosis

55. Which of the following is true regarding long-term prognosis with juvenile rheumatoid arthritis?

A. Life-long exacerbations and remission normally occur.

B. Sixty percent of patients have active disease as adults.

C. Patients are usually left with crippling joint deformities.

D. Life expectancy is considerably shortened in these patients.

E. Most patients have complete remission and resume normal function.

56. Which of the following should be part of the initial care for a child who ingests a button (watch) battery?

A. Immediate esophagoduodenoscopy

B. X-ray to identify the location of the battery

C. Induce vomiting with serum of ipecac

D. Surgical removal of the battery

E. Administration of laxatives to hasten passage of the battery

57. A 10-year-old male presents with muscle weakness in his lower extremities and clumsiness with walking for the past 2 days. This began several days after a trip to northern Wisconsin where the family spent a lot of time outside hiking around the countryside. The child is afebrile. Other than the identified weakness, gait ataxia, and absent lower extremity reflexes, the physical examination reveals a tick in her scalp that is removed. Laboratory testing, including CSF analysis, is normal. Which of the following is true regarding this patient's condition?

A. The patient most likely has tick paralysis and removal of the tick is curative.

B. The patient has meningitis and should be started immediately on IV antibiotics.

C. The mortality rate for this disease is 40%.

D. CT scan of the brain will reveal characteristic findings to confirm the diagnosis.

E. The patient most likely has tick paralysis and full recovery is unlikely.

58. An 8-year-old boy presents with poison ivy on his legs. He has mild erythema and itching associated with this rash, which is linear and has a few small vesicles associated with it. No other areas of skin are involved. Which of the following is the most appropriate therapy?

A. Oral prednisone 1 mg/kg for 7 days

B. Desensitization therapy for poison ivy

C. Oral antihistamines for 2 weeks

D. Topical corticosteroids until resolution of the rash

E. Oral cephalexin 40 mg/kg twice daily for 5 days

59. A 15-year-old male with type 1 diabetes mellitus will be participating in track next year. He will be participating in running events. He ordinarily has very good glucose control and is wondering about his diabetes as it relates to exercise. Which of the following is true regarding diabetes and exercise?

A. Exercise should be discouraged in diabetic children.

B. Exercise will impair peripheral utilization of glucose and cause hyperglycemia.

C. The patient will likely need to increase his carbohydrate intake to avoid hypoglycemia.

D. The patient will likely need to increase his insulin dose to avoid hyperglycemia.

E. He should inject his insulin into his thighs to hasten absorption to prevent hyperglycemia.

60. The mother of a 1-year-old boy expresses concerns that her baby is chubby. She feeds him table foods, baby foods, and has just switched him to whole milk. She and his father are of normal height and weight. His weight is at the 75th percentile as is his height, and his physical examination and development are normal. She would like to place him on a low-fat diet at this time and restrict his eating. Which of the following is true regarding this patient?

A. He should be placed on skim milk and a low-fat diet.

B. He should not be taking solid foods at this stage.

C. Obesity in infants is not predictive of adult obesity.

D. He is most likely hypothyroid.

E. She should replace milk in his diet with juices.

61. While you are examining a 2-week-old male, you note laxity and a definite click while performing Ortolani's maneuver. The child is otherwise normal and had an unremarkable prenatal course and delivery. This child is diagnosed with developmental dysplasia of the hip. Which of the following is true regarding this condition?

A. The condition is always detectable at birth.

B. Double diapering the child is effective therapy.

C. If not detected until 18 months of age, surgery is usually required.

D. Ultrasound and standard x-ray examination are not useful in confirming the diagnosis.

E. Maintenance of hip adduction is required for effective treatment.

62. A 12-year-old male in your practice is diagnosed with Marfan's syndrome. Which of the following cardiac conditions should be routinely assessed in following this patient?

A. Mitral stenosis

B. Coarctation of the aorta

C. Atrial septal defect

D. Aortic root dilatation

E. Ventricular septal defect

63. Which of the following cardiac conditions is associated with cyanosis?

A. Ventricular septal defect

B. Atrial septal defect

C. Pulmonic stenosis

D. Patent ductus arteriosis

E. Tetrology of Fallot

64. On office follow-up of a newborn at 4 days of age, the infant is noted to be jaundiced. The mother noted the onset of the jaundice at 2 days of age. The mother is breast-feeding and the infant otherwise appears well and had no prenatal or birth-related complications. The bilirubin is 9 mg/dL. In addition to continued monitoring of this patient, you recommend which of the following?

A. Decreasing the frequency of the feedings

B. Supplemental formula feeding

C. Supplementation with water

D. Increasing the duration of the feedings

E. Feeding the infant more frequently

65. A 4-year-old male presents with pruritis in the anal area noted most intensely at night. You suspect he has pinworms. Appropriate therapy would be which of the following?

A. Metronidazole

B. Rifampin

C. Mebendazole

D. Sulfamethoxazole

E. Amoxicillin

66. You are examining a macrosomic newborn in the nursery after a difficult vaginal delivery. You palpate the clavicles for crepitus and deformity and find the examination to be normal. Which of the following, if present, would signal that a clavicular fracture might have occurred?

A. Persistent crying

B. Internal rotation of the arm

C. Grunting respirations

D. Limited arm movement

E. Bruising and swelling in the clavicular region

67. A 13-year-old male expresses concerns that he has not developed any axillary or pubic hair and yet many of his peers have. On physical examination, which of the following signs occurs first in the sequence of pubertal changes for boys?

A. Testicular enlargement

B. Development of pubic hair

C. Penile enlargement

D. Growth of facial hair

E. Development of axillary hair

68. A 2-year-old male is brought to the office with a reluctance to move his left arm. This began when the mother was crossing the street with him, and while holding his hand the mother pulled on his arm to prevent a fall. Examination reveals mild tenderness at the radial head but is otherwise normal. X-rays are ordered and are normal. Which of the following is the most likely diagnosis in this child?

A. Colles' fracture

B. Occult fracture of the radial head

C. Nursemaid's elbow

D. Dislocation of the shoulder

E. Attention-seeking behavior on the part of the child

69. A 7-year-old male presents with persistent purulent rhinorrhea. You suspect sinusitis and start antibiotic therapy. Which of the following is the most appropriate choice for antibiotic therapy?

A. Levofloxacin

B. Cephalexin

C. Erythromycin

D. Tertracycline

E. Amoxicillin

70. Which of the following is an example of positive reinforcement of behavior?

A. Giving a child a cookie for undesired behavior

B. Spanking a child for undesired behavior

C. Placing a child in time-out for undesired behavior

D. Ignoring undesired behavior

E. Taking away privileges (e.g., TV or phone) for undesired behavior

71. A 4-year-old presents with nonbloody diarrhea for 2 days. She has had no vomiting or fever. On examination, she has moist mucous membranes, appears well hydrated, and has hyperactive bowel sounds. Recommendations for treatment should include which of the following?

A. Trimethoprim-sulfamethoxazole

B. Loperamide

C. Clear liquid diet

D. Her usual age-appropriate diet

E. Dicyclomine

72. A 9-month-old female is diagnosed with scabies. Which of the following is the most appropriate treatment of this child?

A. 1% lindane topically

B. 5% permethrin topically

C. Mebendazole orally

D. Mefloquine orally

E. Ivermectin orally

73. A 6-year-old child is brought to your office 18 hours after being stung by a bee. The child was stung on the left arm and was noted to have swelling and erythema on the left arm associated with mild itching and pain. He has no other symptoms and complaints. Other than the erythema and edema at the sting site, his physical examination is unremarkable. Which of the following is the most appropriate therapy for this child?

A. Antihistamines

B. Antibiotics to cover staph and strep

C. Subcutaneous epinephrine

D. Hospitalization to monitor for anaphylaxis

E. Oral steroids (e.g., prednisone)

74. A newborn infant is noted to have bilious vomiting approximately 24 hours after birth. On examination, there are active bowel sounds and some visible peristaltic waves but no abdominal distention. An x-ray is obtained and the radiologist advises you that it shows the "double-bubble" sign. Which of the following would most likely account for this child's vomiting?

A. Volvulus

B. Pyloric stenosis

C. Tracheoesophageal fistula

D. Duodenal atresia

E. Intussusception

75. When evaluating a newborn, you note what appears to be a tooth in the position of the mandibular central incisor. It is not movable and firmly attached. The mother has chosen to bottle feed her infant and the lesion does not appear to bother the child at all. What recommendations should you make to the parents regarding this lesion?

A. Immediate surgical removal

B. Surgical removal at 2 months of age

C. Therapy with nystatin until resolution of the lesion

D. Dental x-ray evaluation

E. No evaluation or treatment is necessary

76. A 4-year-old male presents with a history of nosebleeds for the past 4 months. The nosebleeds occur approximately once per week and spontaneously resolve. The child has no other significant past medical history and the mother reports no history of excessive bruising or other sites of bleeding. Physical examination reveals erythema along the anterior aspect of the septum. The most common cause for nosebleeds in children is which of the following?

A. Bleeding disorder

B. Nose picking

C. Foreign body

D. Osler–Weber–Rendu syndrome

E. Child abuse

77. Which of the following is a true statement regarding strabismus in children?

A. It never spontaneously resolves.

B. Visual evoked responses are required for detection of strabismus.

C. Failure to correct strabismus may result in permanent visual loss.

D. Most cases are due to paralysis of an extraocular muscle.

E. No intervention is required in those with a positive family history for strabismus.

78. Which of the following is associated with excessive tearing in newborn infants younger than 1 month of age?

A. Strabismus

B. Congenital glaucoma

C. Amblyopia

D. Congenital cataracts

E. Subconjunctival hemorrhage

79. Which of the following is a cause for childhood hypochromic microcytic anemia?

A. Sickle cell anemia

B. G6PD deficiency

C. Folate deficiency

D. Lead poisoning

E. Acute blood loss

80. A 3-year-old female presents for routine physical examination. The mother is concerned that she appears pale. On further questioning she notes that the child's diet includes a lot of milk but very little red meat. The hemoglobin is found to be 8.0 with hypochromic and microcytic indices. Appropriate management of this child would now include which of the following?

A. Therapeutic trial of iron

B. Bone marrow biopsy

C. Blood transfusion

D. Endoscopy to evaluate for GI blood loss

E. Once daily multivitamin with iron

81. Which of the following disorders is identified by abnormalities in the prothrombin and/or partial thromboplastin times?

A. Henoch–Schonlein purpura

B. Classic hemophilia

C. Idiopathic thrombocytopenic purpura

D. Glanzmann's disease

E. G6PD deficiency

82. After delivery of an infant, you note the presence of prominent labia with rugal fold and an enlarged clitoris (1.5 cm). In evaluating this infant, which of the following steps is recommended?

A. Do not discuss the concerns with the parents until test results are available.

B. Immediate genetic testing and laboratory evaluation.

C. Hold off on testing and reassess the genitalia as the child develops.

D. The infant should be assigned a gender and named at birth.

E. No intervention is needed.

83. Which of the following is the most common organism causing urinary tract infections in children?

A. *Enterococcus*

B. *Moraxella catarrhalis*

C. *Haemophilus influenzae*

D. *Staphylococcus aureus*

E. *Escherichia coli*

84. Which of the following rotational disorders of the lower extremity should be diagnosed and treated during the neonatal period?
A. Medial tibial torsion
B. Lateral tibial torsion
C. Clubfoot
D. Blount's disease
E. Legg–Perthes disease

85. A 2-year-old male presents because the parents are concerned about his bowlegs. They have noticed progressively increased bowing of his legs since he began to walk. Review of his history reveals that he began walking at 9 months of age and has had normal growth and development. He has no other significant history. Physical examination is normal except for bilateral genu varum and internal tibial torsion. Which of the following is the most common cause of pathologic bowing of the legs?
A. Rheumatoid arthritis
B. Blount's disease
C. Achondroplasia
D. Rickets
E. Slipped capital femoral epiphysis

86. An 8-year-old girl is brought to your office for evaluation of leg pains. She has had three episodes of bilateral pains in the calves that occur at night and awaken her from sleep. Her physical activity during the day is unaffected. She has been afebrile, recalls no injuries, and has been otherwise well. Her past medical history is unremarkable. Her physical examination is unremarkable. Which of the following is the most appropriate next step?
A. Reassurance of child and parents
B. X-ray of lower extremities
C. Bone scan
D. Sedimentation rate and rheumatoid factor
E. Referral to orthopedic surgeon

87. Legg–Calvé–Perthes disease is characterized by which of the following?
A. Elevated white blood cell count
B. Increased uptake in the femoral head on bone scan
C. Decreased uptake in the femoral head on bone scan
D. Characteristic x-ray findings present with disease onset
E. Elevated erythrocyte sedimentation rate

88. A 7-year-old female presents after sustaining an injury to her left ankle. She was playing soccer and severely twisted her ankle in a collision with another player. She has been unable to bear weight since the injury. Examination reveals tenderness and edema laterally with some associated bone tenderness. X-rays are negative. Which of the following injuries is most likely in a child of this age?
A. Ankle sprain
B. Salter–Harris fracture
C. Stress fracture
D. Osteomyelitis
E. Osteosarcoma

89. The day after delivering her new baby boy, the mother develops a rash and fever. You suspect that she has chickenpox.

Regarding management of the infant, which of the following is recommended?
A. No therapy
B. Varicella immunoglobulin
C. Acyclovir
D. Varicella vaccine
E. Acyclovir for 2 weeks, along with the varicella vaccine

90. Which of the following is true regarding migraine headaches and children?
A. The prevalence of migraines increases with age.
B. At all ages, girls are affected more than boys.
C. Sumatriptan is indicated for use in children as young as age 6 years.
D. Narcotics are the mainstay of therapy.
E. Migraine headache is an uncommon form of headache in children.

91. You are assuming care for a newborn whose mother is hepatitis B surface antigen positive. Proper care for this infant should include which of the following?
A. Hepatitis B immunoglobulin only
B. Hepatitis B vaccine only
C. Isolation of the infant
D. Both hepatitis B vaccine and immunoglobulin
E. No therapy is required

92. A 3-year-old presents for routine physical examination. The parents note that he has a slight waddling gait. His past medical history is unremarkable and he achieved his developmental milestones at the normal times. On physical examination, he is alert and has a slight lordotic posture, a positive Gower's sign, and a Trendelenburg gait. Which of the following tests would be helpful in establishing the diagnosis?
A. MRI brain
B. Plain hip x-rays
C. Muscle biopsy
D. Erythrocyte sedimentation rate
E. Electroencephalogram

93. The most common cause of nephrotic syndrome in children is which of the following?
A. Systemic lupus erythematosis
B. IgA nephropathy
C. Chronic hepatitis
D. Diffuse mesangial proliferative glomerulonephritis
E. Minimal change disease

94. A 3-month-old male presents with parental concerns regarding spitting up his "whole bottle" after each feeding. The parents note that the formula comes up effortlessly. They have tried switching formulas but the problem has persisted. The baby has not been fussy and takes the bottle well. He has had normal stools and urine output and no respiratory difficulty. The prenatal and neonatal history is unremarkable. The physical examination, including weight and growth, are normal. Which of the following would you now recommend in caring for this child?
A. Esophagoduodenoscopy
B. Observation as he will outgrow this condition

C. Upper GI series

D. Switching to soy-based formula

E. Metoclopropamide four times daily

95. A 16-month-old male presents to the emergency room with a seizure described by the parents as tonic–clonic-type activity. The child is currently sleepy. He had onset of a URI the preceding day, and then he developed a fever to 103°F. He has no significant past medical history, and his physical examination, other than nasal congestion and being slightly lethargic, is normal. During the emergency room visit, he fully awakens, appears normal, and his laboratory tests are normal. He is diagnosed with a febrile seizure and instructed to follow-up with you. On follow-up, which of the following is recommended with regard to evaluation and treatment of febrile seizures?

A. Electroencephalogram

B. CT scan of the head

C. Acetaminophen with onset of future illness

D. Phenobarbital with onset of future illness

E. Phenytoin daily to achieve therapeutic dose

96. A 4-year-old male presents following an upper respiratory infection with rash and joint aches. On physical examination, he is noted to have a temperature of 100.5°F and scattered petechiae and purpura. Examination of the heart, lungs, abdomen, and joints is normal. On testing, he is noted to have hematuria and heme-positive stools. His WBC is 11.5, with a platelet count of 370,000. He is suspected to have Henoch–Schoenlein purpura (HSP). Which of the following is true regarding this disease?

A. Intussusception can occur as a complication.

B. Seizures commonly occur with HSP.

C. Renal involvement is not commonly found with HSP.

D. HSP is caused by misuse of aspirin.

E. Prognosis for full recovery is poor.

97. A 4-day-old infant is brought to your office for evaluation of possible jaundice. He is the product of a normal term pregnancy and had an uneventful hospital course. There is no significant family history and the mother is on no medications. He is being breast-fed without difficulty and is having 7 or 8 wet diapers daily. On physical examination, he is noted to have scleral icterus and jaundice but otherwise appears well. Which of the following is true regarding jaundice in the newborn?

A. Jaundice is of no concern in otherwise normal term newborns.

B. Switching to bottle-feeding is the only advice necessary.

C. The infant should be hospitalized for monitoring.

D. A serum bilirubin should be obtained.

E. Phototherapy should be initiated.

98. The mother of a 2-year-old child called, stating that her child ingested five 325 mg acetaminophen pills approximately 1 hour ago. The child currently appears well. She estimates that the child weighs 22 pounds. Appropriate advice would include which of the following?

A. Reassurance that acetaminophen is safe and will pose no risk.

B. Schedule an office appointment for the following day.

C. Administer syrup of ipecac and monitor the child at home.

D. Administer a laxative and monitor the child at home.

E. Take the child to the emergency room immediately for evaluation and treatment.

99. Screening for galactosemia may be performed by which of the following tests?

A. Urine testing for ketones

B. Urine testing for reducing substances

C. Measurement of serum anion gap

D. Erythrocyte sedimentation rate

E. Complete blood count

100. Which of the following is a risk factor for sudden infant death syndrome (SIDS)?

A. Primiparous mother

B. Breast-feeding

C. Advanced maternal age

D. Low socioeconomic status

E. Female gender

101. Which of the following is a true statement regarding the effects of maternal substance abuse?

A. Fetal alcohol syndrome is the most common preventable cause of birth defects.

B. Cocaine is a known teratogen.

C. Premature infants are more susceptible to opiate withdrawal than are term infants.

D. Drug and alcohol use affect 2% of pregnancies.

E. Drugs and alcohol may cause premature birth but are not associated with intrauterine growth retardation.

102. A 4-week-old infant is brought to the office for evaluation of repeated nonbilious vomiting over the past week. He has had a slight decrease in weight and number of wet diapers. He has a very good appetite and seems hungry. You determine that the child has pyloric stenosis based on your assessment and examination. Which of the following is true regarding pyloric stenosis?

A. African Americans are more commonly affected than other ethnicities.

B. Lab work will reveal hyperchloremic metabolic acidosis.

C. Most cases resolve with supportive care and H2 blockers.

D. Surgery is recommended treatment.

E. Clinical examination and ultrasound are equally sensitive in diagnosing pyloric stenosis.

103. A mother presents with exacerbation of her allergic rhinitis. She has been on no medications and has not taken anything yet because she wants to be sure any medicine she takes will be safe while she is breast-feeding. Which of the following is not recommended for breast-feeding mothers?

A. Brompheniramine

B. Cetirazine

C. Fenofexadine

D. Loratidine

E. Diphenhydramine

104. A 17-year-old male is brought to the emergency room because of change in behavior. His parents suspect drug or alcohol ingestion. The patient admits to having a couple of sips of beer. On physical examination, he has marked motor incoordination but is alert. What blood level of alcohol would account for these findings?

A. 40 mg/dL

B. 75 mg/dL

C. 150 mg/dL

D. 300 mg/dL

E. 500 mg/dL

105. A 3-month-old male presents with a rash consistent with atopic dermatitis. Which of the following is true regarding atopic dermatitis?

A. Onset prior to 1 year of age is uncommon.

B. In infants, atopic dermatitis predominantly affects the flexural creases.

C. Atopic dermatitis clears by school age in 50% or more of patients.

D. Avoiding certain foods is effective therapy for most children.

E. Atopic dermatitis affects 40% of infants.

106. A 2-month-old presents with a diaper rash that predominantly involves the inguinal folds but also has associated satellite lesions. Appropriate therapy for this rash includes which of the following?

A. Zinc oxide paste topically

B. Oral amoxicillin

C. Nystatin with triamcinolone cream topically

D. Clotrimazole cream topically

E. Bacitracin ointment topically

107. A 2-week-old male presents with a white adherent coating of his tongue and buccal mucosa. There is some associated erythema and the lesion bleeds when you try to remove the white coating. Which of the following is an appropriate step in caring for this infant?

A. Evaluation for immunocompromised state

B. Oral griseofulvin

C. Oral nystatin

D. No therapy needed

E. Frequent brushing or wiping of gums and tongue with toothbrush or gauze

108. A 6-year-old male presents with a wart on his right hand. Which of the following is true regarding warts in children?

A. Cryotherapy, although painful, is always effective.

B. Sixty-five percent of warts clear without treatment in 2 years.

C. *Verrucae vulgaris*, or common warts, commonly occur in the genital region.

D. Warts affect more than 50% of school-age children.

E. Following treatment, 50% of warts will recur.

109. Which organism has been associated with development of acne?

A. *Proprionibacterium acnes*

B. *Pityrosporum orbiculare*

C. *Corynebacterium minutissimum*

D. *Epidermophyton floccosum*

E. *Staphylococcus epidermidis*

110. A 3-year-old male presents with a crusting golden-colored lesion associated with erythema around his nares. The onset of this occurred in association with an upper respiratory infection, which is now resolving. The lesion is slightly tender to touch. No other skin lesions are noted and the patient appears well. Which of the following is the likely diagnosis for this lesion?

A. Furuncle

B. Folliculitis

C. Impetigo

D. Atopic dermatitis

E. Seborrheic dermatitis

111. A 10-year-old girl presents for evaluation of a painful ear. Upon questioning, she reports swimming a great deal recently. She has not been ill recently and has no other medical problems. Examination reveals a tender left tragus but normal appearing skin on the tragus and auricle. The left external canal appears erythematous, edematous, and an exudate is noted in the canal. The left tympanic membrane is slightly dull, but mobile, and has no erythema. Which of the following is the appropriate treatment for this patient?

A. Aggressive ear irrigation to remove the exudates and debris

B. Oral cephalexin

C. Intravenous aminoglycosides and antistaphylococcal penicillin

D. Topical antibiotic and steroid combination

E. Oral fluroquinolone

112. You are serving as the team physician for a football team and one of the players comes off the field after a hard collision in a confused state. He does not lose consciousness but is confused for 10 minutes and then returns to his normal state. He denies any symptoms and is neurologically intact. Which of the following is now recommended for this player?

A. He may return to play.

B. He may again participate after being asymptomatic for 1 week.

C. He must sit out the rest of the season.

D. He should be transported to the hospital for evaluation.

E. He should never again participate in contact sports.

113. The parents of a 5-year-old male present with concerns that their child has developed a tic within the past 6 weeks. He has been noted frequently blinking his eyes. He has been otherwise well and very successfully completed his year in kindergarten. There is no significant family history, and no undue stresses or illnesses have been noted in the family. The child is noted to have frequent eye blinking during the visit but is otherwise neurologically intact. Which of the following is true regarding this patient's condition?

A. The child has Tourette's syndrome.

B. Coprolalia is necessary to diagnose Tourette's syndrome.

C. Symptoms must be present for at least 3 months to diagnose Tourette's syndrome.

D. Tics most commonly occur in adolescent children.

E. Tics occur in up to one-fourth of children.

114. A 10-year-old male presents with a past medical history of asthma and complaints of seasonal rhinorrhea, nasal itching, and sneezing. He is currently on albuterol as needed for mild intermittent asthma. He has no known allergies. His symptoms are worse in the late summer. On examination, he has boggy bluish nasal turbinates and his lungs, ears, and skin are clear. Which of the following is the likely cause for this patient's condition?

A. Vasomotor rhinitis

B. Allergic rhinitis

C. Sinusitis

D. Upper respiratory infection

E. Rhinitis medicamentosa

115. The mother of a 13-month-old child presents with questions regarding varicella vaccine. Which of the following is true regarding this vaccine?

A. The vaccine may not be given with other vaccines.

B. The vaccine is 80% effective in preventing severe disease.

C. Current data suggest that immunity lasts for 20 or more years.

D. Fewer than 1% of vaccines develop a varicella-like rash after the vaccine.

E. Prior to age 13 years, the vaccine must be administered twice.

116. A 10-year-old male presents as a new patient to your practice. The mother had refused MMR vaccines in the past due to concerns about adverse effects of the vaccine. Thus, he has never received an MMR vaccine. He is current on his other vaccines and received a varicella vaccine 2 weeks ago. Which of the following is true?

A. The second MMR is recommended only to boost the immune response that wanes over time.

B. Unimmunized children should receive two MMR vaccines at least 4 weeks apart.

C. MMR should be given during this current visit.

D. Measles vaccine is known to cause autism.

E. Children older than age 10 only require one MMR vaccination.

117. The mother of an 18-month-old presents reporting that the child has had a fever to 103°F for 3 days. He is doing better today with no fever, but he has developed a rash. There are no other localizing symptoms. On exam, he appears well, his temperature is 98.6°F, and his examination is normal except for a maculopapular rash on the trunk and neck along with some shotty posterior cervical lymphadenopathy. Which of the following is the likely diagnosis?

A. Roseola

B. Fifth disease

C. Measles

D. Kawasaki's disease

E. Allergic reaction

118. You have just diagnosed a 6-year-old boy with Fifth disease and the mother tells you she is 24 weeks pregnant. Which of the following is true?

A. The woman should stay away from the child until the rash resolves.

B. The child should avoid contact with other children and adults.

C. There is a 50% chance of fetal death due to hydrops if the mother becomes infected.

D. Serologic testing can be offered to the mother.

E. Fifth disease presents no risk to the mother or her pregnancy.

119. A child is being evaluated in the emergency room with mild stridor and is noted to have retractions, decreased air movement, but normal color and pulse oximetry. He is restless appearing. Which of the following is appropriate treatment for this child?

A. Albuterol by nebulizer

B. Ipratropium by nebulizer

C. Dexamethasone given IM or PO

D. Diphenhydramine orally

E. Ceftriaxone IM

120. Which of the following is true regarding bronchiolitis?

A. Secondhand smoke is more of a risk factor than day care attendance.

B. Steroids are of proven benefit.

C. Antibiotics prevent bacterial complications.

D. The case fatality rate is nearly 10%.

E. Peak occurrence is at 3 years of age.

121. You are evaluating a child and suspect possible Turner's syndrome. Which of the following is associated with Turner's syndrome?

A. Hyperphagia

B. Blindness

C. Precocious puberty

D. Male genotype

E. Webbed neck

122. A 6-year-old male presents with a glucose of 350, bicarbonate 10, potassium 5.5, sodium 131, and pH 7.15. He weighs 55 pounds. He is diagnosed with diabetic ketoacidosis and admitted. Initial treatment should include which of the following?

A. Saline 10 cc/kg bolus

B. Insulin 0.1 unit/kg/hr

C. Sodium bicarbonate 44 mEq IVP

D. Potassium chloride 20 mEq/L in the maintenance fluids

E. Bolus with 1,000 cc of 0.45 NaCl

123. A 4-year-old male presents with a 2-week history of an urticarial rash for the first time. He is not short of breath and has had no new exposures or other recent illnesses. Which of the following is true?

A. Urticaria affects less than 2% of the population.

B. A cause for urticaria is usually found.

C. Urticaria must be present for 6 weeks to be considered chronic.

D. Dietary manipulation frequently causes remission of the urticaria.

E. First-line treatment involves use of corticosteroids.

124. The most common malignancy in children is:

A. Leukemia

B. Wilm's tumor

C. Rhabdomyosarcoma

D. Ewing's sarcoma

E. Neuroblastoma

125. Which of the following is true regarding leukemia in children?

A. Chronic lymphocytic leukemia is the most common form diagnosed in children.

B. Acute lymphocytic leukemia is associated with a cure rate of 80%.

C. Signs and symptoms are generally present for several months before diagnosis.

D. African Americans are affected significantly more often than Caucasians.

E. The CBC is generally normal upon presentation with leukemia.

126. Which of the following is true regarding testicular cancer?

A. It occurs most commonly in children between the ages of 5 and 15 years.

B. Only 1% to 5% of patients with a history of cryptorchid testes develop testicular cancer.

C. Localized disease is curable in approximately 50% of patients.

D. Testicular trauma has been shown to be a risk factor for testicular cancer.

E. Testicular pain is a common complaint with testicular cancer.

127. A 4-year-old male presents for his physical examination and is noted to have slightly elevated blood pressure, microscopic hematuria, and a suspected abdominal mass. You suspect and plan evaluation for possible Wilm's tumor. Which of the following is true regarding Wilm's tumor?

A. Wilm's tumor typically presents in adolescence.

B. Hypertension is present in only 5% to 10% of patients with Wilm's tumors.

C. Wilm's tumor is commonly associated with congenital anomalies.

D. Patients typically present with other symptoms or signs before any mass can be palpated.

E. Hematuria rarely occurs with Wilm's tumor.

128. Which of the following is true regarding Ewing's sarcoma?

A. Ewing's sarcoma refers to tumors arising from bone.

B. The typical presentation is a painless overgrowth of bone.

C. Tumors arising in the pelvis are associated with improved survival.

D. It can present indistinguishable from osteomyelitis, with pain and fever.

E. The diagnosis is established by CT or MRI of the lesion.

129. A 4-year-old is being evaluated for a soft tissue mass. When considering rhabdomyosarcoma in the differential, which of the following is true regarding this type of tumor?

A. Rhabdomyosarcoma typically presents with pain.

B. Rhabodmyosarcoma typically presents with systemic symptoms unrelated to the tumor or its location.

C. Most are resectable at the time of diagnosis.

D. Several months commonly elapse from tumor onset to diagnosis.

E. The most common location is within the gastrointestinal tract.

130. An 18-month-old you have referred for evaluation of a mass is diagnosed with a neuroblastoma. Which of the following is true regarding neuroblastoma?

A. Neuroblastoma is a central nervous system tumor.

B. It is the most frequently diagnosed tumor in infants.

C. The overall cure rate is 90%.

D. Older children are more likely than infants to present with localized disease.

E. These tumors arise from mesenchymal tissue associated with development of striated skeletal muscle.

131. A 13-year-old male presents with a 1-day history of a rash consistent with chickenpox. Appropriate treatment measures would include which of the following?

A. Varicella immunoglobulin and varicella vaccine

B. Varicella immunoglobulin alone

C. Acyclovir

D. Acyclovir and oral steroids

E. Varicella vaccine alone

132. A patient who is 17 years old has established in your practice. He has been previously treated for short stature with recombinant growth hormone but has completed treatment. When following

this patient, which of the following is he at increased risk for as a result of his treatment?

A. Leukemia

B. Creutzfeldt–Jakob disease

C. Diabetes mellitus

D. Hypothyroidism

E. Asthma

133. On routine follow-up, the parent of a 9-month-old notes that when crawling he does not use his legs but does a "commando" crawl. On examination, you note slight scissoring of the lower extremities but the exam is otherwise normal. He is diagnosed with spastic diplegia, a form of cerebral palsy. Which of the following is true regarding this condition?

A. He will likely have an associated seizure disorder.

B. He will likely have impaired intelligence.

C. He will likely have athetoid movement associated with his cerebral palsy.

D. He will have normal upper extremity development with lower extremity disability.

E. Upper extremity involvement generally follows onset of lower extremity disease.

134. A 15-month-old has been ill for the past 12 hours with apparent abdominal discomfort, emesis, and passing bloody mucous per rectum (currant jelly stools). He is slightly pale with increased bowel sounds on examination. His abdominal film shows an obstructive pattern. Appropriate measures now include:

A. Bowel rest and IV hydration until resolution

B. Intravenous antibiotics

C. Barium enema

D. Stool for leukocytes and culture, with treatment pending these results

E. Immediate surgery

135. A 6-year-old male presents for evaluation of repeated absences from school. He will typically complain of a stomach ache and his mother will allow him to stay home. Within an hour, he seems to become asymptomatic. The family is very close-knit and supportive, and there have not been problems reported at home. Which of the following is true regarding school refusal?

A. School refusal most commonly occurs in boys.

B. School refusal is rare, occurring in less than 1% of children.

C. Separation anxiety is a common cause.

D. School refusal is not associated with any long-term consequences.

E. School refusal is more common in intact families than in single-parent families.

136. A mother presents with her newborn for the initial office visit, and on reviewing the newborn laboratory screening you note that the T4 is decreased and the TSH is markedly elevated. When considering the etiology of these findings, the most common is which of the following?

A. Iodine exposure

B. Thyrotropin deficiency

C. Maternal thyrotropin receptor-blocker antibody

D. Thyroid dysgenesis

E. Maternal levothyroxine use

137. When performing a history and physical examination on a 2-year-old, which of the following is a normal finding for age regarding speech development?

A. 50-word vocabulary with two word sentences

B. 250-word vocabulary with three or more word sentences

C. 3- to 5-word vocabulary and can follow one-step commands

D. Discriminate use of "mama" and "dada" and one-word utterances

E. Indiscriminate use of 12 to 15 words

138. You are seeing a 2-month-old African American male for a routine visit. The father has sickle cell trait and the parents are concerned the infant may have sickle cell anemia. Which of the following is true regarding sickle cell anemia in children?

A. Clinical manifestations of the disease are not apparent until after 1 year of age.

B. Up to 10% of children with sickle cell disease suffer a cerebrovascular accident.

C. Detection of sickle cell is not possible in the newborn period.

D. The spleen, bone marrow, and red blood cells are the only affected organs.

E. Painful crises may occur in utero.

139. When evaluating a 12-hour-old infant for sepsis, common organisms to consider as causes for neonatal sepsis include which of the following?

A. *Streptococcus pneumoniae*

B. *Haemophilus influenzae*

C. Group B B-hemolytic streptococci

D. *Staphylococcus aureus*

E. *Neiserria meningitidis*

140. Food allergies are mediated by which of the following types of immunoglobulin?

A. IgG

B. IgM

C. IgA

D. IgE

E. IgD

141. The two most common forms of contact dermatitis in children are:

A. Irritant diaper dermatitis and metal dermatitis

B. Metal dermatitis and Rhus dermatitis

C. Rhus dermatitis and irritant diaper dermatitis

D. Atopic dermatitis and seborrheic dermatitis

E. Atopic dermatitis and metal dermatitis

142. The most common cause of profound hearing loss in children is which of the following?

A. Head trauma

B. Genetic factors

C. Bacterial meningitis

D. Congenital malformations

E. Medications-related adverse effects

143. A child presents with three lesions on the abdomen consistent with a diagnosis of molluscum contagiosum. He is asymptomatic. Which of the following treatments is appropriate for this patient?

A. Surgical excision

B. Electrocautery

C. Observation

D. Topical mupirocin

E. Topical clotrimazole

144. A 2-year-old female with a single documented urinary tract infection presents for follow-up care. When comparing evaluation and treatment of urinary tract infections for adults and children, which of the following is true?

A. Screening cultures are indicated for both adults and children.

B. Tests of cure urine cultures are indicated for both adults and children.

C. Ultrasound is helpful in identifying obstruction or anatomic defects in children but not adults.

D. Vesicocystourethrogram evaluation is useful in identifying reflux in children.

E. Adults and children are equally vulnerable to renal scarring/compromise from infections.

145. A 6-year-old female presents with her mother who has concerns about the girl's weight. Her body mass index is at the 85th percentile for her age. They report a balanced diet but excessive snacking on high-calorie foods between meals. The parents are of average build and there are no obese siblings. Which of the following factors would be least beneficial in helping to prevent obesity in this child?

A. Recommending no further snacking for the girl

B. Advising that she join a sports team

C. Educating the parents on healthy diet

D. Engaging the parents to begin physical activities for the family

E. Encouraging healthy snacking

146. You are contacted by the nurse to evaluate the rash of a newborn in the nursery who is 24 hours old. Other than the rash, the child is doing well. The rash is on the trunk, back, face, and proximal extremities. It is macular with a few papules, vesicles, and pustules. You order a smear and Wright's stain of the material, which shows eosinophils. This rash and associated findings are most consistent with which of the following?

A. Infantile acropustulosis

B. Erythema toxicum neonatorum

C. Transient neonatal pustular melanosis

D. Cutis marmorata

E. Atopic dermatitis

147. In children at normal risk for development of hypertension, at what age should routine blood pressure screening begin?

A. 2 years

B. 3 years

C. 5 years

D. 10 years

E. 15 years

148. Which of the following is indicated routinely in children with no special risk factors at the 5-year physical examination?

A. MMR vaccine

B. DT vaccine

C. Lead screening

D. 23-valent pneumococcal vaccine

E. Hemoglobin testing

149. Which of the following injuries should be considered highly suspicious for potential abuse?
A. Nursemaid's elbow
B. Humeral fracture
C. Clavicle fracture
D. Supraorbital laceration
E. Wrist fracture

150. When evaluating a 15-month-old female, you note that her skull appears elongated. You determine that she has craniosynostosis. Which of the following is the most common cause of craniosynostosis?
A. Nonsyndromic, sporadic
B. Apert's syndrome
C. Pfeiffer's syndrome
D. Crouzon's syndrome
E. Hypothyroidism

151. Topical pimecrolimus is indicated for which of the following?
A. Psoriasis
B. Warts
C. Atopic dermatitis
D. Contact dermatitis
E. Tinea corporis

152. During examination of a 2-month-old female, you note a 2-cm superficial hemangioma on her right thigh. When counseling the parents regarding treatment of this lesion, which of the following is true?
A. Surgery is the treatment of choice.
B. Topical steroids are the most effective therapy.
C. Systemic steroids are the primary form of therapy.
D. Fifty percent of these lesions will spontaneously resolve by age 9 years.
E. Ninety-five percent of these lesions will spontaneously resolve by age 9 years.

153. Which of the following is true about the illicit drug "ecstasy" (3,4-methylenedioxymethamphetamine)?
A. Tolerance does not develop to the "positive" effects of the drug.
B. It is addictive.
C. Paranoid psychosis can occur as a side effect.
D. Toxicity is predictable and dose-related.
E. There are no serious side effects associated with use of ecstasy.

154. The parents of a 6-month-old present with concerns that he sucks his thumb. They are concerned that this will become a hard habit to break and worry about his future dental development. They have tried unsuccessfully to get him to use a pacifier. When counseling these parents, which of the following is true regarding thumb sucking?
A. Less than 10% of children after age 1 engage in thumb sucking.
B. Thumb sucking does not affect dentition.
C. Thumb sucking serves no useful purpose.
D. Pacifiers have lower risks for dental disturbances than thumb sucking.
E. The parents should try to break the habit before eruption of the primary teeth.

155. You are preparing to discharge a 2,000-g infant who was born prematurely at 28 weeks and required an extended neonatal intensive care unit stay. He is doing well and now is 8 weeks old. Which of the following is true regarding care for premature infants?
A. The first hepatitis vaccine should not be given until an infant weighs 2,000 g.
B. Developmental assessment is always based on chronologic age of the child.
C. Most premature infants require no hearing or vision screening.
D. Correction of growth parameters for gestational age continues until 1 year of age.
E. No special feeding formulas/supplement are required.

156. A 14-year-old male with a history of asthma presents with nasal congestion and is noted on physical examination to have a nasal polyp. When recommending therapy for the polyp, which of the following therapies is effective?
A. Cromolyn sodium
B. Intranasal steroid sprays
C. Antihistamines
D. Decongestants
E. Aspirin

157. A 1-month-old female presents with bilious emesis. On evaluation, an upper GI reveals a double-bubble sign. Which of the following is the most likely diagnosis in this child?
A. Volvulus
B. Duodenal atresia
C. Intussusception
D. Gastroenteritis
E. Pyloric stenosis

158. Which of the following is a common complication of cystic fibrosis?
A. Conjunctivitis
B. Inflammatory bowel disease
C. Pancreatitis
D. Orchitis
E. Infertility

159. Which of the following populations of patients has the highest incidence of cystic fibrosis?
A. Asians
B. African Americans
C. Amish
D. Native Americans
E. Native Africans

160. A 4-month-old male presents with fever and lethargy. He undergoes lumbar puncture as part of the evaluation and is noted to have WBCs and gram-positive organisms on staining of the fluid. Which of the following is appropriate as initial therapy in this patient?
A. Ampicillin
B. Vancomycin
C. Vancomycin and ceftriaxone
D. Ceftriaxone
E. Levofloxacin

161. Which of the following is true regarding childhood sexual abuse?
A. Up to 40% of males have been sexually abused by age 18 years.
B. Sexual acting out by the child is specific as an indicator of abuse.

C. Female relatives are common perpetrators.

D. Most abused children have physical findings diagnostic of abuse.

E. Most children voluntarily reveal that abuse has occurred.

162. An 18-month-old with an unremarkable past medical history is seen for a well child visit and the mother reports that he has not yet begun to speak. He is walking and rolled and sat at the appropriate ages. He does not appear to have any visual or hearing difficulties. The physical examination is normal and no dysmorphic features are noted. After a normal hearing evaluation, you suspect possible mental retardation. Which of the following is true regarding mental retardation?

A. Without grossly dysmorphic features, mental retardation is unlikely.

B. Normal motor milestones make mental retardation unlikely.

C. Testing for mental retardation cannot be done in children this young.

D. Up to 90% fall into a category of mild mental retardation.

E. The etiology is identifiable in more than 75% of cases.

163. With regard to pediatric dental health care and prevention of dental caries, which of the following is true?

A. By age 9, 10% of children have dental caries.

B. Juice can be given to children in bottles during the day.

C. Fluoride provides a mechanical barrier against bacteria.

D. Toothpaste should not be used until 4 years of age.

E. Dental caries is an infectious disease caused by mutans streptococci.

164. Which of the following is true regarding infant botulism?

A. Ninety percent of affected children are between 1 and 3 years of age.

B. The majority of cases are diagnosed in Third World countries.

C. Thirty percent of affected children require mechanical ventilation.

D. Up to 90% of infants diagnosed with botulism are breast-fed.

E. Botulism toxin and *Clostridium botulinum* species are found in many foods, including milk.

165. The parents of a 6-week-old male note that during the past few weeks their son has had loud breathing associated on occasion with increased respiratory effort. He has been otherwise well. On examination he is noted to have an inspiratory stridor that is more pronounced in the supine position and when he cries. Which of the following is the most common cause for chronic stridor in children?

A. Laryngomalacia

B. Croup

C. Choanal atresia

D. Foreign body

E. Asthma

166. A 7-year-old female is brought to see you after an episode of loss of consciousness. The mother reports that the patient got her ears pierced and then became pale, diaphoretic, and lost consciousness. When she was unconscious, the mother noted some tonic–clonic activity but no loss of bowel or bladder and no injuries were noted. She has been awake and alert since the episode with no complaints. Which of the following is the most likely cause for her loss of consciousness?

A. Breath-holding spell

B. Arrhythmia

C. Seizure

D. Vasodepressor syncope

E. Valvular heart disease

167. A 12-year-old female presents with a rash bilaterally on her trunk and proximal extremities. The lesions are 1 or 2 cm in size, oval in shape, and have a ring of fine scale along the edges. One of the lesions is 4 cm in size and similar in appearance. The patient has had no prior skin problems and is asymptomatic with this rash. Which of the following is the most likely diagnosis?

A. Lichen planus

B. Herpes zoster

C. Pityriasis rosea

D. Keratosis pilaris

E. Warts

168. You are seeing a 15-year-old male who complains of palpitations. His ECG shows a shortened PR interval and slurring of the upstroke of a slightly prolonged QRS complex. Which of the following is true regarding his condition?

A. Only one-half of patients with this condition will ever experience symptoms.

B. PR prolongation is a typical finding in these patients.

C. Seventy percent of these cases are associated with underlying cardiac disease.

D. Wide complex tachycardias are the most common presentation.

E. These findings are consistent with septal hypertrophy.

169. A 13-year-old male presents with recurrent episodes of bloody diarrhea. Cultures are negative and he is ultimately diagnosed with ulcerative colitis. Which of the following is true regarding ulcerative colitis?

A. Onset of disease most commonly occurs between 5 and 10 years of age.

B. Cigarette smoking is protective against developing ulcerative colitis.

C. Family members are at no increased risk for inflammatory bowel disease.

D. Risk for colon cancer does not increase until age 40 years.

E. Ulcerative colitis may affect any portion of the gastrointestinal tract.

170. Which of the following children should undergo evaluation for immunodeficiency?

A. A child with a past history of meningitis who develops osteomyelitis

B. A child with four episodes of otitis media

C. A child who develops *Streptococcal pneumoniae* meningitis

D. A child with two episodes of cellulites

E. A child with six URIs in the past year

171. A 6-year-old patient is admitted to the hospital with acute renal failure. He is undergoing evaluation for the underlying cause.

Which of the following would be an indication for hemodialysis in this patient?
A. Creatinine value of 3.1 mg/dL
B. Anemia
C. Metabolic alkalosis
D. Hypotension
E. Hyperkalemia

172. Which of the following dietary guidelines applies to growing children with chronic renal failure?
A. Carbohydrate intake should be restricted.
B. Protein should be provided at 0.8 g/kg/day.
C. Water-soluble vitamins should be restricted.
D. Fat intake should be restricted.
E. Vitamin D supplementation is generally necessary.

173. Which of the following is true regarding AIDS and HIV infection in children?
A. It is most commonly acquired by blood transfusion.
B. Clinical evidence of infection is present at birth.
C. Disease progression is more rapid in children than in adults.
D. IgG antibody tests are reliable indicators of HIV status after 6 months of age.
E. The latency period after acquiring the infection is generally 5 to 10 years.

174. An 8-year-old presents for follow-up after being diagnosed with a seizure disorder. The parents have many questions regarding his condition. Which of the following is true?
A. Most seizure disorders are associated with definite causes.
B. Twenty percent of seizure disorders begin in childhood.
C. Seizures are uncommon, occurring in only 1% of the population.
D. Approximately 90% of patients with seizure disorder are well controlled with medication.
E. Surgical treatment is generally necessary to control seizures with onset in childhood.

175. An otherwise healthy 4-year-old male develops osteomyelitis and has group A streptococci on culturing of the biopsy specimen. He responds well to antibiotic therapy and clinically improved after 3 days. With regard to osteomyelitis in children, which of the following is true?
A. 6 weeks of intravenous antibiotic therapy is needed for treatment.
B. Antibiotic treatment for 6 weeks must be provided with either oral or intravenous medication.
C. Osteomyelitis in this patient most likely occurred due to trauma.
D. Seventy-five percent of cases of osteomyelitis in children occur before the age of 5 years.

E. Group A streptococci is the most common cause for osteomyelitis across all age groups.

176. Which of the following is true regarding apnea of prematurity?
A. It usually resolves by 6 months of age.
B. It is predictive of future SIDS.
C. Caffeine is used as a medication treatment.
D. It is associated with a poor long-term prognosis.
E. Airway obstruction is the mechanism for developing the apneas.

177. Which of the following is most specific for diagnosing acute Ebstein–Barr infection?
A. Atypical lympocytosis
B. Viral capsid antigen IgM antibodies
C. Heterophil antibody test
D. Early antigen IgG antibody
E. Clinical examination (history and physical)

178. A 2-year-old male presents with a decline in growth and slight weight loss. He has been anorexic and been noted to have chronic diarrhea. Initial lab studies reveal a mild anemia and a slight decrease in serum albumin. You suspect celiac disease. Which of the following tests would be most helpful in establishing the diagnosis?
A. Antigliadin antibody
B. IgA endomysial antibody
C. Antinuclear antibody
D. Serum trypsinogen level
E. Stool culture

179. Which of the following is true regarding fragile X syndrome?
A. Fifty percent of males with fragile X mutations are clinically abnormal.
B. Fragile X is the second most common genetic cause for mental retardation.
C. Women are never affected by this syndrome.
D. Decreased testicular size is a common feature.
E. Males cannot transmit or carry this genetic defect.

180. Which of the following is typically present in individuals affected by Prader–Willi syndrome?
A. Thin body habitus
B. Ataxic gait
C. Hypogonadism
D. Tall stature
E. Seizures

Chapter 2

Answer Key

1. A	43. C	85. B	127. C	169. B
2. C	44. A	86. A	128. D	170. A
3. D	45. C	87. C	129. D	171. E
4. E	46. B	88. B	130. B	172. E
5. D	47. B	89. B	131. C	173. C
6. C	48. A	90. A	132. A	174. D
7. A	49. D	91. D	133. D	175. D
8. C	50. C	92. C	134. C	176. C
9. A	51. D	93. E	135. C	177. B
10. C	52. A	94. B	136. D	178. B
11. D	53. E	95. C	137. A	179. B
12. D	54. B	96. A	138. B	180. C
13. D	55. E	97. D	139. C	
14. B	56. B	98. E	140. D	
15. A	57. A	99. B	141. C	
16. D	58. D	100. D	142. B	
17. E	59. C	101. A	143. C	
18. C	60. C	102. D	144. D	
19. A	61. C	103. B	145. A	
20. B	62. D	104. C	146. B	
21. A	63. E	105. C	147. B	
22. C	64. E	106. D	148. A	
23. D	65. C	107. C	149. B	
24. D	66. D	108. B	150. A	
25. D	67. A	109. A	151. C	
26. A	68. C	110. C	152. E	
27. C	69. E	111. D	153. C	
28. C	70. A	112. A	154. D	
29. C	71. D	113. E	155. A	
30. C	72. B	114. B	156. B	
31. C	73. A	115. C	157. A	
32. D	74. D	116. B	158. E	
33. A	75. D	117. A	159. C	
34. A	76. B	118. D	160. C	
35. B	77. C	119. C	161. B	
36. C	78. B	120. A	162. D	
37. C	79. D	121. E	163. E	
38. C	80. A	122. B	164. D	
39. A	81. B	123. C	165. A	
40. B	82. B	124. A	166. D	
41. B	83. E	125. B	167. C	
42. D	84. C	126. B	168. A	

Chapter 2

Pediatrics Answers

1. A

Mothers infected with syphilis may transmit the disease to their children either by direct contact of an active lesion or through the bloodstream, transplacentally. In most instances, the children will have a normal physical examination and diagnostic testing must be performed to determine whether the child has been infected. In adults, the VDRL test is a sensitive test for diagnosing syphilis and is generally confirmed by obtaining an FTA-ABS. In the newborn, the VDRL may be positive either falsely or because of maternal infection and thus is not useful in screening the newborn. The FTA-ABS is a test specific for syphilis that would be positive in the infant with congenital syphilis and would not be affected by maternal infection unless the disease had been transmitted to the infant; however, there are no currently available recommended commercial tests for FTA-ABS IgM. Thus, in the infant, VDRL titers exceeding those of the mother, along with risk of infection based on the maternal history and findings, determine the need for further testing or treatment. Other findings that support a diagnosis of congenital syphilis include physical or x-ray findings of congenital syphilis, positive CSF VDRL, or elevated CSF cell count or protein. VDRL titers can be followed to determine response to therapy, and with successful therapy should decline. Blood or swab cultures are not helpful in diagnosing syphilis. Dark field microscopy is a useful test for diagnosing syphilis and must be prepared from active lesion (e.g., nasal discharge), the placenta, or the umbilical cord.

2. C

Urinary tract infection (UTI) must be considered in the differential of any febrile child without an apparent source of infection. When evaluating young children for possible UTI, proper specimen collection is critical to obtaining reliable and meaningful results on which to diagnose and treat the child. Acceptable methods for urine collection in children unable to provide clean catch specimens include transurethral catheterization and suprapubic aspiration. Bag specimens are reassuring only if negative and cannot be relied on for accurate urinalysis or cultures. Definitions of positive cultures depend on the method of collection. Catheter specimens with greater than 100,000 bacterial colonies and suprapubic aspirates with any colony count are considered positive and should be treated.

3. D

Fungal skin infections can generally be treated with topical antifungal medications with the exception of tinea capitus and tinea unguim. These latter two infections affect deeper structures, namely the hair follicle and root of the nailbed. Topical medications are unable to penetrate these areas and eradicate the infection. Thus, tinea capitus responds poorly to topical antifungal agents, and oral griseofulvin is the recommended therapy. Steroids, either topical or oral, do not provide therapy to eradicate fungal infection and may worsen the infection. When there is a significant inflammatory component to the infection, steroids may be used along with antifungal therapy for more prompt symptom relief and to limit the scarring resulting from the inflammation.

4. E

In the child presented, signs of dehydration include weight loss, decreased urine output, tachycardia, and dry mucous membranes. The degree of dehydration is consistent with a moderate dehydration and could be quantified, based on weight change, as approximately 8% to 10%. Since the underlying disease process is ongoing and the child has been unable to maintain hydration by oral intake, intravenous therapy is appropriate. Initial rehydration should be provided as a weight-based bolus of 20 cc/kg of normal saline. A bolus of 500 cc would be too large a quantity for this size infant. Providing D5 0.45 or normal saline at 50 cc/kg/day would be insufficient to provide even maintenance fluids in this child, who would require a maintenance rate of 100 cc/kg/day. Following the initial bolus, replacement of the remainder of the volume deficit, along with maintenance fluids and electrolytes, can then be administered the following 16 hours.

5. D

Kawasaki's disease is the most common cause of acquired heart disease in children in the United States. Diagnosis is based on clinical findings and this disease should be suspected in children who have a fever for 5 days or longer. Four of the following findings along with fever support the diagnosis of Kawasaki's disease: rash, conjunctivitis, lymphadenopathy, strawberry tongue, oropharyngeal erythema, and digital desquamation. Laboratory findings consistent with Kawasaki's disease include elevated white blood cell count, sedimentation rate, and C-reactive protein. The primary concern with Kawasaki's is prevention and detection of cardiac complications, which develop in more than 50% of patients. Myocarditis occurs most commonly—in up to one-half of patients. Coronary aneurysms, which are associated with coronary thrombosis or rupture, and myocardial infarction develop in an additional 20% of patients. Prompt therapy with intravenous immunoglobulin and aspirin lessen the risk for developing these cardiac complications. Included in the differential diagnosis for Kawasaki's disease are scarlet fever, toxic shock syndrome, drug reactions, measles, Stevens-Johnson syndrome, and juvenile rheumatoid arthritis.

6. C

Otitis media is a common pediatric diagnosis requiring antibiotic therapy. Many antibiotics are effective in providing coverage for *Streptococcus pneumoniae*, *Haemophilus influenzae*, and *Moraxella catarrhalis*, the major pathogens associated with acute otitis media. Antibiotics that are active against these pathogens include amoxicillin, sulfonamides, second-generation cephalosporins, and macrolides. Cephalexin, a first-generation cephalosporin, does not provide adequate coverage for these pathogens. In addition to effectiveness, appropriate antibiotic selection should consider the cost of the medication and promotion of bacterial resistance. Increasing use of more expensive broad-spectrum antibiotics has led to increasing bacterial resistance to antibiotics. Thus, amoxicillin remains the first-line antibiotic choice for otitis media and other classes of antibiotics should be reserved for those with suspected bacterial resistance (i.e., persistent or recurrent infections) and those with allergies to penicillins. Risk factors for patients being infected with penicillin-resistant bacteria include day care attendance, recurrent otitis media, and multiple recent courses of antibiotics.

7. A

Sexually transmitted diseases (STDs) commonly occur in adolescents and young adults. Studies have shown that chlamydia infection occurs in up to one-third of sexually active adolescents. Many of these chlamydia infections are asymptomatic and coexist with other STDs, thus increasing the risk for further spread of this disease. When providing care for adolescent patients, a sexual history should be obtained. In those who are sexually active, HIV counseling and counseling about contraception and condom use should be

provided. When STDs are identified, treatment of partners should be provided along with appropriate pharmacologic therapy. Neither ceftriaxone, penicillin, nor metronidazole are effective therapies for chlamydia. Treatment of chlamydia infections may be provided with use of azithromycin, doxycycline, or erythromycin. Azithromycin, although more expensive, has the advantage of single-dose therapy, thus enhancing compliance with treatment, an important consideration in the adolescent population. Following treatment, a repeat cervical swab for chlamydia PCR analysis or cultures should be obtained to document success of therapy. See Table 2.1.

8. C

Enuresis is defined as the involuntary passage of urine. When the enuresis occurs at night and the child has never had previous periods of dryness, it is termed primary nocturnal enuresis. Children who have been dry for at least 6 months and then begin to experience enuresis have secondary enuresis. Primary enuresis is common and occurs more commonly in males than females. In many cases, there is a positive history of enuresis, although no pattern of inheritance has been defined. Initial analysis should document that there is no underlying urinary tract infection that may be contributing to

Table 2.1 STDs

Condition	Recommended Regimens*
Gonococcal cervicitis or urethritis	Ceftriaxone 125 mg IM in a single dose,
	OR ciprofloxacin 500 mg orally in a single dose,
	OR levofloxacin 250 mg orally in a single dose,
	PLUS, IF CHLAMYDIAL INFECTION IS NOT RULED OUT,
	Azithromycin 1 g orally in a single dose,
	OR doxycycline 100 mg orally twice a day for 7 days.
Non-gonococcal urethritis or cervicitis	Azithromycin 1 g orally in a single dose,
	OR doxycycline 100 mg orally twice a day for 7 days,
	OR erythromycin base 500 mg orally four times a day for 7 days,
	OR erythromycin ethylsuccinate 800 mg orally four times a day for 7 days,
	OR levofloxacin 500 mg once daily for 7 days.
Vaginal candidiasis	Intravaginal agents
	Clotrimazole 1% cream 5 g intravaginally for 7–14 days,
	OR miconazole 2% cream 5 g intravaginally for 7 days,
	OR other topical azoles
	Oral agent
	Fluconazole 150 mg oral tablet, one tablet in a single dose.
Bacterial vaginosis	Metronidazole 500 mg orally twice a day for 7 days,
	OR metronidazole gel 0.75%, one full applicator (5 g) intravaginally, once a day for 5 days,
	OR clindamycin cream 2%, one full applicator (5 g) intravaginally at bedtime for 7 days.
Trichomonas vaginalis	Metronidazole 2 g orally in a single dose,
	OR metronidazole 500 mg bid for 7 days.

Table 2.1 (continued)

Condition	Recommended Regimens*

Syphilis
   Benzathine penicillin G 2.4 million units IM, in a single dose.

Lymphogranuloma venerum
   Doxycycline 100 mg orally twice a day for at least 3 weeks
   OR trimethoprim-sulfamethoxazole one double-strength (800 mg/160 mg) tablet orally twice a day for at least 3 weeks,
   OR ciprofloxacin 750 mg orally twice a day for at least 3 weeks,
   OR erythromycin base 500 mg orally four times a day for at least 3 weeks,
   OR azithromycin 1 g orally once per week for at least 3 weeks.

Chancroid
   Azithromycin 1 g orally in a single dose,
   OR ceftriaxone 250 mg IM in a single dose,
   OR ciprofloxacin 500 mg orally twice a day for 3 days,
   OR erythromycin base 500 mg orally three times a day for 7 days.

Herpes
   Acyclovir 400 mg orally three times a day for 7–10 days,
   OR acyclovir 200 mg orally five times a day for 7–10 days,
   OR famciclovir 250 mg orally three times a day for 7–10 days,
   OR valacyclovir 1 g orally twice a day for 7–10 days.

*Tetracyclines should not be used in children younger than age 8 years and fluoroquinolones should not be used in children with open epiphyses.

the lack of bladder control. When the patient is asymptomatic, the physical examination is normal, and the urinalysis and culture are negative, no further workup is indicated with primary enuresis. With expectant management, 10% to 15% of children per year will have resolution of their bedwetting. Urology or psychiatric referrals would not be warranted for primary enuresis but may be indicated for cases of secondary enuresis for which an underlying cause is more likely. Children with enuresis are aware of the problem and may be ashamed and suffer from low self-esteem. Thus, punishment would not be an appropriate recommendation. For parents and children who desire treatment, bed alarms and behavioral modification programs are one of the most successful therapies. Medications, such as DDAVP and tricyclic antidepressants, may also be of benefit. Sertraline is not indicated for treatment of enuresis.

9. A

The most common cause for thrombocytopenia in children is acute idiopathic thrombocytopenic purpura (ITP), a viral-related autoimmune destruction of platelets. The classic presentation is the occurrence of petechiae following a viral infection. Patients are typically asymptomatic and have a normal physical examination but are found to have an isolated decreased platelet count on laboratory evaluation. In most patients, the platelet count returns to normal in less than 6 months. However, up to 20% of patients will have persistent thrombocytopenia, which is then termed chronic ITP. In patients with acute ITP who have no signs of bleeding and platelet counts above 20,000, no therapy may be necessary. In these patients, platelet counts should be monitored until they return to normal. When the platelet count is less than 20,000, or

there is bleeding or excessive bruising, then therapy is generally indicated. Intravenous immunoglobulin and/or corticosteroids are used to raise platelet counts. Since malignancy is also a cause for thrombocytopenia, bone marrow examination should be performed prior to use of corticosteroids, which may mask an underlying malignancy. Intravenous immunoglobulin does not have any effects on malignant disease and thus may be used without need for a bone marrow biopsy before treatment. Immunoglobulin therapy will raise platelet counts within 48 to 72 hours and can assist in confirming the diagnosis. If during the clinical examination the patient is found to have lymphadenopathy, splenomegaly, or symptoms suggestive of underlying disease, then a bone marrow evaluation is warranted. Finally, persistent thrombocytopenia, other abnormal cell lines (i.e., WBC and RBC), and uncertainty regarding the diagnosis also should prompt consideration of performing a bone marrow biopsy.

10. C

All infants and children younger than age 2 years should receive the heptavalent pneumococcal vaccine. The 23-valent pneumococcal vaccine should not be given to infants since it is not immunogenic in infants. High-risk children older than the age of 2 years, such as those with sickle cell disease or asplenia, should also receive the heptavalent vaccine and the vaccine may be offered to lower risk children older than the age of 2 years. The 23-valent vaccine is recommended for high-risk children after age 2 along with the heptavalent vaccine. High-risk children also require booster doses of the 23-valent vaccine every 3 to 5 years after the initial dose. For lower risk children who are older than the age of 2 years, the heptavalent or 23-valent vaccine may be given as a single dose. When administering a heptavalent vaccine series, all repeat doses of the vaccine should be given at least 6 to 8 weeks apart. The heptavalent vaccine may be given concurrently but at different sites than MMR, varicella, and poliovirus vaccines. Children with sickle cell disease or asplenia require antibiotic prophylaxis up to the age of 5 years even if they have received the pneumococcal vaccines. After age 5, those who have been vaccinated may discontinue antibiotic prophylaxis.

11. D

Cystic fibrosis is characterized by elevated sweat chloride, pancreatic insufficiency, and chronic pulmonary disease. Cystic fibrosis is an autosomal recessive disorder that occurs most commonly in Caucasians. An abnormal gene that may cause cystic fibrosis is present in 5% of Americans. Because carriage of the gene is so common, most patients have no family history of cystic fibrosis. Common presentations include difficult passage of stool, meconium ileus, prolonged neonatal jaundice, failure to thrive, and recurrent respiratory or sinus infections. These patients require increased caloric consumption due to increased expenditure associated with their respiratory infections and malabsorption. Thus, the typical patient with cystic fibrosis has a good appetite and fails to thrive despite consuming large numbers of calories. *Staphylococcus aureus*, *Haemophilus influenzae*, and *Pseudomonas aeruginosa* are common respiratory pathogens, and infections with these organisms should heighten one's suspicion for the presence of cystic fibrosis. Sweat testing and genetic testing are the preferred diagnostic tests. Less than 1% of patients with cystic fibrosis have normal sweat chloride. Genetic testing identifies abnormal cystic fibrosis genes in 95% of patients. Diagnosis of cystic fibrosis can be made with the presence of typical clinical features along with positive sweat chloride or genetic testing.

12. D

The significance of group A streptococcal pharyngitis lies in its association with the complications of rheumatic heart disease, glomerulonephritis, and, rarely, peritonsillar abscess. Treatment of the pharyngitis does not significantly shorten the course of the illness but can limit development of complications. Treatment within 10 days of onset prevents development of rheumatic heart disease. Antibiotic therapy may also lessen the likelihood of peritonsillar abscess, but it has no effect on the occurrence of glomerulonephritis. Penicillin is the first-line choice for antibiotic therapy of streptococcal pharyngitis. Penicillin-allergic patients with group A streptococcal pharyngitis may be treated with erythromycin, newer macrolides, or clindamycin. Cephalosporins may be used in those with an insignificant past reaction to penicillins when other choices are also limited. Cephalosporins do exhibit a crossover sensitivity with penicillins, so in those with a history of more severe allergic reactions, such as anaphylaxis, cephalosporins should generally be avoided. Sulfonamides can be used as prophylaxis for those with a past history of rheumatic fever but are not effective as primary treatment for group A streptococcal pharyngitis. Prophylaxis against group A strep is indicated for patients who develop rheumatic fever with or without carditis. Asymptomatic family members require no testing or therapy unless the index case has glomerulonephritis or rheumatic fever. Patients are no longer contagious after 24 hours of antibiotic therapy and if they feel well enough may return to school or day care.

13. D

Neisseria meningitidis is a common cause for serious illness and death due to bacteremia and meningitis. It is a gram-negative diplococcus that is spread from person to person by respiratory droplets. Patients with identified disease are hospitalized and receive intravenous antibiotic therapy. Therapy should also be provided prophylactically to close contacts of patients with invasive disease. At-risk persons include household members, day care or nursery school attendees, and health care workers exposed to respiratory secretions of patients with active disease. Prophylactic therapy should also be provided to carriers of the meningococcal bacteria. Rifampin administered orally for 2 days, a single intramuscular dose of ceftriaxone, or a single oral dose of ciprofloxacin are antibiotics recommended for prophylaxis. Ciprofloxacin should not be given to children with open epiphyses. A meningococcal vaccine is also available as a prophylactic therapy but would not provide the immediate protection needed to those exposed to patients with active disease.

14. B

Failure to thrive (FTT) is present when growth fails to meet the expected age-determined norms. When a child is failing to thrive, initially the weight will drop below the previous growth curves. When the weight has dropped below the fifth percentile or has crossed two quartiles, this should prompt assessment for FTT. Chronic FTT will then result in diminished height and, finally, head circumference. The pattern of "head sparing" follows the pattern seen with intrauterine growth retardation. Other symptoms or signs that support the diagnosis of FTT include failure to meet developmental milestones, muscle or fat wasting, recurrent infections, and alopecia. All of the listed choices may cause FTT, but the most common cause is psychosocial. Children living in poverty, living in families with significant discord, or depression in the caregiver are common psychosocial reasons for a child failing to thrive.

15. A

This child has mild intermittent asthma, which according to current guidelines warrants only short-acting B2 agonist therapy to control the infrequent daytime symptoms. Inhaled steroids are indicated for those with persistent asthma—those with more than two episodes per week or with nocturnal symptoms. Cromolyn sodium or monteleukast are recommended as options for patients with mild persistent asthma. Long-acting B2 agonists may also be used for those with persistent asthma and are particularly useful in those with nocturnal symptoms. See Table 2.2.

16. D

Reassurance would be the appropriate management of this patient since she has signs of both breast and pubic hair growth, which signify the presence of estrogen and sensitivity to androgens. As part of this reassurance, she should be told that menarche typically follows thelarche by approximately 2 years and that the average age of menarche is 12.5 to 13 years of age.

When menses do not occur by age 16 years, primary amenorrhea is present. This condition affects 2% to 3% of adolescent girls and should prompt evaluation. Initial evaluation for primary amenorrhea should document normal anatomy, including the presence of the uterus and a patent vagina. In some instances, in order to obtain a thorough exam, anesthesia or pelvic ultrasound may be necessary. For those patients without a uterus or without normal breast development, hormonal levels and genetic karyotyping are indicated. Bone age, as determined by x-ray evaluation, can also be

Table 2.2 Stepwise approach to asthma management

	Long-Term Control	**Quick Relief of Symptoms**
Step1: Mild intermittent	*No daily medication*	Short-acting inhaled **beta₂-agonist** *(If used >2 times/wk, may need to initiate long-term treatment)*
Step 2: Mild persistent	*One daily medication:* **Inhaled corticosteroids** (Low dose) or **Cromolyn** or **Nedocromil** or **Leukotriene** modifiers	Short-acting inhaled **beta₂-agonist** (Increasing *use* or Daily *use may indicate the need for additional long-term control therapy.*)
Step 3: Moderate persistent	*Two daily medications* **Inhaled corticosteroids** (Low–medium dose) and **Long-acting Bronchodilators** (salmeterol *sustained-release theophylline, or* long-acting beta₂-agonist tablets) or Leukotriene modifier or *One daily Medication:* **Inhaled corticosteroids** (Med. to high dose)	(Increasing *use* or Daily *use may indicate the need for additional long-term control therapy.*) Short acting inhaled **beta₂-agonist**
Step 4: Severe persistent	Daily medications: **Inhaled corticosteroids** (High dose) and **Long-acting Bronchodilators** (salmeterol *sustained-release* theophylline, or long-acting beta₂-agonist tablets) or Leukotriene modifier and **Oral corticosteroids** (daily dose of 2 mg/kg) (**max. dose 60 mg/day**)	Short-acting inhaled *beta₂-agonist* (Increasing *use* or Daily *use may indicate the need for additional long-term control therapy.*)

useful since pubertal development should begin at an approximate bone age of 11 years. In those with a bone age less than chronologic age, a constitutional delay in growth and pubertal development should be suspected. Secondary amenorrhea is the cessation of menses after the patient has experienced menarche. Evaluation for underlying causes is indicated and initially serum TSH and prolactin are commonly ordered as initial testing to evaluate these patients. Serum TSH and prolactin may also be useful in patients with primary amenorrhea and normal anatomy. After pregnancy has been ruled out, administration of progesterone to induce a withdrawal bleed can be provided to document normal estrogen priming of the uterus and an intact outflow tract.

17. E

Since a critical part of treatment for allergies involves allergen avoidance, allergy testing can be very useful both diagnostically and therapeutically. When considering allergy testing, clinical correlation, including consideration of the patient's age, should dictate the specific allergens tested and is required to interpret the results of any testing. Radioallergosorbent testing (RAST) tests the patient's serum for the presence of IgE for the allergens tested. Skin testing is performed by administering percutaneous or intradermal injections of the allergens and searching for a physiologic response to the allergens injected. Skin testing is more sensitive and specific than RAST. However, RAST is indicated in certain clinical situations. For example, RAST is indicated in those patients with a history of severe anaphylactic reaction, severe skin disease, or the inability to discontinue medications that would interfere with skin testing results (e.g., antihistamines and antidepressant medications). Both RAST and skin testing may be performed in any age patient.

18. C

Although rare, sudden cardiac death is catastrophic when it occurs in young athletes. Cardiovascular deaths occur in 1 of every 200,000 athletes. The incidence is significantly (five times) higher in males than females. The most common cause of sudden cardiac death in student athletes is hypertrophic cardiomyopathy. Screening measures in young athletes should focus on the family history, any symptoms the patient may be experiencing, and a thorough cardiovascular exam. Risk factors for cardiac disease include a family history of premature death, coronary disease before age 50, or specific conditions (hypertrophic cardiomyopathy, Marfan's syndrome, or prolonged QT syndromes or arrhythmias). Significant risk factors in the athlete include a history of hypertension, murmurs, inappropriate fatigue, shortness of breath, chest pain, or syncope. The physical examination should include assessment for Marfan's syndrome, lower extremity pulses, blood pressure, and cardiac auscultation in the supine and upright positions. Electrocardiography and echocardiography are not currently recommended as routine screening tests for student athletes.

19. A

Breast milk provides the optimal nutrition for infants and requires no vitamin supplementation in the term newborn. Formulas also provide adequate nutrition and do not require supplementation, but they lack the benefits of breast-feeding in lowering the occurrence of respiratory and gastrointestinal infections. Either breast milk or formula should be provided to all infants for the first year of life, after which time whole milk may be introduced. When the breast-fed infant reaches the age of 4 to 6 months, iron, fluoride, and vitamin D should be provided as supplements. This age also correlates with introduction of cereals and baby foods and thus, iron-containing foods, fluorinated water, and adequate sunlight are common sources for this supplementation. Pumped breast milk may be refrigerated for 48 hours and frozen indefinitely.

20. B

Lateral curvature of the spine occurs commonly in adolescent patients, and when the curvature is 10 degrees of more, the condition is termed scoliosis. Up to 4% of adolescents are affected by scoliosis, and the incidence is equal in males and females. Scoliosis is associated not only with pain and physical deformity but also with neurologic and pulmonary complications. More severe disease is associated with continued progression of the curvature and complications. Risk factors for progression have been identified and include female gender, skeletal immaturity, sexual immaturity, and higher degrees of curvature. Periods of rapid skeletal growth are high-risk periods for progression or worsening of the scoliosis. During adolescent growth spurts, curves may progress by up to 2 degrees per month. Once growth is completed, those patients with milder degrees of scoliosis (less than 30 degrees) are at low risk for disease progression. Those with curves greater than 30 degrees may have continued disease progression. Serial x-ray evaluation of adolescents with scoliosis should be performed to monitor for increasing degrees of scoliosis. Orthopedic referral should be provided for those with pain, curves greater than 20 degrees, progression of the curve by 5 degrees or more, or abnormal neurologic findings.

21. A

In order to document an acute urinary tract infection in children, sterile collection of urine for culture and sensitivity must be performed. During the acute infection, renal ultrasound is performed to assess renal anatomy and for the presence of obstruction, and renal nuclear dimercaptosuccinic acid (DMSA) scans can be performed acutely to document pyelonephritis. After resolution of infection, DMSA scans may be performed to assess for scarring. Another form of nuclear scan, renal nuclear glucoheptonate scans, can be performed following resolution of the infection to assess renal function, particularly in those with recurrent infections or renal scarring. Voiding cystourethrograms (VCUGs) are performed following treatment of the acute infection, while still on suppressive therapy, to assess for the presence of reflux. Therapy should be completed prior to performance of the VCUG since infection may be a cause for reflux. The VCUG can help determine the need for continued medical therapy, surveillance, or surgical intervention. Indwelling Foley catheter drainage would not be indicated unless there was urinary retention as a contributing factor. Cystoscopy is not routinely performed in acute urinary tract infections in children and urethral cultures would not be helpful.

22. C

The two most common causes for short stature are familial short stature and constitutional delay in growth. Patients with familial short stature are genetically destined to have a short stature. Patients with familial short stature have short parents, normal growth velocity, and normal onset of puberty. Their bone age is equal to their chronologic age. Patients with a constitutional delay have a family history of delayed growth and sexual maturity. They have normal growth in the first years of life, followed by a slowing of growth around ages 2 to 4 years, followed by a resumption of a normal growth rate. Their bone age is less than their chronologic age and they are delayed in sexual maturity. They will continue to grow until their bone age catches up to their chronologic age and their ultimate height will be normal or consistent with that predicted based on parental height. Neither of these conditions require therapy.

23. D

Kawasaki syndrome is an acute inflammatory condition of unknown cause that affects medium and large arteries. This vasculitis may affect the coronary arteries, leading to thrombosis or aneurysm formation. Diagnostic criteria for Kawasaki syndrome set forth by the Centers for Disease Control and Prevention include fever for 5 or more days along with at least four of the following: conjunctivitis, polymorphous rash, oral lesions (fissuring lips, strawberry tongue, and pharyngeal erythema), erythema or desquamation of the palms and soles, and cervical adenopathy.

Laboratory findings that support the diagnosis include elevated erythrocyte sedimentation rate, leukocytosis, thrombocytosis, mild anemia, increased liver enzymes, and elevated C-reactive protein. When there is cardiac involvement, the chest x-ray may show cardiomegaly and PR prolongation, reduced voltages, and ST-T wave changes may be present on electrocardiography. Aneurysms may be seen when echocardiography is performed. Intravenous gamma-globulin, aspirin, and close monitoring for cardiac complications are the mainstays of therapy. An elevated ASO titer is seen with group A streptococcal infections. A positive monospot test is consistent with a diagnosis of mononucleosis. These latter two tests are not features of Kawasaki syndrome.

24. D

Accidents are the leading cause of childhood deaths in the United States. Accidents and injuries account for approximately one-half of deaths that occur in children. The leading forms of accidents are motor vehicle accidents and drowning. Distressingly, homicide and suicide are the next two most common causes for childhood deaths, accounting for 13% and 10% of deaths, respectively. With the advent of antibiotic therapy and immunizations, mortality from infectious causes has declined. Malignancy, pulmonary disease, and HIV-related disease cause significant childhood illness and death but are not as common as accidents, homicide, and suicide. Although cardiovascular disease is the leading cause of death in adults, it is not a major cause for childhood mortality.

25. D

Concerns about vaccination of infants, especially preterm infants, are common discussions in primary care offices. An adverse reaction in a family member or friend of the family often is the trigger for this concern. Discovering the cause for the concern and providing patient education can help in allaying the reluctance to provide the necessary vaccines. Current recommendations state that vaccines should be administered to premature infants on the same schedule as term infants, beginning 2 months after birth. Family history of medical disease or adverse events does not impact the decision to administer a vaccine, although it will play a role in providing additional counseling and reassurance for anxious parents. Contraindications and precautions in administering the DtaP vaccine have been defined. See Table 2.3.

Table 2.3 Contraindications and precautions for DTaP use

Contraindications	Precautions
History of anaphylaxis to vaccine	Fever ≥40.5°C within 48 hours of prior dose of vaccine
Encephalopathy within 7 days of receiving prior dose	Hypotonia, hyporesponsiveness, or inconsolable crying (more than 3 hours) within 48 hours of prior dose
Seizures within 3 days of prior dose	

26. A

The most important element in deciding on additional therapy or referral for persistent middle ear effusions is the impact the effusions are having on hearing. Thus, an evaluation of hearing is warranted, which could be achieved with either audiometry or brain stem auditory evoked responses (BAER) testing. BAER testing is used for neonatal hearing screening but can also be used to screen hearing in younger children (≤3 years) who are too young to cooperate with audiometry. Middle ear effusions affect the results of these tests, but BAER is not generally used to assess hearing loss with middle ear effusions. Audiometry is the preferred test and can document hearing loss that would indicate a need for further therapy or referral for tympanostomy tube placement. Although tympanometry can confirm the presence of effusion, it has no role in determining the need for additional therapy or referral. Electronystagmography is useful for evaluating vertigo, but it does not evaluate middle ear effusions. Most middle ear effusions resolve spontaneously within 2 or 3 months. Bilateral effusions that persist for more than 4 to 6 months and that are associated with bilateral hearing deficits of 20 decibels or more are indications for tympanostomy tube placement.

27. C

Asthma is a chronic inflammatory condition that results in increased reactivity of the airways. The components of therapy for patients with persistent disease include not only bronchodilators for the airway reactivity but also anti-inflammatory therapy to treat the underlying inflammation. The patient presented has moderate persistent asthma and requires further therapy. Antibiotic therapy is generally not part of asthma therapy unless pneumonia or another bacterial complication is documented. Inhaled corticosteroid therapy would be the next component of therapy added, to address the airway inflammation characteristic of asthma. Long-acting B2 agonists may also be of benefit in helping manage his airway reactivity and to lessen the frequency of use of the shorter acting B2 agonists. Inhaled anticholinergic medications are not currently one of the mainstays of outpatient therapy but are sometimes used in sick hospitalized patients. Oral antihistamines can be used in treating the broader spectrum of allergic disease but are not generally considered an integral part of treating asthma.

28. C

When childhood development falls outside the normal range in one or more areas, a child may have underlying cognitive, physical, or psychological disease causing the developmental lag. Developmental screening tests can identify children who fall outside of the expected normal range in reaching developmental motor, cognitive, and communication milestones and need further evaluation to determine the underlying cause. Many different instruments have been developed to systematically evaluate a child's development relative to a standardized peer group (e.g., Denver Developmental Screening Instrument). When developmental delay is identified, the physician can then initiate the evaluation by making any necessary referrals for a formal assessment of the particular concerns. Developmental screening tests do not diagnose mental retardation, behavioral disorders, genetic disorders, or learning disabilities. See Table 2.4.

29. C

Chlamydial infection is transmitted from an infected mother to her newborn during the birth process. When newborns develop chlamydial infections, including conjunctivitis, a larger percentage of these infants are then colonized with Chlamydia and carry the

Table 2.4 Developmental milestones

Age	Gross Motor	Fine (Visual) Motor	Language	Social
1 month	Raises head slightly from prone	Follows with eyes to midline only; tight grasp	Alerts/startles to sound	Fixes on face
2 months			Smiles responsively	Recognizes parent
3 months	Holds head up, steady	Hands open at rest	Coos	Reaches for familiar objects or people
4–5 months	Rolls front to back, back to front; sits well supported	Grasps with both hands together	Orients to voice	Enjoys observing environment
6 months	Sits well unsupported	Transfers hand to hand; reaches with either hand	Babbles	Recognizes strangers
9 months	Crawls, cruises, pulls to stand	Uses pincer grasp; fingerfeeds	Begins to use "dada/mama"; understands "no"	Plays pat-a-cake
12 months	Walks alone	Throws, releases objects	1–8 words other than "dada/mama"; follows one-step commands	Imitates; comes when called; cooperates with dressing
15 months	Walks backward; creeps upstairs	Builds 2-block tower; scribbles		
18 months	Runs	Feeds self (messily) with utensils	Points to body parts when asked	Plays around (not with) other children
21 months	Squats and recovers	Builds 5-block tower	Two-word combinations	
24 months	Walks well up and down stairs	Removes clothing	Understands 2-step commands; stranger understands ½ of speech	Parallel play
30 months	Throws ball overhand		Appropriate pronoun use	Knows first, last names
3 years	Pedals tricycle	Draws a circle	3 word sentences; past tense; uses plurals; stranger understands ¾ of speech	Group play; shares
4 years	Alternates feet going down stairs; skips	Catches ball; dresses alone	Knows colors	Imaginative play
5 years		Ties shoes	Prints first name	Plays cooperative games; understands "rules" and abides by them

Table 2.5 Cholesterol levels in children and adolescents 2 to 19 years old*

Category	Total Cholesterol (mg/dL)	LDL Cholesterol (mg/dL)
Acceptable	Less than 170	Less than 110
Borderline	170–199	110–129
High	200 or greater	130 or greater

*HDL levels should be ≥35 mg/dL and triglycerides should be ≤150 mg/dL.
From www.americanheart.org

bacteria in the nasopharynx. Without systemic treatment, these infants are at risk for developing chlamydial pneumonia. Topical medications may treat the conjunctivitis but are not considered appropriate therapy for chlamydial conjunctivitis because they do not eliminate carriage of the bacteria in the nasopharynx. Oral erythromycin can treat the conjunctivitis and help eradicate the organism from other sites but must be provided as a 14-day course of therapy. Topical aminoglycosides or sulfonamides have no role in treating chlamydial conjunctivitis.

30. C

Cholesterol values in children are not predictive of future adult values and hence make cholesterol screening in children a source of some debate. Nonetheless, cholesterol screening is currently recommended for children older than 2 years of age with a family history of premature cardiovascular disease (≤55 years old) in the parents or grandparents, or a parental history of hypercholesterolemia. When screening is performed, values less than 170 mg/dL are considered normal, values of 170 to 199 mg/dL are considered borderline abnormal, and values higher than 200 mg/dL are considered elevated. Cholesterol values can be variable over time and are affected by diet and level of physical activity; thus, any elevated values should be confirmed. See Table 2.5.

31. C

Normal 6-month-old infants sleep approximately 14 hours per day, of which 11 hours occur at night. Generally, infants this age require two daytime naps. Infants this age should be able to sleep through the night without feeding. All infants will have arousals during sleep; however, they should learn by 4 to 6 months of age to provide self-comfort and get themselves back to sleep. When infants are consistently put to bed asleep, either in association with feeding or rocking or being held, they do not learn these self-comforting skills. Thus, when they awaken at night, they are not able to get themselves back to sleep and cry until they are provided with the comforting measure that they associate with sleep. The mother should be provided with instructions to put the infant to bed when he is sleepy but still awake. In addition, she must be educated that he has learned this association and must now develop the skills to fall asleep on his own, including during the nighttime arousals. This should not be considered normal since 40% of children who have sleep problems during infancy continue to have sleep problems at the age of 3 years. She should not awaken him to feed, and when he does awaken and cry, she should refrain from picking him up or feeding him. She should not ignore the crying but respond and briefly reassure him. The response should be brief and avoid stimulating the infant.

32. D

Understanding the cognitive development of children and their abilities to understand and relate with their environment can allow physicians to more effectively communicate with pediatric patients at their level. Jean Piaget outlined a well-accepted schema for childhood cognitive development. Children in the birth to 2-year age group experience the world through sensations and their bodily movements, termed the sensorimotor stage. Children in the 2 to 6 year age group are egocentric and engage in fantasy play and exhibit magical thinking. Piaget labeled this stage preoperational. The next stage, ages 6 to 11 years, is called concrete operational stage, and at this stage children can distinguish between self and non-self and relate many of their mental processes to real objects. The final stage is called formal operations, and at this point in development the child has developed the ability to think in abstract terms. Other developmental milestones are presented in Table 2.4.

33. A

Viewpoints regarding routine circumcision have changed over the years and currently the opinion appears to be almost evenly divided between those who advocate routine circumcision and those who have no opinion either for or against routine circumcision. The uncircumcised state can be associated with the development of several complications, such as phimosis, UTIs, paraphimosis, balanitis, and possibly penile cancer. These complications may be indications for circumcision. Phimosis refers to the inability to retract the foreskin in an uncircumcised male. Phimosis is considered normal and physiologic up to the age of 6 years, by which time 90% of uncircumcised males have retractable foreskins. Many physicians advocate circumcision for those with persistent phimosis past the age of 10 years. Medical management prior to recommending circumcision may include use of topical steroid cream for 4 to 6 weeks to help in promoting retractability of the foreskin. UTIs, particularly recurrent infections, are an indication for circumcision. UTIs occur more frequently in uncircumcised males in association with colonization of the foreskin by pathogenic bacteria. Paraphimosis refers to inability to return the retracted foreskin to the unretracted state. The foreskin then acts as a tourniquet and obstructs lymphatic flow leading to swelling and further increased difficulty replacing the foreskin. This too is an indication for circumcision. Balanitis is an inflammation or infection of the glans often caused by yeast (candida) or gram-negative bacteria. Balanitis occurs almost exclusively in uncircumcised males and if recurrent is an indication for circumcision. There is an association between penile cancer and

Recommended Childhood and Adolescent Immunization Schedule UNITED STATES • 2006

Vaccine ▼ / Age ▶	Birth	1 month	2 months	4 months	6 months	12 months	15 months	18 months	24 months	4–6 years	11–12 years	13–14 years	15 years	16–18 years
Hepatitis B[1]	HepB	HepB		*HepB[1]*		HepB					HepB Series			
Diphtheria, Tetanus, Pertussis[2]			DTaP	DTaP	DTaP		DTaP			DTaP	Tdap	Tdap		
Haemophilus influenzae type b[3]			Hib	Hib	*Hib[3]*	Hib								
Inactivated Poliovirus			IPV	IPV	IPV					IPV				
Measles, Mumps, Rubella[4]						MMR				MMR	MMR			
Varicella[5]						Varicella					Varicella			
Meningococcal[6]							Vaccines within broken line are for selected populations			MPSV4	MCV4	MCV4	MCV4	
Pneumococcal[7]			PCV	PCV	PCV	PCV				PCV	PPV			
Influenza[8]					Influenza (Yearly)					Influenza (Yearly)				
Hepatitis A[9]										HepA Series				

This schedule indicates the recommended ages for routine administration of currently licensed childhood vaccines, as of December 1, 2005, for children through age 18 years. Any dose not given at the recommended age should be administered at any subsequent visit when indicated and feasible.

▓▓▓ Indicates age groups that warrant special effort to administer those vaccines not previously administered. Additional vaccines may be licensed and recommended during the year. Licensed combination vaccines may be used whenever any components of the combination are indicated and other components of the vaccine are not contraindicated and if approved by the Food and Drug Administration for that dose of the series. Providers should consult the respective ACIP statement for detailed recommendations. Clinically significant adverse events that follow immunization should be reported to the Vaccine Adverse Event Reporting System (VAERS). Guidance about how to obtain and complete a VAERS form is available at: www.vaers.hhs.gov or by telephone, 800-822-7967.

▓ Range of recommended ages
▓ 11–12-year-old assessment
▓ Catch-up immunization

FOOTNOTES ON REVERSE SIDE

DEPARTMENT OF HEALTH AND HUMAN SERVICES
CENTERS FOR DISEASE CONTROL AND PREVENTION
SAFER • HEALTHIER • PEOPLE™

CDC Immunization

The Childhood and Adolescent Immunization Schedule is approved by:
Advisory Committee on Immunization Practices www.cdc.gov/nip/acip
American Academy of Pediatrics www.aap.org
American Academy of Family Physicians www.aafp.org

More information regarding vaccine administration can be obtained from the websites above or the CDC-INFO contact center:
800-CDC-INFO
ENGLISH & ESPAÑOL – 24/7
[800-232-4636]

Keep track of your child's immunizations with the CDC Childhood Immunization Scheduler
www.cdc.gov/nip/kidstuff/scheduler.htm

FOOTNOTES

1. **Hepatitis B vaccine (HepB).** *AT BIRTH:* All newborns should receive monovalent HepB soon after birth and before hospital discharge. **Infants born to mothers who are HBsAg-positive** should receive HepB and 0.5 mL of hepatitis B immune globulin (HBIG) within 12 hours of birth. **Infants born to mothers whose HBsAg status is unknown** should receive HepB within 12 hours of birth. The mother should have blood drawn as soon as possible to determine her HBsAg status; if HBsAg-positive, the infant should receive HBIG as soon as possible (no later than age 1 week). **For infants born to HBsAg-negative mothers,** the birth dose can be delayed in rare circumstances but only if a physician's order to withhold the vaccine and a copy of the mother's original HBsAg-negative laboratory report are documented in the infant's medical record. *FOLLOWING THE BIRTH DOSE:* The HepB series should be completed with either monovalent HepB or a combination vaccine containing HepB. The second dose should be administered at age 1–2 months. The final dose should be administered at age ≥24 weeks. It is permissible to administer 4 doses of HepB (e.g., when combination vaccines are administered after the birth dose); however, if monovalent HepB is used, a dose at age 4 months is not needed. **Infants born to HBsAg-positive mothers** should be tested for HBsAg and antibody to HBsAg after completion of the HepB series at age 9–18 months (generally at the next well-child visit after completion of the vaccine series).

2. **Diphtheria and tetanus toxoids and acellular pertussis vaccine (DTaP).** The fourth dose of DTaP may be administered as early as age 12 months, provided 6 months have elapsed since the third dose and the child is unlikely to return at age 15–18 months. The final dose in the series should be administered at age ≥4 years.

   Tetanus and diphtheria toxoids and acellular pertussis vaccine (Tdap – adolescent preparation) is recommended at age 11–12 years for those who have completed the recommended childhood DTP/DTaP vaccination series and have not received a Td booster dose. Adolescents aged 13–18 years who missed the age 11–12-year Td/Tdap booster dose should also receive a single dose of Tdap if they have completed the recommended childhood DTP/DTaP vaccination series. Subsequent **tetanus and diphtheria toxoids (Td)** are recommended every 10 years.

3. *Haemophilus influenzae* **type b conjugate vaccine (Hib).** Three Hib conjugate vaccines are licensed for infant use. If PRP-OMP (PedvaxHIB® or COMVAX® [Merck]) is administered at ages 2 and 4 months, a dose at age 6 months is not required. DTaP/Hib combination products should not be used for primary immunization in infants at ages 2, 4 or 6 months but can be used as boosters after any Hib vaccine. The final dose in the series should be administered at age ≥12 months.

4. **Measles, mumps, and rubella vaccine (MMR).** The second dose of MMR is recommended routinely at age 4–6 years but may be administered during any visit, provided at least 4 weeks have elapsed since the first dose and both doses are administered beginning at or after age 12 months. Children who have not previously received the second dose should complete the schedule by age 11–12 years.

5. **Varicella vaccine.** Varicella vaccine is recommended at any visit at or after age 12 months for susceptible children (i.e., those who lack a reliable history of chickenpox). Susceptible persons aged ≥13 years should receive 2 doses administered at least 4 weeks apart.

6. **Meningococcal vaccine (MCV4).** Meningococcal conjugate vaccine (MCV4) should be given to all children at the 11–12-year-old visit as well as to unvaccinated adolescents at high school entry (aged 15 years). Other adolescents who wish to decrease their risk for meningococcal disease may also be vaccinated. All college freshmen living in dormitories should also be vaccinated, preferably with MCV4, although **meningococcal polysaccharide vaccine (MPSV4)** is an acceptable alternative. Vaccination against invasive meningococcal disease is recommended for children and adolescents aged ≥2 years with terminal complement deficiencies or anatomic or functional asplenia and for certain other high-risk groups (see *MMWR* 2005;54 [RR-7]:1-21; use MPSV4 for children aged 2–10 years and MCV4 for older children, although MPSV4 is an acceptable alternative.

7. **Pneumococcal vaccine.** The heptavalent **pneumococcal conjugate vaccine (PCV)** is recommended for all children aged 2–23 months and for certain children aged 24–59 months. The final dose in the series should be administered at age ≥12 months. **Pneumococcal polysaccharide vaccine (PPV)** is recommended in addition to PCV for certain high-risk groups. See *MMWR* 2000; 49(RR-9):1-35.

8. **Influenza vaccine.** Influenza vaccine is recommended annually for children aged ≥6 months with certain risk factors (including, but not limited to, asthma, cardiac disease, sickle cell disease, human immunodeficiency virus [HIV], diabetes, and conditions that can compromise respiratory function or handling of respiratory secretions or that can increase the risk for aspiration), healthcare workers, and other persons (including household members) in close contact with persons in groups at high risk (see *MMWR* 2005;54[RR-8]:1-55). In addition, healthy children aged 6–23 months and close contacts of healthy children aged 0–5 months are recommended to receive influenza vaccine because children in this age group are at substantially increased risk for influenza-related hospitalizations. For healthy persons aged 5–49 years, the intranasally administered, live, attenuated influenza vaccine (LAIV) is an acceptable alternative to the intramuscular trivalent inactivated influenza vaccine (TIV). See *MMWR* 2005;54(RR-8):1-55. Children receiving TIV should be given a dosage appropriate for their age (0.25 mL if aged 6–35 months or 0.5 mL if aged ≥3 years). Children aged ≤8 years who are receiving influenza vaccine for the first time should receive 2 doses (separated by at least 4 weeks for TIV and at least 6 weeks for LAIV).

9. **Hepatitis A vaccine (HepA).** HepA is recommended for all children at 1 year of age (i.e.,12–23 months). The 2 doses in the series should be administered at least 6 months apart. States, counties, and communities with existing HepA vaccination programs for children 2–18 years of age are encouraged to maintain these programs. In these areas, new efforts focused on routine vaccination of 1-year-old children should enhance, not replace, ongoing programs directed at a broader population of children. HepA is also recommended for certain high-risk groups (see *MMWR* 1999; 48[RR-12]1-37).

Figure 2-2. This schedule indicates the recommended ages for routine administration of currently licensed childhood vaccines, as of December 1, 2001, for children through age 18 years. Any dose not given at the recommended age should be given at any subsequent visit when indicated and feasible. The striped bars indicate age groups that warrant special effort to administer those vaccines not previously given. Additional vaccines may be licensed and recommended during the year. Licensed combination vaccines may be used whenever any components of the combination are indicated and the vaccine's other components are not contraindicated. Providers should consult the manufacturer's package inserts for detailed recommendations. From www.cdc.gov.

the uncircumcised state; however, the exact causative factors are unclear. Infection with human papilloma virus may play a significant role. Although penile cancer occurs more commonly in uncircumcised males, it is still a relatively rare form of cancer, and prevention of penile cancer is not considered to be an indication for circumcision in older males. Tinea cruris, a yeast infection in the inguinal region, plays no role in determining the need for circumcision. Proper hygiene leads to cleanliness in both the uncircumcised and the circumcised states. Cosmetic appeal is a common reason that circumcisions are performed, but this does not constitute a medical indication for the procedure.

34. A

Supplemental foods are generally not added to an infant's diet until 4 to 6 months of age. Introduction of solid foods at too early an age is associated with obesity as well as increased incidence of food allergies. There are several indicators that supplementation with solid foods is necessary and appropriate. The infant needs to be developmentally able to sit and support her head. The infant's weight should be at least double her birth weight, and the infant should be consuming more than 32 ounces of formula per day. An infant who seems unsatisfied and hungry despite this amount of formula or who requires more than 8 to 10 feedings per day is a candidate for introduction of solid foods. When solids are introduced, iron-fortified cereals are the typical first foods, followed by fruits or vegetables. Meats may be introduced after 6 months of age. Limited amounts of juices may also be introduced at this time. As a rule, one new food may be introduced per week.

35. B

Normal language development in a 3-year-old child would include at least a 250-word vocabulary and the ability to form sentences. In addition, 75% or more of this language should be understandable by strangers. The child represented in this case has language development commensurate with a child younger than 2 years of age. Hearing impairment is one of the most common causes for delay in language acquisition. Many children suffer unrecognized hearing loss until the age of 2 or 3 years. Even when a problem is first suspected, delays in evaluation and therapy are common. In this otherwise normal appearing child, the initial step in evaluation would include a hearing assessment. The type of testing performed will depend on the age of the patient and may include brain stem auditory evoked response, behavioral audiometry, or pure-tone audiometry.

36. C

The childhood immunization schedule is presented in Figure 2-2. In children who have fallen behind in receiving the proper immunizations, every opportunity should be made to provide as many vaccines as possible in an effort to get the child up-to-date. This includes providing vaccines on visits during which children present with mild upper respiratory infections. The immune response is not inhibited by simultaneous administration of vaccines. Thus, there is no limit to the number of vaccines that may be administered. Two or more live vaccines may be given at the same time. However, if the child receives a live vaccine, there should be a 30-day interval before receiving another live viral vaccine. After the age of 5, the *Haemophilus* vaccine (Hib) is no longer recommended.

37. C

In order to detect conditions associated with trisomy 21, children with trisomy 21 require some additional screening measures in addition to the routine childhood care. Congenital heart disease occurs in up to 50% of children with Down's syndrome, and thus in the newborn period, ECG, echocardiogram, and chest x-ray are routinely recommended in these children. If normal, then subsequent need for performing these tests is based on the development of symptoms or findings on physical examination. Congenital hypothyroidism is present in 1% of these children and acquired hypothyroidism occurs commonly. Thyroid screening should occur in the newborn period and then annually during childhood. Ocular anomalies and hearing loss are common findings and warrant evaluation in the newborn period and annually throughout childhood. Atlantoaxial instability is a common musculoskeletal anomaly that places the child at risk for cervical cord injury, particularly during sporting activities that may involve neck flexion. Cervical spine films with flexion and extension views are recommended prior to sports participation in order to detect this and to make any recommendations regarding participation. Annual chest x-rays and ECGs are not necessary in providing routine care for children with trisomy 21.

38. C

Parents who express concern about sibling rivalry and fighting should be reassured that this behavior is normal but should also be provided with constructive ways to handle their concerns. Each child should be treated as an individual and should be provided with his or her own unique possessions and time with the parents. The children should be complimented for positive interactions and allowed or encouraged to vent any negative feelings. The limits of acceptable or unacceptable behavior between siblings should be defined, and physical or verbal abuse should be considered unacceptable. The parents need to be cautious in taking sides. In many instances, the older child is always saddled with the blame. Situations that may foster rivalry should be anticipated, and when conflict does arise the children should be encouraged to help resolve the conflict if this is possible.

39. A

There are increasing pressures for children to be toilet trained at an earlier age. Some of these revolve around parental concerns and the convenience of not having to change diapers and others around enrolling the child in preschools that require toilet training before entry. The age at which most children in the United States are toilet trained is between 2.5 and 3.0 years. Girls generally are trained at a slightly younger age and most achieve bowel and bladder control simultaneously. The child must be developmentally mature enough and interested in using the toilet for successful toilet training to occur. Developmental maturity is indicated by lengthening periods of dryness (more than 2 hours), the ability to recognize and signal the need to eliminate, and the ability to follow simple commands. Introduction to a potty seat, encouraging dryness and cleanliness by more frequent changing, and helping the child understand the connections between his or her signaling the need to use the toilet and cleanliness and dryness can assist in stimulating interest in the child for toilet training. Punishment, especially physical punishment, should never be used.

40. B

In children younger than 36 months who are febrile without an apparent source, the risk of occult bacteremia is 3% to 5%. In those who are bacteremic and do not receive antibiotic therapy,

Table 2.6 Recommendations for treatment/intervention with elevated lead levels

Blood Lead Level (μg/dL)	Intervention
<25	Environmental assessment
25–44	Environmental assessment and consider chelation therapy if persist after environmental intervention
45–69	Assess for enteral lead (abdominal x-ray); chelation therapy
≥70	Consider hospitalization and consultation for chelation therapy

From: www.cdc.gov.

20% remain bacteremic and are at risk for meningitis or other localized infections. The age of the child, the severity of the illness, the laboratory findings, and the reliability of the parents influence management of these children. In children with temperatures over 102.2°F (39°C) and WBC counts over 15,000, the risk for bacteremia increases fourfold. Neonates require hospitalization and empiric antibiotic therapy pending culture results (which usually includes CSF). Children between 1 and 3 months of age will undergo laboratory workup that includes CBC, blood cultures, urinalysis, lumbar puncture, and usually chest x-ray. These children will usually be hospitalized and empirically treated pending test and culture results. However, if the child does not appear ill, all of the laboratory findings are within normal limits, and the patient can be reliably followed up, then these patients may not require hospitalization. In older children who are ill appearing, hospitalization is again warranted. In children 3 to 36 months who are not ill appearing, a CBC, urinalysis with culture, chest x-ray, and blood cultures should be obtained and intramuscular ceftriaxone may be given with reevaluation in 24 hours. Again, the decision regarding hospitalization depends on the appearance of the child and reliability of the parents.

41. B
Soy-based formulas account for approximately 25% of formula sales in the United States. Soy-based formulas have been used for a variety of different feeding problems; however, the true indications for the need to use a soy-based formula are narrow. Indications for soy formulas include lactose intolerance, allergy to cow's milk protein, and galactosemia. Soy formulas are also commonly used during or following a bout of gastroenteritis to manage feeding during the relative lactase-deficient phase. Many parents also use soy formulas in attempts to treat the apparent formula intolerance associated with colic. Contraindications to use of soy formulas include soy allergy, prematurity, and cystic fibrosis. Of those infants with cow's milk protein allergy, 20% will also be allergic to soy and must then use hydrolyzed protein formulas.

42. D
Lead is a heavy metal that is part of the environment in which we live in varying levels. Exposure to excessive amounts of lead can be detrimental to the developing brain in children, causing lower IQ and other behavioral effects. Blood levels greater than 10 μg/dL are considered significant and warrant evaluation. Levels less than

this are considered normal and require no evaluation. Historically, the heaviest exposures have been through the lead in gasoline and paints. In 1978, lead was banned from all paints, and in 1995 lead was no longer present in gasoline. When screening parents regarding possible lead exposure, the age of the home, other children in the building with elevated lead levels, and inquiry about parental occupation and hobbies should be included. See Table 2.6.

43. C
Up to one-third of children will be part of a family in which the parents divorce. Invariably, primary care physicians will become aware of children in this situation due to parents' questions about how to handle various issues, due to physicians' questions about the family, or when children present with behavioral concerns. As a rule, the children should be told of the divorce and living arrangements. They should not be asked their opinion about whether the parents should get divorced, and they should not be put in the position of having to choose loyalties and living arrangements. Disputes between the parents should be kept between the parents, and the children should not be used as a messenger or sounding board to vent negative feelings or anger. The household rules, schedules, and sleeping arrangements should be maintained as intact as possible. The child should not begin sleeping with the custodial parent and symbolically "replacing" the absent parent. Children should be encouraged to discuss their feelings and should be made aware that they are not responsible for causing or correcting the problems that led to divorce. If children or families are having difficulties adapting, then referral for individual or family counseling may be beneficial.

44. A
Death is a difficult concept to explain to a child and difficult for children to understand. When explaining death, it should be presented in a factual way and not that someone is "sleeping," has "passed away," or is "lost." Children's questions should be answered at the time, but they generally do not require a long speech. Children may discuss the death over the ensuing several weeks or months with spontaneous "out of the blue" questions. Depending on their age and stage of development, children may say things that are insensitive and upsetting to the parents. Correcting any undesirable behavior along with setting limits should be consistently enforced. Resuming the usual schedule and rules will help children to cope and feel secure as they move forward. Experts agree that children should be allowed to attend the funeral of a family member. Asking a more distant relative or friend to chaperone younger children can be helpful to grieving parents as well as the children.

45. C

Encopresis is defined as the involuntary passage of stool in anatomically normal children older than the age of 4 years. Encopresis occurs in approximately 2.5% of boys and 1.3% of girls. The most common underlying cause for encopresis is chronic constipation. When there is obstruction of the colon, then liquid stool will leak around the obstruction and be involuntarily passed. When evaluating patients for chronic constipation, the workup should include consideration of Hirschsprung's disease, neurologic disease, hypothyroidism, and rectal or anal lesions. Therapy should not include punishment but should focus on initially clearing the colon of stool using enemas, suppositories, and laxatives. Once the colon is clear, then maintaining regular bowel movements with stool softeners, fiber, and regular time on the toilet are essential. A reward system is often helpful in achieving regular toilet time. With treatment and follow-up, 90% will improve significantly over 6 months and 65% will be in remission.

46. B

In general, the age of majority when adolescents are considered adults is 18 years. At this age, they may consent for their own care regardless of the living situation or who is paying for the care. For children younger than 18 years of age, parental consent may be required depending on the age of the child and the circumstances necessitating medical care. For example, every state has a statute allowing minors to seek care for sexually transmitted diseases without parental consent. Most states also allow minors to independently seek care for substance abuse and mental health services. Emancipated minors may also give their own consent. A minor may be emancipated if he or she is married, in the armed forces, pregnant, or has been legally declared emancipated. Emergency care in situations in which the child may suffer permanent injury or death can be provided without parental consent. For the cases presented, only the 15-year-old with a penile discharge would clearly not require parental consent for evaluation and treatment.

47. B

Adolescence is a time of defining one's identity, including sexual orientation. During this time, there is an increasing awareness and experience that may involve sexual experimentation. One's sexual orientation is not defined by any one action but evolves over time and is defined by patterns of behavior. Some have suggested that sexual orientation lies along a continuum between homosexuality and heterosexuality and that this may change over time. The data suggest that up to 17% to 30% of males and 6% to 20% of females have had a homosexual experience. An estimated 5% of the population is defined as homosexual. Thus, the individual presented should not be categorized or labeled but reassured and provided with facts about the evolution of sexual identity. Adolescents who choose to be sexually active should be counseled about the risks of sexual activity, including sexually transmitted diseases that may be spread through oral, anal, or genital sex. Unless this individual seems overly distressed by this incident or has signs or symptoms of psychiatric disease, referral for psychotherapy would not be indicated.

48. A

Adverse effects of oral contraception (OCP) have been well publicized; however, the beneficial effects are not well-known by patients. The primary adverse effects of concern are the risk of thrombophlebitis and myocardial infarction (increased in women older than age 35, especially those who smoke). Rare liver adenomas or carcinoma have been reported. Weight gain may occur but

not consistently. Breast cancer risk may be minimally elevated with use of OCPs. Beneficial effects include regulation of menstrual cycles, less menstrual flow, lower risk for anemia, and improvement in dysmenorrheal. In addition, OCPs may be helpful in treating acne, endometriosis, and ovarian cysts, and they lower the risk for ovarian and uterine cancer. OCPs do not prevent sexually transmitted diseases but do protect against development of pelvic inflammatory disease. See Table 2.7.

49. D

Anorexia nervosa and bulimia nervosa are two of the major eating disorders that may occur. Anorexia nervosa is characterized by severe weight loss, restricted eating, and body image distortion. Bulimia differs in that the body weight may be in the normal range and the hallmark is binge eating with compensatory behaviors to prevent weight gain (e.g., self-induced vomiting and laxatives). Both occur more commonly in women than men, and the age of onset is most commonly adolescence and young adulthood. The average age of onset for bulimia is between 17 and 25 years and is present in up to 15% of college-age women. Anorexia nervosa has an average age of onset between 14 and 18 years and is present in approximately 1% of girls. Psychiatric comorbidities are very common with both of these entities, with depression being present in up to 50% of patients with eating disorders. See Table 2.8.

50. C

Suicide is the second most common cause for death in teenagers, with accidents being the most common cause. Although girls make more attempts at suicide, boys die more often as a result of suicide. Underlying psychiatric disease, such as mood disorders, conduct disorders, or borderline personality, increase the risk for suicidal behavior. In addition, substance abuse, history of violent acts, history of abuse, and family history of suicide place the teenager at increased risk for suicide.

51. D

The testicle normally descends from its original intra-abdominal position by the time of birth. Three percent of term males and 20% of preterm males will have an undescended testis. The undescended testicle must be distinguished from a retractile testicle through careful physical examination in a warm room with warm hands. If, on one occasion, this distinction is not possible, then having the child return for re-examination may be necessary. Eighty percent or more of undescended testes will spontaneously descend by 1 year of age. Return of the testes to the scrotum is important in order to have two functioning testes and to limit the risk for testicular cancer. A testicle in the intra-abdominal position is subjected to higher temperatures and after 2 or more years will begin to show degenerative changes. Intra-abdominal testes are also at 40-fold increased risk for testicular cancer, and return to the normal scrotal location can lower this risk. Surgery would not be indicated immediately but would be indicated if the testicle had not descended by 1 year of age. Hormonal therapy with human chorionic gonadotropin or gonadotropin-releasing hormone may be successful in some cases; however, the exact percentage of success is controversial.

52. A

Indirect inguinal hernias are by far the most common hernias found in children younger than the age of 10 years. Indirect hernias are considered congenitally acquired by failure of the processus

Table 2.7 Failure rates for various contraceptive methods

Method	Percent of Women Who Become Pregnant	
	Theoretical Failure Rate	Actual Failure Rate
No method	85.0	85.0
Periodic abstinence	—	20.0
Calendar	9.0	
Ovulation method	3.0	
Symptothermal	2.0	
Postovulation	1.0	
Withdrawal	4.0	18.0
Lactational amenorrhea	2.0	15.0–55.0
Condom		
Male condom	2.0	12.0
Female condom	6.0	21.0–26.0
Diaphragm with spermicide	6.0	18.0
Cervical cap	6.0	18.0
Sponge		
Parous women	9.0	28.0
Nulliparous women	6.0	18.0
Spermicide alone	3.0	21.0
IUDs		
Progestasert	2.0	2.0
Paraguard copper T	0.8	0.7
Combination pill	0.1	3.0
Progestin-only pill	0.5	3.0–6.0
Norplant	0.09	0.09
Depo-Provera	0.3	0.3
Tubal ligation	0.2	0.4
Vasectomy	0.1	0.15

*Adapted from Speroff L, Darney P. *A Clinical Guide for Contraception*. 2nd ed. Baltimore: Williams & Wilkins; 1996:136.

Table 2.8 Characteristics of anorexia and bulimia

Anorexia Nervosa	Bulimia Nervosa

Two types
  Restrictive
  Purging
	Two types
	  Purging
	  Nonpurging

Low body weight	Normal or above average weight
Denial of disorder	Aware of eating disorder
Psychological problems	Low self-esteem displaced onto food
Body image disturbance	Eating triggers guilt, depression, and compensatory behaviors

vaginalis to close, thus allowing abdominal contents to descend through the inguinal ring. Hernias contain abdominal viscera, most commonly small intestine in boys and ovaries and fallopian tube in girls. Hydroceles are related in that they are also caused by a patent processus vaginalis, but they contain fluid and not abdominal viscera. Two to five percent of boys will develop inguinal hernias. Hernias occur much more commonly in boys than girls, and one-third are diagnosed before 6 months of age and more than one-half are diagnosed by 1 year of age. Hydroceles may be observed during the first year of life and may resolve with closure of the processus vaginalis. If a reducible hernia develops, then it should be repaired within the next 2 to 4 weeks to limit development of complications, such as incarceration or strangulation. In children presenting with incarcerated hernias, prompt operative repair should be performed.

53. E

Detection of hematuria by dipstick examination of the urine should prompt microscopic evaluation of the urine. More than 3 to 5 RBCs/hpf is considered significant for hematuria and should be evaluated. Initial evaluation should include analysis of the urine for persistence of the hematuria as well as checking for proteinuria. The finding of proteinuria or RBC casts suggests the presence of intrinsic renal disease (e.g., glomerulonephritis). Other testing to initially evaluate hematuria should include a serum creatinine to evaluate renal function, a urine culture to detect an infectious cause, and a urine calcium to creatinine ratio (normal is less than 0.18) to determine the presence of hypercalciuria. Imaging studies, such as ultrasound and voiding cystogram, should be performed to evaluate for anatomic causes of hematuria. If no causes are identified, then continued surveillance of hematuria and renal function is warranted. For patients with identified abnormalities or with gross hematuria, consultation is recommended.

54. B

Although this child's blood pressure is high normal by adult standards, using pediatric tables his blood pressure would be considered as severe hypertension and above the 99th percentile. To determine whether the blood pressure is normal or elevated, the child's height percentile must be obtained. The percentile for the blood pressure reading is obtained by combining the reading along with the child's age and height percentile (see Table 2.9). Normal blood pressure readings are less than the 90th percentile. Greater than the 99th percentile is severe hypertension. Prior to adolescence, secondary causes are the most common causes for

Table 2.9 BP levels for boys by age and height percentile (through age 5 years)

Age (years)	BP Percentile	SBP (mmHg) Percentile of Height							DBP (mmHg) Percentile of Height						
		5th	10th	25th	50th	75th	90th	95th	5th	10th	25th	50th	75th	90th	95th
1	50th	80	81	83	85	87	88	89	34	35	36	37	38	39	39
	90th	94	95	97	99	100	102	103	49	50	51	52	53	53	54
	95th	98	99	101	103	104	106	106	54	54	55	56	57	58	58
	99th	105	106	108	110	112	113	114	61	62	63	64	65	66	66
2	50th	84	85	87	88	90	92	92	39	40	41	42	43	44	44
	90th	97	99	100	102	104	105	106	54	55	56	57	58	58	59
	95th	101	102	104	106	108	109	110	59	59	60	61	62	63	63
	99th	109	110	111	113	115	117	117	66	67	68	69	70	71	71
3	50th	86	87	89	91	93	94	95	44	44	45	46	47	48	48
	90th	100	101	103	105	107	108	109	59	59	60	61	62	63	63
	95th	104	105	107	109	110	112	113	63	63	64	65	66	67	67
	99th	111	112	114	116	118	119	120	71	71	72	73	74	75	75
4	50th	88	89	91	93	95	96	97	47	48	49	50	51	51	52
	90th	102	103	105	107	109	110	111	62	63	64	65	66	66	67
	95th	106	107	109	111	112	114	115	66	67	68	69	70	71	71
	99th	113	114	116	118	120	121	122	74	75	76	77	78	78	79
5	50th	90	91	93	95	96	98	98	50	51	52	53	54	55	55
	90th	104	105	106	108	110	111	112	65	66	67	68	69	69	70
	95th	108	109	110	112	114	115	116	69	70	71	72	73	74	74
	99th	115	116	118	120	121	123	123	77	78	79	80	81	81	82

From www.nhlbi.nhi.gov.

sustained hypertension. In adolescents and adults, primary hypertension is most common. Among the secondary causes, renal parenchymal disease is most common from infancy to 6 years of age. Underlying renal disease may include renal scarring from repeated infections, cystic renal disease, and glomerulonephritis. Renal artery stenosis would be a consideration in younger or older adult patients but would be uncommon in children. Bronchopulmonary dysplasia may be a consideration in the newborn period, and pheochromocytoma is a rare disease at any age.

55. E
Juvenile rheumatoid arthritis (JRA) is the most frequent of the major rheumatologic disorders that occurs in childhood. JRA may present in basically three different ways: (a) oligoarthritis—affecting one or few joints; (b) polyarthritis—affecting five or more joints; and (c) systemic onset with high fever, rash, and visceral involvement. Onset of disease, by definition, is before the age of 16 years. At disease onset, fewer than 4% of patients are rheumatoid factor (RF) positive and 40% are antinuclear antibody (ANA) positive. These factors, along with the type of disease presentation, are useful in establishing the patient's prognosis. Oligoarthritis is the presentation of 60% of patients and is in general associated with a good prognosis. Those with oligoarthritis, however, are more prone to being affected with uveitis, thus making regular ophthalmologic exams of vital importance. Patients with oligoarthritis who are ANA positive are at higher risk for eye disease, and those who are RF positive have a poorer prognosis from a musculoskeletal standpoint. Patients present with polyarthritis in 30% of cases, and this presentation has an overall good prognosis, except in those who are RF positive. Ten percent of patients present with systemic disease, and the prognosis will vary depending on the pattern of joint involvement, with a better prognosis for those with few involved joints. Overall, 70% to 90% of patients with JRA can be expected to enter adulthood without active disease and with minimal or no disability. Fewer than 1% of patients with JRA die as a result of the disease (generally, systemic onset type) and thus life expectancy is not usually affected.

56. B
Ingestion of a battery poses risks of esophageal or intestinal obstruction. In general, button batteries, such as those used for watches, are small enough to spontaneously pass through the gastrointestinal tract. If the battery should become lodged, then potential complications of pressure necrosis and caustic injury from leakage of alkaline material from the battery may occur. If the battery passes through the esophagus and pylorus, then it should pass through the remainder of the bowel without difficulty. Initial management of this type of ingestion should include x-ray examination to determine the location of the battery. Those found to be in the esophagus and airway should be removed. Those in the stomach or intestines may be followed and expected to pass. If the battery is identified in the stool, then no further follow-up in the clinically well child is needed. If the battery is not identified, then a follow-up x-ray in 1 week may be performed to document clearance. Esophagoduodenoscopy and surgery would only be performed in those with complications or failure of the foreign body to pass. Induction of vomiting would be contraindicated and administration of laxatives unnecessary in this situation and may place the child at risk for additional injury.

57. A
Tick paralysis occurs due to a neurotoxin released in the saliva of an attached female tick. The toxin is believed to block the release of acetylcholine at the neuromuscular junction and thus leads to development of a paralysis. Other undefined actions may also occur since in many instances patients are also described as having cerebellar symptoms, such as ataxia. Onset of symptoms is generally 4 to 7 days after the tick attaches and begins with restlessness, irritability, and an ascending flaccid paralysis and possibly ataxia. Deep tendon reflexes are lost and the symptoms can rapidly progress over a few days, causing respiratory depression and bulbar paralysis. Patients with progressive disease may die unless the tick is removed. Removal of the tick is curative, with resolution of symptoms in anywhere from a few to 48 hours. Laboratory evaluation is unremarkable and CT findings would be expected to be normal. Finding this constellation of symptoms with an associated tick is virtually diagnostic. The mortality rate from this disease is approximately 10%, with most cases occurring in children. The normal CSF findings, the absence of fever, and clinical presentation do not support a diagnosis of meningitis. Antibiotics have no role in the therapy of tick paralysis.

58. D
Poison ivy, or Rhus contact dermatitis, is the most common form of contact dermatitis encountered by primary care physicians. This reaction occurs when the skin comes into contact with the sap from poison ivy or poison oak plants. Typically, hours to days later the patient will develop erythema and often vesiculation in the area of contact with the plant. The initial lesions are commonly linear resulting from the leaf or plant material tracking across the skin in what is typically incidental contact. The sap may then be spread from clothing or the original skin point of contact to other areas. The fluid within the vesicles will not spread poison ivy to other areas. Once the skin and clothing are washed, further spread should not occur. However, confusion may occur since not all lesions will appear at the same time and clothing such as shoes may be overlooked and not washed. Shoes that are not washable should be set aside in a ventilated area for 2 weeks to allow evaporation of the resin. For patients with extensive involvement, especially when the face is involved, oral steroids are commonly used. Oral steroids are not generally recommended for patients with limited disease, as in this patient. Topical steroids are recommended for patients with limited disease. Desensitization therapy is not available for poison ivy. Oral antihistamines are used to treat the itching and are used on an as-needed basis. Antibiotics would be warranted only in those cases with suspected secondary infection.

59. C
Exercise is of benefit to diabetic patients in a number of ways and should be encouraged. In addition to the cardiovascular and psychosocial benefits, exercise will improve peripheral utilization of glucose and may lead to a decrease in insulin needs. In well-controlled diabetics, hypoglycemia is a risk due to increased peripheral glucose utilization and insulin absorption associated with exercise. Although absorption of insulin may increase with injections at any site, in order to limit the effects of this increased absorption, injection should occur at a site not being actively exercised (i.e., in this patient, not the thighs or legs). The patient should monitor the glucose more frequently. He will likely need to take an additional carbohydrate exchange before exercise and should have glucose available during and after exercise. In many instances, the dose of insulin may need to be reduced on the day of exercise in order to avoid hypoglycemia. In contrast, patients who are poorly

controlled will have insufficient insulin to counteract the increased counterregulatory hormones present during exercise. In these individuals, hyperglycemia and ketoacidosis may result.

60. C

Obesity in adults and children has been increasing in prevalence in the United States. This has been accompanied by increases in some related health problems, such as early onset of type 2 diabetes mellitus. Many infants and toddlers appear overweight due to the relatively increased adipose tissue present in infants. As the child matures and becomes more active, the body composition changes and the child often appears less "chubby." Utilization of growth curves, including those developed for body mass index (Figure 2-3), can help in determining the appropriateness of a child's weight as well as height. This child is height and weight proportionate and falls within the growth chart at the 75th percentile. The parents can be reassured and should not alter his diet in any way. They should be encouraged to continue with whole milk and solid foods and educated about the benefits of healthy eating and exercise. The fact that the parents are of normal height and weight would place the child at lower risk for obesity. In addition, obesity in early childhood is not predictive of adult obesity. Hypothyroidism is unlikely given the normal growth and development of this child.

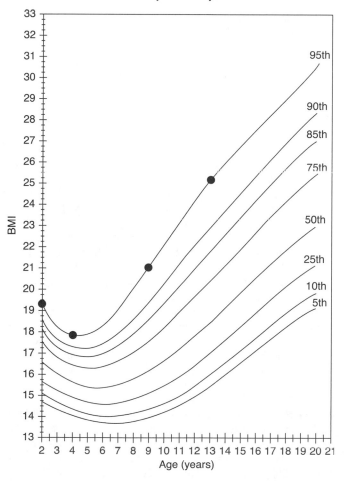

Boys: 2 to 20 years

Figure 2-3. Sample growth curve for body mass index. From www.cdc.gov.

61. C

The term developmental dysplasia of the hip (DDH) is used to encompass congenital dislocation, subluxation, and acetabular dysplasia of the hip. These conditions are often detectable at birth by performing Ortolani's or Barlow's maneuvers. However, some infants may have initially normal examinations and be found to have DDH months or even up to 1 or 2 years later. Thus, examination of the child's hip should be part of the physical examination during the first 2 years of life. To establish or confirm the diagnosis, standard x-ray and ultrasound may be helpful. The goal of therapy is to reseat the femoral head into the acetabulum until the capsular tissue has contracted and the acetabulum has developed to cover the femoral head. This requires placing the child's hip in abduction. Initially, the newborn may be double diapered. This therapy cannot be used beyond a few days since the child will gain increasing strength and tone. At this point, the adductor strength is too much for the diapering to be effective therapy and a device such as the Pavlik harness must be used. The later the age at which the DDH is detected, the longer the necessary time of therapy. If not detected until 18 to 24 months, then operative therapy will usually be needed.

62. D

Marfan's syndrome is a defect in the production of elastin that is inherited as an autosomal dominant trait with nearly complete penetrance. Marfan's syndrome affects 1 in 10,000 births. The diagnosis is made clinically by findings of skeletal, cardiovascular, and ocular abnormalities. Some of the findings are age dependent and thus diagnosis is frequently not made in the neonatal period but, rather, later in childhood. Findings suggestive of the diagnosis include tall stature with disproportionate increase in the distance from pubis to heel, arm span greater than height, long thin fingers, pectus excavatum, and ligamentous laxity as evidenced by hyperextensible joints. Complications associated with Marfan's include ocular lens dislocation, scoliosis, spontaneous pneumothorax, aortic root dilatation, and mitral valve prolapse. The life span of individuals with Marfan's is shortened due to cardiovascular complications. These individuals should have regular ophthalmologic and cardiovascular exams, including echocardiography as part of their follow-up.

63. E

Tetrology of Fallot is a congenital heart lesion associated with cyanosis as one of its features. Tetrology of Fallot consists of (a) right ventricular outflow obstruction, (b) ventricular septal defect, (c) dextroposition of the aorta with overriding of the aorta over the septum, and (d) right ventricular hypertrophy. Cyanosis occurs because venous blood that returns to the heart is shunted to the overriding aorta and into the systemic circulation because of the right ventricular outflow obstruction. The other lesions alone do not result in cyanosis. Pulmonic stenosis generally presents with right-sided heart failure. In the newborn with severe pulmonic stenosis and a patent foramen ovale, cyanosis may occur. Atrial septal defect, ventricular septal defect, and patent ductus arteriosis cause shunting of blood from left to right, with already oxygenated blood returning to the pulmonary circulation.

64. E

Jaundice occurs in 60% or more of term infants and 80% of preterm infants. Hyperbilirubinemia occurs in virtually all newborns during the second to fourth day of life. This is termed physiologic jaundice and is most likely due to a combination of increased red blood cell turnover and immaturity of hepatic metabolism. Evaluation of nonphysiologic causes of hyperbilirubinemia should be considered for those infants who develop jaundice in the first 24 hours of life, who have increases in bilirubin of more than 5 mg/dL/24 hours, and for those with persistent jaundice. Values of bilirubin over 25 mg/dL are associated with kernicterus. As the values approach these levels, intervention such as phototherapy is generally recommended. Breast-fed infants have higher bilirubin levels associated with physiologic jaundice and should be fed frequently to avoid significantly elevated levels. True breast milk jaundice begins at approximately 7 days of life and is caused by an as yet unidentified protein. Cessation of breast-feeding results in a prompt decrease in bilirubin values. Breast-feeding may then be resumed without further increases in bilirubin.

65. C

Pinworm infestation is caused by the organism *Enterobius vermicularis*. It is the most common parasitic nematode in the United States. The infestation occurs when eggs are ingested and then pass to the small intestine, where they hatch and then migrate to the colon. Female pinworms lay their eggs on the perianal skin at night. An allergic response to nematode proteins may trigger itching, which then leads to perianal scratching and autoinfection or transmission of the eggs to others. In addition, the eggs may survive in clothing, bedding, and in house dust for up to 2 weeks. Diagnosis of pinworm infection may occur through visual identification of the worm (1 cm and threadlike) in the stool or perianal area or by the "Scotch tape" test. The Scotch tape test is performed by applying Scotch tape to the perianal area in the morning before passing stool or bathing. The tape is then applied to a slide and viewed under a microscope to identify eggs. Repeated testing increases sensitivity. Treatment requires use of medications effective against nematode parasites and the current preferred agents are mebendazole or pyrantel pamoate. Pyrantel pamoate is available as an oral suspension that is dosed according to weight. Mebendazole is available as a chewable tablet and the same dose is used for all patients. Re-treatment 2 weeks after the initial dose is recommended to destroy any surviving pinworms that hatched following the first dose. In addition, family members should also be treated and clothing and bedding should be washed in hot water to prevent reinfection. The other choices listed are antibiotics effective against a variety of bacteria.

66. D

Clavicular fractures are the most common fractures occurring during childbirth, representing more than 90% of fractures that occur. Infants will typically present either without signs or symptoms or with limited movement and use of the affected extremity. In some instances, the fracture is not discovered until a bony callus is identified signifying healing of the clavicle. Treatment involves immobilization for approximately 2 weeks, commonly by pinning the affected arm sleeve to the shirt, creating a sling type of effect. Affected infants do not seem to experience significant pain and do not exhibit excessive crying. If noted, other causes of crying or respiratory symptoms should be sought. Internal rotation and lack of use of an extremity occur with Erb's palsy, a brachial plexus injury that can occur with stretching and injury to the brachial plexus during difficult births.

67. A

Secondary sexual characteristics normally develop in males between the ages of 9 and 14 years. Onset of sexual development occurs earlier in girls, between ages 8 and 13 years. The initial sign of onset in boys is testicular enlargement, and in girls it is breast bud development. In boys, following testicular enlargement, the penis increases in size; pubic, axillary, and facial hair develop; and then growth accelerates. In girls, after development of breast buds, they develop sexual hair, have accelerated growth, and then have menarche. Menarche generally occurs 2 to 2.5 years after onset of breast development. Delayed onset of puberty is present if there is no breast budding in girls by age 13 or no testicular enlargement in boys by age 14 years. See Table 2.10.

68. C

Nursemaid's elbow is the most common upper extremity injury in children younger than 6 years of age. Nursemaid's elbow is a subluxation of the radial head that occurs when a child is swung or pulled by the extended and pronated arm. The injury is most common in children 2 or 3 years of age. The typical presentation is that of a child who holds the arm at the side, lightly flexed and pronated. The child will not use the arm and may be resistant to movement of the arm. With the appropriate history and absence of significant tenderness, swelling, or ecchymosis, x-rays are unnecessary and reduction of the subluxation may be attempted. Following reduction, the child will usually use and move the arm painlessly within minutes. In cases with significant swelling, ecchymosis, or persisting symptoms after reduction attempts, x-rays should be obtained. Colles' fracture is a fracture of the distal radius that occurs with falling and attempting to break the fall with the outstretched hand. An occult fracture of the radial head is certainly a possibility but would be less likely than nursemaid's elbow. Dislocation of the shoulder occurs most commonly in adolescents and older individuals and is uncommon at younger ages. The history and location of the tenderness that is typical of nursemaid's elbow make attention-seeking behavior unlikely in this case.

69. E

Therapy for sinusitis should be directed at the most common respiratory pathogens, namely *Streptococcus pneumoniae*, *Haemophilus influenzae*, and *Moraxella catarrhalis*. Amoxicillin is the most reasonable first-line agent in individuals who have not had chronic or recurrent symptoms. Those who have had persistent or recurrent symptoms may be more likely to be infected with resistant organisms and thus may benefit from treatment with amoxicillin-clavulanic acid or a second- or third-generation cephalosporin. Fluoroquinolones are contraindicated in children younger than 18 years of age due to their effects on growing cartilage and the potential for causing arthropathies in those exposed. Tetracyclines can have adverse reactions on the dentition of children younger than age 8 years and thus should be avoided. Erythromycin and cephalexin do not have the spectrum of coverage for the organisms that cause sinusitis. For a child allergic to penicillin, an extended spectrum macrolide, such as azithromycin, or trimethoprim-sulfamethoxazole are alternative first-line medications.

70. A

Positive reinforcement is the provision of some form of reward for a behavior. The behavior itself may be positive or negative, and the positive reinforcement will reward and encourage repetition of the behavior. Many parents mistakenly reinforce unwanted behavior by providing positive reinforcement. For example, if a child is misbehaving in the doctor's office and the mother gives him cookies to quiet him, then this is positive reinforcement. This rewards the misbehavior. Spanking children should not be encouraged and is a

Table 2.10 Secondary sex characteristics: Tanner

Breast Development

Stage I	Preadolescent; elevation of papilla only
Stage II	Breast bud; elevation of breast and papilla as small mound; enlargement of areolar diameter (11.15 ± 1.10)
Stage III	Further enlargement and elevation of breast and areola; no separation of their contours (12.15 ± 1.09)
Stage IV	Projection of areola and papilla to form secondary mound above level of breast (13.11 ±1.15)
Stage V	Mature stage; projection of papilla only due to recession of areola to general contour of breast (15.33 ± 1.74)

Note: Stages IV and V may not be distinct in some patients.

Genital Development (Male)

Stage I	Preadolescent; testes, scrotum, and penis about same size and proportion as in early childhood
Stage II	Enlargement of scrotum and testes, skin of scrotum reddens and changes in texture; little or no enlargement of penis (11.64 ±1.07)
Stage III	Enlargement of penis, first mainly in length; further growth of testes and scrotum (12.85 ± 1.04)
Stage IV	Increased size of penis with growth in breadth and development of glans; further enlargement of testes and scrotum and increased darkening of scrotal skin (13.77 ± 1.02)
Stage V	Genitalia adult in size and shape (14.92 ±1.10)

Pubic Hair (Male and Female)

Stage I	Preadolescent; vellus over pubes no further developed than that over abdominal wall (i.e., no pubic hair)
Stage II	Sparse growth of long, slightly pigmented downy hair, straight or only slightly curled, chiefly at base of penis or along labia (Male: 13.44 ± 1.09; Female: 11.69 ± 1.21)
Stage III	Considerably darker, coarser and more curled; hair spreads sparsely over junction of pubes (Male: 13.9 ± 1.04; Female: 12.36 ±1.10)
Stage IV	Hair resembles adult in type; distribution still considerably smaller than in adult. No spread to medial surface of thighs (Male: 14.36 ± 1.08; Female: 12.95 ±1.06)
Stage V	Adult in quantity and type with distribution of the horizontal pattern (Male: 15.18 ± 1.07; Female: 14.41 ± 1:12)
Stage VI	Spread up linea alba: "male escutcheon"

form of negative reinforcement. A recommended form of negative reinforcement is the use of time-out for undesirable behavior. In this case, the child is placed in his or her time-out location for a few minutes and then receives no attention as a result of the undesired behavior. Ignoring the child's behavior may, in some instances, serve the same purpose as a time-out. However, in general, in order to lessen undesired behaviors, they need to be acknowledged consistently with negative reinforcement (along with provision of positive reinforcement of positive behaviors).

71. D

This child has an acute diarrheal disease and no signs of dehydration are noted. The most likely etiologic agents responsible for these types of illness are self-limited viral infection. In well-hydrated children and after rehydration in mild-moderately dehydrated children, recommendations are to provide the usual age-appropriate diet, including lactose-containing foods. The children should be monitored for signs of malabsorption, such as worsening or persisting diarrhea. In children who are unlikely to be monitored, who have had lactose intolerance in the past, or who are malnourished, a reduced-lactose or lactose-free diet should be provided. There is no role for antibiotics in the patient described. If the diarrhea persists, or the nature of the stools changes, then re-evaluation including stool examination and culture should be performed. A differential diagnosis for diarrhea in children is presented in Table 2.11. Loperamide use is discouraged in those with acute diarrhea but may be used for convenience and symptom management in some cases of chronic diarrhea. Although increased clear liquid intake should be encouraged to replace and maintain hydration, this should not be the only nutrition provided. Data from various studies indicate that

Table 2.11 Differential diagnosis of diarrhea in children

Acute Diarrhea	Chronic Diarrhea
Intraintestinal Infections	**Renal**
Viral gastroenteritis	Hemolytic uremic
Rotavirus	syndrome
Enterovirus	
Adenovirus	**Vasculitis**
Norwalk agent	Henoch–Schönlein *purpura*
Bacterial enterocolitis	
Shigella	**Infectious**
Salmonella	Parasites
Yersinia	Amoebiasis
Campylobacter	Giardiasis
Escherichia coli	*Cryptosporidium*
(enteroinvasive/	
enteropathogenic)	**Gastrointestinal**
Clostridium difficile	Cow/soy milk intolerance
Neisseria gonorrhoeae	Overfeeding
Chlamydia Trachomatis	Ulcerative colitis
	Crohn disease
Extraintestinal infections	Hirschsprung disease
Otitis media	Lactase deficiency
Urinary tract infection	Irritable bowel disease
	Encopresis
	Excessive fructose intake
Gastrointestinal	Cystic fibrosis
Intussusception	Celiac sprue
Appendicitis	
Hyperconcentrated	
infant formula	**Allergy**
Cystic fibrosis	Food allergies
Toxic ingestion	
Iron, mercury, lead,	
fluoride ingestion	
Medication induced	
Any antibiotic,	
chemotherapeutic agents	

early feedings are beneficial in reducing stool output and hastening recovery. Antispasmodic agents, such as dicyclomine, are indicated for irritable bowel syndrome but would play no role in this acute viral gastroenteritis.

72. B
Permethrin is a very effective and very safe topical therapy used for patients of all ages who are diagnosed with scabies. It is applied topically from the neck down and left on for approximately 12 hours. Lindane may also be used in older children but has fallen into disfavor in infants due to the potential for neurotoxicity. It is applied and left on the body in a manner similar to permethrin. Effectiveness is essentially equivalent to that of permethrin.

Other agents that may be used include topical sulfur preparations and oral ivermectin. The topical sulfur is compounded in petrolatum, has an unpleasant odor, and must be left on for 24 hours for 3 consecutive days of therapy. Ivermectin is available only for adult use. Mebendazole is an oral agent used to treat pinworms, and mefloquine is an antimalarial. Another important aspect of treatment is prevention of reinfection. Reinfection may occur from other family members or contaminated clothing or bedding. Family members should also be treated for scabies. To prevent reinfection by clothing or bedding, these items should be washed in hot water, which kills the scabies mite.

73. A
This child is experiencing a local reaction to a hymenoptera or bee sting. This is a reaction to the venom and is not an allergic reaction that requires any treatment other than symptomatic therapy. Antihistamines may help with the itching and local application of ice or cold compresses may limit pain and swelling, especially if applied soon after the sting occurs. Antibiotics are not necessary since this is not an infectious process. Subcutaneous epinephrine, oral steroids, and hospitalization would only be warranted for suspected systemic allergic reaction to the sting. Manifestations that should raise this suspicion include pruritis and swelling distant from the site of the sting, urticaria, angioedema, and signs or symptoms of respiratory obstruction, laryngeal edema, or bronchospasm. Often, these reactions develop within minutes of the sting.

74. D
Duodenal atresia is a failure in canalization of the lumen of the duodenum. Thus, there is a very proximal small bowel obstruction that will present within the first day of life with bilious vomiting associated with a nondistended abdomen. X-ray findings supporting the diagnosis are the finding of the "double-bubble" sign representing distention and air in the stomach and proximal duodenum. The distal duodenum and the remainder of the bowel are devoid of gas. Normally, there is evidence of gas within the small intestines and colon by 1 to 3 hours of age. Children with duodenal atresia must be evaluated thoroughly for associated anomalies. Nasogastric suction, provision of intravenous fluids, and surgery are required for survival. Volvulus can present at any time in life and will have findings consistent with a bowel obstruction, including abdominal distention. Pyloric stenosis generally presents between 3 weeks and 5 months of age with projectile nonbilious vomiting after eating. The infant has a voracious appetite but, because of the vomiting, will lose weight and become dehydrated if not diagnosed and treated. Tracheoesophageal fistula (TEF) is a connection between the esophagus and trachea that may take one of several forms. This condition should be suspected when attempts to pass a gastric tube are unsuccessful, when eating is associated with coughing, when there are excess oral secretions, and when the pregnancy is complicated by polyhydramnios. TEF is associated with other anomalies and the VACTERAL syndrome—vertebral, anorectal, cardiac, tracheoesophageal, renal, radial, and limb anomalies. Intussusception occurs most commonly in infants 6 to 12 months of age. Intussusception is an infolding of the intestine within itself resulting in colicky abdominal pain, vomiting, and the passing of bloody stools often described as currant jelly-like.

75. D
The lesion described is a natal tooth, which occurs in approximately 1 in 300 children. Natal teeth are present at the time of birth and most commonly represent premature eruption of a

primary tooth. Most commonly, they occur in the mandibular central incisor location. Natal teeth may be loose due to poorly developed roots. Dental x-rays should be performed to assess whether the natal tooth represents a supernumerary tooth. Natal teeth require no special care except cleaning unless they are loose, causing pain in the breast-feeding mother or child, or supernumerary. Loose teeth may represent a risk of aspiration and thus should be removed. Painful teeth likewise can be removed. Supernumerary teeth that are left in place will lead to crowding when the primary teeth erupt. On the other hand, removal of a primary natal tooth may lead to shifting of the remaining primary teeth, which can lead to misalignment and crowding when the permanent teeth erupt. Nystatin would have no effect on a natal tooth.

76. B

Most nosebleeds that occur in children are anterior nosebleeds resulting from inflammation in Kiesselbach's plexus on the anterior nasal septum. The inflammation most commonly results from nose picking or in association with upper respiratory infections. Allergic rhinitis, other forms of trauma, foreign bodies, bleeding disorders, blood vessel disorders (e.g., Osler–Weber–Rendu syndrome), and tumors are other potential causes for nosebleeds, but they occur much less commonly. Most children with nosebleeds require no evaluation other than obtaining a history and physical examination. Those with a history of recurrent nosebleeds, severe or prolonged nosebleeds, or with other areas of bleeding or bruising may warrant evaluation of hemoglobin and coagulation studies. Therapy for nosebleeds generally involves measures to treat the associated dryness that is present with antibiotic ointments, saline nasal sprays, and humidifiers. Persistent or recurrent nosebleeds may warrant referral for ENT evaluation.

77. C

Strabismus in children may take one of several forms and up to 75% of normal children will have transient neonatal strabismus that resolves with CNS maturity during the first 3 months of life. Up to 3% of children will have other forms of strabismus that require intervention. In this latter group, up to 50% have a family history of strabismus. Most cases are nonparalytic in nature, due to infantile esotropia or exotropia, cataracts, or refractive errors. Identification of the child with strabismus involves screening by performing the corneal light reflex test or cover–uncover test. The corneal light reflex test involves shining a penlight toward the eyes and noting the location of the light reflex on the cornea. Normally, the light shines on the same location in each eye. If this does not occur, then deviation of one eye is present. The cover–uncover test involves having the patient focus on an object and covering an eye and then the other. Normally, when an eye is uncovered, it is focused on the object. An abnormal response is found when the eye must refocus to find the object. Children with suspected strabismus should be referred for ophthalmologic evaluation to detect underlying conditions and to prevent the permanent visual loss (ambylopia) that can occur with untreated disease.

78. B

Strabismus is a misalignment of the eyes that results in dysconjugate gaze and is not associated with excessive tearing. Ambylopia is the visual loss that can occur as a result of strabismus or other conditions leading to nonuse of the affected eye. Congenital cataracts are opacities of the lens that compromise vision and warrant ophthalmologic evaluation and referral as well as assessment for any associated anomalies. Subconjunctival hemorrhage is a benign and self-limited condition occurring as a result of the birth process. Congenital glaucoma refers to an increase in intraocular pressures, generally from abnormalities in the iridocorneal angle that prevent normal flow of aqueous humor. The resultant pressure causes breakdown and irritation of the corneal epithelium, which lead to excessive tearing. Surgery is commonly required for treatment and urgent ophthalmologic consultation should be obtained to prevent optic nerve damage and visual loss.

79. D

Lead poisoning is one of the causes of hypochromic microcytic anemia. Other causes include iron deficiency, thallasemia, and anemia of chronic disease. G6PD deficiency and sickle cell anemia cause anemia due to intrinsic RBC defects and are associated with normochromic, normocytic anemia. Folate deficiency and vitamin B12 deficiency are common causes for hyperchromic, macrocytic anemia. See Table 2.12.

80. A

In children who appear well and have a normal physical examination, laboratory confirmation should be performed to document the anemia. Following this, a therapeutic trial of iron is recommended as initial therapy for suspected iron deficiency anemia. Iron is administered at 6 mg/kg/day divided into two doses and response to therapy should be evident within 1 week. A multivitamin with iron would provide insufficient iron to correct iron deficiency. Evidence of response should be monitored by checking for a reticulocytosis and increase in hemoglobin in response to the iron therapy. Common historical factors that suggest insufficient dietary iron intake are excessive milk intake as well as little or no meat consumption. In children with anemia refractory to therapy, as evidenced by no reticulocyte response, bone marrow evaluation may be warranted. Blood transfusion should be reserved for those with aplastic anemia, evidence of cardiovascular compromise, or severe anemia along with ongoing blood loss. Endoscopic evaluation should be undertaken in those with evidence of blood loss (i.e., heme positive stools and increased reticulocyte count).

81. B

Classic hemophilia is an X-linked hereditary disorder that results in a deficiency of factor VIII. It is the most commonly diagnosed factor deficiency and results in the finding of a prolonged partial thromboplastin time. Affected children often present with multiple ecchymoses, oral or nasal bleeding, and bleeding into joints. Life-threatening bleeding, such as CNS or retroperitoneal bleeding, may also occur. Von Willebrand's disease is a related disorder that is also genetically transmitted. Von Willebrand's disease is a deficiency of von Willebrand factor (vWF), which is responsible for effective platelet adherence to damaged endothelium. It also serves as a carrier for factor VIII. Thus, deficiency of vWF may result in prolongation of the bleeding time as well as the partial thromboplastin time. Henoch-Schoenlein purpura is a vasculitis that does not affect coagulation times. Idiopathic thrombocytopenic purpura is an autoimmune platelet destruction that will prolong bleeding times. Glanzmann's disease is a receptor defect on platelets that results in altered platelet aggregation and prolongation of the bleeding time. G6PD deficiency is an inherited red blood cell enzymatic defect making the RBCs more susceptible to oxidative stress.

Table 2.12 Differential diagnosis of common anemias defined by mean corpuscular volume

Anemia	Differential Diagnosis
Microcytic anemias	Iron deficiency
	Severe lead poisoning
	Thalassemia syndromes
	Sideroblastic anemia
	Chronic disease
Macrocytic Anemias	
Megaloblastic	Vitamin B_{12} deficiency
	Folate deficiency
	Orotic aciduria
Nonmegaloblastic	Aplastic anemia
	Diamond–Blackfan anemia
	Bone marrow infiltration
	Hypothyroidism
	Fanconi anemia
	Liver disease
Inherited hemolytic anemias	Abnormal hemoglobins
	Sickle cell disease
	Thalassemia
	Red blood cell enzyme disorders
	G6PD deficiency
	Pyruvate kinase deficiency
	Red blood cell membrane disorders
	Hereditary spherocytosis, elliptocytosis
Acquired hemolytic anemias	Antibody-mediated anemias
	Autoimmune hemolytic anemias
	Isoimmune hemolytic anemias
	Microangiopathic hemolytic anemias
	Hemolytic uremic syndrome
	Disseminated intravascular coagulation
	Paroxysmal nocturnal hemoglobinuria
Normocytic Anemias	
Chronic inflammation[a]	
Acute blood loss	
Splenic sequestration	
Transient erythroblastopenia of childhood	
Chronic renal disease	

[a]Seventy-five percent of anemias of chronic illness are normocytic; 25% are microcytic.

82. B
Ambiguous genitalia occurs in 1 in 3,000 births and may be due to one of several causes. Female pseudohermaphrodism is the most common disorder and is often due to congenital adrenal hyperplasia. Other causes for ambiguous genitalia include androgen insensitivity, true hermaphrodism, and mixed gonadal dysgenesis. When ambiguous genitalia are present, the parents will often be aware and this finding should be discussed with them. Genetic testing and laboratory evaluation should be promptly performed so that answers can be provided to the parents and so that a gender can be assigned and a name given. Initial testing should include determination of the karyotype, serum electrolytes, and screening for congenital adrenal hyperplasia by measurement of serum 17-hydroxyprogesterone and urinary 17-ketosteroids and pregnanetriol. Very often, results can be obtained within 48 hours. If the initial tests are inconclusive, then further testing is warranted.

83. E
Urinary tract infections are common in infants and children. Bacteruria occurs in 1% to 2% of newborns, infants, and girls. After infancy, bacteruria is uncommon in males. The most common organism isolated in the urine of individuals with urinary tract infections is *Escherichia coli*, which is present in up to 80% of cases. Other organisms that may cause urinary tract infections include *Proteus mirabilis*, *Klebsiella*, *Enterobacter*, enterococci, and *Staphylococcus saprophyticus*. *Moraxella catarrhalis*, *Haemophilus influenzae*, and *Staphylococcus aureus* are not common urinary pathogens.

84. C
Clubfoot is present and recognizable at birth, whereas the other conditions listed as options usually do not present until later in childhood. The constellation of findings that cause the clubfoot deformity are forefoot varus, heel varus, and ankle equines. Untreated, clubfoot will result in permanent deformity and disability. Treatment generally begins at birth with manipulation and serial casting. Surgery is ultimately required in three-fourths of infants.

85. B
During normal childhood development, the lower extremities will have a normal sequence of angular alignment. For example, from birth through approximately age 2 years, the tibia and femur show a slight varus alignment such that varus deformity may be present. From ages 3 through 7 years, the lower extremities have a valgus alignment that may persist into adulthood. These normal variants are referred to as physiologic bowing and physiologic knock-knees. A distinguishing feature of physiologic variants and pathologic conditions is that physiologic changes occur at the previously noted ages and the femur and tibia are involved. Pathologic angular deformities may occur at other ages, and the deformity does not involve both the femur and the tibia and is asymmetric. Blount's disease is the most common cause for pathologic bowing of the legs and is most commonly seen in children 1 to 3 years of age. It occurs most commonly in overweight children who walk at an early age. A growth disturbance involving the proximal tibial epiphysis results in a sharp angulation at the proximal tibia. Rickets is less common and may cause either pathologic bowing or knock-knees depending on the age and physiologic angulation of the legs at the time the process develops. Rheumatoid arthritis is associated with knock-knees in older children, and achondroplasia is a rare condition

that may cause bowlegs. Slipped capital femoral epiphysis typically affects adolescents and is a separation of the proximal femoral growth plate resulting in external rotation of the femur and limb shortening (Figure 2-4).

86. A

Growing pains is the term used to describe idiopathic leg pains that affect up to 15% to 30% of children between the ages of 3 and 12 years. The exact etiology is unclear. The history is typical and includes the development of intermittent nocturnal leg pains and restlessness that may awaken the child from sleep. The pains may occur in the calves or thighs but spare the joints. The pain is brief and the children then usually go back to sleep. Daytime activities are unaffected and the physical examination is normal. In children with the classic symptoms, as well as normal growth, development, and physical examination, advice recommending supportive measures, such as application of heat and massage, may be helpful. Laboratory or x-ray evaluation is not indicated in these instances. X-ray, laboratory testing, or orthopedic referral may be indicated in children with limitations in activity, joint involvement, prior trauma, or abnormal growth, development, or physical examination.

87. C

Legg–Calvé–Perthes disease is an avascular necrosis of the femoral head that develops for unknown reasons. It most commonly affects children ages 4 to 8 years and boys more often than girls (5:1). Early in the disease, there may be pain with movement, particularly internal rotation and abduction. Following resolution of the synovitis that is present early on, the child will have a painless limp. Early in the disease, both x-ray and bone scan findings may be normal. However, subsequent bone scans will show decreased uptake, indicating decreased blood flow, in the affected femoral head. Plain x-rays of the hip will subsequently show patchy areas of radiolucency and density followed by flattening of the femoral head. White blood cell counts and sedimentation rates would be expected to be normal with this disease. Treatment involves orthopedic consultation and immobilization of the affected hip to maintain the femoral head in the acetabulum in an effort to maintain normal contour of the femoral head. Prognosis is good for children affected prior to age 6 and worse for those diagnosed after age 8 years. Legg–Calvé–Perthes disease increases the risk for subsequent development of osteoarthritis of the hip, often at an early age (i.e., 40 to 50 years).

88. B

In children with open epiphyses (growth plates) who present with an injury in the region of a growth plate, injury to the growth plate should be suspected. In the growing musculoskeletal system, the epiphysis is structurally the weakest point. Fractures that involve the growth plates have been defined using the Salter–Harris classification. Because of the radiolucency of the epiphysis, many Salter-Harris fractures may occur without radiologic findings. Inability to bear weight, along with bone tenderness and open epiphyses, suggests that a fracture is the most likely injury in this child. Sprains may also occur in children; however, severe sprains are uncommon because the epiphysis is more likely to give way first. Stress fractures occur as a result of repetitive microtrauma. Osteomyelitis is a bone infection and would not occur acutely in association with a soccer injury. Osteosarcoma is a malignant bone disease and also would not be a result of this acute injury.

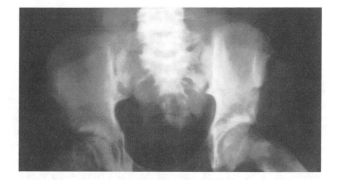

Figure 2-4. *Radiograph of a slipped capital femoral epiphysis. Frog-leg view in this 13-year-old boy demonstrates increased radiolucency of the left femoral epiphysis with medial and perhaps posterior angulation of the femoral head on the neck.*

89. B

The chickenpox virus is a member of the herpesvirus family. In normal adults and children, the disease is associated with a fever and diffuse vesicular rash. However, infection at susceptible times in utero or in the neonatal period may lead to either congenital varicella or overwhelming infection and possibly death. Maternal infection and transfer of the virus to the infant in the first trimester may lead to varicella embryopathy (congenital varicella). Infants can have abnormalities of the limbs, CNS, and eyes, as well as scarring of the skin. During the second trimester, an inapparent infection may occur. If the mother contracts the disease more than 5 days prior to delivery, then maternal antibody is formed and transferred to the infant and confers protection. Maternal infection less than 5 days before or 2 days after delivery results in lack of antibody transfer to the infant along with a significant viral exposure that may result in overwhelming neonatal infection and death. Treatment recommendations are to provide the infant with varicella immunoglobulin (VZIG). In the absence of active infection, acyclovir is not indicated. The varicella vaccine is recommended for children after the age of 12 months.

90. A

Migraine headaches are the most frequent type of headache encountered in the pediatric population. They are associated with a positive family history of migraine headaches and occur in 4% of children between the ages of 7 and 15 years. Migraine headaches increase in prevalence with increasing age, and up to 15% to 20% of adult women suffer from migraine headaches. In adolescence and adulthood, women are affected more commonly. At younger ages, boys are more commonly affected. Sumatriptan is indicated for use in individuals older than the age of 18 years. Narcotics should be avoided as treatment for migraines. Effective therapies for children include nonnarcotic analgesics and antiemetics for acute attacks, and beta-blockers, calcium channel blockers, tricyclic antidepressants, cyproheptadine, and topiramate as prophylactic therapies.

91. D

Hepatitis B can be transmitted perinatally from mother to infant. Up to 90% of those infected will develop chronic hepatitis B. Administration of hepatitis B immunoglobulin and hepatitis B vaccine within 12 hours of birth can prevent transmission in up to 95% of infants exposed. Completion of the vaccine schedule should then occur as recommended for all infants. Neither the infant nor the mother needs to be isolated. Universal precautions should be practiced to prevent potential exposure to the virus.

92. C

These findings are most consistent with muscular dystrophy. Of the muscular dystrophies, Duchenne and Becker muscular dystrophies are most common. These diseases are transmitted as X-linked recessive hereditary diseases and affect approximately 1 in 3,500 boys. They manifest as onset of proximal muscle weakness in the toddler years. Children may exhibit a lordotic posture and a positive Gower's sign. Gower's sign is when the child must use the upper extremities and a tripod-type position in order to move from sitting on the floor to standing. This occurs due to proximal muscle weakness, which also leads to development of the Trendelenburg gait. These diseases are associated with progressive muscular weakness, cardiomyopathy, and premature death. The diagnosis may be suggested by EMG and elevated CPK levels, but to be definitively diagnosed muscle biopsy must be performed. MRI, electroencephalogram, hip x-rays, and erythrocyte sedimentation rate would not be helpful in diagnosing muscular dystrophy.

93. E

Ninety percent of children with nephrotic range proteinuria have idiopathic nephrotic syndrome. Of those with idiopathic nephrotic syndrome, 85% have minimal change disease. Boys are affected more commonly. These children will present between the ages of 2 and 6 years with edema. On evaluation, they are found to have significant proteinuria and may also have evidence of hematuria. In children without significant pleural effusions or ascites, outpatient therapy may be initiated without renal biopsy. Prednisone is the cornerstone of therapy along with dietary modification to regulate sodium intake. Diuretics may also be of benefit in managing this disease. Following steroid treatment, the child may go into remission, as evidenced by the absence of proteinuria. Steroids are then tapered over approximately 6 months. For those not responding to steroids, re-evaluation should be pursued and alternative medications, such as cyclophosphamide,

Table 2.13 Causes of nephrotic syndrome

Primary
Minimal change disease
Focal segmental glomerulosclerosis
Membranoproliferative glomerulonephritis
Membranous glomerulonephritis
Secondary
Acute viral illness
Alport's syndrome
Bacterial endocarditis
Congestive heart failure
Hemolytic–uremic syndrome
Hypertension
Medications
Postinfectious glomerulonephritis
Systemic lupus erythematosis

may be considered. Long-term prognosis for those responding to steroids is good, with resolution of the disease by age 20 and normal renal function. Causes for nephrotic syndrome are listed in Table 2.13.

94. B

Gastroesophageal reflux is common in infancy, occurring in up to 20% of infants. The condition may be physiologic or pathologic. Physiologic gastroesophageal reflux is characterized by brief, asymptomatic, and self-limited episodes. Pathologic gastroesophageal reflux is persistent and symptomatic. Symptoms may include respiratory difficulty, decreased feeding, anemia, and weight loss. Pathologic reflux is found more commonly in children with neurologic disease and is more common in male infants. Evaluation of children with suspected pathologic reflux may include esophagogastroduodenoscopy, upper GI series, and pH monitoring. Therapy may include optimal positioning of the infant with the head elevated 30 degrees, thickened feedings, and H2 blockers. Changing to a soy-based formula would be of no benefit. The child presented has no signs or symptoms suggestive of pathologic reflux, and observation would be recommended. At least 80% of infantile reflux will resolve by 18 months of age.

95. C

Febrile seizures affect up to 5% of children and in most cases are idiopathic, associated with no significant underlying neurologic or systemic disorders. Febrile seizures occur rarely before 9 months of age or after 5 years of age. The peak occurrence is between 14 and 18 months of age. Febrile seizures are often familial and are associated with a rapid rise in temperature. Evaluation, such as CT scans or EEG testing, is warranted if atypical features are present or abnormalities are identified on examination. Atypical features include seizures lasting longer than 15 minutes, focal seizures, and recurrent seizures. The future risk of developing epilepsy is 1% in those with typical febrile seizures and increases to 9% in those with atypical features or when febrile seizures occur in children younger than 9 months of age. Treatment is directed at minimizing the rate of temperature rise through use of antipyretics with onset of illness. Thus, acetaminophen and/or ibuprofen are the recommended treatments. Chronic phenytoin use or phenobarbital at onset of illness would not be beneficial or indicated in this case.

96. A

Henoch-Schoenlein purpura (HSP) is an immune complex vasculitis affecting the small blood vessels that has no identifiable underlying causative factor. It commonly develops following an upper respiratory infection in children between the ages of 2 and 8 years. Males are affected more often than females. The disease manifests itself as low-grade fever and fatigue in association with a rash that initially is pink and maculopapular but subsequently develops into petechiae and purpura. The rash may appear in crops every 3 to 10 days over as long as a 3-month period. Arthritis is present in up to two-thirds of patients with joint effusions, most commonly in the knees and ankles. Laboratory findings consistent with HSP are mild anemia; elevated platelet count, white blood cell count, and sedimentation rate; and the presence of immune complexes. Gastrointestinal complications include development of mucosal edema, abdominal pain, hemoccult positive stools, diarrhea, and intussusception. Renal involvement occurs in 25% to 50% of patients and manifests as hematuria, pyuria, and proteinuria. Severe renal impairment may occur in 1% of patients, and 0.1% may have chronic renal impairment as a result. Seizures are a rare occurrence. The disease is self-limited and the overall prognosis is excellent. Most patients only require supportive care and monitoring for complications. Patients with gastrointestinal complications may benefit from treatment with corticosteroids.

97. D

Up to 60% of term newborns will have clinical jaundice in the first week of life. Hyperbilirubinemia can be associated with underlying illness and thus should be evaluated. Significantly elevated bilirubin levels are associated with kernicterus and the associated neurologic complications of cerebral palsy, retardation, and hearing loss. Physical examination may identify jaundice but is not reliable in predicting bilirubin levels. After completing a history and physical examination, assessment often includes determination of the serum bilirubin. In term healthy newborns without risk factors, this value is usually less than 12 mg/dL. Risk factors for developing hyperbilirubinemia include maternal–child blood type incompatibility, breast-feeding, medications, prematurity, infections, and birth trauma. Following determination of the bilirubin value, further evaluation may include fractionating the bilirubin into direct and indirect fractions, hemoglobin determination, and evaluating for hemolysis, infection, and other underlying causes. Prior to altering the diet or hospitalization, the bilirubin level should be determined. Normal values are determined based on age. Phototherapy and exchange transfusion are the two principal therapeutic modalities. Phototherapy may be used in infants younger than 48 hours of age as bilirubin values exceed 12 mg/dL and in older children with values over 15 mg/dL. Exchange transfusion is used if phototherapy fails or for values over 25 mg/dL in infants younger than 48 hours of age or values over 30 mg/dL in older infants. See Figure 2-5.

98. E

Acetaminophen is associated with hepatic toxicity and overdose may result in hepatic injury and failure. The risk for developing hepatic injury depends on the amount ingested. In children, ingestion of more than 75 to 150 mg/kg is of concern and requires emergent assessment and possibly treatment. Adults ingesting more than 4 g in association with chronic alcohol use, malnourishment, or concomitant medications affecting acetaminophen metabolism are at risk. Ingestion of more than 7.5 g per 24-hour period in otherwise well adults places the patient at risk. Assessment of the patient presenting with acetaminophen overdose involves checking a serum drug level and hepatic enzymes. Elevation of either places the patient at higher risk. Treatment of acetaminophen overdose to avert hepatic injury involves use of activated charcoal immediately and a series of doses of oral N-acetylcysteine initiated within 8 hours of ingestion.

99. B

Galactosemia results from an autosomal recessive disorder of galactose metabolism that results in accumulation of galactose in the blood and tissues. Lactose, the main sugar present in milk, is made up of glucose and galactose. Infants with galactosemia will present with symptoms within a few days after initiating a milk-containing diet. Symptoms that may occur include failure to thrive, vomiting, diarrhea, jaundice, and organomegaly. Untreated, cataracts may develop within several weeks and mental retardation may occur in up to one-third of patients. Screening for galactosemia

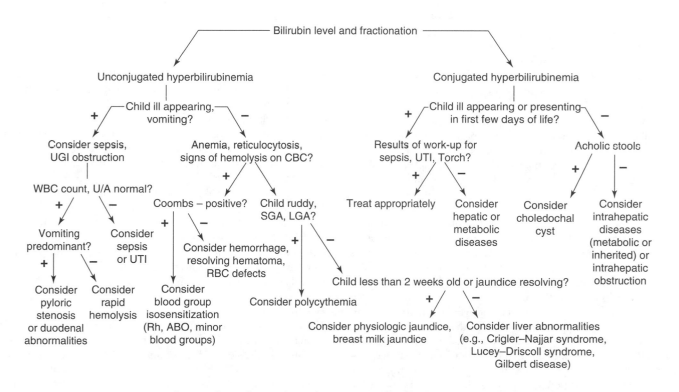

Figure 2-5. *Evaluation of a newborn with jaundice. CBC, complete blood cell count; LGA, large for gestational age; RBC, red blood cell; SGA, small for gestational age; TORCH, toxoplasmosis, other (congenital syphilis and viruses), rubella, cytomegalovirus, and herpes simplex virus; U/A, urinalysis; UGI, upper gastrointestinal; UTI, urinary tract infection; WBC, white blood cell.*

occurs by measurement of serum galactose by blood spot tests done as part of universal newborn screening. In children who have not had a milk-containing diet or who have not eaten for several hours before testing, false-negative results may occur. Urine testing for reducing substances is another common means used to screen for galactosemia. If reducing substances are present, then further testing to confirm the presence of galactosemia and to identify the specific defect can be performed. Early treatment can lessen the long-term impact of this disease.

100. D

Sudden infant death syndrome (SIDS) is the most common cause of death in infants between 1 month and 1 year of age in developed countries. It accounts for almost 50% of deaths in these infants. The peak incidence of SIDS is at 2 to 4 months of age, and 95% of cases have occurred by 6 months of age. Autopsy findings are usually consistent with asphyxia. Risk factors for SIDS have been identified and include maternal factors such as smoking or drug use, increased parity, decreased age, decreased education, and low socioeconomic class. Infant risk factors include family history of SIDS, premature birth, intrauterine growth retardation, bottle-feeding, male gender, and sleeping in the prone position. The most effective strategy that has resulted in a reduction in SIDS in the United States has been the introduction of the "Back to Sleep" campaign to promote having infants sleep in the supine and not the prone position. This has resulted in a 35% decline in SIDS occurrence.

101. A

Substance abuse during pregnancy is very common; however, the exact prevalence of this problem is unknown. Studies have reported rates from 15% to more than 30% of drug and alcohol use by pregnant women. The effects of substance abuse vary by drug and may include prematurity, intrauterine growth retardation, placental abruption, fetal demise, spontaneous abortion, and birth defects. Alcohol is the most common substance used during pregnancy and fetal alcohol is the most common preventable cause for birth defects. Fetal alcohol syndrome may result in cognitive and developmental impairments, craniofacial abnormalities, and cardiovascular, urogenital, or gastrointestinal defects. Cocaine is another commonly abused drug during pregnancy and may result in growth retardation or placental abruption, but it has no known teratogenic effects. Opiates may cause prematurity, intrauterine growth retardation, and neonatal abstinence syndrome. Term infants are more susceptible to the abstinence syndrome due to differences in brain maturation.

102. D

Hypertrophic pyloric stenosis is a gastric outlet obstruction from overgrowth of the pyloric musculature that creates a stenosis. It occurs in approximately 3 in 1,000 births in the United States. This disease affects whites, males, and first-born children more commonly. The exact cause is unknown. Affected children present around 3 weeks of age with nonbilious vomiting that follows each feeding. The child is otherwise well and will be hungry and want to feed again. As the vomiting continues, dehydration may occur along with a hypochloremic metabolic alkalosis. The diagnosis may be obtained clinically through the history and physical examination findings of a palpable olive-shaped hard nodule in the pyloric region. In addition, gastric peristaltic waves may be visible across the abdomen after feeding. Clinical diagnosis is thought to be 60% to 80% sensitive. Ultrasonography can aid in diagnosis by visualization of the abnormal pyloris. Ultrasound is reported to be 90% sensitive. Medical therapies have been tried in the past but are

associated with a slower resolution of symptoms and a higher mortality rate. Treatment involves surgery, namely, a pyloromyotomy in which the pyloris muscle is split. Metabolic abnormalities correct promptly following surgery.

103. B

Many medications may be excreted into breast milk in sufficient quantities to affect the infant. Prior to prescribing medications to mothers who are breast-feeding, the safety and effects on breast-feeding should be reviewed. Some medications have not been sufficiently proven to be safe for use, whereas others may safely and confidently be prescribed to lactating mothers. Of the medications listed, cetriazine does not have sufficient safety data with breast-feeding and should not be taken while breast-feeding.

104. C

Alcohol consumption is common among adolescents who may be experimenting, recreationally drinking, or have chronic alcohol use and dependence. Legal intoxication is defined as a level of 80 to 100 mg/dL depending on the state in which one resides. Prior to achieving these levels, approximately 40% to 50% of individuals will exhibit decreased inhibitions and slurred speech. Significant motor incoordination occurs at levels between 100 and 200 mg/dL. Profound lethargy and stupor occur at levels of 300 mg/dL, and coma with depressed vital signs and possibly even death may occur at levels of 500 mg/dL. This individual is likely to have a level of approximately 150 mg/dL and can be sent home under the care of his parents. Additional drug screening should also be performed to detect the presence of other substances. If alcohol is the only substance present, then the patient should clear the alcohol from his blood at a rate of 16 mg/dL/hour, or in 9 or 10 hours. Attention to any psychosocial issues that may relate to the ingestion should be addressed and, if necessary, referral for counseling and outpatient care should be provided.

105. C

Atopic dermatitis is a common condition that affects 10% or more of children. Of those affected, 60% will have onset of disease between 2 and 6 months of age. In infants, typically the face and extensor surfaces are the affected areas by this pruritic, dry scaling rash. Fifty percent or more of children will have resolution of the disease by school age. An additional 25% resolve by puberty, and the remaining 25% continue to have atopic dermatitis into adulthood. During adolescence and adulthood, the sites of predilection for atopic dermatitis shift to involvement of the flexural creases. Treatment involves use of emollients, antipruritics, and, in those with inflammatory lesions, topical corticosteroids. An additional available therapy for children older than 2 years of age for short-term or intermittent use is the topical immunosuppressants tacrolimus and pimecrolimus. Dietary therapy is generally not helpful and benefits only a small percentage of children.

106. D

The two major forms of diaper rash are primary irritant contact dermatitis and candidal infections. Irritant dermatitis occurs due to contact of the skin with urine and stool. These substances contain ammonia and other irritants that cause erythema of the exposed surfaces that come into contact with the diaper, thus sparing the folds. Candidal infections, on the other hand, most commonly affect the inguinal folds and skin creases. This rash is erythematous with sharp borders and satellite lesions. Treatment of candidal diaper dermatitis involves the use of topical antifungal preparations. Combination products that include potent steroids such as triamcinolone should be avoided because this is an occluded area and skin atrophy may result. Oral antibiotics may actually promote development of fungal infections. Topical bacitracin is an antibiotic and would likely have no treatment effect. Zinc oxide is a barrier treatment used for treating and preventing irritant dermatitis.

107. C

Oral candidiasis, or thrush, is a common finding in newborn infants. It may develop due to exposure to maternal vaginal candidiasis, gastrointestinal colonization of the infant, or as a result of antibiotic usage. Evaluation for immunocompromised state may be warranted in rare circumstances of a complicated, recurrent, or indolent infection, but for typical thrush, no further evaluation is necessary. Treatment is provided through use of oral nystatin suspension. For persistent cases, gentian violet may be applied. Oral griseofulvin is used for tinea infections, most commonly tinea capitus. Frequent brushing or wiping of the lesions may lead to additional irritation and not resolution of the infection.

108. B

Warts are caused by one of approximately 50 subtypes of papillomavirus. Warts affect approximately 10% of school-age children, with peak occurrence in adolescence. Warts may occur on any area of the body but are most commonly found on the hands and feet. Genital warts in younger children should raise the suspicion for possible sexual abuse. Treatment will vary depending on the age of the child. Without therapy, up to 65% of warts will resolve within 2 years. Following therapy, there is a 10% recurrence rate. No single form of treatment is uniformly effective. Treatment options include cryotherapy, topical salicyclic acid preparations, topical retinoic acid, topical cantharidin, topical podophyllin (for genital warts), intralesional bleomycin, and laser therapy. Cimetidine, an oral H2 blocker, has also been used orally with some success.

109. A

Proprionibacterium acnes is the bacterium associated with acne. It is thought to act through enzymatic cleavage of triglycerides present in sebum releasing free fatty acids and other materials that are irritating to the follicles. Effective therapies for acne commonly include one or more agents that are active against *P. acnes*. Benzoyl peroxide, tetracyclines, erythromycin, and clindamycin are active against this organism. *Pityrosporum orbiculare* is the organism associated with seborrheic dermatitis. *Corynebacterium minutissimum* is the causative agent for erythrasma. *Epidermaphyton floccosum* is a fungus that can cause tinea infections. *Staphylococcus epidermidis* is a common skin colonizer that rarely can cause skin infections such as cellulitis or folliculitis.

110. C

Impetigo is the most common bacterial skin infection in children. It is a superficial infection of the skin with erythema and vesicles that rupture to form honey-colored crusts. This infection is caused by either *Staphylococcus aureus* or *Streptococcus pyogenes*. Folliculitis is a bacterial infection of the hair follicle that manifests as a pustule associated with erythema that is centered around a hair follicle. The predominant organisms are the same as for impetigo, with *Staphylococcus* occurring more commonly. Gram-negative

organisms may also cause folliculitis. With extension, deeper follicular infections may develop into abscesses that are termed furuncles. Atopic dermatitis is a chronic skin condition that would not develop so acutely. Typically, the lesions are dry, scaly, and pruritic, but they may also become exudative and have some similarities in appearance to impetigo. Seborrheic dermatitis is a mildly erythematous, scaly rash that would not be associated with crusting or scabs. See Table 2.14.

111. D

The history and examination suggest that this patient has otitis externa. This infection may be either bacterial or fungal. The most common organism responsible is *Pseudomonas aeruginosa*. *Staphylococcus aureus*, other gram-negative organisms, and the fungi *Aspergillus* and *Candida* are other causative organisms. Otitis externa is thought to occur as a result of a loss of the sebaceous and ceruminous secretions in the external canal in association with moisture and swimming. Excess moisture may also cause edema of the epithelium and then any manipulation or trauma may allow invasion of organisms. Treatment includes topical antibiotics in association with steroids as anti-inflammatories. If the infection extends beyond the external canal, systemic antibiotics may be necessary. In this case, intravenous coverage should be provided for pseudomonas and Staphylococcus. However, the patient presented had localized disease and does not warrant intravenous therapy. Oral cephalexin would provide inadequate coverage and oral fluoroquinolones are contraindicated in children. Although removal of debris for full visualization may be necessary, manipulation of the external canal should be kept to a minimum.

112. A

This patient has suffered from a concussion without loss of consciousness and with resolution of symptoms in less than 15 minutes. There are different systems for grading concussions along with different recommendations. The American Academy of Neurology system would consider this a grade 1 concussion and would allow the player to return to play. A grade 2 concussion is defined as symptoms lasting longer than 15 minutes and would require the patient to sit out for 1 week and then return to play provided he remains asymptomatic and he has a normal neurologic examination. A grade 3 concussion involves loss of consciousness. Patients with grade 3 concussions should be transported to the hospital for evaluation and then, provided they remain asymptomatic and have a normal neurologic examination, may return to play after 1 or 2 weeks. See Table 2.15.

113. E

Tics occur in up to one-fourth of children and may manifest as motor or vocal tics. Tics are usually of insidious onset and occur in children between the ages of 4 and 10 years. The most common form of tic is the transient tic disorder, which is self-limited. Whenever tics occur, many physicians and parents may express concerns about possible Tourette's syndrome. This disorder is of unknown etiology but is thought to be a disorder involving dopamine metabolism and the basal ganglia. Tourette's syndrome cannot be diagnosed until symptoms have been present for at least 1 year. The constellation of symptoms is more than just tics and includes other behavioral and learning disorders, most commonly attention deficit disorder. Coprolalia, the utterance of obscene words, is not required for the diagnosis of Tourette's and, in fact, is present in less than 25% of patients.

Table 2.14 Diagnostic testing and treatment of common skin infections

Infection	Diagnostic Test	Treatment
Impetigo	Clinical exam	Topical mupirocin, oral dicloxacillin, cephalexin
Cellulitis	Clinical exam, blood or wound cultures	Oral or intravenous dicloxacillin, cefazolin, cephalexin
Furuncles	Clinical exam, culture of drainage	Incision and drainage, antibiotics
Herpes simplex	Clinical exam, Tzanck smear, culture	Antivirals: acyclovir, famciclovir, valacyclovir
Chickenpox, herpes zoster	Clinical exam, culture, serology	Antivirals as for herpes above
Warts	Clinical exam, biopsy	Electrocautery, cryotherapy, topical salacylic acid or imiquimod
Molluscum contagiosum	Clinical exam, biopsy	Curettage, cryotherapy, Retinoin, salacylic acid
Fungal infections	Clinical exam, Wood light, KOH microscopy, culture (fungal media)	Topical or oral antifungals; nails and hair require oral therapy
Scabies	Clinical exam, microscopy	Topical lindane, permethrins, crotamiton, sulfur; clothing and bedding washed in hot water; treat close contacts
Lice	Clinical exam, microscopy	Topical lindane, permethrins, pyrethrins, malathion; must treat twice and remove nits

Table 2.15 Concussion treatment

Grade	Diagnosis	Initial	Repeat Episodes
1	No loss of consciousness; symptoms for less than 15 minutes	May return to play same day provided symptoms resolved and normal exam	May return after 1 week provided symptoms resolved and normal exam
2	No loss of consciousness; symptoms for more than 15 minutes	May return to play in 1 week provided symptoms resolved and normal exam	May return to play in 2 weeks provided symptoms resolved and normal exam
3	Loss of consciousness	May return after 1 or 2 weeks provided symptoms resolved and normal exam	Must sit out for at least 1 month

114. B

The patient presented has signs and symptoms consistent with allergic rhinitis. The seasonal nature of the symptoms along with itching and sneezing, hallmarks of allergic symptoms, support the diagnosis. Asthma is commonly a disease that precedes the diagnosis of allergic rhinitis, and eczema may be another associated disease. Common seasonal allergens include tree pollens in the spring, grass pollens in the summer, and weed pollens in the late summer or fall. Perennial allergens include animal dander, dust, mold, and cockroach allergens. Vasomotor rhinitis is seen in adults and is rare in children. The recurrent nature of the symptoms, itching, and atopic history do not lend support for either sinusitis or upper respiratory infections as the cause. Rhinititis medicamentosa is a rebound congestion that may occur with withdrawal from chronic use of nasal decongestants. Routine use of nasal decongestants would suggest rhinitis medicamentosa as a potential cause for the chronic nasal congestion.

115. C
Varicella vaccine is a live attenuated vaccine preparation that should be given subcutaneously as a one-time immunization for children aged 12 months to 12 years. In this group of children, more than 95% develop an immune response. The vaccine should be given twice, 4 weeks apart, to individuals 13 years or older. Seroconversion rates in this group are 80% after one dose and 99% after two doses. Current data from Japan suggest that the immunity with this vaccine lasts 20 years or more. The vaccine is 85% to 90% effective for prevention of varicella infection and 100% effective for preventing severe disease. The vaccine can be given with other vaccines. The vaccine is safe and reactions are primarily local at the injection site. From 3% to 5% will develop a generalized varicella-like rash. More serious reactions are rare.

116. B
Measles is a live attenuated vaccine that is administered subcutaneously as a two-shot series, at 12 months of age and at 5 to 10 years of age. Those who seroconvert after one shot are thought to maintain their immunity. Recommendations for a second MMR vaccine came about due to outbreaks that were thought to occur due to low immunization rates coupled with a 5% vaccine failure rate with the single immunization scheme. Thus, in order to lessen the vaccine failure rate, a second vaccine was recommended, and this results in greater than 99% seroconversion rates. Previously unimmunized older children should be provided with two MMR vaccines 4 weeks apart. In the child presented, the vaccine will need to be given on another visit because it is recommended that live viral vaccines, varicella and MMR in this case, be given either simultaneously or at least 4 weeks apart. Although there have been reports publicized about a link between MMR and autism, there have been no medical data supporting any link between the two.

117. A
Roseola, due to human herpes virus 6 or 7, affects primarily children younger than the age of 3 years. Manifestations include fever, often to 103°F and cervical adenopathy. When the fever remits, patients frequently develop a maculopapular truncal rash. Other symptoms are more variable and include respiratory or gastrointestinal symptoms. Fifth disease typically is associated with a prodromal illness with low-grade fever followed by a rash described as a "slapped cheek" appearance. Measles is associated with coryza, conjunctivitis, cough, and Koplik's spots. Kawasaki's disease likewise has other manifestations, including conjunctivitis, mucosal involvement, and rash with desquamation involving the palms and soles. An allergic reaction would not typically present with fever and there is often a past medical history of prior allergic reactions.

118. D
Fifth disease is caused by parvovirus B19 and is characterized by mild systemic symptoms and the characteristic rash. The rash frequently involves the face and is described as a "slapped cheek" appearance with intensely red cheeks and circumoral pallor. On the trunk, the typical rash is maculopapular, "lace-like," and symmetrical and may be pruritic. Infection during pregnancy is associated with a risk of fetal infection, which can cause hydrops and fetal death. The risk for fetal death is approximately 2% to 6%, and the risk is greatest during the first half of pregnancy. Studies indicate that patients are infectious before onset of illness, and that by the time the rash develops they are no longer infectious. Children with the rash may attend school and do not need to avoid any particular groups of individuals. The mother in this case has already been exposed and at this point need not stay away from her child. The low risks of problems can be explained to the mother and she should be offered serologic testing to determine if she is already immune and thus not at risk. More than 50% of children are seropositive by age 15.

119. C
Croup is a narrowing of the subglottic trachea resulting from inflammation and secretions due to viral infection. The most common viruses implicated are parainfluenza, respiratory syncytial, influenza, and rhinovirus. Children between the ages of 6 months and 6 years may be affected, with the peak occurrence at age 2 years. Treatment may include the use of mist, nebulized racemic epinephrine, dexamethasone (IM or PO), or nebulized budesonide. Antibiotics have no role in the treatment of croup. If the child responds well to epinephrine therapy, remains stable for 2 hours of observation, and follow-up care is reliable, then the patient may be discharged and not admitted. Patients who are still symptomatic or have recurring symptoms require admission for continued therapy and monitoring. A croup score can assist in making some of these decisions. A score of 4 or more may indicate the need for hospitalization and close monitoring, and a score of 7 or greater may indicate the need for intensive care unit admission. The addition of steroids to treatment of croup, either dexamethasone given IM or PO or nebulized budesonide, has resulted in a decrease in the number of children requiring intubation and the number of days of intensive care.

120. A
Bronchiolitis is a viral infection that affects the smaller airways, resulting in fever, dyspnea, wheezing, and difficulty feeding. Children younger than 2 years of age are most commonly affected, with peak occurrence being at 6 months of age. The most common virus causing this disease is respiratory syncytial virus. Risk factors include diminished lung function (e.g., bronchopulmonary dysplasia), exposure to secondhand smoke, day care attendance, and crowded living conditions. Exposure to secondhand smoke is associated with a higher risk than day care attendance. Treatment is supportive, and antibiotics and steroids play no role. Nebulized beta agonists are useful in some cases. The case fatality rate is less than 1%, with most occurring in children with heart or lung disease or who are immunocompromised.

121. E
Turner's syndrome results from a chromosomal anomaly where the patient is of the 45X karyotype. This results in gonadal dysgenesis and female phenotype, short stature, webbed neck, low-set ears, and sexual immaturity. Turner's syndrome is associated with a variety of malformations, including musculoskeletal, cardiac, and renal anomalies. Several disorders are increased in prevalence in patients with Turner's syndrome, including Hashimoto's thyroiditis, rheumatoid arthritis, and inflammatory bowel disease. Up to one-half of patients have nerve deafness and one-fifth are reported to be mentally retarded. Hyperphagia is not a feature of Turner's syndrome, but it is a prominent feature of Prader–Willi syndrome.

122. B

Diabetes mellitus in children is typically type 1 and is thought to result from viral and/or autoimmune destruction of the endocrine pancreas resulting in insulin deficiency. In its most extreme form, insulin deficiency results in diabetic ketoacidosis. In addition to searching for and treating the underlying cause, treatment involves restoring intravascular volume by aggressive use of fluids, providing insulin, and monitoring glucose and electrolytes. With the glucose-induced diuresis, most patients are dehydrated and are potassium deficient. Generally, a saline bolus of 20 mg/kg is provided initially, along with an insulin drip at 0.1 unit/kg/hour. Serum potassium levels may be normal despite the patient being in a deficit state. This is due to the shift of potassium out of cells to help buffer the acidosis that develops. Replacement of potassium in the maintenance fluids should begin when the potassium is high normal. Bicarbonate therapy does not need to be provided if the serum pH is ≥ 7.0.

123. C

Urticaria is a skin disorder characterized by well-circumscribed erythematous, raised skin lesions of various sizes that may be located on various parts of the body. The individual lesions resolve over 24 to 48 hours and new ones may appear in other locations. Urticaria is an allergic-type reaction that is either IgE or complement mediated. This disorder affects 20% of the population at some point in their lives and the cause is not found in the vast majority of cases. Typically, the disease is self-limited, but when it has been present for 6 weeks, it is termed chronic urticaria. Treatment is symptomatic, with the mainstay of therapy being use of antihistamines. Steroids are used only in extreme cases due to the generally self-limited nature of the condition and the potential toxicity of this class of medication. Dietary manipulation is rarely of any benefit.

124. A

Cancer is one of the leading causes of death in children, accounting for 10% of deaths in children younger than the age of 15 years. The most commonly diagnosed malignancy is leukemia, with acute lymphocytic leukemia being the most common form. Brain tumors are the second most common malignancy, followed by lymphoma and neuroblastoma. Neuroblastoma is the most common soft tissue tumor not of CNS origin and accounts for approximately 8% of childhood cancers. Soft tissue sarcomas (Ewing's and rhabdomyosarcoma) and Wilm's tumors occur slightly less frequently. Incidence rates for cancers are presented in Table 2.16.

125. B

Leukemia is the most common cancer diagnosis in children, and acute lymphocytic leukemia accounts for 75% of leukemia cases. The incidence of this disease is about two times more in Caucasians than in African Americans. Most commonly, children will present within 4 weeks of disease onset with symptoms that may be nonspecific in nature, such as anorexia, irritability, or lethargy. Some patients may present with what appears to be a persisting viral infection or with pallor or petechiae. On examination, lymphadenopathy is often present and 60% will have splenomegaly. Laboratory examination will reveal an anemia and thrombocytopenia in most patients, and examination of the peripheral smear will show the presence of blast cells. Bone marrow evaluation is needed for definitive diagnosis. The overall cure rate for acute lymphocytic leukemia is 80%.

Table 2.16 Childhood age-adjusted invasive cancer incidence rates* and 95% confidence intervals by primary site, United States[†]

Cancer	14.5 (14.2–14.8)	16.1 (15.8–16.4)
Bones and joints	0.7 (0.6–0.8)	0.9 (0.8–1.0)
Brain and other nervous system	3.2 (3.0–3.3)	2.9 (2.8–3.0)
Hodgkin lymphoma	0.5 (0.5–0.6)	1.2 (1.1–1.3)
Kidney and renal pelvis	0.8 (0.7–0.9)	0.6 (0.6–0.7)
Leukemia	4.5 (4.4–4.7)	4.1 (4.0–4.2)
Acute lymphocytic	3.4 (3.3–3.6)	3.0 (2.9–3.1)
Acute myeloid	0.6 (0.6–0.7)	0.7 (0.6–0.8)
Non-Hodgkin lymphoma	0.9 (0.8–1.0)	1.1 (1.0–1.2)
Soft tissue	1.0 (0.9–1.0)	1.0 (0.9–1.1)
Other	2.9 (2.8–3.1)	4.3 (4.1–4.4)

*Rates are per 100,000 persons and are age-adjusted to the 2000 U.S. standard population (19 age groups; Census P25-1130).

[†]Data are from selected statewide and metropolitan area cancer registries that meet the data quality criteria for all invasive cancer sites combined. Rates cover approximately 93% of the U.S. population.

From www.cdc.gov.

126. B

Testicular cancer represents 1% of all cancers diagnosed in males, but it is the most common malignancy in men between the ages of 15 and 35 years. The risk is increased 40 times for those with a history of cryptorchidism; however, this represents a 1% to 5% risk for the individual male with a history of cryptorchidism. Testicular trauma is not a risk factor for developing testicular cancer. The most common presentation is that of a painless testicular mass or enlargement. Testicular ultrasound can aid in diagnosis. When patients present with localized disease, more than 80% are curable.

127. C

Wilm's tumor is a renal neoplasm that occurs in children with a median age of 3 years. It affects all races and both sexes equally. In up to 10% of cases it is associated with congenital anomalies, most commonly of the genitourinary system. It is also part of two genetic conditions, WAGR syndrome and Beck-Wiedeman syndrome, that are associated with defects on chromosome 11. The parents or physician may incidentally note an abdominal mass that is usually asymptomatic. Besides the mass, hypertension is present in up to 60% and microscopic hematuria in 25% of children with Wilm's tumor. Ultrasonography may be used to assist with diagnosis; however, CT scan of the abdomen and chest may provide the most useful information for delineation of the mass and staging. Treatment initially involves surgical removal of the affected kidney.

128. D

Ewing's sarcoma is a family of tumors that may arise from bone and soft tissue and also includes peripheral primitive neuroectodermal tumor. These tumors generally present with pain, swelling, tenderness, and limited motion of the involved area. Patients may also have systemic symptoms, such as fever and weight loss; thus, they are often treated for infections such as osteomyelitis before the diagnosis is made. Radiographic evaluation reveals a lytic bone lesion and on CT or MRI there is often an associated soft tissue mass. Diagnosis requires biopsy, which may be CT guided. Treatment requires a multidisciplinary approach including surgery, radiation, and chemotherapy. Tumors that arise peripherally have a better prognosis than those involving the pelvis.

129. D

Rhabdomyosarcoma is the most common pediatric soft tissue sarcoma. These tumors are thought to arise from the same embryonic mesenchyme as striated skeletal muscle. Rhabdomyosarcoma may arise in any location but is most commonly found in the head, neck, genitourinary tract, or extremities. These tumors may be painful but most commonly produce symptoms by a mass effect on adjacent structures, such as respiratory or swallowing difficulty with nasopharyngeal tumors. Because of the lack of pain and systemic symptoms, these tumors are commonly present for several months before being diagnosed. This results in most tumors not being completely resectable at the time of diagnosis. Those with resectable tumors have an 80% to 90% long-term disease-free survival.

130. B

Neuroblastoma is the most common solid tumor diagnosed outside the central nervous system. It affects younger children and is the most common neoplasm diagnosed in infants. It arises from neural crest cells in the peripheral sympathetic nervous system. Most often, neuroblastoma develops in the abdomen; however, 30% arise in the cervical, thoracic, or pelvic ganglia. Diagnosis is by biopsy, commonly after discovery of a mass and evaluation by CT or MRI. Infants tend to present with more localized disease, whereas older children more often have disseminated disease. Overall survival is reported to be 55%.

131. C

Generally, management of chickenpox in children involves symptomatic care, such as acetaminophen and diphenhydramine. Individuals who should be considered for additional therapy in the form of antiviral therapy are those who are immunocompromised, receiving steroids or aspirin therapy, with chronic skin or respiratory illness, and those older than the age of 12 years. Thus, in this individual, oral antiviral therapy should be considered. Viral replication stops within 72 hours after onset of the rash; thus, the medication must be started early in the illness, preferably within the first 24 hours. Immunoglobulin along with the vaccine are provided to unimmunized at-risk individuals who have been exposed to chickenpox but do not yet have the disease. Steroids are not indicated in chickenpox but, although controversial, have been used in treatment of shingles with the goal of lessening the likelihood of developing postherpetic neuralgia.

132. A

Patients with growth hormone deficiency and some patients with short stature have undergone treatment with growth hormone administered subcutaneously 6 or 7 days per week for variable periods of time—possibly for several years. The risks of this therapy include development of pseudotumor cerebri, slipped capital femoral epiphysis, gynecomastia, worsening of scoliosis, and a twofold increased risk of leukemia. A reversible hypothyroidism may develop during therapy but is not seen after completion of therapy. Diabetes mellitus develops only rarely during treatment. Creutzfeldt-Jakob disease does not develop in those with recombinant growth hormone but is a risk for those who received growth hormone obtained from cadavers. There is no association between asthma and therapy with growth hormone.

133. D

Spastic diplegia is a bilateral spasticity of the legs with sparing of any involvement of the upper extremities. Children usually develop normally and when they begin to crawl are noted to drag the legs. Scissoring is a common exam finding, along with brisk lower extremity reflexes, ankle clonus, and bilateral Babinski signs. Walking and use of the lower extremities are affected, but upper extremity development and intelligence are usually normal. Seizures and athetoid movements rarely occur with this form of cerebral palsy. Other forms of cerebral palsy include spastic hemiplegia, spastic quadriplegia, and athetoid cerebral palsy, all of which tend to have poorer prognoses for normal intellectual function. See Table 2.17.

134. C

Intussusception is the most common cause for intestinal obstruction in children younger than the age of 6 years. Sixty percent are younger than 12 months of age and 80% are younger than 2 years of age. Obstruction occurs due to telescoping of the intestine upon itself and trapping a segment of intestine within an adjacent segment. The pressure on the trapped segment can cause vascular compromise and edema of the intestinal wall, and in many instances there is some associated blood loss. Characteristically, the blood is mixed with mucous and the term "currant jelly" stools has been used to describe the bloody mucous that is passed.

Table 2.17 Types of cerebral palsy

Type	Frequency	Characteristics
Spastic	70%–80%	Muscles are stiffly and permanently contracted. Type of spastic cerebral palsy is based on which limbs are affected. Scissors gait occurs when both legs are affected. With spastic hemiparesis, may experience hemiparetic tremors, in which uncontrollable shaking affects the limbs on one side of the body.
Athetoid, or dyskinetic	10%–20%	Uncontrolled, slow, writhing movements affecting the hands, feet, arms, or legs and, in some cases, the face and tongue, causing grimacing or drooling. Movements often increase during periods of emotional stress and disappear during sleep.
Ataxic	5%–10%	Poor coordination; walk unsteadily with a wide-based gait and experience difficulty when attempting quick or precise movements, such as writing or buttoning a shirt. May also have intention tremor.
Mixed forms		Symptoms of more than one of the previous three forms. The most common mixed form includes spasticity and athetoid movements, but other combinations are also possible.

The clinical picture along with obstruction on abdominal radiographs should prompt consideration of intussusception as a possible diagnosis. Barium enema will not only confirm the diagnosis but also may be curative in up to 80% of cases. For patients seen after 48 hours, the success rate lessens. Surgery is necessary for those not successfully reduced by barium enema. The other choices listed will lead to delay in appropriate treatment and increase the chances of the patient needing surgical intervention. Untreated intussusception is fatal.

135. C
School refusal is a common problem affecting up to 5% of children. Boys and girls are affected equally. Psychiatric disease is more common in children who are repeatedly absent from school. The most common diagnoses are conduct disorder, depression, anxiety, separation anxiety, and social phobias. Family dysfunction also appears to play a role. Although single-parent families are overrepresented in this group of children, many of these children come from intact families. Families that are overly close, or enmeshed, also appear to have more problems with school refusal. Seeking appropriate therapy is important since long-term sequelae have been identified. Long-term sequelae include lower levels of academic achievement, lower rates of employment, lower socioeconomic status, and higher rates of psychiatric disease as adults.

136. D
Congenital hypothyroidism is generally recognized during the newborn period as a result of state-mandated newborn screening. Although there are many potential causes, thyroid dysgenesis accounts for 90% of cases. In these instances, there is failure of the thyroid to develop and minimal or no thyroid tissue is present. Therapy is generally instituted with thyroxine before clinical symptoms are manifest. During the newborn period, infants are

generally asymptomatic. One clinical clue is the presence of an enlarged posterior fontanelle (greater than 0.5 cm). During the first few weeks of life, prolonged physiologic jaundice, feeding difficulties, sluggishness, and somnolence may be present. As the child grows older, myxedema, stunted growth with enlargement of the head, and developmental delay will be present. Delay in therapy can lead to long-term mental impairment. An algorithm for diagnosis of hypothyroidism is presented in Figure 2-6.

137. A
Speech begins to develop at approximately 8 or 9 months of age when the infant may indiscriminately use the words "mama" and "dada." Discriminate use of these words and formation of new words begins at approximately 1 year of age. At 1 year of age, the infant may be able to say 3 to 5 words and should be able to follow one-step commands. During the second year of life, the vocabulary expands, and by age 2 most children will know approximately 50 words and be able to combine the words into two-word sentences. At this point, 50% of the speech should be intelligible by strangers. By age 3 years, most children will have a 250-word vocabulary and be able to put together 3-word sentences. At this point, 75% of the speech should be intelligible by strangers. At school entry, speech should be readily understood by strangers.

138. B
Sickle cell disease is an alteration of the normal hemoglobin structure by substitution of glutamic acid in the beta chains by valine. This leads to a deformed hemoglobin in the deoxygenated state that is destroyed and can cause occlusion of smaller blood vessels in various organs. Sickle cell disease can be diagnosed prenatally or postnatally and is part of many neonatal screening programs. The earliest clinical manifestations can be present in the first 2 or 3 months of life when a hemolytic anemia develops as the fetal

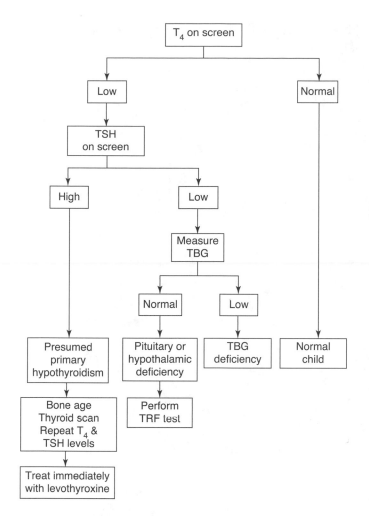

Figure 2-6. *Algorithm for the diagnosis of hypothyroidism. Reproduced with permission from Marino B, Snead K, McMillan J.* Blueprints in Pediatrics. *2nd ed. Malden, MA: Blackwell Science, Inc.; 2001:211.*

hemoglobin is replaced by adult hemoglobin. By 5 or 6 months of age, symptoms due to vaso-occlusion of bone and bone marrow vessels in the hand may cause pain and swelling in the hands, termed hand-foot syndrome. Sickle cell disease may ultimately affect virtually any organ, and up to 10% of children will suffer from cerebrovascular accidents as a result of this disease. These vaso-occlusive episodes are generally very painful and are often referred to as "painful crises." Painful crises and clinical symptoms do not appear until after the fetal hemoglobin is replaced by the abnormal adult hemoglobin and thus do not occur in utero. Acute treatment includes oxygen, intravenous fluids or transfusion, and pain medication.

139. C

Neonatal infection affects 1 to 5 per 1,000 live births. Up to 5% to 10% of newborns will undergo evaluation for infection or receive antibiotics. Neonatal sepsis is most commonly caused by organisms that colonize the maternal genital tract. The organisms most commonly responsible include group B B-hemolytic streptococcus, gram-negative organisms (most commonly *Escherichia coli*), and Listeria monocytogenes. Listeria is most commonly associated with later disease onset than in this infant, commonly around 1 week of age. Up to 25% of infants with positive blood cultures will also have

positive CSF cultures. The organisms responsible for bacterial infections, sepsis, and meningitis change as the child ages, and in children beyond the first 6 weeks of life, *Streptococcus pneumoniae*, *Haemophilus influenzae*, *Staphylococcus aureus*, and *Neiserria meningitidis* begin to appear as causes for infection. However, these organisms rarely cause disease in the immediate newborn period.

140. D

Food allergies are estimated to affect 2% to 8% of the pediatric population. The most common food allergies are type I immediate hypersensitivity reactions mediated by IgE directed toward the food allergen. The most common allergens are milk, peanuts, soy, eggs, wheat, fish, and nuts. The symptoms may include anaphylaxis, rhinitis, urticaria, and atopic dermatitis as well as vomiting, diarrhea, and failure to thrive. A common difficulty in diagnosing food allergies is distinguishing them from food intolerance, which is not an allergic phenomenon. RAST may be performed or referral to an allergist for skin or oral challenge testing may help in achieving a diagnosis. The primary therapy is patient education and avoidance of the particular food and any cross-reactive foods.

141. C

The most common forms of contact dermatitis in children are Rhus dermatitis and irritant diaper dermatitis. Irritant diaper dermatitis must be distinguished from other forms of diaper dermatitis, most notably candidal infection. A major distinguishing feature is the tendency for irritant dermatitis to affect the exposed surfaces of skin, whereas candidal infections tend to preferentially affect the skin folds. Treatment for irritant dermatitis includes avoiding contact with urine and stool through frequent diaper changes and applying a barrier cream or ointment to the skin. Rhus dermatitis occurs due to a reaction from exposure to plant resin from poison ivy or poison oak. The classic presentation is the presence of linear vesicular erythematous lesions on exposed surfaces during work or hiking in an area with plants. The rash is pruritic. Treatment includes topical steroids, antihistamines, and calamine lotion or Burow's soaks. If there is extensive or facial involvement, then oral steroids may be warranted. Advice to prevent re-exposure by bathing and washing the clothing that may have contacted the plant should be provided. See Figure 2-7.

142. B

Genetic factors account for 50% or more of cases of profound hearing loss, and most of these are sporadic isolated cases without a known cause. In these instances, the hearing loss may be conductive, sensorineural, or mixed. The recurrence rate for siblings is 10% when the cause is unknown. Other causes for hearing loss include head trauma, noise trauma, bacterial meningitis, congenital malformations, hyperbilirubinemia, and medication toxicity. Hearing loss is also associated with Down's and other syndromes. Early identification of hearing loss leads to earlier intervention and more normal language development. Universal neonatal screening for hearing loss is currently recommended.

143. C

Molluscum contagiosum is an infection of the skin caused by poxvirus that is characterized by multiple discrete 2- to 5-mm skin-colored papules with a central umbilication. It can spread by person-to-person contact or by autoinoculation. Diagnosis is generally made clinically, but laboratory evaluation of stained material curreted from the lesions can confirm the diagnosis. Observation

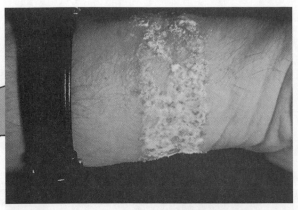

From leather watch band.

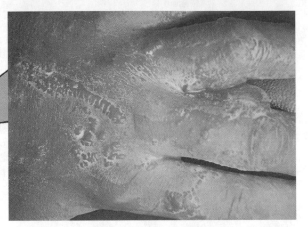

From poison ivy. Note linear vesicles.

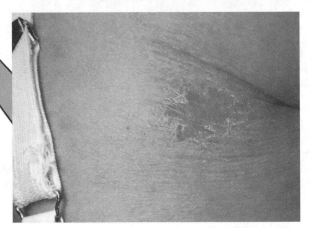

From nickel metal in garter strap.

Figure 2-7. *Contact dermatitis. From Burroughs Wellcome Co.*

for resolution of the lesions in 6 to 9 months is one option for managing these lesions. However, many parents are disturbed by the presence of the lesions and potential for spread and want something done. Treatment options include use of cantharidin, tretinoin, and salicylic acid as well as curettage or cryosurgery. Trichloroacetic acid and laser therapy have also been used. Surgical excision and electrocautery are not recommended, and nonscarring treatments are used for this self-limited disease. See Figure 2-8.

144. D

Urinary tract infections in children require a different approach to evaluation and management than is generally provided in adults due to the vulnerability of the still growing renal system to infection and permanent scarring and renal compromise. Imaging of girls younger than age 5 years and all boys for a single infection is indicated to assess the anatomy and for the occurrence of reflux. During an acute infection, ultrasound may be performed to assess anatomy and for obstruction. Ultrasound is also useful for these same

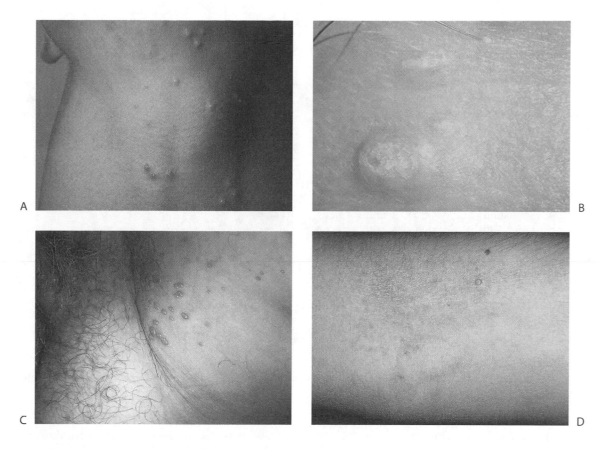

Figure 2-8. *Molluscum contagiosum. From Glaxo Dermatology.*

purposes in adults with repeated or complicated infections. Tests of cure and screening cultures are commonly performed in children in order to ensure eradication of the infection and to detect any recurrence. These tests are not done in asymptomatic adults. Following acute treatment and while still on suppressive therapy (generally 6 weeks after onset), a vesicocystourethrogram is performed to assess for reflux of urine from the bladder into the ureters and kidney. This testing is not generally part of the evaluation for adults.

145. A

Obesity is a nationwide problem on the rise for both adults and children. The potential long-term complications for obesity include diabetes, cardiovascular disease, and hypertension. It is estimated that up to one-third of adults and 14% of children are significantly overweight. A common means to define obesity and overweight status is use of the body mass index (BMI), which is the weight in kilograms divided by the height in meters squared. A BMI between the 85th and 95th percentiles for age in children places them at risk for becoming overweight, and being overweight is defined as a BMI greater than the 95th percentile. Another significant risk factor is having parents who are obese. Children with normal-weight parents are at lower risk. Efforts to treat children who are at risk for being overweight or obese must include the parents and family. The only effective and safe measures are lifestyle modifications that increase physical activity and promote healthy eating habits. Activities that involve sports teams and family physical activities are more likely to be successful than recommending individual exercise. A healthy diet may include snacks that are also healthy.

146. B

Erythema toxicum neonatorum is a very common rash seen in up to 50% of newborns. The rash appears anytime within the first few weeks of life, most commonly in the first 2 days. The lesions consist of macules, papules, vesicles, and pustules on the trunk, face, and proximal extremities, sparing the palms and soles. The lesions resolve within 3 or 4 days. The classic finding that confirms the diagnosis is eosinophils on staining of a smear of the vesicle or pustule. No therapy is required. Transient neonatal pustular melanosis is a rash most commonly seen in African American infants in the first few days of life and resolves in 3 or 4 days without treatment. The individual lesions are pustules with polymorphonuclear cells but no organisms. The palms and soles may be involved with this rash. Infantile acropustulosis is a similar rash to transient pustular melanosis, but it involves only the extremities and has its onset at 3 to 12 months of age. This rash may recur with new lesions every 2 to 4 weeks, persisting until 3 years of age. Cutis marmorata refers to the skin changes of "mottling" associated with cooling of the extremities of infants. Atopic dermatitis generally does not develop in the neonatal period and is a scaling, erythematous, macular rash commonly involving the cheeks and extremities in infants and younger children.

147. B

Current recommendations for routine blood pressure screening begin at age 3 years. Blood pressure increases with age and blood pressures above the 95th percentile for age define hypertension. Blood pressures between the 90th and 95th percentiles are considered high-normal and should be monitored more closely. Up to

5% of children may have an elevated blood pressure on initial readings. Only 1% have continued elevations on follow-up. The higher the blood pressure, the more likely the repeat readings will be elevated as well. Causes for hypertension in children compared to adults are more likely to be secondary. Not until adolescence is primary hypertension the most common form. In younger children, renal causes are most common, with coarctation and endocrine-related disease also causing secondary hypertension. When a child is found to have hypertension, a search for underlying disease must be pursued.

148. A

Routine screening at the 5-year visit should include vision and hearing assessment, vaccination with MMR, DtaP, and IPV, along with physical examination. Anticipatory guidance, with focus on injury and accident prevention, is also very important. Hemoglobin and lead screening are recommended for younger and at-risk children. Pertussis would only be omitted from vaccination for those children who had adverse reactions in the past. The 23-valent pneumococcal vaccine should be provided to high-risk children, such as those with functional or anatomic asplenia.

149. B

The most common manifestations of child abuse are soft tissue injuries and fractures. Fractures are present in most abused children and when present in a child younger than age 3 years, abuse should be suspected. There is no one fracture that is pathognomonic of abuse, but certain fractures are more commonly associated with abuse. For example, fractures in children younger than age 1 year and bilateral or multiple fractures, especially of different ages, are highly suspicious for abuse. Humeral fractures and femur fractures in young children (younger than 3 years) are also highly suspicious. Other clues that may suggest abuse are an inconsistent history, delay in seeking care, history of repeated injuries, and evasiveness on the part of the parents. Although any of the injuries listed could occur due to abuse, humeral fracture is most suspicious. Nursemaid's elbow is a dislocation of the radial head that often occurs incidentally when playing or preventing a fall in a toddler. Clavicle fracture occurs commonly as a result of falling and is the most common childhood fracture. Wrist fractures also commonly occur with accidental falls. A supraorbital laceration would occur due to a collision or falling.

150. A

Craniosynostosis is the premature fusion of the cranial skull sutures. Normally, the separation of the sutures allows for new bone growth and deposition of bone to allow for the growing brain. When a suture prematurely closes, the remainder of the skull will continue to grow and the shape will become asymmetrical or misshapen depending on which suture fuses early. Approximately 90% of cases are sporadic and nonsyndromic. The most common suture that fuses prematurely is the sagittal suture and results in elongation of the skull, termed scaphocephaly. Girls are affected slightly more often than boys. There is elevation of the intracranial pressure, but there are usually no associated neurologic deficits. Treatment involves surgical separation of the sutures. Syndromes that are associated with craniosynostosis include Apert's, Pfeiffer's, and Crouzon's syndromes; however, these are much less common than sporadic, nonsyndromic cases. Hypothyroidism commonly causes a delay in suture closure, and enlargement of the posterior fontanelle is a clinical clue to the presence of hypothyroidism.

151. C

Pimecrolimus is part of a relatively new class of topical medications useful for the treatment of mild-moderate atopic dermatitis in children as young as age 2 years. These medications are immune modulators that inhibit the inflammatory response rather than treating the inflammation once it has developed. The safety of the medication with long-term use has been questioned because of an association with the development of lymphoma or skin cancers. For short-term or intermittent use, the safety profile appears to be excellent, with the primary contraindications for use including hypersensitivity to the medication, immunocompromised status, or an actively infected skin lesion.

152. E

Superficial hemangiomas are common skin lesions that appear within the first few months of life. Occasionally, they may be present at birth, but more commonly they are heralded by a bluish or pale area, which subsequently develops a vascular pattern. These lesions may occur on any part of the body and initially undergo expansion before spontaneously involuting. Sixty percent will be resolved by age 5 years and 90% to 95% will be gone by age 9 years. Unless they become ulcerated, infected, or are inhibiting function (e.g., larger facial lesion that obstructs vision or interferes with eating), treatment is expectant observation. In those cases that require therapy, laser, surgery, prednisone (intralesional or oral), and interferon have been used.

153. C

Ecstasy is the popular name for 3,4 methylenedioxymethamphetamin (MDMA), which is a drug commonly used at dance parties. The desired effects on the user are euphoria, intimacy, and a closeness to others. There is a tolerance to these effects and frequent use will lessen the effects; thus, many users space out their use of this drug (e.g., every 2 weeks). There is no evidence that MDMA is addictive. Common side effects include post-use drowsiness, muscle aches, depression, and difficulty concentrating. Other more serious side effects include hypertensive crisis, intracerebral hemorrhage, cardiac arrhythmias, hepatitis, memory impairment, rhabdomyolysis, hyperthermia, and paranoid psychosis. The adverse effects are not predictable or dose related.

154. D

Thumb sucking is a common habit of children that is used for self-comforting, soothing, and as a pleasurable activity. Up to 90% of newborns, 40% of 1- to 3-year-olds, and 25% of 5-year-olds continue with the thumb-sucking habit. Thumb sucking can affect dentition, as well as speech, and is considered more harmful than pacifiers due to the softer nature of pacifiers and the countertraction exerted by the plastic shell of the pacifier on the teeth and mouth. When children become more physically active, their time spent thumb sucking decreases. Efforts to break this habit should attempt to use praise for not sucking and should commence around the age of 4 years. A goal would be to break the habit before the eruption of secondary dentition.

155. A

Infants who were born prematurely and are being discharged should continue to be followed closely for appropriate growth and development. Feeding may require special formulas or human milk fortifier until the infant is at his or her term date. Vitamins may be needed until the infant is taking 32 ounces of formula or if he or she is being breast-fed. Iron supplementation is often advised until 12 to 15 months of age. Vision and hearing screening should be performed on all neonatal intensive care unit infants and is done prior to discharge. The primary physician should be aware of any necessary follow-up exams. Vaccinations should be given on a schedule following the infants' chronologic age with the exception of hepatitis B. It is recommended to wait until the infant is at least 2,000 g prior to the first hepatitis B vaccine. Growth and development are both corrected for the gestational age, and special growth charts are available for preterm infants. After 2 years of age, standard growth charts are used.

156. B

Nasal polyps are thought to occur as a result of chronic inflammation of the nasal mucosa in combination with a genetic predisposition. Nasal polyps are found in association with cystic fibrosis, asthma, aspirin sensitivity, and rhinitis, but they are not found with greater frequency in those with allergies. Options for therapy include medication and surgery. Medications that are effective include oral, intranasal, and direct injection of steroids into the polyp. Cromolyn sodium, antihistamines, and decongestants have no effect on polyps. For larger lesions, oral steroids may initially be used and then tapered and converted to intranasal sprays. For those that are refractory to medical therapy, polypectomy may be required. Recurrence is common, and maintenance intranasal steroids are commonly recommended to prevent nasal polyp recurrences.

157. A

Volvulus commonly occurs in association with malrotation, which occurs in 1 in 500 births. Of those with malrotation, volvulus will eventually develop in 75%, and 75% of these cases will present within the first month of life. The presentation is that of a sudden onset of bilious emesis and abdominal distention. Less acute presentations and lack of abdominal distention do not exclude the diagnosis. Abdominal films will show signs of obstruction with air-fluid levels and dilated loops of bowel. The classic finding, also seen in duodenal atresia, is the double-bubble sign, which represents dilation of the stomach and the proximal duodenum. Duodenal atresia presents within the first 24 hours of life and is seen generally in newborn nurseries. See Figure 2-9.

158. E

Cystic fibrosis is a multisystem disease resulting from abnormalities in cellular sodium and chloride transport that cause changes in the secretions from various organs that ultimately lead to their malfunction or destruction. In the lungs, mucous is abnormally viscous and not easily cleared, leading to obstruction of airways, recurrent infections, and respiratory failure. In the pancreas, obliteration of the ducts leads to exocrine pancreatic insufficiency. However, pancreatitis is identified only rarely, in less than 1% of patients. The sinuses are prone to recurrent infections due to poorly cleared mucous. Children with cystic fibrosis have bulky sticky stools that are more difficult to pass. This, along with increased intra-abdominal pressures associated with frequent coughing, leads to rectal prolapse in 20% of children. In males, 98% have obstruction of the vas deferens and azoospermia. Up to 20% of women with cystic fibrosis are infertile, either due to changes in the cervical mucous that prevent sperm penetration or due to anovulation associated with their chronic lung disease. Orchitis, inflammatory bowel disease, and conjunctivitis have no particular association with cystic fibrosis.

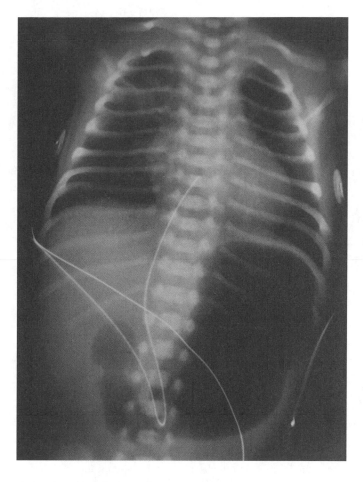

Figure 2-9. *"Double-bubble" sign of duodenal atresia.*

159. C

Cystic fibrosis is an autosomal recessive trait that results from mutations at a single locus located on chromosome 7. The white population is affected much more commonly than blacks. One in 2,500 live births to white parents has cystic fibrosis compared to 1 in 17,000 for blacks. A high incidence has been reported in the Amish, and the Ohio Amish are affected with cystic fibrosis at a rate of 1 in 569 births. The carriage rate for the cystic fibrosis gene mutation in the white population has been reported to be as high as 5%. Cystic fibrosis is rare in Asians, Native Americans, and black Africans.

160. C

The presentation of meningitis in infants can be very nonspecific. Fever, altered feeding, lethargy, and tachypnea may occur. In this 4-month-old with fever and lethargy, a sepsis evaluation, including blood cultures, and cerebrospinal fluid analysis and culture are indicated. The organisms responsible for infection in the neonatal period (birth to 30 days of age) are commonly group B streptococcus and gram-negative organisms, predominantly *E. coli*. After this period, *S. pneumoniae*, *N. meningitidis*, and *H. influenzae* increase in prevalence and need to be considered in providing antibiotic coverage. Prior to the emergence of resistant *S. pneumoniae*, coverage was commonly provided with a second- or third-generation cephalosporin (e.g., ceftriaxone or cefotaxime) alone. With the emergence of resistant *S. pneumoniae*, vancomycin should be provided until antibiotic sensitivities are known.

161. B

Up to one-fourth of girls and 10% of boys are victims of sexual abuse by the time they reach the age of 18 years. Perpetrators are commonly relatives or nonrelatives known to the family, and most are male. Most children will not voluntarily present this information to parents or physicians, and most have no physical findings that are diagnostic of abuse. Thus, a high index of suspicion and consideration of the possibility of abuse are needed in the differential of children presenting with behavioral changes, such as regression, sleep disturbances, and sexual acting out. Sexual acting out has been shown to be a specific indicator of potential abuse. Other possible presentations of victims of abuse include trauma related to the abuse and unexplained physical complaints, such as abdominal pain.

162. D

Mental retardation can be difficult to diagnose in young children. Up to 2% or 3% of children are mentally retarded either as part of a syndrome or as an isolated finding. In up to 50% of cases, no definite etiology is identified. When evaluating a child for developmental delay in one or more areas, many physicians will overlook the diagnosis of mental retardation because a child does not look dysmorphic, the child is ambulatory, or because they believe that testing is not feasible in young children. Parental concerns about developmental delay accurately target the majority of children with developmental problems and should be addressed. Up to 90% of children diagnosed with mental retardation will fall into the mild category and may present with normal motor achievements and speech delay as a manifestation. Referral to a developmental assessment team or clinic should be considered as soon as developmental delay is identified. These clinics often utilize a multidisciplinary approach including speech, hearing genetics, neurology, ophthalmology, psychiatry, and developmental pediatrics in order to arrive at a possible diagnosis and can help in providing parents with education and resources needed in caring for their child.

163. E

Dental caries develop in more than 50% of children by age 9 years. Dental decay and cavities are thought to be largely caused by mutans streptococci, thus making dental caries an infectious and transmissible disease. Fluoride is bacteriostatic against these bacteria and has been important in decreasing the rates of dental decay in children. Increased attention to preventive dental care can lessen a child's risk for dental decay. On gums and newly erupted teeth, cleansing can be done with moistened gauze or a soft bristled toothbrush without toothpaste. After 1 year of age, a toothbrush can be introduced and at 2 years toothpaste (pea-sized amount) may be used. Children should not be put to bed with bottles, and juices should be provided from cups and not bottles. Routine dental care can be started as early as 1 year of age and should not be delayed past 3 years of age.

164. D

Infant botulism is a rare disease worldwide and most cases are diagnosed in the United States. The disease occurs secondary to a toxin produced by *Clostridium botulinum* that is found in soil or honey products. The toxin is ingested and absorbed, causing a gradual-onset paralytic disease by blocking acetylcholine receptors at the neuromuscular junctions. More than 90% of affected infants are younger than 6 months of age and more than 70% eventually require mechanical ventilation. Interestingly, 70% to 90% of affected infants are breast-fed. The reason for this association is unclear, but

it may be due to a slower onset of disease allowing for diagnosis before the disease is fatal. Treatment is supportive, and prevention by avoiding feeding honey-containing products to infants should be part of anticipatory guidance to parents.

165. A

The most common cause for chronic stridor in young children is laryngomalacia. This condition is characterized by congenital deformities or laxness of the cartilage making up the larynx. This laxness leads to collapse of the walls of the larynx on inspiration and resultant stridor. Males are affected more often than females by a 2.5:1 ratio. Symptoms are worsened in the supine position. Feeding may be difficult in more severe cases. No specific therapy is needed in most cases. Those more severely affected may require smaller, more frequent feedings and, in rare instances, tracheostomy. The condition resolves by 18 months of age, although some children may develop recurrent stridor with crying or respiratory infections. Choanal atresia is a lack of canalization of a nare or, less commonly, both nares that may cause stridor. This condition is rare. Croup causes an acute stridor. Foreign bodies also most commonly cause acute dyspnea and stridor, although on rare occasion they may cause chronic symptoms. Foreign body aspiration most commonly occurs in children 1 or 2 years of age. Asthma is a chronic recurrent airway obstruction associated with expiratory wheezing.

166. D

This episode represents a classic description of vasodepressor syncope, also commonly referred to as vasovagal syncope. This form of syncope results from autonomic dysfunction often in response to standing still in a warm environment or a noxious stimulus, such as a blood draw or ear piercing. The heart rate slows and the blood pressure drops, leading to a decrease in cerebral perfusion, resulting in syncope. Usually, there are premonitory symptoms of pallor, diaphoresis, and an uneasy feeling that precede the event and allow for self-protection. During a syncopal episode, up to 50% of patients will have brief tonic contractions of the muscles of the face, trunk, and extremities that result from neuronal discharge from the reticular formation and are not true seizures. Patients with recurrent episodes of vasodepressor syncope may warrant tilt-table testing and treatment with beta-blockers. Most patients with one or rare episodes should be counseled regarding the warning symptoms and self-protection. Breath-holding spells are voluntary efforts on the part of a child to not breathe and cause cyanosis and may result in syncope. These are usually a means to seek attention. Cardiac syncope needs to be considered in any individual with an episode of syncope. Cardiac syncope occurs without aura or prodromal symptoms, other than possibly a history of palpitations.

167. C

This rash is typical of pityriasis rosea, a common, benign, and self-limited rash of unknown etiology. The rash most commonly affects teens and young adults, but it may occur at virtually any age. The rash typically begins with a larger lesion, termed the "herald patch." The lesions of pityriasis rosea are oval, pink, and flat and have a ring of fine scale around the edges. Individual lesions may be mistaken for ringworm. The distribution of lesions on the trunk parallels the skin lines and gives the appearance of the "Christmas tree" pattern. The disease clears spontaneously in 1 to 3 months. Many patients are asymptomatic; however, there may be associated pruritis for which symptomatic therapy may be needed. Lichen planus is a pruritic rash consisting of violaceous papules on the extremities. Lesions may also occur on the mucous membranes, and the nails may be affected. Herpes zoster is a reactivation of chickenpox along one or two dermatomes. These lesions are vesicular and have the appearance of chickenpox lesions. Keratosis pilaris is a follicular hyperkeratosis that presents as flesh-colored papules on the anterior thighs and extensor surfaces of the extremities, often in association with atopic dermatitis. Warts are skin-colored papules resulting from infection with the human papilloma virus. See Figure 2-10.

168. A
Wolff–Parkinson–White (WPW) syndrome is the most common accessory pathway syndrome affecting the heart. The classic features are a shortened PR interval and a slurring of the upstroke of the QRS complex, called the delta wave, that leads to prolongation of

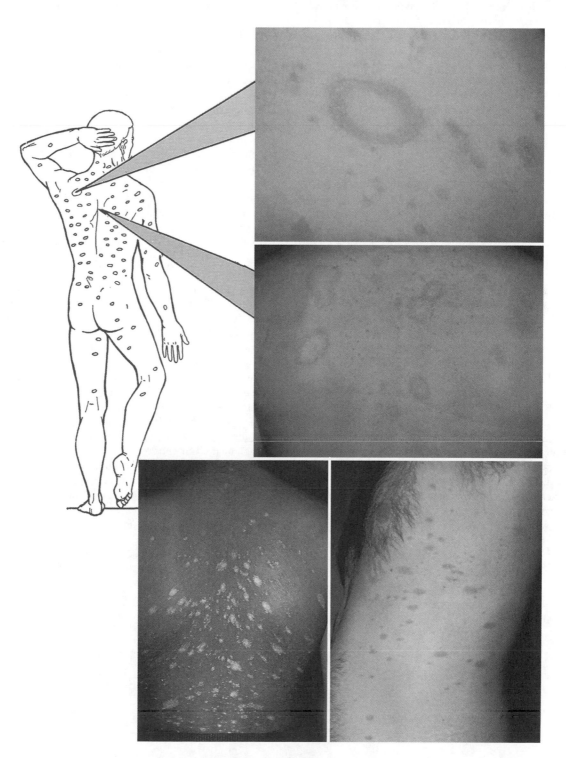

Figure 2-10. *Pityriasis rosea. Bottom left photograph is of a black man. From Westwood Pharmaceuticals.*

the QRS to greater than 0.10 seconds. Approximately 70% of individuals with this condition have no underlying cardiac disease. Only 50% of patients will ever experience symptoms. Symptoms that most commonly occur are related to supraventricular tachycardias that may occur due to participation of the accessory pathway in a re-entrant circuit. The most common tachycardias that present are narrow complex tachycardias where normal conduction occurs through the AV node and retrograde conduction occurs through the accessory pathway (orthodromic tachycardia). Wide complex tachycardias may also occur where the antegrade conduction is through the accessory pathway and retrograde conduction occurs through the AV node (antidromic tachycardia). Amiodarone or procainamide are the recommended treatments for wide complex tachycardias since medications that act on the AV node may enhance conduction through the accessory pathway. Electrophysiologic study of patients with WPW may allow for ablation of the accessory pathway and elimination of the associated arrhythmias. See Figure 2-11.

169. B

Crohn's disease and ulcerative colitis are inflammatory bowel diseases that are chronic in nature and of undetermined etiology. Crohn's disease affects any portion of the gastrointestinal tract, whereas gastrointestinal involvement with ulcerative colitis is limited to the colon. Both are associated with extraintestinal manifestations. The most common times for disease onset for inflammatory bowel disease are during adolescence and young adulthood. Environmental and genetic factors are thought to be factors leading to development of inflammatory bowel disease and family members are at increased risk. Interestingly, cigarette smoking has been found to be protective against development of ulcerative colitis, but it is a risk factor for Crohn's disease. Colon cancer risk is slightly elevated in Crohn's disease but markedly elevated with ulcerative colitis. After 10 years of disease, the risk increases by 1% per year. Recommendations for caring for individuals with ulcerative colitis include colonoscopy every 1 or 2 years after the patient has had the disease for 10 years.

170. A

Infectious diseases are one of the most common reasons for children to visit their primary care physician. Deciding what constitutes "too many" or "severe" infections that warrant evaluation for possible immunodeficiency can be challenging. Some guidelines that have been recommended include evaluation for immunodeficiency if a child has an unusual or opportunistic infection (e.g., Aspergillus), infection in an unusual site (e.g., brain abscess), two or more systemic bacterial infections, three or more serious respiratory or documented bacterial infections, and infections with common pathogens but of unusual severity. Initial screening may include a CBC with differential, sedimentation rate, peripheral smear, and serum immunoglobulin and complement levels. If all screening tests are normal but immunodeficiency is still suspected, then referral to an immunologist may be warranted.

171. E

Acute renal failure is an uncommon but potentially life-threatening problem that children may present with. In the newborn period, congenital abnormalities, sepsis, and other conditions that may cause shock and hypotension are the most common causes. In older children, glomerulonephritis, intravascular coagulation disorders (e.g., hemolytic–uremic syndrome), acute tubular necrosis due to drugs, chemicals, or hypotension, and acute interstitial nephritis are renal causes for renal failure. Prerenal factors, such as dehydration and acute blood loss, may also cause acute renal failure, as may postrenal factors that obstruct flow of urine. While evaluating the child for underlying causative factors, some children may require dialysis to prevent complications. Indications for dialysis include acidosis, hyperkalemia, or hypertension that is refractory to initial therapies. Anemia is not an indication for dialysis.

172. E

The primary nutritional factor that is required for growth and that impacts renal function is dietary protein. Thus, in chronic renal failure dietary restriction of protein intake is advised. However, the needs for protein in a growing child greatly exceed those of an adult, and thus the recommended protein intake is 2.5 g/kg/day in a growing child with chronic renal failure compared to the recommendation for adults with chronic renal failure of 0.8 g/kg/day. Carbohydrates should not be restricted solely on the basis of chronic renal failure and in fact may need to be supplemented along with fats to ensure enough calories for adequate growth. Water-soluble vitamins commonly need to be supplemented in children undergoing dialysis. Vitamin D supplementation is also recommended since impaired renal function will lead to decreases in hydroxylation of vitamin D and decreased vitamin D activity. Other fat-soluble vitamins do not need to be supplemented.

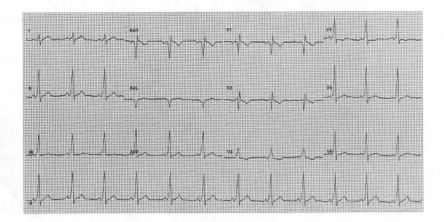

Figure 2-11. Pre-excitation (WPW syndrome). The PR interval is short, and the QRS is slightly widened. Slurring of the upstroke of the QRS is apparent in multiple leads (I, aVL, and V leads); this is the delta wave.

173. C

Most cases of HIV in children are acquired perinatally from an HIV-infected mother. A smaller percentage acquire the disease through breast-feeding and a very small percentage are infected through blood products. When children reach the teen years, they may acquire the disease in the same way as adults. Clinical evidence of infection is not present at birth and IgG antibody screening is not reliable before the age of 18 months. In children with suspected HIV who are younger than 18 months, viral detection testing, such as HIV DNA PCR, HIV culture, and HIV antigen testing, may be useful in achieving the diagnosis. The disease follows a more aggressive course than in adults. In up to 25% of infants, the disease is rapidly progressive, causing recurrent infections and death within 9 months of birth. Sixty to eighty percent of infants have a slower course with median survival times of 6 years. Less than 5% of infected infants are long-term survivors. This pattern of disease contrasts with adult infections, in which the clinical latency often lasts up to 12 years.

174. D

Seizures occur in up to 5% of the pediatric population and epilepsy is diagnosed in 1% of children. Most (60%) cases of epilepsy are diagnosed in childhood and most have no underlying cause for the epilepsy and thus are diagnosed with idiopathic epilepsy. Ninety percent of patients are well controlled with medication, and only 10% have seizures that are refractory to medical therapy. Factors that may worsen previously well-controlled seizures include infection, fever, excessive fatigue, stress, and medications such as phenothiazines, theophylline, and methylphenidate. For patients who are refractory to medical therapy, surgery may be beneficial, particularly for those with focal seizures.

175. D

Osteomyelitis in otherwise healthy children occurs from hematogenous seeding of the bone by the offending bacteria. Trauma and complications of surgical procedures can also lead to development of osteomyelitis, but these occur less commonly. *Staphylococcus aureus* is the most common organism responsible for patients of all ages. In neonates, group B strep and gram-negative organisms may also cause osteomyelitis. In older children, group A streptococci are a common cause, and in children older than age 6 who suffer puncture wounds to the foot, *Pseudomonas aeruginosa* must be considered as a pathogen. Initial treatment must consider the potential pathogens, and when cultures identify the organism, specific therapy should be provided. Guidelines for treatment duration have been modified throughout the years. In children who are clinically responding well to therapy, antibiotics may be switched to oral medication, provided an appropriate antibiotic is available in oral form. In those with a good clinical response and normalization of the sedimentation rate who are infected with group A strep, *Haemophilus*, or *S. pneumoniae*, 2 weeks total of antibiotics may be adequate. A minimum of 3 weeks of antibiotics should be provided for staphylococcal infections.

176. C

Idiopathic apnea of prematurity occurs in the absence of underlying causes. It may exhibit features of obstructive apnea, central apnea, or be mixed. Most commonly, it is mixed, with short apneas occurring due to central apnea and longer pauses being obstructive. Apnea of prematurity generally resolves by 36 weeks postconceptional age. In the interim, infants with apnea are monitored with apnea monitors and may be treated with oxygen and with theophylline or caffeine. Episodes of apnea may be treated with cutaneous stimulation or bag and mask ventilation. Apnea of prematurity is not predictive of future episodes of SIDS and, in the absence of other conditions associated with prematurity, does not affect long-term prognosis.

177. B

Epstein–Barr virus (EBV) infection is best known for causing infectious mononucleosis but has also been associated with X-linked and post-transplantation lymphoproliferative disorders, Burkitt's lymphoma, nasopharyngeal carcinoma, and B cell lymphoma. In many cases, the diagnosis of EBV is made by combining the clinical presentation with a positive heterophile antibody test. These tests are convenient and readily available, but they are nonspecific. An increase in atypical lymphocytes is also supportive of the diagnosis of EBV infection, but again it is nonspecific. Antibodies to early antigen are often produced early on in the infection but may persist for up to several years, which limits the usefulness of this test in diagnosing acute EBV infection. IgM antibody to viral capsid antigen is the most specific indicator for acute EBV because it is produced early and is detectable for 4 to 12 weeks. An algorithm for serologic workup of mononucleosis is presented in Figure 2-12.

178. B

Celiac disease is a malabsorptive disorder in which the small bowel is damaged as a result of permanent sensitivity to dietary gluten. Patients will present with this disorder between the ages of 6 months and 2 years, which coincides with introduction of gluten into the diet. This disease is present in 1 in 10,000 live births in the United States. Genetic and environmental factors are thought to contribute to the development of the sensitivity to gluten, specifically the gliadin fraction of gluten, which sensitizes lymphocytes and leads to surface epithelial damage, villous atrophy, and crypt hyperplasia. Clinically, these result in malabsorption, diarrhea, poor weight gain, or weight loss and anorexia. Diagnosis can

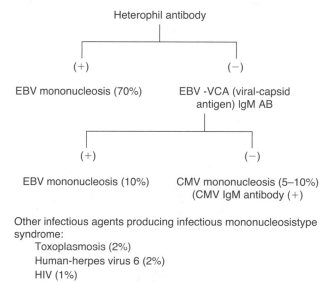

Figure 2-12. Algorithm for serologic workup of mononucleosis syndromes.

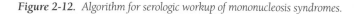

definitively be made with small bowel biopsy; however, noninvasive testing can also be performed using the IgA endomysial antibody, which has near 100% sensitivity and specificity. Antigliadin antibody can also be performed but is not reliable. Antinuclear antibody is not useful for celiac disease. Serum trypsinogen is useful in establishing pancreatic insufficiency as a cause for malabsorption.

179. B

Fragile X is a genetic mutation that results in mental retardation in affected individuals. It may affect 1 in 1,500 males and is the second most common genetic cause for mental retardation, with Down's syndrome being most common. Other features of the syndrome include a long face with a large mandible, macro-orchidism, and large everted ears. The syndrome undergoes amplification with successive generation leading to some unusual characteristics of this X-linked disease. For example, 20% of males with this gene are clinically normal, termed "transmitting" males, and 50% of carrier females are affected with mental retardation. These features confused geneticists initially, but the process leading to these characteristics was subsequently defined.

180. C

Prader–Willi syndrome is a genetic disorder resulting from deletion of a band of the long arm of chromosome 15 that results in a syndrome with mental retardation, short stature, hypotonia, obesity, small hands and feet, and hypogonadism. Interestingly, the defect has been traced to a deletion of the paternal chromosome 15, and deletions of the maternal chromosome 15 in the same region result in a different syndrome, termed Angelman syndrome. This syndrome is characterized by ataxic gait, seizures, and inappropriate laughter. Thus, the parent of origin of certain deletions may affect the expression of a particular genetic defect.

Obstetrics Questions

1. A 22-year-old G1P0 presents for routine prenatal visit at 36 weeks of gestation. She has a history of mood disorders but discontinued medication early in her pregnancy. Her psychiatrist has suggested that she resume this medication after delivery. She would like to breast-feed her baby for at least 6 months. Which of the following medications requires caution when prescribed for a breast-feeding woman?

A. Amitriptyline

B. Buproprion (Wellbutrin)

C. Paroxetine (Paxil)

D. Trazodone (Desyrel)

E. Lithium

2. A male infant presents for his 2-week checkup. His vaginal birth was unremarkable and his parents express no concerns. The infant is exclusively breast-fed, feeding about every 4 hours. He has about four wet diapers daily and stools once a day. His weight today is 7 lbs 2 oz compared to a birth weight of 7 lbs 12 oz. His skin is anicteric, and he does not have signs of dehydration. The parents are very motivated to continue breast-feeding. Given this information, what advice would you offer his mother regarding breast-feeding?

A. Stop breast-feeding altogether.

B. Begin formula supplementation but continue breast-feeding every 4 hours.

C. No changes in breast-feeding are necessary.

D. Breast-feeding should be "on demand."

E. Breast-feed every 1 or 2 hours around the clock.

3. A 25-year-old woman presents for preconception counseling. She wants to know more about nutrition, particularly about folic acid. She has read a lot about it in magazines. You can tell her that:

A. Folic acid supplementation is associated with an increased level of alpha-fetoprotein in maternal serum.

B. She needs to take either a prenatal vitamin or a supplement that provides at least 4 mg (4,000 µg) of folic acid.

C. She needs to start folic acid supplementation as soon as her pregnancy test is positive.

D. Most women get enough folic acid through their diet.

E. Folic acid requirements are higher in women with type 1 diabetes mellitus.

4. Weight, nutrition, and exercise are common areas of concern in pregnancy. Which of the following is correct?

A. Body mass index (BMI) is not important to assess in early pregnancy because outcomes are not related to BMI.

B. Pregnancy requires 500 extra kcals per day, which can be increased based on activity levels.

C. Infertility is more strongly associated with being underweight (BMI less than 19) than with being obese (BMI greater than 30).

D. Being underweight (BMI less than 19) is a not a risk factor for preterm birth.

E. Weight gain recommendations during pregnancy are based on BMI, with 25 to 35 lbs recommended for normal weight women.

5. A couple comes to you for a preconception visit. You take a thorough history. Which of the following would prompt you to refer to a geneticist?

A. The woman's sister was born with a congenital heart defect.

B. The woman has mild persistent asthma under good control.

C. The couple has had one miscarriage in the past.

D. The man has a brother with hemophilia.

E. The mother worked in a hospital for 5 years.

6. A 33-year-old G1P0 presents to your office for the first time, stating that her period is late and that she had a positive home pregnancy test. You confirm the pregnancy in the office, and the patient is nervous but happy about the pregnancy. You measure her blood pressure as 140/100, with other vital signs normal. The urinanalysis reveals no protein. Last menstrual period (LMP) and ultrasound date the pregnancy at 13 weeks, with a single intrauterine fetus seen. Follow-up blood pressure in a week is 142/96. She has not seen a physician for a while and denies a history of hypertension or other health problems. She is a nonsmoker, exercises 3 or 4 times a week, and works in an office. You diagnose her with:

A. Pre-eclampsia

B. Renal artery stenosis

C. Chronic hypertension

D. Pregnancy-induced hypertension

E. Anxiety

7. This same patient returns for subsequent follow-up visits with a blood pressure of 160/110. She has no protein or glucose in her urine. Other vital signs are stable, and she has no complaints. What is the medication of choice in pregnant patients with hypertension?

A. Atenolol (Tenormin)

B. Enalapril (Vasotec)

C. Hydralazine (Apresoline)

D. Methyldopa (Aldomet)

E. Hydrochlorothiazide (HCTZ)

8. Using Nägele's rule, the estimated delivery date for a patient with menarche age 12, regular menses, and an LMP of March 25 is:

A. December 28

B. December 31

C. January 1

D. January 2

E. January 18

9. A 17-year-old woman presents complaining of absent menses. She has had irregular periods since menarche. She does not recall the date of her last period. On physical examination a mass is felt extending from the lower abdomen to just below the umbilicus. A urine pregnancy test is positive and fetal heart tones are present. Assuming a singleton pregnancy, what is your best estimate of gestational age?

A. 6 weeks

B. 10 weeks

C. 14 weeks

D. 18 weeks

E. 22 weeks

10. A patient presents for confirmation of her first pregnancy. Her menstrual dates place gestational age at 10 weeks. Which of the following sets of symptoms and signs are consistent with these menstrual dates?

A. Fatigue, nausea, temperature 99°F, chloasma

B. Fatigue, urinary frequency, spider veins, soft cervix

C. Nausea, urinary frequency, temperature 99°F, soft cervix

D. Fatigue, breast tenderness, spider veins, soft cervix

E. Nausea, breast tenderness, chloasma, temperature 97°F

11. An elementary school teacher, 24 weeks pregnant, complains of intermittent lightheadedness. This symptom can occur at any time but is most noticeable at work. What is the most likely cause of this symptom?

A. Vasovagal reactions

B. Bradycardia of pregnancy

C. Vertigo due to hormonal vestibular stimulation

D. Hypoxia of pregnancy

E. Hypotension due to hypovolemia

12. The emergency room physician calls regarding your patient, a 43-year-old pregnant female, whom he is evaluating for chest pain. The patient presented with a burning substernal pain for 1 hour. Her past medical history and family history are negative for cardiac disease. Physical examination is unremarkable except for the cardiac exam, which reveals a grade 2/6 systolic murmur heard loudest at the left sternal border and a loud S3. Her fundal height is 34 cm (consistent with dates). CPK is normal. ECG shows normal sinus rhythm at a rate of 90 bpm with left axis deviation and nonspecific ST changes. Her symptoms have resolved. Based on these findings, what is the most likely diagnosis?

A. Angina

B. Cardiomyopathy

C. Mitral valve stenosis

D. Gastroesophageal reflux disease

E. Hyperthyroidism

13. A 26-year-old female with asthma undergoes pulmonary evaluation with pulmonary function testing and ABG measurement during the second trimester of pregnancy. Which one of the following best describes her results during pregnancy?

A. FEV1 increased, tidal volume increased, PO_2 decreased, PCO_2 decreased

B. FEV1 unchanged, tidal volume decreased, PO_2 decreased, PCO_2 increased

C. FEV1 decreased, tidal volume increased, PO_2 decreased, PCO_2 decreased

D. FEV1 unchanged, tidal volume increased, PO_2 increased, PCO_2 decreased

E. FEV1 increased, tidal volume increased, PO_2 increased, PCO_2 increased

14. A 40-year-old woman is ecstatic when she becomes pregnant. She is 7 weeks from her last menses. You are not surprised that she has nausea but become worried when the patient starts to have painless brown discharge. On exam, the uterus seems to be growing larger than expected. An ultrasound demonstrates a "snowstorm" pattern. Which one of the following is the most appropriate step in managing her condition?

A. Awaiting fetal heart activity with a hand-held Doppler prior to making any decisions

B. Treating with promethazine (Phenergan) IM for the nausea and bed rest

C. Performing a chest x-ray and a uterine evacuation

D. After termination, advising the patient to wait 2 months prior to attempting another pregnancy

E. Checking the alpha-fetoprotein level as this correlates to outcome

15. Which of the following is true regarding development of hyperemesis gravidarum?

A. Hydatidiform mole and multiple gestations are a risk factors.

B. It occurs in more than 20% of pregnancies.

C. It is commonly seen in older mothers.

D. Hypothyroidism is a risk factor.

E. It is most common during the second trimester.

16. A mid-third trimester screening ultrasound reveals oligohydramnios. This is most likely associated with which anomaly?

A. Esophageal atresia

B. Polycystic kidneys

C. Broncho-esophageal fistula

D. Duodenal atresia

E. Urinary tract dysplasia

17. A patient of yours works as an x-ray tech at the local hospital. When she becomes pregnant, she is concerned about continuing her work. She is currently at 10 weeks gestation. Regarding radiation, what do you tell her?

A. Radiation exposure is associated with fetal demise in 10% of women.

B. Her greatest risk from radiation, at this stage, is fetal growth retardation.

C. Radiation most often results in intestinal damage and mucosal sloughing.

D. A single CT scan results in threatening levels of radiation, greater than 100 cGy.

E. The risk of radiation is greatest during the last trimester, when rapid growth is expected.

18. A 25-year-old G1P0 at 28 weeks gestation is involved in a motor vehicle accident. She was the belted driver and does not think her abdomen was struck. She reports no uterine contractions

and wants to go home. The ER calls you for a disposition. Your management includes:
A. Place her in an observational bed on labor and delivery for electronic fetal monitoring; if stable, she may go home in 4 hours.
B. Admit to the antenatal ward for strict bed rest, monitoring, and serial pelvic exams.
C. Discharge home with instructions to follow up first thing in the morning.
D. Perform a biophysical profile in the ER and, if normal, send patient home.
E. Have the patient walk for 1 or 2 hours and then monitor; if there are no contractions, then the patient may go home.

19. The Kleihauer–Betke stain is helpful in pregnant patients to:
A. Evaluate the risk of congenital anomalies
B. Establish the risk of imminent delivery
C. Determine the volume of maternal–fetal hemorrhage
D. Determine if Rh immune globulin is required prophylactically at 28 weeks gestation
E. Investigate the need for magnesium sulfate infusion

20. Postpartum depression is often associated with which one of the following comorbid conditions?
A. Psychosis
B. Mania
C. Substance abuse
D. Obsessions
E. Catatonia

21. Which of the following is a risk factors for fetal macrosomia?
A. Female fetus
B. Small mother
C. Maternal diabetes
D. Nuliparous mother
E. Hypertension of pregnancy

22. When performing a routine prenatal visit on a 28-year-old G2P1 at 38 weeks gestation, you suspect the fetus weighs nearly 10 pounds. There is no history of diabetes. You order a stat ultrasound to evaluate for fetal weight, which they estimate as 4,800 g. Your management includes:
A. Immediate induction of labor because you are certain of her dates and want to avoid shoulder dystocia
B. Plan on a vaginal delivery with adequate staffing in case shoulder dystocia ensues
C. Place the patient on a calorie-restricted diet and follow her twice weekly
D. Schedule her for an elective caesarean section in 1 week to minimize risk of dystocia
E. Transfer the patient to a high-risk center for immediate double setup delivery

23. Which one of the following HIV-positive patients who is pregnant is most likely to transmit HIV to her newborn?
A. CD4 count 500 and viral load 1,000,000
B. CD4 count 20 and viral load 12,000
C. CD4 count 420 and viral load 28,000
D. CD4 count 100 and viral load 100,000
E. CD4 count 500 and viral load less than 500

24. Which of the following is appropriate for the care of the pregnant woman and fetus whose prenatal lab shows a positive hepatitis B surface antigen (HBSAg)?
A. Advise her it is not safe to breast-feed.
B. Give her hepatitis B immune globulin (HBIg) at the beginning of the second trimester.
C. Determine if she has been immunized against hepatitis B.
D. Give her newborn HBIg within 12 hours of delivery.
E. Check for concurrent hepatitis A infection.

25. Which of the following statements regarding Rh-negative patients and antibody screening during pregnancy is true?
A. Hemolysis from isoimmunization may cause erythroblastosis fetalis.
B. Anti-Lewis antibody is clinically significant to the fetus.
C. Rh-negative mothers should be offered Rho (D) immune globulin (RhoGAM) during the first trimester.
D. RhoGAM should not be given to Rh-negative patients involved in a motor vehicle accident.
E. HIV transmission is a risk of the administration of RhoGAM.

26. Which of the following is true regarding erythroblastosis fetalis?
A. It is caused by anti-Lewis isoimmunization hemolysis.
B. Treatment is not recommended until after delivery.
C. Fetal ascites can be detected by ultrasound.
D. It occurs most commonly in primagravida women.
E. Preventative treatment should be given early in the pregnancy.

27. Pregnant women with HIV should not be offered which of the following treatments?
A. Pneumovax to prevent pneumococcal infections
B. Trimethoprim-sulfamethoxazole for *Pneumocystis carinii* pneumonia (PCP) prophylaxis for CD4 count less than 200
C. Acyclovir to prevent herpes infection
D. Rubella vaccine if not immune to rubella
E. Antiretroviral regimens

28. Which of the following is suspicious for active hepatitis in the pregnant patient?
A. Jaundice
B. Known HIV infection
C. Hyperemesis gravidarum
D. Elevated transaminases
E. All of the above

29. Which of the following is true regarding urine cultures in pregnancy?
A. Asymptomatic bactiuria is present in 25% of pregnant women.
B. Asymtomatic bactiuria should be treated in pregnancy.
C. Pyridium (phenazopyridine HCl) is contraindicated during pregnancy.
D. Pregnant patients are less likely to develop ascending urinary tract infections.
E. A urine culture should be done as a screen in the third trimester.

30. A 31-year-old G3P2 patient has just delivered a 3,152-g baby after an oxytocin induction and vacuum-assisted delivery. The placenta spontaneously detaches and delivers 6 minutes after delivery of the baby. After the placenta delivers there is a significant blood loss. What is the most likely immediate cause for the postpartum bleeding?

A. Multiparity
B. Retained placenta tissue
C. Instrumented delivery
D. Uterine atony
E. Oxytocin induction

31. Which of the following drugs is contraindicated with breast-feeding?

A. Ergotamine (Migranal)
B. Metronidazole (Flagyl)
C. Fluconazole (Diflucan)
D. Ketorolac (Toradol)
E. Azithromycin (Zithromax)

32. A 25-year-old G2P2 female presents to your office 2 weeks postpartum after delivering a 3,325-g male infant. She is concerned about her breast milk supply. She did not have any difficulties with milk supply with her first child. She breast-fed the baby 10 times in the last 24 hours. His weight in the office today is 3,100 g. Which of the following is a cause of decreased milk production?

A. Breast engorgement
B. Use of a breast pump
C. Exclusive breast-feeding
D. Frequent breast-feeding
E. Retained placental tissue

33. A woman who is 28 weeks pregnant calls to inform you that she baby-sat a neighborhood child several days ago who has now come down with chickenpox. She calls to ask if there is anything she needs to do. You check her prenatal record and note that she never had a varicella antibody test done with her initial prenatal labs. What is your next step?

A. IgG varicella serology
B. Varicella zoster immunoglobulin (VZIG) within 96 hours of exposure
C. Varicella vaccination after she delivers if seronegative
D. Prophylactic treatment with acyclovir to prevent fetal transmission
E. Counseling on the signs and symptoms of varicella

34. A women at 35 weeks estimated gestational age (EGA) presents for a routine obstetrical appointment. She notes a pruritic rash that began on her abdomen and spread to her thighs and buttocks within several days. The face and periumbilical region are both spared. What is your next step?

A. Reassure her and provide symptomatic relief with topical steroids.
B. Biopsy the lesions to ensure proper diagnosis.
C. Begin treatment with systemic oral corticosteroids.
D. Admit the patient to the hospital for induction of labor.
E. Begin weekly antepartum testing to ensure fetal well-being.

35. A 26-year-old G2P1 woman at 29 weeks EGA presents complaining of contractions. Cervical examination reveals advanced dilation. History is significant for delivery of her first pregnancy at

31 weeks secondary to preterm labor. Which of the following is a risk factor for preterm labor?

A. Caucasian race
B. Singleton pregnancy
C. Higher socioeconomic status
D. Substance abuse (alcohol, tobacco, drugs)
E. Gestational diabetes

36. A 24-year-old G1P0 at 40 5/7 weeks EGA was admitted to the hospital in labor several hours ago. Her cervix was last checked an hour ago and was 5 cm dilated, 100% effaced at -1 station. She is contracting every 1 to 2 minutes and has good pain control with epidural anesthesia. You plan to recheck her cervix momentarily. What is the minimum dilation that you will expect in this women after 1 hour in active labor in order to document adequate progression?

A. 0.5 cm/hour
B. 1.0 cm/hour
C. 1.1 cm/hour
D. 1.2 cm/hour
E. 1.5 cm/hour

37. A 28-year-old G3P2 at 10 weeks presents for her initial OB visit. Her first pregnancy resulted in a normal spontaneous vaginal delivery, but her second resulted in C-section secondary to fetal distress. The operative report is available and documents a lower transverse vertical incision. She inquires regarding the option of vaginal birth after C-section (VBAC). Which one of the following statements reflects the most appropriate advice?

A. The use of oxytocin is contraindicated.
B. The success rate of VBAC is approximately 50%.
C. Cytotec (misoprostol) is the preferred agent if induction or augmentation is needed.
D. Uterine dehiscence and rupture are rare complications occurring less than 1% to 2% of the time.
E. If her baby is more than 4,000 g estimated fetal weight, she will be disqualified from a trial of labor.

38. A 25-year-old G1P0 at 33 6/7 weeks EGA presents complaining of contractions for several hours that were not relieved by rest and hydration. You direct her to Labor and Delivery, where, upon examination, her cervix is noted to be dilated 2 cm with 50% effacement. Her cervix, when examined several weeks earlier, had been long and closed. What is the most appropriate next step?

A. Initiation of therapy with terbutaline (Brethine)
B. Initiation of therapy with magnesium sulfate
C. Sterile speculum exam to assess for rupture of membranes and to collect cultures for chlamydia, gonorrhea, and group B streptococcus
D. Administer steroids to promote fetal lung maturity
E. Perform ultrasound to establish estimated fetal weight

39. A 32-year-old G2P2 woman presents 8 weeks postpartum for her routine checkup. She complains that since her delivery she has noted loss of what she considers excessive amounts of her hair. She is upset because her normally thick and healthy mane has thinned considerably. Further questioning reveals no other symptoms in her review of systems that would be of concern. What response is most appropriate?

A. She needs a thyroid panel immediately.
B. Reassure her that hair growth will reoccur 6 to 15 months postpartum.

C. Reassure her that her hair will return to its previous thickness.
D. Hair loss may occur for up to 12 months.
E. You will prescribe Rogaine if she is interested.

40. A 26-year-old G2P1 at 31 weeks EGA presents complaining of contractions. Her history is unremarkable and pregnancy to this point has been uncomplicated. Examination reveals intact membranes, normal KOH and wet prep, and cervix dilation of 3 to 4 cm with 25% effacement. Which of the following is least appropriate in her management?
A. Corticosteroids
B. Labetolol (Normodyne)
C. Nifedipine (Procardia)
D. Magnesium sulfate
E. Ampicillin

41. Low levels of maternal serum alpha-fetoprotein (MSAFP) are affiliated with what fetal disorder?
A. Open neural tube defect
B. Gastroschisis
C. Cystic hygroma
D. Omphalocele
E. Trisomy 18

42. Which steroid hormone is measured on maternal serum triple screen?
A. Unconjugated estriol
B. Follicle-stimulating hormone
C. Estradiol
D. Luteinizing hormone
E. DHEA

43. What week of gestation is appropriate to perform genetic amniocentesis?
A. 12 weeks
B. 16 weeks
C. 20 weeks
D. 26 weeks
E. 28 weeks

44. Which of the following medications is contraindicated to treat hypertension in pregnancy?
A. Methyldopa (Aldomet)
B. Nifedipine (Procardia)
C. Labetalol (Normodyne)
D. Hydralazine
E. Captopril (Capoten)

45. Which of the following would be the recommended choice of medication for scabies in the pregnant woman?
A. Lindane (Kwell)
B. Crotamiton (Eurax)
C. Mebendazole (Vermox)
D. Permethrin (Elimite, Nix)
E. Piperazine (Antepar)

46. Which of the following regimens is contraindicated in the treatment of chlamydia during pregnancy?

A. Ofloxacin (Floxin) 300 mg PO bid ×7 days
B. Erythromycin 500 mg PO bid ×7 days
C. Amoxicillin (Amoxil, Timox) 500 mg PO tid ×10 days
D. Clindamycin (Cleocin) 450 mg PO qid ×7 days
E. Azithromycin (Zithromax) 1 g PO ×1 dose

47. Which of the following is a sign of severe pre-eclampsia?
A. Systolic blood pressure 150 mmHg
B. 24-hour urine protein of 6500 g
C. Urine output of 80 cc/hour
D. Uric acid of 4.2
E. Platelets = 200,000/mL

48. Magnesium sulfate is the drug of choice for severe pre-eclampsia. What is the goal of the therapy?
A. To cure pre-eclampsia
B. To raise the seizure threshold and prevent eclampsia
C. To lower the blood pressure
D. To raise platelets
E. To improve symptoms such as abdominal pain and headache

49. Which of the following is a risk factor for gestational diabetes?
A. Age younger than 30 years
B. Family or personal history of diabetes
C. Caucasian race
D. Hypothyroidism
E. Hypertension

50. You have just received lab results on your patient, a 32-year-old G2P1. She has 1-hour 50-g glucose tolerance test of 165. What is the next step?
A. Start the patient on insulin therapy.
B. Send the patient to a dietician for diabetic diet counseling.
C. Do nothing; the test is normal.
D. Order a 3-hour glucose tolerance test.
E. Begin checking blood sugars at home qid.

51. Tocolysis in preterm labor is indicated in which of the following situations:
A. Intrauterine growth restriction (IUGR)
B. Prolonged preterm rupture of membranes (PPROM)
C. Chorioamnionitis
D. Vaginal bleeding
E. Fetal death

52. Which of the following is true regarding placental abruption?
A. Cocaine use decreases the risk of abruption.
B. The classic presentation is painless vaginal bleeding.
C. It occurs when the placenta separates from the uterine wall.
D. The patient is not at risk for shock or DIC.
E. Ultrasound is highly sensitive for abruption.

53. Which one of the following is true regarding postpartum depression?
A. Selective serotonin reuptake inhibitors are relatively contraindicated in postpartum depression.
B. The incidence is approximately 50%.

C. Postpartum depression always begins within the first few days postpartum.

D. There does not have to be a past history of depression prior to pregnancy.

E. If untreated, 20% will progress to psychosis.

54. Which maneuver is contraindicated with a shoulder dystocia?

A. McRoberts maneuver (flexing thighs onto maternal abdomen)

B. Suprapubic pressure

C. Fundal pressure

D. Episiotomy

E. Remove the posterior arm of the fetus

55. Which of the following statements represents current medical advice to schizophrenic patients who are planning a pregnancy?

A. Continue psychotropic drugs throughout pregnancy.

B. If possible, stop using the drugs before trying to conceive.

C. Avoid medication use during the third trimester of pregnancy.

D. If medications are needed, use only newer psychiatric medications.

E. Psychiatric disorders generally improve during pregnancy.

56. Which of the following conditions increases the risk of postpartum psychosis?

A. Previous episode of postpartum psychosis

B. Pre-eclampsia

C. Gestational diabetes

D. Marijuana use in pregnancy

E. Family history of depression

57. Which of the following statements about postpartum psychosis is true?

A. It usually occurs in the first 7 days after delivery.

B. Patients are not at increased risk of suicide.

C. Infanticide does not occur with this condition.

D. Home treatment is preferred.

E. The condition requires hospitalization.

58. After examining a patient at 32 weeks gestation, you note that her fundal height is only 28 cm, the same as her last visit. Your immediate plan includes:

A. Send the patient for an urgent ultrasound to determine biometric measurements of the fetus.

B. Have the patient increase her dietary fat and return to the office in 1 week for a recheck.

C. Measure both parents' heights and extrapolate appropriate fetal growth.

D. Admit the patient to the hospital for a non-stress test and biophysical profile.

E. Consider induction after steroid administration.

59. In determining whether a fetus suffers chronic uteroplacental insufficiency, the best ultrasound measurement is:

A. Amniotic fluid index

B. Biparietal diameter

C. Head circumference

D. Femur length

E. Abdominal circumference

60. A 22-year-old woman presents to your office with a positive home pregnancy test. After confirming the results, you take a thorough history. She is a recent immigrant from Mexico. All routine prenatal labs are performed and the only abnormality is a very low IgG titer to rubella, indicating nonimmunity. You advise her that:

A. She should avoid all children for the duration of the pregnancy.

B. IVIG is available should she be exposed to someone with rubella.

C. She will be immunized after giving birth but remains susceptible during this pregnancy.

D. She can be immunized with an MMR at the next visit, but a booster may be needed after the delivery.

E. Rubella can be contracted in the third trimester without risk of fetal injury.

61. The greatest risk factor for the development of pyelonephritis in pregnant women is:

A. Glycosuria

B. Increased urine volume

C. Leukorrhea of pregnancy

D. Asymptomatic bacteriuria

E. Decreased bladder tone

62. A 26-year-old G2P1001 presents to the office at 27 weeks gestational age complaining of chills, cramping pain, and nausea. Her exam is significant for a temperature of 101°F but little else. The fundal height and fetal heart tones are appropriate. Her urine analysis reveals blood, ketones, protein, and leukocyte esterase. Your treatment would include:

A. Antidiarrheals for the impending gastroenteritis and a specimen cup given to collect a stool sample

B. Admission to the antepartum floor for tocolysis with terbutaline and serial exams

C. Transfer to the ER for IV fluids and perchlorperazine (Compazine) per rectum

D. Admission to the antepartum unit for IV hydration and empiric antibiotic therapy for pyelonephritis

E. Seeing the patient again in 1 or 2 days to determine if symptoms have improved

63. Induction of labor is absolutely contraindicated in which clinical scenario?

A. 25-year-old G1P0 who is at estimated gestational age of 40 weeks and has developed pregnancy-induced hypertension (PIH)

B. 28-year-old G2P1 who is found to have a fundal height greater than dates at 41 weeks; an ultrasound demonstrates polyhydramnios

C. 30-year-old G1P0 who underwent a transmural myomectomy prior to conceiving, now at 41 weeks gestation

D. 19-year-old G1P0 who is at 42 weeks with a floating fetal head

E. 32-year-old G5P4 at 41 weeks with an ultrasound-confirmed breech presentation

64. You make the decision to induce labor in a 27-year-old G2P1 because she is nearing 42 weeks gestation. Her first baby was also post dates and required a caesarian section when the induction failed. She has stated her desire to have another try at a vaginal delivery and understands all the risks and benefits. During the examination, you note that the fundal height is 39 cm and the fetal heart tones are 130. The patient has good fetal movement but no contractions at all. Her cervical exam reveals a Bishop score of 4.

Which of the following would be the most optimal method to induce labor in this patient?
A. Oxytocin (Pitocin) drip at a low dose through the IV
B. Dinoprostone insert (Cervidil) placed intravaginally overnight, with fetal monitoring
C. Misoprostol (Cytotec) 200 g given orally with oxytocin induction in the morning
D. Cervical membrane stripping performed in the office, serially if needed
E. Low-dose misoprostol (Cytotec) 25 g inserted vaginally with fetal monitoring

65. Indications for use of vacuum at delivery include:
A. Dense epidural analgesia, normal fetal heart tones
B. Nulliparous woman with no analgesia pushing for 1 hour
C. Brow presentation
D. Fetal scalp pH demonstrating mild acidosis
E. A multiparous woman with an epidural pushing for 2 hours

66. Electronic fetal monitoring (EFM) has been shown to:
A. Increase the rate of caesarian section
B. Improve newborn Apgar scores
C. Reduce the occurrence of cerebral palsy
D. Diagnose fetal distress
E. Facilitate maternal positioning

67. The most ominous abnormality of fetal heart rate on electronic fetal monitoring is:
A. Early decelerations to 90 bpm with return to baseline of 130 bpm
B. Fetal bradycardia with a rate of 105 bpm
C. Normal variability but late decelerations down to a rate of 110 bpm
D. Rate of 130 bpm with no beat-to-beat variability
E. Normal variability with variable decelerations to 100 bpm

68. Early decelerations are different from late deceleration because:
A. Precontraction acceleration or "shoulder" occurs
B. Cervical dilation is less at the time of the deceleration
C. Fetal gestation age is less than 32 weeks when the decelerations occur
D. Mechanism consists of increased fetal vagal stimulation
E. Decelerations are persistent

69. A 26-year-old G1P0 is in active labor but progressing slowly. When her cervix is at 5 cm and fetal head is at station -1, amniotomy is performed and an intrauterine pressure catheter is introduced. Her Montevideo units are over 200. After 3 hours, her cervix is reexamined and she remains at 5 cm with as station of -1. Options for her care include:
A. Caesarian section for "failure to progress," likely cephalopelvic disproportion
B. Starting oxytocin (Pitocin) augmentation for inadequate uterine contractions
C. Giving the patient IV narcotic analgesia to relax her pelvis
D. Placement of fetal scalp electrode to monitor tolerance of contractions
E. Forceps-assisted descent of the fetal head to improve chances of vaginal delivery

70. What are the recommended standards for a patient whose fetus is intolerant to labor regarding a caesarian section in a hospital with a labor and delivery?
A. Immediately because there should be 24-hour in-house coverage
B. One hour from the time that anesthesia is called, to allow placement of the epidural
C. Within 20 minutes of the first deceleration to prevent fetal compromise
D. The patient should be on the table within 30 minutes, with incision within 45 minutes
E. The incision should occur 30 minutes after the decision is made to perform a caesarian section

71. A 30-year-old Italian American female presents to your office for preconception counseling. After a thorough history and physical, which of these screening tests would you offer?
A. Complete blood count
B. Sickle cell smear
C. HIV
D. A and C
E. All of the above

72. The same 30-year-old Italian American female is not up to date on her immunizations. Which of the following should *not* be given less than 1 month prior to conception?
A. Hepatitis B
B. Mumps
C. Tetanus and diphtheria
D. Influenza
E. Meningococcal

73. During your review of the medical history with a newly pregnant 32-year-old G1P0 patient, she admits to a history of deep vein thrombosis 4 years prior. Which of the following medications is indicated during pregnancy?
A. Warfarin (Coumadin)
B. Low–molecular-weight heparin (Lovenox)
C. Enteric-coated aspirin (Ecotrin)
D. Dipyridamole (Aggrenox)
E. Clopidogrel (Plavix)

74. A patient presents to your office at 12 weeks of gestation with a pre-pregnancy BMI of 18; she weighs 122 lbs and is 69 in. tall. What is her recommended weight gain for this pregnancy?
A. greater than 18.2 kg (greater than 40 lbs)
B. 12.7 to 18.2 kg (28 to 40 lbs)
C. 11.4 to 16 kg (25 to 35 lbs)
D. 6.8 to 9.1 kg (15 to 20 lbs)
E. less than 6.8 kg (less than 15 lbs)

75. Which of the following statements about thyroid disease and function in pregnancy is correct?
A. Maternal hypothyroxinemia is most significant in the third trimester.
B. Low maternal free T4 levels may interfere with normal neurodevelopment of the fetus.
C. The mother is the sole source of thyroid hormone throughout the pregnancy.

D. Hypothyroidism during pregnancy most often stems from iodine deficiency.

E. Routine screening for thyroid disease is recommended for pregnant women.

76. A 27-year-old G1P0 reports to your clinic at 18 weeks gestation. Physical exam reveals a fundal height of 23 cm. You decide to perform an ultrasound to investigate further. What amniotic fluid index measurement would make you concerned about the diagnosis of polyhydramnios?

A. One large pocket measuring 10 cm

B. Three pockets measuring 5, 6, and 6 cm, respectively

C. Four pockets measuring 7, 8, 6, and 6 cm, respectively

D. Four pockets measuring 3, 1, 2, and 1 cm, respectively

E. I am not concerned about polyhydramnios in this patient

77. Your ultrasound exam reveals a single fetus and an amniotic fluid index measurement consistent with oligohydramnios. Which of the following is in the differential diagnosis of oligohydramnios?

A. Diabetes

B. Twin gestation

C. Trisomy 18

D. Renal anomalies

E. Fetal skeletal disorders

78. A 32-year-old G4P2012 presents to Labor and Delivery at 32 weeks complaining of vaginal bleeding. She denies pain but was alarmed by the amount of blood she saw. To evaluate the cause of bleeding, you would perform:

A. Sterile vaginal exam

B. Nitrazine test, followed by a fern test

C. Speculum exam followed by cerclage

D. Transabdominal ultrasound

E. Kleihauer–Betke test

79. Your patient, a 27-year-old G2P1 woman at term, has had a normal prenatal course and is in active labor. Her first baby weighed 4,100 g (approximately 9 lbs). She has been pushing for 3 hours and is exhausted. The baby's heart rate dropped to below 90 beats per minute that lasted for more than 1 minute and you decide to attempt an assisted delivery. Which of the following statements is true?

A. If you can deliver the head, there is no risk for shoulder dystocia.

B. A bladder (indwelling) catheter is required prior to vacuum or forceps usage.

C. Vacuum and forceps deliveries carry an equal risk of cephalo hematomas.

D. Vacuum can be used for some malpositions but not for malpresentations.

E. Vacuum can be used if the cervix is 8 cm dilated, but forceps can only be used if the cervix is completely dilated.

80. A healthy 25-year-old nulliparous patient comes to you for a well woman exam. She was married approximately 9 months ago and she and her husband are planning to try to get pregnant some time in the next few months. She has heard about use of folic acid during pregnancy but is unclear about recommendations. Regarding folic acid:

A. Supplementation during pregnancy has been associated with a decrease in sudden infant death syndrome (SIDS) after the baby is born.

B. The recommended dose is 400 µg daily for women at average risk of neural tube defects.

C. The recommended dose is unchanged for women who have a personal history of spina bifida.

D. Folic acid is a B vitamin that is found in abundance in unsupplemented foods that we eat.

E. Women should wait until the end of the first trimester before starting folic acid because of the risk to the fetus during organogenesis.

81. Patients or couples with which of the following disorders are recommended to have preconception genetic counseling?

A. Women with a history of gestational diabetes

B. Women with a single previous first trimester loss

C. Patients with a distant relative with Down's syndrome

D. Previous infant with Down's syndrome

E. Previous pregnancy affected by Sheehan's syndrome

82. A 23-year-old G1P0 woman presents for prenatal care. She is fairly certain that the first day of her LMP was 7 weeks and 4 days ago. She had not been on oral contraceptives or other hormonal contraception prior to getting pregnant. On exam, her uterus is palpable just above the symphysis pubis and fetal heart tones are heard in the 160s. Which of the following statements is true?

A. The physical exam confirms her dates, so ultrasound examination is not needed at this time.

B. If her menses were regular and every 26 to 30 days apart, ultrasound examination is not necessary.

C. Ultrasound examination should be performed since clinically her size is less than dates.

D. Ultrasound examination should be performed to confirm a 12 or 13 week gestation or the possibility of a pelvic mass.

E. Persistent corpus luteum cyst may explain the size–date discrepancy.

83. A 17-year-old G4P0030 patient comes in for evaluation. She has had three elective first trimester abortions. She does not recall having a menses since her most recent abortion 4 months ago. She has had no cramping or bleeding since that time. Examination reveals the fundus to be palpable halfway to the umbilicus and fetal heart tones are heard in the 150s. Which of the following is true?

A. Ultrasound examination is not necessary since the date of her abortion is equivalent to her LMP.

B. Ultrasound examination should be deferred until the patient is 20 to 22 weeks gestation in order to obtain an adequate structural survey.

C. Ultrasound examination is not necessary at this time because she has had no vaginal bleeding.

D. Ultrasound examination is recommended to confirm her dates, since the time to return to ovulation following an abortion is unpredictable.

E. Both A and C are correct.

84. Today you are seeing a new obstetrical patient. This is her first pregnancy, and she wants to know the schedule for office visits for routine prenatal care. The correct schedule is:

A. Monthly visits until 30 weeks, every 3 weeks until 36 weeks, and then weekly until delivery

B. Monthly visits until 32 weeks, every 2 weeks until 36 weeks, and then weekly until delivery

C. Monthly visits until 28 weeks, every 2 weeks until 36 weeks, and then weekly until delivery

D. Monthly visits until 30 weeks, every 2 weeks until 36 weeks, and then twice weekly until delivery

E. Monthly visits until 32 weeks, every 2 weeks until 36 weeks, and then twice weekly until delivery

85. On an initial obstetrical history and physical the patient admits to smoking a pack of cigarettes a day for the past 10 years. At this time, she does not want to quit. Which of the following complications are associated with smoking?

A. Low birth weight

B. Breech presentation

C. Post-date delivery

D. Gestational diabetes

E. Uterine rupture

86. During your initial prenatal visit, you discover a 28-year-old G4P2012 smokes only about one-half of a pack per day. She states that during the past month she has attempted to quit several times and has been unsuccessful. She is asking for assistance in quitting. The least appropriate treatment modality for this patient would be:

A. Enroll patient in a quit smoking program.

B. Offer a prescription for buproprion (Zyban).

C. Encourage patient to begin a nicotine replacement program.

D. Help patient establish a quit date and offer short follow-up visits.

E. Assess partner's smoking status and readiness to quit.

87. A 42-year-old African American G2P0101 at 36 weeks presents to Labor and Delivery complaining of painful contractions. She admits that her first delivery was a C-section secondary to fetal intolerance of labor. What are her risk factors for preterm labor?

A. African American race

B. Age older than 40

C. History of preterm birth

D. Uterine surgery

E. All of the above

88. An obstetrical patient presents at 42 weeks EGA. She has not felt any painful contractions and is beginning to worry about risks to her baby. Which answer is a true statement if the pregnancy is truly post date?

A. There are no risks to the baby.

B. Perinatal mortality is the same as before 40 weeks.

C. Placental insufficiency is present in one-third of post-date births.

D. Infants develop a thick subcutaneous fat layer.

E. Post-date births have been associated with prior preterm births

89. Which of the following is true regarding medications taken during pregnancy?

A. All natural products are considered safe during pregnancy.

B. Category D medications are safe to take during pregnancy.

C. Category medications have been through controlled human studies.

D. The risk factors associated with the various categories during pregnancy also can be used for assigning risk during lactation.

E. Category E medications can be associated with fetal anomalies.

90. You have a 32-year-old G3P2 patient who has been treated successfully for depression using Prozac (fluoxetine) 40 mg. She is 8 weeks pregnant. What do you advise her regarding her depression?

A. She should reduce her dose to 20 mg.

B. Most depression spontaneously improves during pregnancy. She will probably require no medications.

C. Prozac (fluoxetine) is a category D medication and should be discontinued during pregnancy.

D. She should discontinue the Prozac (fluoxetine) until her second trimester, when it can be safely resumed.

E. The maternal benefits of Prozac (fluoxetine) must be weighed against the potential fetal risk.

91. Which of the following statements about depression and pregnancy is true?

A. The incidence of depression is lower in pregnant than in non-pregnant women.

B. The risk of depression postpartum is lower than the risk during pregnancy.

C. Most tricyclic antidepressants and selective serotonin reuptake inhibitors appear to be teratogenic.

D. Women with severe chronic depression are at risk of morbidity with relapse if medication is discontinued.

E. Use of monoamine oxidase inhibitors is recommended during pregnancy.

92. Which of the following is true regarding treatment of psychosis during pregnancy?

A. Chronic schizophrenia rarely relapses when medication is discontinued during pregnancy.

B. Lithium, Depakene (valproic acid), and Tegretol (carbamazepine) are all safely used in the treatment of bipolar disorder during pregnancy.

C. Haldol (haloperidol) is the most teratogenic antipsychotic medication.

D. It is very beneficial to provide prophylaxis against postpartum relapse in patients with a history of bipolar disorder.

E. Most psychopharmacologic agents do not cross the placenta.

93. Which of the following is a risk factor for preterm labor?

A. Caucasian race

B. Bacterial vaginosis

C. Singleton gestation

D. Alcohol use

E. Inaccurate dating

94. A 26-year-old primagravida is 14 weeks pregnant. One of her kindergarten students has developed chickenpox. Your patient is uncertain if she had chickenpox in the past. You should:

A. Administer the varicella vaccine.

B. Advise the patient to terminate the pregnancy due to the teratogenic effects of varicella infection.

C. Obtain IgA serology and, if positive, administer VZIG.

D. Obtain IgA serology and, if negative, administer VZIG.

E. Reassure the patient that varicella is nonthreatening during pregnancy.

95. A 17-year-old primagravida is positive for chlamydia cervicitis. Which of the following treatment regimes is indicated?
A. Amoxicillin (Amoxil, Timox) 500 mg three times daily for 10 days
B. Erythromycin 333 mg three times daily for 10 days
C. Doxycycline (Vibramycin) 100 mg two times daily for 10 days
D. Clindamycin (Cleocin) vaginal cream, one applicator full for 7 days
E. Ciprofloxacin (Cipro) 250 mg one-time dose

96. A 33-year-old G3P2 is 9 weeks pregnant. She presents to your office with a pruritic thick white vaginal discharge. You diagnose yeast vaginitis. Which of the following treatments would you offer her?
A. Miconizole (Monistat) 7 vaginal cream, one applicator full for 7 days
B. Clindamycin (Cleocin) vaginal cream, one applicator full for 7 days
C. Clindamycin (Cleocin) 150 mg orally, four times daily for 7 days
D. Metronidazole (Flagyl) 500 mg orally, two times daily for 7 days
E. Fluconazole (Diflucan) 100 mg orally, one dose

97. Your patient is 36 years old and has essential hypertension. She is planning to conceive. Currently, her hypertension is well controlled on captopril (Capoten) 50 mg twice daily. What should you advise her regarding her blood pressure and pregnancy?
A. There are no anti-hypertensives considered safe during pregnancy.
B. Her blood pressure will most likely improve spontaneously during pregnancy and she will not need any medication.
C. She should continue her current anti-hypertensive regime.
D. She should change medications to methyldopa (Aldomet) 250 mg four times daily.
E. She should change medications to hydrochlorothiazide 25 mg once daily.

98. Which of the following regarding hydatidiform mole is true?
A. The incidence in the United States is 1 in 250.
B. Patients with a history of molar pregnancy are not at higher risk of subsequent molar pregnancy.
C. Most complete hydatidiform moles have a 46,XX chromosomal pattern arising from the father.
D. It is unusual for a patient with a molar pregnancy to have vaginal spotting.
E. It is difficult to identify a molar pregnancy with ultrasound.

99. Which is true regarding the treatment of hydatidiform mole?
A. Embolization of trophoblastic tissue is a risk during suction aspiration.
B. Most molar pregnancies pass spontaneously and do not require evacuation of the uterus.
C. It is important to follow BHCG levels until they begin to fall.
D. Most patients require chemotherapy as part of their management.
E. All patients should be encouraged to undergo hysterectomy in order to eliminate future risk of malignancy.

100. A 24-year-old G1P0 woman at 33 weeks gestation was the unrestrained driver of a sedan. She was struck from behind and sustained facial, chest, and abdominal trauma. She did not have loss of consciousness. Which of the following is true?
A. She is at increased risk of placenta previa.
B. She is at increased risk of placental abruption.

C. At 33 weeks, her fetus is well protected by an amniotic fluid cushion and thus the pregnancy is not at risk.
D. Uterine rupture is a frequent complication of motor vehicle accidents.
E. If the mother's vital signs are stable, complications are unlikely.

101. Your 39-year-old G4P3 patient is 8 weeks pregnant. She presents to your office with bright red vaginal bleeding. She tearfully tells you that 2 days ago she tripped and fell down a short flight of stairs. You tell her:
A. Vaginal bleeding is common during the first trimester and probably does not indicate a risk to the pregnancy.
B. Her recent fall is most probably not related to her current vaginal bleeding.
C. If she adheres to strict bed rest, she will be able to avert a miscarriage.
D. Miscarriage is inevitable at this point.
E. Trauma such as she sustained in her fall often leads to miscarriage.

102. You have a 31-year-old patient at 38 weeks gestation. She presented with spontaneous rupture of membranes 3 hours ago. She has not had any contractions. This is an example of:
A. Preterm premature rupture of membranes (PPROM)
B. Imminent preterm delivery
C. Premature rupture of membranes (PROM)
D. Spontaneous onset of labor at term
E. Failure to progress

103. Corticosteroids are administered to mothers between 24 and 34 weeks gestation in preterm labor in order to reduce which of the following fetal complications?
A. Hyaline membrane disease
B. Sepsis
C. Intraventricular hemorrhage
D. Meconium aspiration
E. A and C

104. Which of the following is true regarding tocolytic therapy for patients in preterm labor?
A. Short-term tocolytic therapy has been shown to significantly improve neonatal outcomes.
B. Oral magnesium therapy is ineffective in preventing preterm labor.
C. Indomethacin has been shown to decrease neonatal morbidity.
D. Oral terbutaline following subcutaneous or intravenous tocolysis results in prolonged pregnancy.
E. Tocolytic therapy can frequently delay labor for up to several weeks.

105. Which one of the following is true regarding polyhydramnios?
A. It is an indication for urgent delivery.
B. It is defined on ultrasound as an amniotic fluid index of greater than 25 cm.
C. It is best assessed using transvaginal ultrasound.
D. It is common in multiple gestation.
E. It can be successfully treated with amnioinfusion.

106. Which of the following are ultrasound findings of fetal demise?
A. No cardiac activity
B. Oligohydramnios
C. Abnormal lie

D. Subcutaneous edema

E. All of the above

107. Which of the following is true regarding oligohydramnios?

A. In a post-date pregnancy, oligohydramnios is generally an indication for delivery.

B. Oligohydramnios is defined on ultrasound by an amniotic fluid index of less than 10 cm.

C. Amnioinfusion rarely improves the fetal heart tone tracing.

D. Amnioinfusion using normal saline can lead to fetal electrolyte imbalance.

E. It increases the risk of cord prolapse.

108. A 28-year-old G2P1 at 36 weeks gestation presents for routine prenatal care. She mentions that she has noted diminished fetal movement over the past week. Which of the following would be the appropriate initial evaluation of her complaint?

A. A digital exam of her cervix

B. Ultrasound

C. Turbidity test

D. Non-stress test

E. Contraction stress test

109. Which of the following is part of the clinical assessment of a woman at 32 weeks who presents with uterine contractions every 7 minutes?

A. Speculum exam to assess pooling of fluid

B. Fetal monitor strip for 10 minutes

C. McRoberts maneuver

D. A and C

E. All of the above

110. You have a 37-year-old G2P1 patient who has well-controlled chronic hypertension. Which of the following circumstances would prompt you to hospitalize her?

A. Pyelonephritis

B. A grade II/VI systolic murmur

C. New onset of proteinuria (greater than 1 g/24?)

D. A and C

E. All of the above

111. A 15-year-old G1P0 patient at 36 weeks presents to your office complaining of headaches, blurry vision, and increased swelling for the last 3 days. Her blood pressure is 150/94 and her weight is up 6 lbs from your visit 2 weeks ago. Her fundal height measures 36.5 cm and fetal heart tones are in the 150s. She has 2+ protein in her urine. You make a diagnosis of pre-eclampsia. Which of the following is true of pre-eclampsia?

A. It is responsible for the majority of maternal morbidity and mortality in the United States in the 21st century.

B. It can be effectively prevented by taking low-dose aspirin (81 mg daily) throughout the second and third trimesters (starting after 14 weeks gestation).

C. It is responsible for the majority of neonatal morbidity and mortality in the United States in the 21st century.

D. The diagnosis can clearly be differentiated from pregnancy-induced hypertension on the basis of the presence of lower extremity edema.

E. It is more common among women who are nulliparous than those who are multiparous.

112. A 37-year-old G2P1001 patient at $39\frac{2}{7}$ weeks presents for routine prenatal visit. She is asymptomatic but her blood pressure is 142/86 and urine dip shows 1+ protein. Fundal height is 38 cm and fetal heart tones are heard in the 130s. Her cervix is 3 cm/60%/-1 station and soft. Which of the following statements is correct regarding pre-eclampsia?

A. Women older than the age of 35 years are at lower risk than women younger than the age of 18 years.

B. If a woman had pre-eclampsia with her first pregnancy, she is no more likely to have pre-eclampsia with her second pregnancy.

C. Vasospasm is not an underlying mechanism of pre-eclampsia.

D. Delivery is the treatment of choice for pre-eclamptic patients at term.

E. Ten percent to 15% of pregnancies are complicated by pre-eclampsia.

113. A 19-year-old G1P0 patient at $37\frac{3}{7}$ weeks gestation presents for her routine prenatal visit. Her pregnancy has been uncomplicated until this point except for poor weight gain (12 lbs during pregnancy prior to this visit). You review her chart before you enter the exam room and notice that her weight is up 8 lbs from her last visit 2 weeks ago (20 lbs for total pregnancy). Noticing this weight gain, you review the signs and symptoms of pre-eclampsia. Which of the following would make you suspect pre-eclampsia?

A. Fatigue

B. Sporadic contractions

C. Elevated blood pressure

D. Decreased fetal movement

E. Glucosuria

114. A 22-year-old G1P0 patient is at 37 weeks. Her pregnancy has been uncomplicated but you noted on her initial physical that she had inverted nipples. When reviewing her birth plan, she indicates that she wants to breast-feed. Which one of the following will you recommend?

A. Nipple shields starting now, to help prepare her nipples for breast-feeding

B. Breast-feeding every 3 or 4 hours to allow significant milk accumulation to occur between feedings

C. Breast shells worn daily, under bra

D. Late third trimester pumping with an electric pump to help evert the nipples

E. No changes in her care

115. A 17-year-old G1P0 woman presents to you for prenatal care at $10\frac{2}{7}$ weeks gestation. Her history and physical examination are unremarkable and her uterine size is consistent with dates. You order routine lab work and educate her about her pregnancy. She is undecided about breast-feeding. You encourage her to breast-feed by pointing out the benefits of breast-feeding, including which of the following?

A. Decreased risk of infections in the infant

B. Decreased risk of infections in the mother

C. Prevents the transmission of HIV from mother to child

D. Increases risk of food allergies in the infant

E. Increases the chances of conception

116. A 27-year-old G1P0 patient presents for initial prenatal care. She has been trying to get pregnant for approximately the past 7 months and has been keeping track of her menstrual periods in a pocket calendar. Menarche was at age 12. Her menses have a light flow and last 3 days. She has regular menses every 32 to 34 days. She has no history of sexually transmitted diseases. She was on oral contraceptives until 1 year ago when she married. In determining her gestational age and estimated date of confinement (EDC), you inquire about her LMP. Which of the following accurately describes Nägele's rule?

A. To determine the patient's EDC, take the LMP, add 9 months, and subtract 7 days.

B. To determine the patient's EDC, start with the LMP, add 3 months, subtract 7 days, and add 1 year.

C. Nägle's rule assumes regular menstrual cycles and cycle interval of 26 to 30 days.

D. Nägle's rule is more accurate than ultrasound determination in the first trimester.

E. Nägle's rule should not be used in this patient because of her history of hypomenorrhea.

117. An 18-year-old G1P0 patient presents at 16 weeks gestation for routine prenatal care. Her past medical and surgical history are unremarkable. She drank 5 or 6 bottles of beer (total) during the first 8 weeks of her pregnancy; she discontinued when she found out she was pregnant. She was formerly smoking 1 pack per day (ppd) but cut back to $\frac{1}{2}$ppd when she found out she was pregnant. Regarding her current tobacco use, which of the following statements is true:

A. Nicotine replacement (e.g., patches) is considered category A during pregnancy.

B. Smoking cessation advice and behavioral modification are effective for women who are pregnant.

C. If this patient continues to smoke throughout her pregnancy, you should start a nicotine patch when she is admitted in labor since she will be unable to smoke in the labor and delivery suite.

D. Since she has already cut back to $\frac{1}{2}$ppd, she is smoking a safe number of cigarettes.

E. Buproprion, although effective for smoking cessation, is contraindicated during pregnancy (category X).

118. A 17-year-old G3P2002 patient presents for prenatal care. Both her previous pregnancies were complicated by preterm delivery at approximately 35 or 36 weeks and her infants were small for gestational age. Her most recent delivery was 3 months ago and she has not had a menses since. She broke up with the father of the baby of her last child during her pregnancy and has been involved with a new boyfriend for about 2 months. Her gynecologic history is unremarkable, with menarche at age $11\frac{1}{2}$ and regular menses every 28 to 30 days prior to her first pregnancy 2 years ago. She has had normal Pap smears with each of her previous pregnancies. She had chlamydia with her most recent pregnancy (which was treated) but no other sexually transmitted diseases. She smokes one pack per day but denies alcohol or drug use. After completing her exam, you review smoking cessation with her. Which of the following is a risk of smoking during pregnancy?

A. Smoking during pregnancy is a risk factor for post-date delivery and macrosomia.

B. Smoking during pregnancy is a risk factor for the mother to develop pre-eclampsia.

C. Smoking during pregnancy is a risk factor for the mother to develop gestational diabetes.

D. Infants of smokers have a higher risk of SIDS and higher risk of respiratory infections.

E. Smoking during pregnancy is a risk factor for the infant to develop type 1 diabetes mellitus.

119. Breech presentation at term:

A. Is less common than a face presentation at term

B. Is associated with an increased rate of congenital anomalies

C. Requires immediate delivery by caesarean section

D. Is unlikely to convert spontaneously to a vertex presentation if diagnosed after 34 weeks

E. Is another term for the occiput posterior position ("sunny side up baby")

120. A 31-year-old G4P3003 patient at $37\frac{2}{7}$ weeks comes in for routine prenatal care. Her pregnancy has been uncomplicated and her culture for group B streptococcus was negative. She has no complaints. She has had rare contractions. Her blood pressure is 110/70; her fundal height is 38 cm; her urinalysis shows trace protein, negative glucose, and 1+ leukocyte esterase; and fetal heart tones are heard in the 150s. Cervical exam reveals her to be 2 cm dilated, 30% effaced, presenting part high. By Leopold's and cervical exam, you believe the fetus to be in a breech presentation and bedside ultrasound confirms this. You begin to discuss options for management of breech presentation. Which of the following statements is true about breech presentation at term?

A. Polyhydramnios is an uncommon co-existing condition.

B. Footling breech is a contraindication to external cephalic version (ECV).

C. Because of the risk to the fetus, ECV should only be attempted if a patient refuses elective C-section.

D. Because of the risk to the fetus, ECV should only be attempted if the patient is in labor.

E. When performed by an experienced operator, ECV has few risks and is effective 60% to 70% of the time.

121. A 30-year-old G1P0 patient presents to your office for a routine prenatal visit at $39\frac{5}{7}$ weeks. She reports no contraction, no vaginal bleeding, and no loss of fluid. She has only felt the fetus move once yesterday and once today but was not concerned because she thought the fetus was "resting" to prepare for the birth. Decreased fetal movement late in the third trimester:

A. Indicates an intrauterine fetal demise

B. Is a reassuring symptom of fetal well-being

C. Is a sensitive but not specific symptom of fetal non–well-being

D. Can be evaluated with a contraction stress test

E. Is very common and does not require medical evaluation

122. A 16-year-old G1P0 patient at 39+ weeks presents as a walk-up to your office, asking when her baby is going to be born. She has missed her last four appointments with you, despite numerous calls and letters from you and your office staff. Her prenatal care began at 16 weeks and her dates were determined by a 17-week ultrasound. She has had five previous prenatal visits, the last one at 32 weeks. All of her blood work has been normal. When you start to see her, she says that she has had no contractions, no vaginal bleeding, no leakage of fluid, and rare (1 or 2 times per day) fetal movement for the last 2 weeks. She is normotensive, her fundal height is 38.5 cm, her urine dip is negative for protein and glucose, and fetal heart tones in the 150s are heard. Her cervix is soft, mid position, 2 cm dilated, 70% effaced, and 0 station and presenting part is vertex. Which of the following would be your next step in the management of her pregnancy?

A. Performing a non-stress test

B. Performing a contraction stress test

C. Performing a biophysical profile

D. Reassuring the patient, educating her on kick counts and labor precautions, and scheduling her for an appointment in 1 week

E. Consideration of induction of labor given your concerns with her compliance

123. A 36-year-old G1P0 woman presents for a routine prenatal visit at 38 weeks by LMP (confirmed with 6-week ultrasound). Her pregnancy has been uncomplicated except for weight gain of approximately 48 pounds. She feels "swollen" but otherwise has no complaints. She has normal fetal movement and has had irregular contractions for the past 2 days. At today's visit, her initial blood pressure is 140/80 with a repeat of 138/92 after sitting for 10 minutes. No previous blood pressure reading had been elevated. Her weight is 48 pounds above her pre-pregnancy weight. She has 2+ LE edema, unchanged from the previous visit. Fundal height is 39 cm. Fetal heart tones are in the 150s. Urinalysis dip in your office reveals 1+ protein and negative glucose. Her cervix is soft, anterior, 2 cm dilated, 80% effaced, -1 station, and presenting part is vertex. Which of the following is true:

A. She should be delivered by immediate C-section.

B. You should give her labor precautions and see her in 1 week.

C. You are unable to accurately evaluate her without knowledge of her baseline systolic and diastolic blood pressures.

D. You should check lab work, a non-stress test, and consider inducing her labor with oxytocin.

E. The patient should be admitted for IV magnesium sulfate therapy. If there is cervical change, her labor should be induced with oxytocin.

124. Which of the following groups of women should be screened for gestational diabetes mellitus (GDM)?

A. Women who are members of ethnic groups with a low prevalence of GDM

B. Women who have no known diabetes in their first-degree relatives

C. Women who are older than 25 years

D. Women who are not obese prior to pregnancy

E. Women who have no history of poor obstetric outcome

References

Question 4: Gabbe SG, Niebyl JR, Simpson JL, eds. Obstetrics—normal and problem pregnancies. 4th ed. New York: Churchill Livingstone; 2002.

Question 13: Gabbe SG, Niebyl JR, Simpson JL, eds. Obstetrics—normal and problem pregnancies. 4th ed. New York: Churchill Livingstone; 2002. These are from MD Consult.

Question 14: Imaged MD from Tamimi H. Atlas of Clinical Gynecology: Gynecologic Pathology. Philadelphia: Current Medicine; 1998.

Question 37: Gabbe SG, Niebyl JR, Simpson JL, eds. Obstetrics—normal and problem pregnancies. 4th ed. New York: Churchill Livingstone; 2002. These are from MD Consult.

Question 53: Gabbe SG, Niebyl JR, Simpson JL, eds. Obstetrics—normal and problem pregnancies. 4th ed. New York: Churchill Livingstone; 2002. These are from MD Consult.

Question 64: Gabbe SG, Niebyl JR, Simpson JL, eds. Obstetrics—normal and problem pregnancies. 4th ed. New York: Churchill Livingstone; 2002. These are from MD Consult.

Question 79: G Gabbe SG, Niebyl JR, Simpson JL, eds. Obstetrics—normal and problem pregnancies. 4th ed. New York: Churchill Livingstone; 2002. These are from MD Consult.

American College of Obstetricians and Gynecologists (ACOG). Operative Vaginal Delivery. Practice Bulletin No. 17. Washington, DC: ACOG; 2000.

Chapter 3

Answer Key

1. E	43. B	85. A
2. E	44. E	86. C
3. E	45. D	87. E
4. E	46. A	88. C
5. A	47. B	89. C
6. C	48. B	90. E
7. D	49. B	91. D
8. C	50. D	92. D
9. D	51. B	93. B
10. C	52. C	94. D
11. E	53. D	95. B
12. D	54. C	96. A
13. D	55. B	97. D
14. C	56. A	98. C
15. A	57. E	99. A
16. E	58. A	100. B
17. B	59. E	101. B
18. A	60. C	102. C
19. C	61. D	103. E
20. D	62. D	104. B
21. C	63. C	105. B
22. B	64. B	106. E
23. A	65. E	107. A
24. D	66. A	108. D
25. A	67. D	109. A
26. C	68. D	110. D
27. D	69. A	111. E
28. E	70. E	112. D
29. B	71. D	113. C
30. D	72. B	114. E
31. A	73. B	115. A
32. E	74. B	116. C
33. A	75. B	117. B
34. A	76. C	118. D
35. D	77. D	119. B
36. D	78. D	120. E
37. D	79. D	121. C
38. C	80. B	122. A
39. B	81. D	123. D
40. B	82. D	124. C
41. E	83. D	
42. A	84. C	

Chapter 3

Obstetrics Answers

1. E

Amitriptyline, buproprion, paroxetine, and trazodone appear in breast milk at low concentrations. While no immediate adverse effects are recognized, the long-term developmental and behavioral effects of exposure to these psychoactive substances are unknown. In contrast, lithium is a water-soluble substance that passes easily into breast milk. Serum lithium levels in the infant are one-third to one-half the maternal level. Breast-fed infants whose mothers are treated with lithium must be monitored closely for signs of toxicity. The American Academy of Pediatrics classifies lithium as a drug that should be used with caution in nursing mothers.

2. E

The infant in this question shows several signs of inadequate nutrition but does not seem in acute danger. At 2 weeks of age, he should have regained his birth weight. In addition, by 5 days of age, a breast-fed infant should pass at least three stools daily and urinate at least 5 times. Most infants must be breast-fed 8 to 12 times daily in order to meet these goals, whereas this infant is eating only 6 times a day. Breast-feeding should not be stopped, but the frequency needs to be increased. The increased feeding will have the added benefit of increasing the mother's milk supply. Once the child's parents can recognize adequate nutrition, breast-feeding on demand can be instituted. If the parents are encouraged to start formula supplementation, the mother's milk supply will diminish due to the decreased demand. In addition, there may be nipple confusion resulting from the very different sucking action needed to drink milk from a bottle. Often, patients such as these will benefit from a lactation consultant.

3. E

Women with insulin-dependent diabetes are at significantly higher risk of neural tube defects (NTDs) and require 4 mg daily supplementation. Folic acid has been proven to reduce the risk of NTDs. On a maternal serum panel, elevated alpha-fetoprotein levels are associated with open NTDs; therefore, folic acid is associated with normal levels. Folic acid requirements for all women who may become pregnant are 400 μg. The only patients who need 4 mg are women who are at high risk for fetal NTDs, such as those who have given birth to an infant with an NTD previously, those on anticonvulsants, and those with type 1 diabetes mellitus. Since the neural tube closes 4 weeks after fertilization, the need for folic acid is greatest prior to the first missed menses. Waiting until the pregnancy test is positive is too late. More than two-thirds of women do not get enough folic acid in their diet. Folic acid has been proven to prevent 50% or more of neural tube defects, which include anencephaly and spinal bifida. The other half of NTDs are multifactorial or genetic. One month prior to conception and through the first trimester, women should avoid folic acid antagonists such as aminopterin, pyrimethamine, trimethoprim, triamterane, sulfasalazine, methotrexate, and anticonvulsants (e.g., valproic acid and carbamazepine).

4. E

Pregnancy surprisingly does not require many extra calories. Only 100 more kcals per day is recommended in the first trimester and then 300 kcals extra per day in the last two trimesters. Breast-feeding requires 500 extra calories a day. Body mass index (BMI) is a very helpful tool in risk assessment of the pregnant patient. A starting BMI of 30 or above has an odds ratio of 2.8 for term stillbirth. Conversely, a starting BMI of 19 or less is associated with preterm births, both small for gestational age (odds ratio, 1.69) and normal for gestational age (odds ratio, 1.34). Both natural and assisted conception are markedly reduced in even moderately overweight women (BMI greater than 27). If the woman's BMI is 35 or greater (very obese), her fecundity odds ratio is only 0.5 compared to individuals with normal weight. Weight gain recommendations are indeed based on preconception BMI. Both the American College of Obstetricians and Gynecologists (ACOG) and the Institute of Medicine have similar recommendations. Those with BMIs less than 19 should gain 28 to 40 lbs and women with normal BMIs (19 to 26) should gain 25 to 35 lbs. Overweight women (BMI 26 to 29) should gain 15 to 25 lbs and obese women (BMI greater than 29) should aim for 15 lbs or less. Weight loss in pregnancy, however, is not recommended. See Table 3.1.

5. A

All pregnant women have a 2% to 4% risk of congenital anomalies; however, there are couples who have an increased need for genetic counseling. Congenital heart defects often have a genetic component. Any personal or family history of heart defects should be investigated. Hemophilia is an X-linked disorder. If the man does not have hemophilia, he cannot be carrying the abnormal gene. However, if the woman had a brother with hemophilia, she would require counseling because she may be a carrier. Any couple with a history of two or three miscarriages should be counseled. About one-half of all first trimester abortions are due to chromosomal abnormalities. If there have been multiple losses or a malformed fetus, the risk of a balanced chromosomal transposition is 4% for either parent. If the transposition is Robertsonian, involving chromosome 21, the risk of Down's syndrome is significant. There are other indications for genetic counseling, including a maternal age older than 35 at the time of delivery, a family history of neural tube defects or genetic diseases, delivery of a previous infant with congenital abnormalities, and certain environmental exposures at the workplace. Women from ethnic groups with higher risk of genetic disease such as Italians, Greeks, Phillipinos, Ashkenazi Jews, Cajun or French Canadians, and those of African ancestry should

Table 3.1 Summary of recommended dietary allowances for women aged ≥25 to 50 years, changes from nonpregnant to pregnant, and food sources

Nutrient	Nonpregnant	Pregnant	Percentage Increase	Dietary Sources
Energy (kcal)	2,200	2,500	+13.6	Proteins, carbohydrates, fats
Protein (g)	50	60	+20	Meats, fish, poultry, dairy
Calcium (mg)	800	1,200	+50	Dairy products
Phosphorus (mg)	800	1,200	+50	Meats
Magnesium (mg)	280	320	+14.3	Seafood, legumes, grains
Iron (mg)	15	30	+100	Meats, eggs, grains
Zinc (mg)	12	15	+25	Meats, seafood, eggs
Iodine (μg)	150	175	+16.7	Iodized salt, seafood
Vitamin A (μg RE)	800	800	0	Dark green, yellow, or orange fruits and vegetables, liver
Vitamin D (IU)	200	400	+100	Fortified dairy products
Thiamin (mg)	1.2	1.5	+36.3	Enriched grains, pork
Riboflavin (mg)	1.3	1.6	+23	Meats, liver, enriched grains
Pyridoxine (mg)	1.6	2.2	+37.5	Meats, liver, enriched grains
Niacin (mg NE)	15	17	+13.3	Meats, nuts, legumes
Vitamin B12 (μg)	2.0	2.2	+10	Meats
Folic acid (μg)	180	400	+122	Leafy vegetables, liver
Vitamin C (mg)	60	70	+16.7	Citrus fruits, tomatoes
Selenium (μg)	55	65	+18.2	

From National Academy of Sciences. *Recommended Dietary Allowances*. 10th ed. National Academy Press: Washington, DC; 1989.

be counseled. After conception, women who have abnormalities on ultrasound or an abnormal maternal serum triple screen should be referred.

6. C

Chronic hypertensive disease of pregnancy is defined as blood pressure greater than 140/90 seen before the 20th week of pregnancy. Many women receive medical care only when pregnant, so a history of high blood pressure with a previous pregnancy may actually be chronic hypertension. In women who do not meet the blood pressure criteria but have a diastolic blood pressure persistently greater than 80 mmHg before the 20th week, chronic hypertension is likely because there is a natural decrease in baseline blood pressure during the first and second trimester. A history of chronic renal disease or any other cause of secondary hypertension should also alert the family practitioner. Management can be continued by the family physician but would warrant obstetrical or perinatology involvement because of the risks of growth retardation, placental insufficiency, and superimposed pre-eclampsia.

7. D

Methyldopa remains the drug of choice in treating chronic hypertension in pregnancy, although other therapies with beta-blockers such as labetalol, which has selective alpha-1 blocking activity, have increasingly been used. Interestingly, atenolol is currently not recommended in pregnancy because of studies that indicate an increased risk of intrauterine growth restriction (IUGR) with this particular beta-blocker. Hydralazine may also be used and is the drug of choice in England. However, the multiple dosing regimen may lead to decreased compliance. ACE inhibitors such as enalapril are contraindicated in pregnancy since they have been shown to cause fetal and neonatal death during the second and third trimesters. Hydrochlorothiazide is also contraindicated because of the risk of fetal malformations and electrolyte abnormalities.

8. C

To use Nägele's rule for estimated delivery date (EDD) calculation, add 7 days and subtract 3 months from the last menstrual period (LMP). In this example, March 25 plus 7 days is April 1 (31 days in March) minus 3 months yields January 1 as the EDD. The date of menarche is not involved in calculation of EDD. Nägele's rule is based on the assumption of a 280-day pregnancy

9. D

In a normal pregnancy, fundal height increases as pregnancy progresses. The fundus should be palpable above the pelvic brim by 12 to 14 weeks and level with the umbilicus at 20 weeks. Between 20 and 36 weeks, the fundal height in centimeters roughly equals gestational age of the fetus within 1 or 2 weeks. Urine pregnancy tests are very sensitive, confirming pregnancy by 4 or 5 weeks. Using a handheld Doppler, fetal heart tones are detectable at 8 to 10 weeks gestation.

10. C

Chloasma (mask of pregnancy) and spider veins are common skin changes seen in the second trimester of pregnancy. Nausea, vomiting, fatigue, urinary frequency, and breast tenderness are common complaints in the first trimester of pregnancy. Mild temperature elevation and cervical changes, including softening and bluish color change, also occur in early pregnancy.

11. E

There are several characteristic changes in cardiovascular physiology during pregnancy. The heart rate increases by 10 to 15 bpm above baseline. Cardiac output increases during the second trimester. This increase is primarily dependent on increased stroke volume, rather than increased heart rate. The symptom of lightheadedness in the second trimester is most often caused by inadequate fluid intake. This hypovolemia leads to hypotension from inadequate cardiac output to meet physiologic demand. A vasovagal reaction is an abnormal physiologic reaction to stress, in which excessive autonomic stimulation leads to hypotension and often syncope. The vestibular system does not change in response to hormonal stimulation. Pregnancy leads to elevated PO_2, not hypoxia.

12. D

The patient's cardiac findings of a flow murmur and S3 and ECG findings with left axis deviation and nonspecific ST changes are all normal for this phase in pregnancy. Hyperthyroidism would be more likely to present with tachycardia. Peripartum cardiomyopathy and mitral valve stenosis would be more likely to present with shortness of breath and fatigue. Although chest pain in women can present in an atypical manner, given the patient's age and phase of pregnancy, the most likely cause of her pain is gastroesophageal reflux disease.

13. D

Physiologic changes in pregnancy lead to an increased tidal volume with slightly increased PO_2 and decreased PCO_2. Before the uterus enters the abdominal cavity, there is already the sensation of dyspnea related to this increase in tidal volume and subsequent alkalosis. The effect is thought to be centrally mediated by progesterone. Even when the uterus is large, diaphragmatic excursion is thought to remain unchanged because the intra-abdominal cavity pressure remains low. In addition, airway resistance decreases with pregnancy. Women may undergo pulmonary function testing for increasing dyspnea or worsening lung disease, such as asthma. For this patient, it is important to note that the FEV1 is not changed by pregnancy. Thus, the FEV1 and peak flow measurements remain useful for treating the pregnant patient with asthma. See Figure 3-1 and Table 3.2.

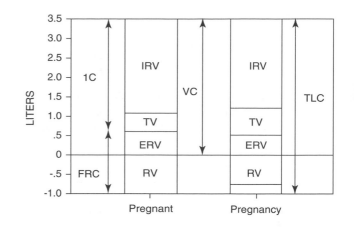

Figure 3-1. Lung volumes in nonpregnant and pregnant women. TLC, total lung capacity; VC, vital capacity; IC, inspiratory capacity; FRC, functional residual capacity; IRV, inspiratory reserve volume; TV, tidal volume; ERV, expiratory reserve volume; RV, residual volume. Reproduced from Cruickshank DP, Wigton TR, Hays PM. Maternal physiology in pregnancy. In Gabbe SG, Niebyl JR, Simpson JL, eds. Obstetrics: normal and problem pregnancies. 3rd ed. New York: Churchill Livingstone; 1996:94, with permission.

14. C

This is a classic case of molar pregnancy. Molar pregnancies come under the classification of gestational trophoblastic disease and are benign. If there is no fetal tissue, then it is a complete mole; if there is fetal tissue or an amnionic sac, then it is classified as a partial mole. Patients at the extremes of age are most at risk. Early symptoms include hyperemesis gravidarum, painless vaginal bleeding, uterine size greater than dates, and no fetal heart tones on Doppler exam. Later in pregnancy, hypertension, anemia from hemorrhage, and thyrotoxicosis may occur. Treatment is aimed at immediate evacuation of the mole with special attention paid to possible metastasis, notably to the lungs. Follow-up continues for a year, in which serial beta human chorionic gonadotropin levels are measured to ensure that there is no recurrence. Patients should not become pregnant for a full year because the risk of developing malignant trophoblastic disease with the next pregnancy is increased. See Table 3.3.

15. A

While the routine nausea and vomiting of pregnancy occurs in about 50% of women, less than 2% have hyperemesis gravidarum, which is vomiting that causes electrolyte disturbance, ketonuria, starvation, and dehydration. The etiology may be related to elevated levels of estrogen and beta human chorionic gonadotropin (HCG). Since hydatidiform moles, multiple gestation, and hyperthyroidism can elevate HCG, they are often seen with this hyperemesis. Because HCG can also act as a thyroid-stimulating hormone, it is possible to have a transient hyperthyroidism as a result of hyperemesis. Symptoms are most severe between weeks 8 and 12 and generally are completely resolved by week 20.

16. E

Oligohydramnios is almost always associated with an abnormality. It is determined by ultrasound examination if the largest pocket of fluid is less than 2 × 2 cm. During the end of pregnancy, an amniotic fluid index (AFI) may be determined by adding the vertical depth of the largest pocket in all four quadrants of the uterus. An AFI less than 5 is considered oligohydramnios. This finding is

Table 3.2 Lung volumes and capacities in pregnancy

Measurement	Definition	Change in Pregnancy
Respiratory rate (RR)	Number of breaths per minute	Unchanged
Vital capacity (VC)	Maximum amount of air that can be forcibly expired after maximum inspiration (IC + ERV)	Unchanged
Inspiratory capacity (IC)	Maximum amount of air that can be inspired from resting expiratory level (TV + IRV)	Increased 5% to 10%
Tidal volume (TV)	Amount of air inspired and expired with normal breath	Increased 30% to 40%
Inspiratory reserve volume (IRV)	Maximum amount of air that can be inspired at end of normal inspiration	Unchanged
Functional residual capacity (FRC)	Amount of air in lungs at resting expiratory level (ERV + RV)	Decreased 20%
Expiratory reserve volume (ERV)	Maximum amount of air that can be expired from resting expiratory level	Decreased 15% to 20%
Residual volume (RV)	Amount of air in lungs after maximum expiration	Decreased 20% to 25%
Total lung capacity (TLC)	Total amount of air in lungs at maximal inspiration (VC + RV)	Decreased 5%

From Cruickshank DP, Wigton TR, Hays PM. Maternal physiology in pregnancy. In: Gabbe SG, Niebyl JR, Simpson JL, eds. *Obstetrics: normal and problem pregnancies.* 3rd ed. New York: Churchill Livingstone; 1996:95.

Table 3.3 Complete mole versus partial mole

	Partial Mole	Complete Mole
Karyotype	Triploidy (>90%) Tetraploidy	46,XX (>90%) 46,XY
Presence of fetal tissue	Present	Absent
Hydropic villi	Limited and focal	Extensive
Trophoblastic hyperplasia	Focal without mild atypia	Extensive with significant atypia

associated with disorders of the renal system, including renal agenesis, outflow obstruction, or collecting system abnormality. It is also associated with severe intrauterine growth restriction and fetal demise. Because amniotic fluid plays a role in lung development, fetal movement, and possibly nutrition, oligohydramnios portends poor prognosis if present early. If found later in pregnancy, delivery is indicated.

17. B

Many women are afraid of radiation or work in radiology departments. Counseling them on the risks of radiation is crucial to a successful pregnancy outcome. Radiation poses the greatest threat during organogenesis, which lasts from 2 to 9 weeks. After this, any further risk from exposure seems to be mild, mainly growth restriction. However, heavy doses of radiation may affect the central nervous system. Radiologic studies can be safe, especially if appropriate abdominal shielding is used; it leads to abortion less than 1% of the time. Even high-risk studies such as an abdominal CT scan deliver between 20 and 50 mGy, below the minimum reported threshold of 50 to 100 mGy. If the exposure is greater than 100 cGy, then injury can be expected.

18. A

Trauma is the most common complication a pregnant patient will experience. Trauma affects 7% of pregnancies, whereas diabetes affects only 3%, and hypertension affects only 6% of all pregnancies. Even mild trauma can cause fetal morbidity and mortality. Because a family practitioner cannot determine if there is any injury without a period of observation, all patients, regardless of the severity of injury, should be monitored with external electronic fetal monitoring on labor and delivery. A Kleihauer–Betke (KB) stain should be performed to search for any evidence of maternal–fetal hemorrhage. During the period of observation, the warning signs of vaginal bleeding, abdominal pain, uterine contraction, or non-reassuring fetal heart tones would necessitate keeping the patient and obtaining a specialist consultation. If none of these signs are present, the patient may go home after 4 hours with clear instructions.

19. C

The KB stain is useful in determining if maternal–fetal hemorrhage occurred and in what quantity. A stain of maternal blood containing 5,000 to 10,000 red blood cells is performed and the number of fetal cells is counted. The final result is a percentage of fetal red blood cells in maternal blood. Because both fetal circulating volume and the maternal red blood cell count are known, an estimate of the bleed can be made. This is useful in evaluating trauma patients, those with signs or symptoms of abruption, and those with uterine rupture. The decision to administer Rh immune globulin (RhoGAM) at 28 weeks gestation is based on the maternal blood type and not the KB test.

20. D

Postpartum depression affects 10% to 15% of women in the first year after childbirth. For many women, it is the first episode of mental illness, although a previous history of depression increases the risk of postpartum depression by 30%. Other risk factors include depression during the pregnancy, poor support, and childbirth complications. Among the reasons postpartum depression is underdiagnosed are patient shame, physician dismissal of symptoms, and failure of physicians to inquire about symptoms. Women with postpartum depression have a high rate of anxiety, obsessional thoughts, and panic attacks. In addition to supportive therapy, selective serotonin reuptake inhibitors (SSRIs) are very effective in treating this problem because they treat both the depression and anxiety component. Postpartum psychosis is the most severe form of depression and thought to be a manifestation of bipolar disorder. It occurs in 0.1% of women.

21. C

Both maternal and fetal factors contribute to fetal size. Diabetes, obesity, post-date pregnancy, previous infant with macrosomia, and maternal height all increase the risk of macrosomia. Mutiparity and advanced maternal age are risk factors for both gestational diabetes and obesity, and hence macrosomia. Hypertension and vascular disease are risks for intrauterine growth restriction. The weight of male fetuses is usually 150 g more than females, and this translates to 65% higher incidence of macrosomia in male infants. A rare cause of macrosomia is Beckwith–Wiedemann syndrome, which causes pancreatic islet cell hyperplasia.

22. B

Fetal macrosomia is defined as a birth weight greater than 4,500 g (9 lbs 14 oz). It is difficult to judge fetal weight prior to birth, and an ultrasound has a 10% to 15% error rate, making it more accurate in the exclusion of macrosomia than in the diagnosis. There is no evidence that early delivery or calorie restriction will reduce the complications of macrosomia. Some retrospective studies have advocated elective C-section for those infants suspected to be greater than 4,500 g, but there is not enough evidence to recommend this approach. Although practitioners may electively induce labor, there is data that this approach only increases the C-section rate and does not reduce complications. If the mother has diabetes, special consideration is due to infants presumed to have macrosomia because shoulder dystocia can occur at a lower weight (i.e., 4,000 g). The complication most associated with macrosomia is shoulder dystocia, an obstetrical emergency. Other complications associated with macrosomia, such as hypoglycemia and polycythemia, are presumed to be due to maternal diabetes. During the delivery, the physician and staff should be ready for a shoulder dystocia.

23. A

While CD4 count is an important factor in the severity of HIV and AIDS and the risk of opportunistic infections, viral load is directly correlated to transmission to the newborn. There is no doubt that zidovudine markedly reduces the risk of perinatal transmission. Even with undetectable viral loads, there is a benefit to using zidovudine. However, there is growing evidence that a more aggressive approach with several antiviral agents can provide even more benefits. Monotherapy is no longer considered adequate for a nonpregnant patient and should not be the standard in pregnant ones. A regiment with three or four antivirals, including protease inhibitors, is now recommended by the Centers for Disease Control and Prevention (CDC).

24. D

HBIg is given to the infant and not to the mother during pregnancy. When an infant is born to a mother with HBSAg, the infant should receive the HBIg and the first hepatitis B vaccine within 12 hours of birth. Patients may breast-feed with hepatitis B. In the patient with HBSAg, it is important to discover if the patient has active hepatitis or if it is in the carrier state, as well as to determine if she may also have hepatitis C. Patients previously immunized will have the antibody to HBSAg. It is also wise to screen for other sexually transmitted diseases, including HIV.

25. A

The American College of Obstetricians and Gynecologists recommend that all Rh-negative women should receive RhoGAM at 28 weeks gestation unless the fetus is known to be Rh. 1% to 2% of Rh-negative patients will become sensitized during the third trimester without it. Rh isoimmunization can lead to erythroblastosis fetalis, a potentially life-threatening disorder in the newborn. Anti-Lewis antibodies are commonly picked up on antibody screens but are an IGM antibody and cannot cross the placenta. The fetus cannot bind Lewis antibody to its red blood cells; therefore, the Lewis antibody causes no harm. Trauma places the pregnant patient at risk for maternofetal bleeding and RhoGAM should be given in this situation if the mother is Rh negative. There are no reports of HIV transmission via RhoGAM, despite the fact that it is derived from human blood.

26. C

Hydrops fetalis is the presence of abnormal fluid in two or more fetal compartments, such as the peritoneum, pericardium, skin, placenta, and pleura, caused by the massive hemolysis that occurs when a sensitized mother's anti-D immunoglobulin crosses the placenta and attaches to fetal red blood cells. The hemolysis may cause hepatosplenomegaly and portal hypertension in the fetus, leading to the ascites that is visible on ultrasound. It is recommended to treat hydrops fetalis in utero by intrauterine fetal transfusion in order to prevent death. If a fetus is term or near term, delivery may be an option as well. Isoimmunization against antigen D or Rh factor usually occurs after a first pregnancy in an Rh-negative mother. Ideally, isoimmunization is prevented by administration of RhoGAM to the pregnant Rh-negative mother.

27. D

Rubella immunization during pregnancy may cause congenital rubella syndrome because the vaccine contains live attenuated virus. Pneumovax is considered safe in pregnancy along with the influenza vaccine. PCP prophylaxis is recommended in those with a CD4 count less than 200 because the benefits are believed to outweigh the risks. Pneumocystis pneumonia in pregnancy tends to have a more aggressive course and often leads to both maternal and fetal death. Sulfonamides are usually contraindicated late in pregnancy because it may lead to neonatal jaundice, but in the case of patients with AIDS, the risk of pneumocystis pneumonia is far greater. Other options for PCP prophylaxis, such as dapsone, are even more toxic to the fetus and should be avoided. Acyclovir is acceptable, as are many of the anti-retroviral regimens available to HIV patients.

28. E

All of the following may occur with hepatitis and pregnancy. Viral hepatitis is the most common cause of jaundice in pregnancy; the course of viral hepatitis is not altered by pregnancy. About 15,000 pregnant women are hepatitis B surface antigen positive in the United States each year. If the infection is acquired late in pregnancy, vertical transmission rates are nearly 70%. Treatment of the newborn with immunoglobulin and hepatitis B vaccine can reduce the risk of transmission to less than 3%. Hepatitis C has a variable rate of vertical transmission of near zero to nearly 40%, but no means of preventing transmission is available.

29. B

Asymptomatic bactiuria must be treated in pregnancy because it is associated with maternal and fetal morbidity. A clean-catch specimen is acceptable, although if vaginal bleeding or discharge is present, a catheterized specimen will likely yield more accurate culture results. Urinary tract infection (UTI) is increased in patients with diabetes, previous history of UTI, sickle cell hemoglobin (including trait), and lower socioeconomic status. Asymptomatic bactiuria is estimated to be present in 5% to 10% of pregnant woman, but as many as 25% of these patients will go on to develop pyelonephritis if left untreated. Pregnant patients are more likely to develop pyelonephritis in comparison to their nonpregnant counterparts because of mechanical factors, such as pressure of the uterus on the ureters, and hormonal factors, such as progesterone causing dilation of the ureters. Screening with a urine culture is recommended in the first trimester—ideally at the first prenatal visit. Pyridium is not contraindicated during pregnancy.

30. D

Uterine atony is the most common cause of postpartum bleeding, causing 70% of hemorrhages. Postpartum hemorrhage is the third leading cause of maternal death. Other causes of hemorrhage include retained or invasive placenta, birth trauma, episiotomy, uterine inversion, uterine rupture, and coagulopathies. Multiparity, instrumented delivery, and augmentation all increase the risk of atony or trauma.

31. A

Ergotamine is absolutely contraindicated while breast-feeding because up to 90% of infants exposed to ergotamines in breast milk develop ergotism, a syndrome of vomiting, diarrhea, and convulsion. In addition, the ergotamines are related to bromocriptine, an agent used to suppress lactation. Metronidazole was avoided in the past, but recent American Academy of Pediatrics guidelines do not restrict its use any further. Fluconazole, ketorolac, and azithromycin may be used by the nursing mother. It is an important concept to understand that medications that are teratogenic or prohibited in pregnancy may be safe to an infant who is no longer undergoing organogenesis.

32. E

Breast pumps are an extremely effective method to stimulate or increase milk production. Pumping can be achieved by hand, with a handheld pump, or with an electric pump. In all three methods, the pumping should simulate the suck of an infant, which is a rate of one suck per second or 60 sucks per minute. Pacifier use, as well as the use of bottles, decreases breast-feeding success. The action of the infant's tongue is different when sucking from a bottle or pacifier than from the human breast. Other causes of decreased breast milk supply are stress, infrequent feeding, and retained placenta. This last one can be a common cause of poor milk supply because lactogenesis is stimulated by the delivery of the complete placenta and subsequent rapid decrease in progesterone. A newborn should be nursing 8 to 12 times a day, with multiple soaked diapers and frequent stooling. As a guideline, an infant should regain birth weight by 2 weeks.

33. A

At their first prenatal visit, pregnant women should be asked about their history of varicella and a titer should be checked if the patient has not had chickenpox or is unsure. Approximately 95% of adults will have immunity to varicella, including those who do not recall having a primary infection. If positive, they are not considered at risk for varicella infection. Those who are seronegative should be counseled to avoid exposure during pregnancy. Occasionally, women present to the family practitioner who have been exposed to chickenpox during pregnancy and have not had a titer checked. In that case, one should be checked immediately. If serology is negative, the patient should be offered VZIG. VZIG is most effective when given within 96 hours of exposure. Patients should be counseled on the signs and symptoms of varicella infection. Because acyclovir does not prevent the fetal effects of varicella, it is reserved for serious signs or symptoms of maternal infection. Varicella can lead to significant maternal complications in pregnancy because 10% to 30% of women will develop varicella pneumonia. In the fetus, congenital varicella occurs in 2% to 5% of first trimester exposures. This syndrome is similar to congenital rubella and causes hypoplastic limbs, cutaneous scarring along dermatomes, cataracts, mental retardation, microcephaly, and low birth weight.

34. A

This patient has developed pruritic urticarial papules of pregnancy (PUPP). Her presentation is classic with lesions that began on the abdomen and spread to the legs and thighs. The face is typically spared. The fact that her periumbilical region is spared argues against herpes gestationis, which typically involves the periumbilical region. Early in its course, herpes gestationis and PUPP can look very much alike, thus making differentiation important. Biopsy may be helpful in cases in which the diagnosis is not clear. PUPP typically responds to topical steroids but occasionally systemic corticosteroids will be needed. Herpes gestationis, a variant of bullous pemphigoid, is more likely to require systemic corticosteroids and has been associated with increased fetal morbidity and mortality. Patients with confirmed herpes gestationis should undergo routine antenatal testing.

35. D

Lower socioeconomic status, not higher, puts one at risk for preterm labor. African American women and those who have had a previous history of preterm labor are at increased risk. Smoking, alcohol use, and drug abuse also put women at higher risk. Other risk factors include very low pre-pregnancy weight (less than 100 lbs or BMI less than 19) and anatomic abnormalities such as incompetent cervix, abnormal uterus, or placenta previa. Lack of prenatal care, fetal abnormalities, oligohydramnios, polyhydramnios, multiple gestations, and serious genital or urinary tract infection are among other risk factors.

36. D

In nulliparous women, the fifth percentile for cervical dilation in active phase labor is 1.2 cm/hour. In multiparous women, the fifth percentile is 1.5 cm/hour. Anything less than that is considered a protracted labor. In addition, the fetal descent, which correlates to station, should be greater than 1.0 cm/hour in nulliparous and greater than 2.0 cm/hour in multiparous women. Women in active labor should have their cervix checked periodically to ensure that they are making adequate progress.

37. D

Most patients with prior C-section are potential candidates for a trial of labor. A classic vertical incision is the only absolute contraindication. The success rate of VBAC is between 60% and 80%. Uterine dehiscence (less than 2%) and rupture (less than 1%) are rare events but the cause of significant maternal and fetal morbidity and mortality. Cytotec should not be used in the setting of prior C-section due to increased risk of rupture with hyperstimulation. There is insufficient evidence to recommend against allowing women with suspected macrosomic pregnancy to have a trial of labor. Current standards for VBAC limit it to women with only one prior low transverse scar, at 37 to 40 weeks gestation, vertex position, and in good health. Monitoring and institutional ability to perform an immediate C-section are also recommended. Women outside of these guidelines, such as those who require induction,

have more than one previous C-section, or have an unknown scar, may still undergo a trial of labor but require extensive documented counseling. In the May 22–29, 2002, issue of *JAMA*, a landmark study using the Scottish registry revealed that women undergoing VBAC had a rate of perinatal infant death of 12.9 per 10,000. Although the absolute number is low, it is 11 times higher than a planned repeat C-section, 2 times higher than other multiparous laboring women, and similar to the risk of nulliparous women in labor. Informed consent is essential of any woman undergoing a trial of labor after C-section. See Tables 3.4 and 3.5.

38. C

After confirming that true preterm labor exists, the initial evaluation should include sterile speculum exam to rule out rupture of membranes and infection. Then a tocolytic agent should be initiated if termination of contractions is desired based on history and physical findings. Ultrasound to determine estimated gestational age and fetal weight may be helpful in cases in which dating is unsure or when significant prematurity may require transfer to another facility with a neonatal intensive care unit (NICU). Tocolytics usually cannot stop true labor but will provide a window of time prior to delivery in which to administer steroids and arrange transfer of the mother to a facility with a NICU. Antenatal steroids are effective in promoting fetal lung maturity and improving surfactant manufacture in the neonate. Even one dose of steroids can provide this benefit without increasing the risk of infection. Several studies show that if delivery is averted, repeated doses of steroids are unnecessary and may be harmful.

39. B

Telogen effluvium, or hair loss due to a shift in follicle phase, is commonly seen in the postpartum period. Hair loss typically lasts for 3 or 4 months and patients should be reassured that hair growth will reoccur in 6 to 15 months after delivery. However, patients should be told that their hair might not return to its pre-pregnancy thickness. There is no need to use Rogaine in this situation at this

Table 3.4 U.S. Preventive Services Task Force scoring system for evidence quality

Score	Required Evidence
I	At least one properly designed randomly controlled trial
II-1	Well-designed controlled trial without randomization
II-2	Well-designed cohort or case–control analytic studies, preferably from more than one medical center or research group
II-3	Multiple time series with or without the intervention; dramatic results in uncontrolled experiments
III	Opinion of respected authorities, based on clinical experience, descriptive studies, or reports of expert committees

Adapted from Rosen MG, Dickinson JC, Westhoff CL. Vaginal birth after cesarean: A meta-analysis of morbidity and mortality. *Obstet Gynecol.* 1991;77:465.

Table 3.5 Candidacy for VBAC-TOL: Clinical conditions for which there are insufficient data to make a conclusive recommendation

Condition	Evidence Quality
Prior vertical cesarean (low segment)	II-3
Multiple gestation	II-3
Breech	II-3
EFW greater than 4,000 g (nondiabetic)	II-2
External version	II-2
Prior myomectomy	No data

Adapted from American College of Obstetricians and Gynecologists (ACOG). *Vaginal Delivery after Previous Cesarean Birth.* Practice Bulletin No. 1. Washington, DC: ACOG; 1995.

time. During pregnancy, many women report thicker hair because hair is arrested in the anagen or growth phase due to hormone changes. After pregnancy, these hairs that should have been shed gradually in the preceding months all enter the telogen or rest phase at the same time and are shed approximately 3 months postpartum.

40. B

This patient presents in preterm labor. Labetolol would not be useful in this case. Given prematurity, corticosteroids should be considered in an effort to promote lung maturity. Magnesium sulfate, calcium channel blockers such as nifedipine, and beta agonists such as terbutaline and Ritodrine are all potential tocolytics that might be used in this case. Antibiotic therapy for possible group B strep infection, a potential cause of preterm labor, should be instituted with ampicillin or an appropriate alternative until cultures collected in the examination room are definitive.

41. E

MSAFP will be low in infants with trisomy 18 and 21. Multiple marker screens including human chorionic gonadotropin (HCG) and unconjugated estriol (uE3) along with MSAFP are currently recommended for screening test. MSAFP will be elevated with open neural tube defects and other fetal anomalies, such as gastroschisis, omphalocele, and cystic hygromas, which are benign lymphatic tumors commonly seen in Turner's syndrome.

42. A

Unconjugated estriol (uE3) is measured with a triple screen along with alpha-fetoprotein (MSAFP) and HCG. Estriol will be low in fetuses with trisomy 18 and 21. There are no anomalies associated with an elevated level.

43. B

Genetic amniocentesis is usually recommended between 15 and 18 weeks, in the second trimester. The risk of fetal loss is often quoted as less than 1 in 200, but this risk is likely lower with practiced perinatologists. If the patient desires an earlier diagnosis, chorionic villous sampling (CVS) can be performed in the first trimester between 10 and 13 weeks, with a similar risk of miscarriage of 1 in 200. Amniocentesis may be done in the first trimester but carries a higher risk of fetal loss than the villous sampling or later amniocentesis. Nearer to term, amniocentesis may be performed to determine fetal lung maturity. Both tests have a similar miscarriage rate and are considered gold standards in the detection of chromosomal abnormalities. If there is a concern about neural tube defects, then CVS is not helpful and amniocentesis alone is considered the gold standard.

44. E

Angiotensin converting enzyme inhibitors and angiotensin receptor blockers are contraindicated during pregnancy because of the risk of renal agenensis in the fetus. Nifedipine may be used for hypertension and is also used in some cases for treatment for preterm labor. It may not be used concurrently with magnesium sulfate due to the risk of pulmonary edema. Labetalol is commonly used for treatment of acutely elevated pressures associated with pre-eclampsia and is gaining popularity as a first-line drug. Methyldopa is still considered the first-line therapy because it has the longest track record and proven safety. Hydralazine intravenously is often used acutely to lower blood pressure.

45. D

Permethrin is the only medication listed that is considered acceptable for use in pregnancy. It is applied to the entire body from the neck down and left on for 8 to 10 hours. Lindane is contraindicated due to central nervous system toxicity. The other medications are relatively contraindicated in pregnancy and are not commonly indicated for the treatment of scabies. Another acceptable alternative is to have the pharmacist compound a mixture of 6% to 10% precipitated sulfur in petrolatum (petroleum jelly); this is applied over the entire body for 3 days.

46. A

All of the regiments are acceptable for the treatment of chlamydia. However, ofloxacin is a quinolone and is contraindicated during pregnancy due to cartilaginous anomalies in animal studies. Routine screening for *Chlamydia trachomatis* is performed during pregnancy because it is often asymptomatic and causes significant maternal and fetal morbidity. During the pregnancy, it can cause preterm rupture of membranes and premature labor. Postpartum, it is associated with a higher rate of endometritis. The CDC recommends retesting women 3 weeks after treatment because of the high failure rate. If chlamydia is not treated and an infant is born through an infected cervix, there is risk of perinatal conjunctivitis, oropharyngeal and genital tract infections, and pneumonia. Interestingly, the topical antibiotic ointment placed in all infants' eyes only protects against gonorrhea, so any infant with conjunctivitis within 4 weeks of delivery should be tested and treated for chlamydia. The pneumonia caused by chlamydia presents as cough, hyperinflation, and bilateral diffuse infiltrates on chest x-ray. Infants are usually afebrile. It can occur up to 3 months after delivery. Despite the risks, there are no data to recommend prophylactic antibiotic treatment for infants and no data on the risks of such prophylaxis. Infants born to mothers with untreated chlamydia should be closely monitored to detect any early signs of infection.

47. B

Severe pre-eclampsia is defined by 24-hour urine protein greater than 5 g, blood pressure greater than 160 systolic or 110 diastolic on two occasions at least 6 hours apart, oliguria less than 500 cc/24 hours or less than 30 cc/hour for 3 hours, headache, visual disturbances, epigastric pain, pulmonary edema, hemolysis, elevated liver enzymes, and thrombocytopenia with platelets of 100,000 or less. The treatment is intravenous infusion of magnesium sulfate and urgent delivery of the fetus.

48. B

The goal of magnesium therapy is to raise the seizure threshold. Because seizure is associated with both maternal and fetal hypoxia, it is the most serious consequence of this disorder. Magnesium is clearly proven to be more effective in pre-eclampsia than other anticonvulsants such as phenytoin. Controlling the blood pressure in pre-eclampsia may provide benefits for the mother but does not prevent fetal injury; in fact, it may further compromise perfusion to the fetus. Control of the blood pressure during magnesium therapy is initiated only if the diastolic blood pressure is critical (i.e., over 110 mmHg). The only cure for pre-eclampsia is delivery of the fetus.

49. B

Hypertension may be a concomitant disease but does not lead to gestational diabetes. Gestational diabetes is one of the most common medical complications of pregnancy, affecting 3% to 6% of women. Risk factors include age older than 30 years, ethnicity (African American, Hispanic, and Native American), obesity, family history of diabetes, and prior history of delivery of a macrosomic infant. The pathophysiology of gestational diabetes is similar to type 2 diabetes in that it involves both insulin resistance and relative insulin deficiency. The hormones of pregnancy, such as estrogen, progesterone, prolactin, cortisol, and human placental lactogen, are associated with the insulin resistance. Most women are able to compensate by increasing insulin production. In gestational diabetes, the resistance cannot be met with enough insulin and hyperglycemia ensues. Screening is usually performed at 24 to 28 weeks. Diagnosis is made with a 100 g 3-hour glucose challenge.

50. D

The 1-hour test is a screening tool that is considered positive if the serum glucose exceeds 140 mg/dL. It is estimated that approximately 15% of the population have a positive screen. Patients with abnormal 1-hour glucose screening should have a 100 g 3-hour fasting glucose challenge. It is important to remember that the screening test may miss up to 20% of women with diabetes, so if a woman is at high risk, she should undergo definitive 3-hour testing. It is estimated that 15% of the women taking the 3-hour test will be positive for diabetes, resulting in the estimated 3% of the population with this disorder. Traditionally, the glucose levels for the 3-hour test use the O'Sullivan whole blood levels of 105/190/165/145. Recently, Carpenter and Coustan recalculated these levels for serum with new diagnostic thresholds of 95/180/155/140.

51. B

Pregnancies complicated by preterm rupture of membranes (PROM) without evidence of chorioamnionitis or fetal distress may be continued. If tocolysis is needed, steroids are usually administered to induce fetal lung maturity. There are multiple risk factors for PROM, including preceding uterine contractions, infection, multiple fetuses, and trauma resulting in abruption. Because PROM is usually associated with other complications, delivery is usually imminent either through caesarian section or through vaginal delivery. However, in about 10% of PROM cases, the mother and fetus are stable and a prolonged rupture of membranes or PPROM occurs. There may be a resealing of the membranes. The length of time to delivery is inversely proportional to the gestation age. The other choices contraindicate tocolysis and are indications for delivery. IUGR can be a sign of placental insufficiency and herald fetal non–well-being. Both chorioamnionitis and fetal death require delivery. Vaginal bleeding may herald abruption, which should not be masked by tocolytics.

52. C

Painless vaginal bleeding is consistent with placenta previa. Abruption is usually painful and commonly will show a non-reassuring fetal heart rate pattern. Vaginal bleeding is not always present. Cocaine use is a risk factor, as is multiparity, trauma, domestic violence, hypertension, multiple gestation, polyhydramnios, and tobacco abuse. Abruption occurs in less than 1% of pregnancies but carries a fetal mortality rate close to 20% to 35%. During abruption, there is hemorrhage into the decidua basalis, which separates the placenta from the myometrium and destroys surrounding placenta. Usually, this presents as vaginal bleeding and pain. However, the bleeding may be concealed if the margins of the placenta remain adherent. Besides fetal morbidity and

mortality associated with preterm delivery and hypoxia, the mother may develop shock and disseminated intravascular coagulopathy. Treatment depends on the amount of abruption. About 40% of abruptions are asymptomatic and diagnosed after delivery when a small clot is seen on the placenta. This usually results in uterine irritability but no fetal distress. If there is a larger abruption, then delivery by vagina or caesarian must be performed. Any abruption greater than 50% will result in fetal death unless delivered immediately.

53. D

The time frame for postpartum depression is variable and can begin days to months postpartum. The duration is also variable. SSRIs have been used in lactating mothers without discernable side effects in the neonate. Postpartum depression is very common but may be overlooked. The "blues" postpartum can occur in 50% to 80% of women. True postpartum depression occurs in about 10% of women (range in the literature of 5.8% to 35.4%). Psychosis is rare, with only 0.1% to 0.3% of women experiencing it postpartum. Complicating the diagnosis is that many of the symptoms of depression, such as sleep changes, weight loss, lack of energy, and decreased concentration, are also seen in the nondepressed postpartum woman. If postpartum depression is untreated, infants can suffer cognitive delays and impaired language development. It is known that infants can and do mirror the affect of their mothers. Early diagnosis and treatment are imperative. See Table 3.6.

54. C

Fundal pressure is counterproductive because it further impacts the shoulder into the pubic bone. The other maneuvers all serve to change the relationship of the biacromial diameter within the bony pelvis, increase the functional size of the pelvis, increase the room at the perineum, or decrease the biacromial diameter of the fetus.

55. B

Medication use during pregnancy should be avoided if at all possible. If psychiatric medications are prescribed, it is better to use older medications that have been used in pregnant patients. It is

Table 3.6 Characteristics of antenatal patients that increase the risk for major postpartum depression

Younger than 20 years of age
Unmarried
Medically indigent
Comes from a family of six or more children
Separated from one or both parents in childhood or adolescence
Received poor parental support and attention in childhood
Had limited parental support in adulthood
Has poor relationship with husband or boyfriend
Has economic problem with housing or income
Is dissatisfied with amount of education
Shows evidence of emotional problem, past or present
Has low self-esteem

Data from Posner *et al.*

particularly important to avoid medication during the first trimester of pregnancy because it is the most critical time for fetal organ development. Psychiatric disorders may improve, worsen, or stay the same during pregnancy.

56. A

Women are at increased risk of having a postpartum psychotic episode if they have a personal or family history of postpartum psychosis, schizophrenia, or bipolar mood disorder. Family history of depression, gestational diabetes, pre-eclampsia, and drug use are not known to increase risk. Unlike postpartum depression, which manifests within 3 to 6 months of delivery, psychosis can begin within the first 48 hours of delivery. These mothers will exhibit alternating mood, insomnia, restlessness, and confusion. When interviewing women with postpartum psychosis, there will be disorganized thinking and delusional thought concerning the infant. Women with a previous history of bipolar disorder are at very high risk of relapse, up to 50%. Unfortunately, women with one episode of postpartum psychosis have a 50% to 90% chance of another with subsequent deliveries. The most serious consequence is infanticide, which can occur in 4% of women with psychosis.

57. E

Postpartum psychosis usually occurs within 2 to 4 weeks but may occur up to 3 months postpartum. This condition is a psychiatric emergency best treated with immediate hospitalization. These women need to be hospitalized for their safety and to safeguard their infants because they are at increased risk for suicide and, rarely, infanticide. Some symptoms of psychosis, such as emotional lability, are common in the puerperium. However, the presence of hallucinations or delusions clearly indicates psychosis.

58. A

Intrauterine growth restriction occurs in up to 5% of the pregnant population. Most of these infants are simply small for gestational age, but this is a retrospective diagnosis once all the pathologic causes are ruled out. This mother needs an urgent ultrasound to look at the fetal measurements. Since asymmetrical growth restriction is most ominous, important measures are the biparietal measurement, head circumference, abdominal circumference, and femur length. Brain growth is preserved at the expense of abdominal organs, namely the liver, so the proportion of the head circumference to abdominal circumference will be elevated. If oligohydramnios is also present, it increases the risks to the fetus. Management of IUGR depends on the cause but usually includes treating underlying disease, improved nutrition, and bed rest. Antenatal testing should be instituted, consisting of non-stress testing twice weekly. If that is abnormal, a biophysical profile should be performed. The decision to deliver is based on the risk of prematurity versus the risk of persistent hypoxia.

59. E

The greatest risk of uteroplacental insufficiency is intrauterine growth restriction and chronic hypoxia. The most common cause of uteroplacental insufficiency is hypertensive disorders of pregnancy, especially pre-eclampsia. Ultrasound is a reliable means of determining if growth restriction is present. The definition of IUGR is an estimated fetal weight less than the 10th percentile and an abdominal circumference below the 2.5th percentile. All of the above measurements can be helpful, but the abdominal circumference is the most sensitive indicator. If the abdominal circumference is below the 2.5th percentile, it is more than 95% sensitive for IUGR.

60. C

Rubella, or German measles, is a viral infection spread by contact and respiratory droplets. It is highly contagious but self-limited, often presenting as a maculopapular rash with lymphadenopathy and possible arthralgias. The rubella vaccine contains a live attenuated virus and should not be given to pregnant women or those women who plan pregnancy within 3 months. The vaccine can be given once the infant is born and breast-feeding is not a contraindication. IVIG has not been shown to reduce the risk of congenital infection. The greatest risk of congenital rubella syndrome (CRS) occurs if a susceptible woman contracts rubella during the first 11 weeks of pregnancy; these fetuses have a 90% chance of developing CRS. At 20 weeks the risk drops to 20% to 25%, and in the second half of pregnancy CRS is rare, but these infants may be born with congenital rubella infection rendering them contagious for up to 1 year. The syndrome can cause cataracts, deafness, developmental delay, intrauterine growth retardation, cardiac defects, microcephaly, jaundice, and hepatosplenomegaly.

61. D

One of the screening labs done at the initial visit is the urine culture. This is done because asymptomatic bacteriuria occurs in 10% of pregnant women, leading to increased risk of intrauterine growth restriction, cystitis, preterm labor, and pyelonephritis. Glycosuria occurs frequently and can contribute to bacterial growth. Both the increased urine volume and decreased bladder tone lead to urinary stasis and hence increase the risk of infection. However, none of these causes is as significant as bacteriuria in the development of pyelonephritis.

62. D

This is a classic presentation for pyelonephritis in the pregnant patient, in whom dysuria may not be present and other symptoms such as frequency may be indistinguishable from normal pregnancy-related changes. In order to prevent the complications of pyelonephritis, such as preterm labor, it is necessary to treat early and empirically. Urine cultures should be done immediately, but treatment should also begin immediately. Hospitalization is indicated in any patient who has signs of sepsis, uterine contractions, nausea, vomiting, and dehydration. If none of these signs are present, the patient may be treated as an outpatient with close follow-up. Most antibiotic regiments consist of cefazolin, ampicillin with gentamicin, or ceftriaxone. Parenteral antibiotics are needed until the patient is afebrile, usually 24 to 48 hours. If the patient does not improve on antibiotics, resistant organisms should be suspected. The organisms responsible for pyelonephritis in pregnancy are *Escherichia coli*, *Proteus mirabilis*, *Klebsiella pneumoniae*, and group B streptococcus.

63. C

Induction of labor is performed most often for post-dates pregnancies, defined as labor at or over 42 weeks gestation, which occurs in about 10% of deliveries. Although there are several relative contraindications for induction, the only absolute contraindication listed is the transmural myomectomy. Similarly, a classic uterine caesarian incision would also preclude a woman from having labor induced. Other absolute contraindications include placenta previa, prolapsed cord, active genital herpes, and transverse fetal lie. PIH is not a contraindication to induction unless it is severe.

Polyhydramnios, nonengaged fetal head, and breech are relative contraindications to induction of labor.

64. B

Induction of labor requires that the cervix be ripened and that uterine contractions begin. There are many methods to induce labor, including membrane stripping and amniotomy, and complementary methods such as acupuncture, sexual intercourse, and herbal preparations. The most commonly used methods are pharmacologic. Cervical ripening is mediated by prostaglandins, such as E_2 and F_2 alpha. Dinoprostone is prostaglandin E_2 and misoprotol is a synthetic form of prostaglandin E_1. For "unfavorable" cervixes, those with a Bishop's score less than 8, ripening should be achieved with a prostaglandin. Oxytocin alone may be used if the cervix is favorable. This patient has a relative contraindication to misoprotol, which is a previous caesarian section. This would increase her risk of uterine rupture from the synthetic prostaglandin. See Tables 3.7 and 3.8.

65. E

Vacuum-assisted delivery is a counterpart to forceps, which is easier to learn and requires less skill. This makes it an attractive option for family physicians if assistance is needed in the second stage of labor. Indications for vacuum assistance are similar to forceps and include maternal exhaustion, soft tissue distocia, and prolonged second stage of labor. Primips can have a second stage that lasts 2 hours and up to 3 hours if regional analgesia is used. A multiparous woman's second stage usually lasts for 1 hour and 2 hours if regional analgesia is used. Brow presentation as well as face and breech are contraindications to vacuum extraction. Other contraindications include previous scalp sampling, incomplete cervical dilation, prematurity, known cephalopelvic disproportion, and unengaged fetal head.

66. A

Electronic fetal monitoring which measures fetal heart rate and its variations in relation to uterine contractions was introduced in the 1970s with great hope that it would improve fetal outcomes and reduce cerebral palsy and neonatal seizures. By 1987, the CDC performed a comprehensive review of the literature and found that none

Table 3.7 Assessment of antepartum cervical status by modified Bishop score

Parameter	Score			
	0	1	2	3
Dilatation (cm)	Closed	1–2	3–4	5 or more
Effacement (%)	0–30	40–50	60–70	80 or more
Station	−3	−2	−1 or 0	+1 or +2
Consistency	Firm	Medium	Soft	
Cervical position	Posterior	Midposition	Anterior	

Adapted with permission from Bishop EH. Pelvic scoring for elective induction. *Obstet Gynecol.* 1964;24:266.

Table 3.8 Methods of cervical ripening

Pharmacologic Methods	Nonpharmacologic Methods
Hormonal techniques	Membrane stripping
Prostaglandins Prostaglandin E_2 [dinoprostone (Prepidil)]	Mechanical dilators
Prostaglandin E_1 [misoprostol (Cytotec)]	Hygroscopic dilators (laminaria, lamicel, Dilapan)
Oxytocin	Balloon catheter (alone, with traction, with infusion)
Estrogen	Amniotomy
Steroid receptor antagonists (?)	
RU-486 (Mifepristone)	
ZK98299 (Onapristone)	
Relaxin (?)	
Dehydroepiandrostenedione sulfate (?)	

of these outcomes had materialized. Yet, EFM remains the standard of care in many communities. Intermittent auscultation is a clinically equivalent option but requires nurses or physicians to auscultate fetal heart tones during and after a contraction every 15 to 30 minutes in active labor. Although EFM can alert the physician to possible fetal compromise, it is a screening test and not diagnostic.

67. D

Electronic fetal monitoring is a screening tool to help physicians assess fetal well-being prior to and during labor. Fetal heart rate is determined by both the nervous and cardiac systems. When fetal heart tracings are reassuring, it is likely that the fetus has a pH greater than 7.3 and is not hypoxic. Unfortunately, a non-reassuring fetal heart tracing does not necessarily indicate fetal distress. Interpretation of the tracing requires the physician to assess fetal heart rate, with normal being 120 to 160 bpm. Variability is the term used to describe the constant variations of heart rate seen in a healthy fetus. Short-term variability describes the beat-to-beat variations, usually of 5 to 10 bpm around the baseline. Long-term variability occurs over minutes and has an amplitude of 10 to 25 bpm around the baseline. Loss of short-term variability not associated with fetal sleep cycle, medications, or prematurity is an ominous sign even if the baseline heart rate is normal, especially if associated with late or variable decelerations. Although late decelerations are always non-reassuring, they are not ominous if beat-to-beat variability is intact.

68. D

All decelerations, whether early, late, or variable, are defined by their relationship to uterine contractions. Early decelerations are so named because they occur with the uterine contraction and return to baseline at the end of the contraction. They often look like mirror images of the uterine contraction measured on the tocometer. The mechanism of action is fetal head compression, which increases vagal tone and causes the slowing of the fetal heart. Late decelerations, in contrast, begin with the peak of the contraction and do not return to baseline until after the contraction is over. This is a non-reassuring pattern because it indicates possible uteroplacental insufficiency and the prospect of fetal hypoxia. The depth of the deceleration does not correlate to the severity of the hypoxia, and all late "decels" should be regarded as non-reassuring. Variable decelerations are variable in both shape and relation to contractions; they are thought to occur due to cord compression and are the most common decelerations noted during labor.

69. A

Failure to progress is a generic term that encompasses all the causes of failed labor, including uterine inertia and cephalopelvic disproportion. In this patient, the Montevideo units demonstrate 3 hours of adequate uterine contractions, which would be unlikely to be improved by oxytocin infusion. The failure of the fetal head to become engaged as evident by the station is a strong indicator of cephalopelvic disproportion. When disproportion is present, the fetus will not deliver vaginally and caesarian section is the needed course. Narcotics will not help a patient overcome a pelvic disproportion. Forceps cannot be used prior to full dilation and effacement.

70. E

Caesarian section should be available within a reasonable amount of time for all women at hospitals with maternity care. ACOG has determined that time frame to be 30 minutes. In-house obstetricians and anesthesiologists are not necessary as long as the team can be assembled within the 30-minute time frame.

71. D

Because of the patient's ethnicity, a mean corpuscular volume (MCV) of less than 70 would raise concern for alpha or beta thalassemia. Also, if the patient were anemic you would want to determine the etiology and begin treatment prior to conception. HIV infection is important to diagnose prior to pregnancy because maternal-to-fetal transmission may be reduced from 25.5% to 8.3% with zidovudine (Retrovir) therapy given throughout pregnancy, antepartum, and delivery. Sickle cell smear is not a consideration for routine screening for Mediterranean ethnicity. However, in people of African, Indian, and Middle Eastern descent, it would be considered an appropriate screening test.

72. B

Preconception and prenatal care requires the family physician to evaluate the patient's risk for contracting infections. Despite the high cost of certain infections during pregnancy, mumps, measles, BCG, varicella, and rubella vaccines cannot be given to pregnant patients or those who might become pregnant within the month. Some sources even cite 3 months as the minimum time span from immunization to conception. All of the above vaccines are live attenuated, which makes them contraindicated in or near pregnancy. Hepatitis B may be given during pregnancy and should be administered if the patient is at high risk of blood exposure or sexual transmission. DT and influenza are routinely given during pregnancy. In addition, if circumstances warrant it, meningococcal and rabies vaccines can also be given.

73. B

The patient has approximately a 10% (ranging from 0% to 13% in the literature) chance of developing a recurrence of the deep vein thrombosis during pregnancy. The standard of care is to treat women throughout pregnancy and postpartum for 4 to 6 weeks. The therapy of choice is either heparin or low–molecular-weight heparin (Lovenox), both of which have to be injected once or twice daily. Although aspirin could help prevent deep vein thrombosis, its effects would be overcome by the hypercoagulable state of pregnancy. Dipyridamole has been used in pregnancy for the prevention of pre-eclampsia and clot prevention with mechanical valves without any apparent teratogenic effects. Its use, however, is not indicated in DVT prevention. Clopidogrel is category B but, again, is not indicated in DVT prevention. Coumadin is absolutely contraindicated because of its teratogenic effects consisting of fetal warfarin syndrome, central nervous system defects, miscarriage, and prematurity. The fetal warfarin syndrome can occur if warfarin is taken in the first trimester. It consists of nasal and limb hypoplasia, eye defects, deafness, mental retardation, and small birth weight.

74. B

The recommendations for weight gain during pregnancy by the Institute of Medicine, the ACOG, and AAP are based on BMI. For women who start their pregnancies significantly underweight, such as the patient described, the recommended weight gain is 28 to 40 lbs.

75. B

Maternal hypothyroxinemia or low T4 levels may cause cretinism or impaired neurologic development in the fetus. This risk is most significant in the first trimester since the mother is the sole source of thyroid hormone for the first 12 weeks of gestation. If there is a suspicion of hypothyroidism, it is recommended to measure both TSH and T4 during pregnancy since T4 may be significantly low, even in the setting of a normal TSH. This is because there is often an early transient dip in T4 as the carrier protein, thyroid-binding globulin, increases due to the elevated maternal estrogen, but the thyroid corrects this by increasing hormone production. The most common cause of hypothyroidism in pregnancy is Hashimoto thyroiditis. There is insufficient evidence that screening and early treatment of pregnant women with subclinical hypothyroidism improves subsequent neonatal outcomes. Hypothyroidism causes anovulation, so it is very rare to make an initial diagnosis during pregnancy. Women with treated hypothyroidism should continue on hormone therapy and have TSH levels drawn to measure the adequacy of replacement. Hyperthyroidism occurs in about 0.02% to 0.3% of pregnancies, making it the second most common endocrine abnormality in pregnancy after diabetes. Treatment is with propylthiouracil (PTU) but is difficult because PTU crosses the placenta and can cause a goiter in the fetus.

76. C

Polyhydramnios is greater than normal amniotic fluid volume. Diagnosis is usually made through an ultrasound exam called an amniotic fluid index (AFI). Polyhydramnios is diagnosed if the AFI is greater than 20 cm per AIUM (American Institute of Ultrasound Medicine) standards, although 25 cm has been noted by other sources. The AFI is measured by adding the depth of the largest vertical pocket in all four quadrants of the uterus. In absolute measurements, a fluid volume greater than 2,000 mL makes the diagnosis. Polyhydramnios is associated with an abnormality in

50% to 70% of cases. It is associated with gestational diabetes, multiple gestation, isoimmunization, placental abnormalities, and fetal anomalies such as esophageal atresia, anencephaly, spina bifida, and chromosomal abnormalities. It is important to remember that it does occur in normal pregnancies without any identifiable cause.

77. D

The differential diagnosis of polyhydramnios includes diabetes, twins, trisomy 18, and congenital anomalies such as fetal GI obstructions, fetal neural tube defects, hydrops fetalis, and fetal skeletal disorders. Renal anomalies or agenesis may cause oligohydramnios or a lower than normal amniotic fluid volume diagnosed by an AFI less than 5 cm. Either condition may occur in normal pregnancy, but the finding of polyhydramnios or oligohydramnios should prompt a full anatomic scan if this has not previously been performed.

78. D

All third trimester bleeding, painful or not, should be assumed to be placenta previa until proven otherwise. The safest and most accurate method of diagnosis is on ultrasound. Most of the time, due to routine ultrasound screening in the second trimester, physicians are alerted to the presence of a placenta previa. Risk factors include multiparity, increasing age, previous uterine scar such as previous C-section, and multiple gestation. It is important to remember that abnormal placental adherences such as placenta accreta are strongly associated with placenta previa. A vaginal or rectal exam prior to determining the placental location can start a catastrophic hemorrhage. Nitrazine and fern testing are useful in determining if rupture of the membranes has occurred. Cerclage is needed for cases of incompetent cervix. The KB test can assist in ascertaining if maternal–fetal hemorrhage has occurred and to what extent.

79. D

After a prolonged second stage of labor, if assisted delivery is necessary, it is always important to consider and prepare for shoulder dystocia. The bladder should ideally be empty prior to vacuum or forceps usage. While a straight catheterization may be particularly helpful in women with epidural anesthesia and difficulty voiding, there is no reason for an indwelling catheter to be placed. In fact, it takes up room under the pubic arch. Vacuum deliveries carry a higher risk of cephalohematoma to the baby, whereas forceps carry a higher risk of maternal trauma. For both forceps and vacuum delivery, the cervix must be completely dilated. A vacuum can be placed in case of some malpositions, such as occiput posterior; however, it cannot be utilized for a malpresentation (i.e., breech). See Tables 3.9, 3.10, and 3.11.

80. B

Women at high risk for neural tube defects, including those with a personal history of a neural tube defect or a previous child born with a neural tube defect, should take 4 mg of folic acid per day, prior to conception. Folic acid supplementation (ideally started prior to conception) decreases the risk of neural tube defects, not SIDS. Most unsupplemented foods do not have enough of this B vitamin to give women at least 400 μg per day. Because of our increased understanding of the role of folic acid in preventing neural tube defects, several foods, particularly grain products, are now being supplemented with it. Women who are not protecting themselves from unplanned pregnancies should take a folic acid

Table 3.9 Classification of operative vaginal deliveries

Type of Procedure	Criteria
Outlet forceps	Scalp is visible at the introitus without separating the labia. Fetal skull has reached the level of the pelvic floor. Sagittal suture is in the direct anteroposterior diameter or in the right or left occiput anterior or posterior position. Fetal head is at or on the perineum. Rotation is ≤45 degrees.
Low forceps	Leading point of the fetal skull (station) is +2 or more but has not as yet reached the pelvic floor. 1. Rotation is ≤45 degrees. 2. Rotation is greater than 45 degrees.
Midforceps	The head is engaged in the pelvis but the presenting part is above +2 station.
High forceps	Not included in this classification.

Adapted from American College of Obstetricians and Gynecologists (ACOG). *Operative Vaginal Delivery.* Technical Bulletin No. 196. Washington, DC: ACOG; 1994.

supplement on a daily basis so that they will receive adequate amounts of folic acid prior to conception.

81. D

Sheehan's syndrome affects mothers and not newborns. This syndrome consists of postpartum ischemic necrosis of the anterior pituitary and is usually observed in patients who have experienced severe postpartum hemorrhage with hypotensive shock. Many of these patients are infertile, although spontaneous pregnancies have occurred. Because Sheehan's syndrome is not a genetic abnormality, the patient would not need preconception genetic counseling. Thalassemia trait in both parents would put the fetus at risk for thalassemia. A patient with a family history of a chromosomal abnormality (including in a previous child) makes subsequent pregnancies higher risk for a recurrence. Patients with multiple (three or more) first trimester losses also have a higher risk of a chromosomal abnormality.

82. D

Her size on exam is greater than her gestational age by LMP. Possibilities include inaccurate dates, a pelvic mass, or multiple gestation. Uterine size can be approximated by an orange at 6 weeks gestation, a grapefruit at 8 weeks gestation, or a melon at 10 weeks gestation. At 12 or 13 weeks gestation, the fundus should be palpable abdominally just above the symphysis pubis. Fetal heart tones become easily heard with a handheld Doppler. By 16 weeks, the fundus is palpable halfway between the symphysis and the umbilicus, and by 20 weeks it is palpable at the umbilicus.

Table 3.10 Indications for operative vaginal delivery

Maternal Indications	Fetal Indications	Other Indications	
Maternal exhaustion	Non-reassuring fetal testing	Prolonged second stage of labor	
Inadequate maternal expulsive efforts (such as women with spinal cord injuries or neuromuscular diseases)		Nulliparas: ≥2 hours without regional analgesia, ≥3 hours with regional analgesia	
Need to avoid maternal expulsive efforts (such as women with certain cardiac or cerebrovascular diseases)		Multiparas: ≥1 hour without regional analgesia, ≥2 hours with regional analgesia	
? Lack of maternal expulsive effort		? Elective shortening of the second stage of labor using outlet forceps	

Data from American College of Obstetricians and Gynecologists (ACOG). *Operative Vaginal Delivery*. Technical Bulletin No. 196. Washington, DC: ACOG; 1994.

Table 3.11 Prerequisites for operative vaginal delivery

Maternal Criteria	Fetal Criteria	Uteroplacental Criteria	Other Criteria
Adequate analgesia	Vertex presentation	Cervix fully dilated	Experienced operator who is fully acquainted with the use of the instrument
Lithotomy position	The fetal head must be engaged in the pelvis	Membranes ruptured	The capability to perform an emergency caesarean delivery if required
Bladder empty	The position of the fetal head must be known with certainty	No placenta previa	
Clinical pelvimetry must be adequate in dimension and size to facilitate an atraumatic delivery	The station of the fetal head must be ≥ +2		
Verbal or written consent	The attitude of the fetal head and the presence of caput succedaneum and/or molding should be noted		

83. D

She should have an ultrasound done to confirm her dates since her LMP is unknown and her resumption of ovulation is unpredictable. Deferring the ultrasound to a later gestational age is inappropriate since the dating accuracy decreases with ultrasounds obtained later in pregnancy. Vaginal bleeding is an indication for early ultrasound, but its absence does not preclude the need to do an ultrasound for dating accuracy. A rule of thumb concerning ultrasound accuracy is that they are accurate to within 1 week on either side of the estimated gestational age in the first trimester,

2 weeks in the second trimester, and 3 weeks in the third trimester. It is evident that by the third trimester, the estimated fetal age can be anywhere within a 6-week span. Of course, this is a rule of thumb and the ultrasonagrapher or radiologist will usually give an age range appropriate to that fetus' stage of development.

84. C

The patient should be seen monthly until 28 weeks into the pregnancy, every 2 or 3 weeks until 36 weeks, and then weekly until delivery, as long as the pregnancy is going well. If the pregnancy goes past term, most practitioners will see the patient biweekly and begin antenatal testing. ACOG has traditionally recommended 14 to 16 visits, but a report in 1989 and a study in 1997 support decreasing the number of visits in healthy parous women. The fundal height, weight of the patient, heart tones of the fetus, blood pressure, the presence or absence of edema, and urine screen for protein and glucose must be documented. The pattern of visits is designed especially to alert the practitioner to preeclampsia and allow early intervention. See Figure 3-2.

85. A

Infants of smoking mothers have a fourfold increased rate of being small for gestational age. There are many problems in pregnancy associated with tobacco use, including spontaneous abortion, placental abruption, placenta previa, premature and prolonged rupture of membranes, and IUGR. The carbon monoxide in cigarette smoke reduces oxygen delivery to the infant and nicotine vasoconstricts uterine vessels, diminishing placental flow. Uterine rupture is a poor outcome not associated with tobacco use. There is a higher risk of infertility and ectopic pregnancy. In addition, active and passive smoking are linked to many other negative outcomes, such as maternal depression, SIDS, middle ear effusions, respiratory problems, and allergies. As many as one out of four pregnant women smoke sometime during their pregnancy. The patient should be assessed for readiness to quit and counseled about the morbidity and possible mortality associated with smoking.

86. C

Nicotine replacement, including transdermal patch, spray, and gum, are contraindicated in pregnancy because nicotine is a neural toxin that is harmful to a developing fetus. The Food and Drug Administration has given it a category D rating. In reality, many physicians are using nicotine replacement to help pregnant women quit. There is evidence that for highly addicted smokers, such as women smoking more than a pack of cigarettes per day, nicotine replacement leads to improved quit rates. In addition, there are no other chemicals such as carbon monoxide in nicotine replacement. However, in most moderate and light tobacco abusers, the benefits do not outweigh the risks. The safest scenario would be to establish a quit date, enroll the patient in a smoking cessation program, and continue to see the patient in short interval follow-up visits to monitor her progress. If her partner is willing to quit along with the patient, they both have increased chances of cessation. Buproprion (Zyban) has a category B rating and may be useful in helping both heavy and light smokers quit.

87. E

Preterm labor is defined as cervical change before 37 weeks gestation. Although there are many risk factors for preterm labor, one-half of preterm births occur without an identifiable cause. The leading predictors of preterm birth are history of prior preterm birth, low body mass index, short cervical length, and the presence of fetal fibronectin. Other risk factors include strenuous work, tobacco abuse, age younger than 16 or older than 40 years, cervical infections, urinary tract infection, domestic violence, uterine anomaly, IUGR, and multiple gestation. Preterm labor can not only be difficult to predict and diagnose but also difficult to manage. Tocolytic therapy at best can delay birth 2 to 72 hours. This allows enough time for corticosteroids to increase fetal lung maturity and antibiotic prophylaxis.

88. C

Less than 10% of pregnancies continue past 42 weeks gestation. The cause for post-dates pregnancies is unknown, although it is associated with previous post-dates delivery, primiparity, and certain fetal anomalies. Inaccurate dating can be a common cause, in which case the pregnancy is not truly post-dates. Post-dates pregnancies are associated with an increased risk of shoulder distocia, large for gestation age infant, and eightfold increase in perinatal mortality at 43 weeks. In 35% of cases, meconium staining is present, although not necessarily aspiration. In a true prolonged gestation, postmaturity or dysmaturity syndrome occurs in about one-third of cases. This syndrome includes placental insufficiency, impaired diffusion of oxygen to fetus, loss of subcutaneous fat, excessive hair, dry skin, and long fingernails.

89. C

Five risk factor categories (A, B, C, D, and X) have been assigned to all drugs based on risk to the fetus. These risks refer to teratogenicity and have no relation to breast-feeding risk. Category A is the safest. Controlled human studies on category A drugs have revealed no fetal risk. Category B drugs are those that have either demonstrated no fetal risk in animal studies or shown an adverse effect in animal reproduction studies that has not been confirmed in controlled human studies. Category C drugs are those for which neither animal nor human studies are available or drugs for which animal studies have shown an adverse effect but there are no human studies. Category D drugs are those that have been shown to have adverse human effects but the benefits of using the drugs may outweigh the risks. Category X drugs are contraindicated during pregnancy. Natural products are not evaluated using this protocol.

90. E

Prozac (fluoxetine) is a category C medication. The risks of maternal depression must be weighed against the possible fetal risks. Depression may worsen during pregnancy, and changes in therapy must be carefully considered. Prozac is the SSRI with the longest track record of use during pregnancy. There appears to be no teratogenic effects; in addition, there is at least 7 years of follow-up on children exposed to fluoxetine in utero with no behavioral problems noted. The other SSRIs are presumed to be safe based on the experience with fluoxetine, but there are limited data. Tricyclic antidepressants also have a proven record of safety. Other agents commonly used, including venlafaxine (Effexor) and bupropion (Wellbutrin), have limited data. Monoamine oxidase inhibitors appear not to be safe and cannot be used during pregnancy.

91. D

Onset of major depression tends to occur during the childbearing years. Rates of depression are similar between pregnant and

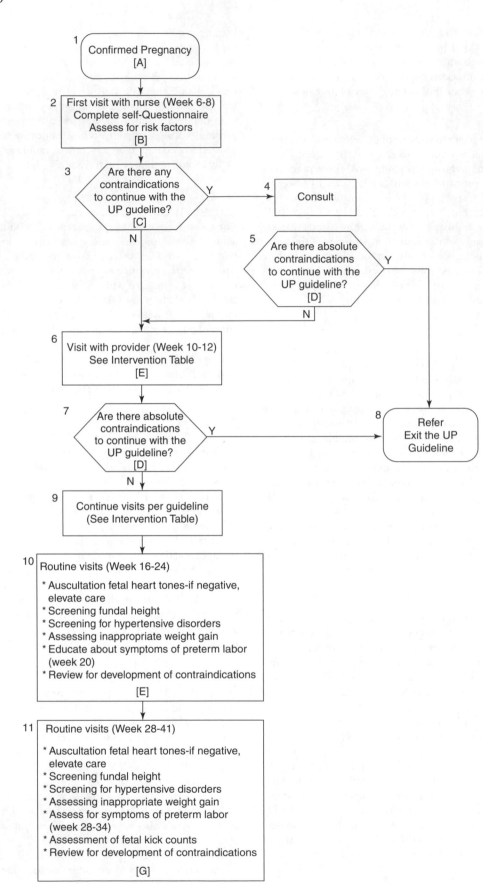

Figure 3-2. Management of uncomplicated pregnancy.

nonpregnant women. Rates of depression postpartum are significantly higher than rates during pregnancy. For patients with a history of severe chronic depression, rates of relapse are high if medication is discontinued. Tricyclic antidepressants and Prozac have been well studied and pose no teratogenic risks. Emerging data on other SSRIs are also encouraging. Monoamine oxidase inhibitors are associated with fetal anomalies and are contraindicated during pregnancy.

92. D

Chronic schizophrenia has a very high rate of relapse when medication is withdrawn. Among the high-potency antipsychotics, Haldol has been the medication most studied and is the preferred choice. It has not been associated with teratogenicity. Unfortunately, the three agents most commonly used in the treatment of bipolar illness—lithium, Depakene, and Tegretol—are known teratogens. Because postpartum relapse rates are so high in bipolar disease, it is advised to initiate treatment prior to delivery or immediately after birth. All psychopharmacologic agents cross the placenta.

93. B

Previous preterm labor is the strongest indicator of future preterm labor. Bacterial vaginosis is frequently associated with preterm labor. Any process that increases uterine size, such as twin gestation, is a risk factor for preterm labor. Poor nutrition, particularly poor protein intake, is common in women with preterm labor, as is a low body mass index. Alcohol is not a factor for preterm labor. Inaccurate dates are a risk for post-date delivery.

94. D

Many cases of varicella are clinically asymptomatic. Prior immunity is indicated by a positive IgA serology. If her serology is negative, the patient should receive VZIG. VZIG is 60% to 80% effective in preventing infection if received within 96 hours of exposure. Varicella vaccine is a live vaccine and is therefore contraindicated during pregnancy. Pregnant women are at higher risk of developing the serious complications of varicella, such as pneumonia. Congenital varicella may be associated with malformations and may lead to miscarriage.

95. B

Erythromycin is safe during pregnancy and effective against chlamydia. Amoxicillin and clindamycin are not indicated in the treatment of chlamydia, although both are safe during pregnancy. Tetracyclines are contraindicated during pregnancy due to adverse effects on fetal teeth and bones. Ciprofloxacin is not recommended therapy during pregnancy due to teratogenicity, especially fetal cartilage and bones.

96. A

Miconizole is the only antifungal agent listed that is appropriate for this patient. Clindamycin and metronidazole are used for bacterial vaginosis in the second and third trimesters. Fluconazole appears to be teratogenic in the first trimester.

97. D

Captopril and other ACE inhibitors are contraindicated during pregnancy because they cause fetal death and spontaneous abortion. ACE inhibitors are also teratogens, causing renal anomalies, anuria, and skull anomalies (fetal calvarial hypoplasia). Thiazide diuretics are not recommended because they cause decreased maternal plasma volume and are associated with low birth weight. Methyldopa has a long safety record and is the most commonly used antihypertensive during pregnancy. Uncontrolled hypertension during pregnancy is associated with increased fetal loss, growth retardation, preterm delivery, and pre-eclampsia.

98. C

Complete moles have no identifiable fetal tissue and are usually 46,XX, arising from paternal origin. If there are fetal parts as well as molar tissue, it is called a partial mole and the chromosomal pattern is usually one of triploidy. Usually, this arises from the fertilization of one egg with two sperm. The U.S. incidence of hydatidiform mole is 1 in 1,000 to 1 in 1,500. Interestingly, Japan has a molar pregnancy rate twice that of other countries. The history of molar pregnancy increases the risk of future molar pregnancy by 1% to 2%. Vaginal bleeding is the most common presenting complaint in molar pregnancy, which can be readily diagnosed with ultrasound.

99. A

Molar pregnancy is most safely treated with suction aspiration, which carries a risk of embolization. BHCG levels must be followed until the titer is zero for 3 weeks. Titers are then followed monthly for 6 to 12 months. Partial molar pregnancies are at low risk for persistent trophoblastic disease. Complete molar pregnancies can be divided into high and low risk. Patients have a higher risk of invasion if the BHCG is over 100,000 mIU/mL, the uterus is of excessive size, or if there are prominent theca lutein cysts. Only 20% of patients with a molar pregnancy require chemotherapy, almost exclusively in the high-risk complete molar group. Hysterectomy is not generally indicated, unless a patient no longer wishes fertility.

100. B

Although the fetus is relatively well protected, placental separation or abruption can occur after blunt trauma to the abdomen. It is important to monitor fetal heart tones and uterine activity for a minimum of 4 hours after trauma because decompensation can occur suddenly despite initially normal maternal vital signs. This is due to the increased circulating blood volume in pregnancy that can mask hypovolemia and internal hemorrhage. The warning signs after trauma are vaginal bleeding, uterine tenderness, nonreassuring fetal heart tones, and uterine contractions. Uterine rupture is not a common complication of trauma, and placenta previa is unrelated to trauma.

101. B

When vaginal bleeding occurs in the first trimester, it often, but not always, indicates inevitable spontaneous abortion. Bed rest will not make a difference in the outcome. Minor trauma, such as falling down several stairs, is not associated with increased risk of first trimester pregnancy loss.

102. C

Premature rupture of membranes refers to rupture of membranes at any gestational age prior to onset of contractions. The patient is at term and, therefore, the delivery will not be preterm. PPROM refers to preterm rupture of membranes but without uterine contractions. These are patients who may be treated with antenatal steroids and tocolytics in the hope that resealing of the membranes will occur. Since part of the definition of labor is painful uterine contractions, this patient is not in labor yet. Failure to progress is a generic term for any intrapartum problem that does not allow adequate descent or dilation and effacement of the cervix.

103. E

Steroids reduce the incidence of hyaline membrane disease, also called respiratory distress syndrome, and intraventricular hemorrhage, both by nearly 50%. Steroids have no effect on sepsis or meconium aspiration. Meconium aspiration does lead to lung disease, but it is a toxic chemical pneumonitis unchanged by the administration of steroids antenatally.

104. B

No oral agents have been proven to reduce preterm labor and delivery. Tocolytic therapy typically delays labor for 24 to 48 hours. The benefit lies in the ability to administer antenatal steroids, which have a demonstrable effect within 24 hours. In some instances, tocolysis may delay labor for up to 7 days. Short-term tocolysis has not been shown to result in improved neonatal outcomes. Likewise, maintenance tocolysis after successful treatment of preterm labor has not been shown to improve fetal outcomes or decrease preterm delivery. Many agents have been used for tocolysis, including betamimetics, indomethacin, magnesium sulfate, and nifedipine. Indomethacin, a nonsteroidal prostaglandin inhibitor, causes constriction of the fetal ductus arteriosus, causes oligohydramnios, and increases fetal morbidity.

105. B

Polyhydramnios is defined as an amniotic fluid index (AFI) greater than 20 to 25 cm. An AFI of 5 to 20 cm is normal, although AFIs less than 10 are considered to be low normal. It is readily seen with transabdominal ultrasound and is measured by adding the lengths of the largest vertical fluid pocket in all four quadrants. Polyhydramnios is often idiopathic, in which case there appears to be no sequelae to the fetus. However, it may also be caused by gastrointestinal anomalies, isoimmunization, diabetes mellitus, and placental abnormalities. Amnioinfusion is a treatment for oligohydramnios.

106. E

All of the above are indicative of fetal demise in utero (FDIU). In addition, there may be gas in the major blood vessels, fetal measurement will be smaller than estimated gestational age, and there may be collapse of the skull. The rates of fetal demise have declined in the United States from 12 per 1,000 in the 1960s to 3 per 1,000 in the early 1990s, mostly due to increased surveillance and prompt delivery. More numbers of fetal death occur prior to 32 weeks, but the risk of fetal death rises sharply after 40 weeks. After 42 weeks, a fetus is 12 times more likely to die in utero than a fetus at 30 weeks. The most common cause of FDIU, accounting for 30%, is asphyxia, caused by placental and cord problems. Maternal complications such as gestational diabetes and pre-eclampsia cause another 30% of fetal deaths, and 15% are due to fetal malformations and anomalies. Only 5% are due to infections. What is important to note is that more than 20% of fetal demises have no identifiable cause. Once FDIU is identified, delivery occurs spontaneously or via induction. The only urgent indication for delivery is the woman with coagulopathy or infection.

107. A

Oligohydramnios is defined on ultrasound as an amniotic fluid index of less than 5 cm. Amnioinfusion is very safe and significantly reduces the incidence of umbilical cord compression with resultant variable decelerations. It is not associated with electrolyte disturbances. Amnioinfusion is performed after rupture of membranes by placing an intrauterine catheter and infusing a physiologically normal solution. Post-date oligohydramnios is usually an indication for prompt delivery because it indicates placental insufficiency. Cord prolapse is a risk in polyhydramnios.

108. D

After checking maternal blood pressure and fetal heart tones, a non-stress test (NST) to monitor uterine activity and concurrent fetal heart tones is indicated. If the NST is not reactive, a biophysical profile (BPP) is indicated. This test consists of ultrasound evaluation of the fetus with two points given for fetal breathing, fetal tone, fetal movement, and amniotic fluid index. A score out of 8 (without NST results) or out of 10 (with NST results) is given with a normal score allowing for lack of one component—that is, 6 out of 8, or 8 out of 10. Fetal breathing is the most sensitive measure of fetal hypoxia on the BPP. An exam of her cervix will not give any information about fetal viability or activity. A turbidity test is performed on amniotic fluid to determine lung maturity of a preterm fetus. The contraction stress test is most appropriately performed in the hospital for women who are post-date to determine the ability of the fetus to tolerate labor.

109. A

A speculum exam is part of the evaluation for rupture of membranes, which is a cause of preterm uterine contractions. All women with preterm contractions should have electronic fetal monitoring (EFM) to determine the exact interval and duration of contractions. In addition, the monitoring will provide fetal heart rate, which can provide information about the fetal well-being. Fetal monitoring should be performed minimally for 30 minutes but would ideally continue until a disposition is established. In addition to a sterile speculum exam and EFM, some family physicians may perform cervical cultures and urine cultures to determine if infection is the etiology of the contractions. A fetal fibronectin test indicates inflammation and can help determine if the woman is at risk for preterm delivery. The McRoberts maneuver is part of the approach for shoulder dystocia.

110. D

Renal insufficiency and pyelonephritis pose significant threats to pregnancy, resulting in preterm delivery, small for gestational age infants, and stillbirth. Renal insufficiency seems to worsen in pregnancy, directly proportional to the level of pre-pregnancy insufficiency. Hypertension is also associated with renal disease in pregnancy. New onset renal insufficiency requires careful workup, including complete history and lab workup focusing on serum electrolytes, creatinine, blood count, and urinalysis, paying special attention to bacteria, protein, and any casts found in the urine. A renal biopsy may be needed. New onset of proteinuria can also be the earliest indication of pre-eclampsia. Low-grade heart murmurs are common in pregnant women due to the increase in circulating volume and cardiac output.

111. E

Risk factors for pre-eclampsia include nulliparity, multiple gestation, chronic hypertension, previous pre-eclampsia, and extremes of maternal age (younger than 18 or older than 35 years). Prematurity is the diagnosis responsible for the majority of neonatal morbidity and mortality in the United States. Intentional and unintentional injury (including homicides, motor vehicle accidents, domestic violence, drug-related deaths, and suicides) is the diagnosis responsible for most of the maternal morbidity and mortality in the United States, especially in urban areas. Injuries account for 38% of deaths to pregnant women. Currently, thromboembolic disease, including pulmonary embolism, causes the highest rate of pregnancy-related maternal mortality. Hypertensive disorders account for 15% of maternal deaths. PIH is hypertension that occurs after 20 weeks gestation but does not have other signs of pre-eclampsia, namely proteinuria. Since edema of the lower extremities occurs in 75% of all pregnant women, it cannot be used to differentiate PIH from pre-eclampsia. There are several randomized prospective trials that clearly show that daily aspirin does not prevent pre-eclampsia.

112. D

Pre-eclampsia that occurs early in pregnancy is more likely to recur in subsequent pregnancies. However, there is no relation to the gestational age at which it appears in the subsequent pregnancies. There may even be some data to suggest it may appear at a later gestational age. Although teens are classically thought of as the patients with pre-eclampsia, older mothers are actually at a slightly increased risk. The incidence is 2% to 7% of all pregnancies. The treatment of choice in pre-eclampsia at term is delivery. If the infant is premature and the degree of pre-eclampsia is mild, then weekly non-stress testing with or without biophysical profile is recommended. This should be done biweekly if there is any concern about oligohydramnios or fetal growth restriction, both signs of placental dysfunction. Laboratory study evaluation of renal function, liver enzymes, platelet counts, and urine protein levels can also aid in monitoring this disease. See Table 3.12.

113. C

Decreased fetal movement, while of concern, is not generally associated with pre-eclampsia. Pre-eclampsia is a syndrome that

Table 3.12 Risk factors for pre-eclampsia

Nulliparity
Pregestational diabetes
Thrombophilia
Nephropathy
Connective tissue disease
Molar pregnancy
Fetal hydrops
Multifetal gestation
Chronic hypertension
Obesity
Prior pregnancy complicated by pre-eclampsia
Antiphospholipid antibody syndrome
Family history of pre-eclampsia or eclampsia
Fetal aneuploidy

Adapted from Scott JR, ed. *Danforth's obstetrics & gynecology.* 8th ed. Philadelphia: Lippincott-Raven Publishers; 1998.

classically includes hypertension, edema, and proteinuria. Symptoms include neurologic symptoms (headache, blurry vision, scotoma, and, in rare cases, lethargy or altered mental status) and gastrointestinal symptoms (nausea, vomiting, and right upper quadrant pain), especially when associated with HELLP syndrome (*h*emolysis, *e*levated *l*iver enzymes, and *l*ow *p*latelets). There is often edema in the lower extremities, hands, and face as well as hyper-reflexia.

114. E

Inverted or flat nipples occur in 10% of all women. It can cause increased difficulty of breast-feeding but by no means prevents it. The inverted nipples are caused by tethered lactiferous ducts that often elongate without any treatment in the third trimester due to breast growth. In fact, most women's nipples will protrude with gentle pressure to the areola, even women with flat or inverted nipples. Because the stimulation of the nipple causes oxytocin release, which may stimulate contractions, any manipulation of the nipples is discouraged prior to term. After delivery, early initial breast-feeding within the first hour of life is associated with fewer breast-feeding problems and longer duration of breast-feeding. Some women may use breast shields, breast shells, or a breast pump initially to help evert the nipple, but only after delivery. Nipple shields are made of silicone and cover the nipple and areola during feeding. They help infants latch on when the mother has inverted nipples, the infant has been bottle fed, or the mother has an overactive let-down reflex. Breast shells are plastic cups worn between feedings that provide gentle pressure on the base of the shortened ducts. A powerful elongator of the nipple is electric pumping. What should be discouraged is breast engorgement, which will cause the nipple to protrude even less. Frequent breast-feeding is essential if the mother has inverted nipples.

115. A

Although the benefits of breast-feeding are multiple, they do not include decreasing the risk of infections in the mother. There is a somewhat higher chance of the mother developing mastitis, although breast-feeding has no impact of the risk of postpartum endometritis Although weight loss is often mentioned as a benefit, this is not universal and some women may actually gain weight while breast-feeding. HIV infection in the mother is a contraindication to breast-feeding. Breast-feeding delays ovulation and therefore increases the interval between pregnancies. See Table 3.13.

116. C

Nägele's rule assumes regular menstrual cycles and cycle intervals of 26 to 30 days. Nägle's rule states that the EDC can be determined by taking the LMP, subtracting 3 months, adding 7 days, and adding 1 year. In this patient, the EDC needs to be adjusted by 5 days since her cycle interval is longer than 30 days. Ultrasound in the first trimester is extremely accurate and the EDC should be changed if it differs from the menstrual dating by more than 5 to 7 days. Beyond the first trimester, ultrasound may be less accurate because of differences in fetal growth.

117. B

Pregnant women are often motivated to make lifestyle changes that they do not make when nonpregnant. Numerous studies have demonstrated the effectiveness of physician advice to stop smoking and behavioral modification techniques. There is no such

Table 3.13

Research in the United States, Canada, Europe and other developed countries, among predominantly middle-class populations, provides strong evidence that human milk feeding decreases the incidence and/or severity of diarrhea, lower respiratory infection, otitis media, bacteremia, bacterial meningitis, botulism, urinary tract infection, and necrotizing enterocolitis. There are a number of studies that show a possible protective effect of human milk feeding against sudden infant death syndrome, insulin-dependent diabetes mellitus, Crohn's disease, ulcerative colitis, lymphoma, allergic diseases, and other chronic digestive diseases. Breast-feeding has also been related to possible enhancement of cognitive development.

Source: Amerian Academy of Pediatrics, Work Group on Breast-feeding. Breast-feeding and the use of human milk. *Pediatrics.* 1997: 1035–1039 [Paragraph includes 39 citations]. Adapted from Scott JR, ed. *Danforth's obstetrics & gynecology.* 8th ed. Philadelphia: Lippincott-Raven Publishers; 1998.

thing as a safe number of cigarettes. Nicotine patches are category C during pregnancy, whereas buproprion is category B. Nicotine should be avoided intrapartum because of its effects on placental blood flow and the risk to the fetus.

118. D

Smoking and nicotine increase the risk for preterm birth, SGA babies, and maternal cervical cancer. In addition, the baby growing up in a household with smokers is exposed to secondhand smoke. The baby has a higher risk of SIDS and of respiratory and ear infections. There is no known association between in utero tobacco exposure and type 1 diabetes mellitus of gestational diabetes.

119. B

Congenital anomalies are more common in fetuses that are malpresented at term. Breech presentation is the most common malpresentation, affecting 3% or 4% of pregnancies at term, whereas face presentation occurs in only 1 in 500 to 1,200 pregnancies. Congenital anomalies occur in approximately 6.2% to 23% of breech presentations (versus 2.3% in vertex presentations), including hip dysplasia and hydrocephalus. Occipital posterior position refers to a fetus that presents with the anterior parts upward and the fetal spine toward the maternal spine. This malposition occurs in about 2% or 3% of term deliveries. Management options for breech presentation at or near term include external cephalic version, breech exercises, C-section, and, rarely, vaginal breech delivery. Due to studies that show decreased morbidity and mortality with C-section delivery of breech babies, C-section is indicated for a patient in labor. It is less common for a breech to spontaneously convert to vertex at 36 weeks, but it does occur at 34 weeks.

120. E

Polyhydramnios and multiparity are common co-conditions with breech presentation. Active labor is a contraindication to attempting external cephalic version. ECV is generally considered safe,

although complications can occur, including non-reassuring fetal heart tones, abruption, fetal or maternal hemorrhage, knotted and/or entangled umbilical cord, fetal mortality, and maternal mortality due to amniotic fluid embolism. Any of these may necessitate immediate C-section at the time of version. Usually, version is attempted at term, with the plan to induce labor as soon as the version is successful.

121. C

Decreased fetal movement is sensitive but not specific for fetal non–well-being. Most cases of compromised infants are preceded by the maternal sensation of decreased fetal movement. The absence of fetal activity requires further assessment before one can conclude that the fetus is compromised. At the same time, the vast majority of women who report decreased fetal movement have normally active fetuses on NST. A nonreactive NST should be followed with a BPP or contraction stress test (CST) and consideration of delivery should be made for these patients. In addition, many family physicians start kick counts at or near term as a way to obtain more objective information about fetal movement. There are at least eight ways to do kick counts, but all involve the patient monitoring and recording any fetal rolls, kicks, stretches, or punches. Patients should be given parameters to call their physician if the movements are decreased. Patients who report decreased fetal movement should always be evaluated because of the risk of IUFD. Most stillborn births occur in women with no risk factors. It may be possible to prevent some demises by early intervention if there is any evidence of compromise.

122. A

Reassurance only would be an inappropriate way of managing this patient given her subjective sense of decreased fetal movement and her noncompliance. Decreased fetal movement is sensitive but not specific for fetal non-well-being. Most cases of compromised infants are preceded by the maternal sensation of decreased fetal movement. The absence of fetal activity requires further assessment before one can conclude that the fetus is compromised. At the same time, the vast majority of women who report decreased fetal movement have normally active fetuses on NST. A nonreactive NST should be followed with a BPP or CST and consideration of delivery should be made for these patients. Patients who report decreased fetal movement should always be evaluated because of the risk of IUFD, and it may be possible to prevent demises by early intervention (i.e., delivery).

123. D

The patient has mild pre-eclampsia and is at term with a ripe cervix. There are no contraindications to delivering her and good reasons to induce her labor. There is significant morbidity to fetus and mother associated with delaying delivery. Delaying evaluation for another week would be inappropriate. Since her cervix is ripe and she does not have severe pre-eclampsia, she does not need immediate C-section. She should be monitored during labor, and if her blood pressure remains elevated and/or her lab tests are abnormal, magnesium sulfate should be started when she is in active labor.

124. C

Since 1998, the recommendation to test all pregnant women for GDM has been changed and women considered to be at low risk no longer require the 50-g glucose load test. Women younger than

25 years old with no other risk factors may be excluded. Also, those excluded should have no history of abnormal glucose metabolism. If patients have a positive screen, which is usually considered to be a glucose of 140 mg/dL, then they must perform the 3-hour glucose tolerance test. This test consists of a 100-g oral glucose load taken fasting after 3 days of a carbohydrate-rich diet. There are two sets of criteria in use for the diagnosis of gestational diabetes. The

National Diabetes Data Group uses a fasting glucose reading of 105, 1-hour postprandial reading of 190, 2-hour postprandial reading of 165, and 3-hour postprandial reading of 145 to make the diagnosis. The American Diabetic Association has lowered its limits to 95/180/155/140 because of increasing evidence that improved glucose control even in women previously labeled as only glucose intolerant significantly reduces infant morbidity and mortality.

Chapter 4

Gynecology Questions

1. What is the most common factor responsible for a couple's infertility?

A. Ovulatory factor

B. Male factor

C. Tubal and peritoneal factor

D. Cervical factor

E. Uterine factor

2. Which of the following is the most common cause of male infertility?

A. Testicular failure

B. Obstruction

C. Low semen volume

D. Varicocele

E. Cryptorchidism

3. Regarding Turner's syndrome, which of the following statements is true?

A. It is caused by complete androgen insensitivity.

B. A karyotype would reveal 47, XXY.

C. Coarctation of the aorta is the most common cardiovascular abnormality.

D. It is always associated with infertility.

E. Patients often exhibit a eunachoid body habitus.

4. Which of the following is a true statement regarding uterine bleeding?

A. Normal menstrual bleeding occurs every 21 to 35 days with an average blood loss of 120 cc.

B. The degree of endometrial shedding is not related to estrogen exposure while the endometrium is proliferating.

C. Greater than three-fourths of dysfunctional uterine bleeding is attributable to anovulation.

D. Carcinoma is the most common cause of uterine bleeding in postmenopausal women.

E. Uterine bleeding in a premenarchal girl is pathognomonic for neoplasm.

5. Which of the following statements is true with regard to bacterial vaginosis?

A. The vaginal pH is less than 3.

B. The discharge is almost always associated with vulvar irritation and inflammation.

C. There is an increased incidence of preterm labor in pregnant women with bacterial vaginosis.

D. The typical discharge is white and thick in appearance.

E. It has not been found to spread to the upper genital tract.

6. Which of the following is an absolute contraindication to the use of oral contraceptive pills?

A. Personal history of smoking in a woman younger than 35 years of age

B. Obesity

C. Hypertension

D. Personal history of diabetes mellitus

E. History of thrombophlebitis

7. With regard to recurrent vulvovaginitis, which is true?

A. *Candida albicans* causes 30% of vulvovaginitis.

B. A full evaluation can be made with visual inspection alone.

C. Since most vaginal discharge is from yeast, evaluation for chlamydia, gonorrhea, and trichomonas is not needed in cases of abnormal vaginal secretions.

D. In cases caused by *Candida albicans*, there is a high incidence of resistance to antifungal therapy.

E. Over-the-counter medications used for treatment of symptoms of vulvovaginitis are frequently misused.

8. When prescribing the medroxyprogesterone acetate (Depo-Provera) method of contraception, which of the following should be discussed with the patient?

A. Possibility of menstrual irregularities including amenorrhea

B. Decreased necessity for the use of barrier methods to protect against sexually transmitted disease (STD)

C. A documented failure rate of approximately 10%

D. Possibility of weight loss

E. Potential worsening of arthritic pain

9. A 30-year-old female is seen by you for increased facial hair. On exam, you also note lower abdominal hair. In the evaluation of this patient, which set of labs would yield the greatest information?

A. CBC, serum testosterone, follicle-stimulating hormone (FSH), luteinizing hormone (LH)

B. Comprehensive metabolic screen, FSH, LH, testosterone

C. FSH, LH, adrenal CT scan, dehydroepiandrosterone sulfate (DHEAS level)

D. Serum testosterone, DHEAS, serum prolactin, 17-OH progesterone

E. Pelvic ultrasound, serum testosterone, DHEAS, fasting glucose

10. An elderly female patient presents to your office to obtain a "second opinion" about the use of a pessary. Your discussion with the patient should include which of the following?

A. Weekly douching and cleaning of the device is recommended

B. Topical estrogen use increases the risk of complications from pessary use

C. Urinary tract infection is a potential complication

D. A pessary should not be used in a woman who plans to become pregnant

E. Vaginal discharge should be expected and is a normal finding

11. When examining a patient after a sexual assault:

A. A history of previous sexual assaults should not be taken to protect patient privacy.

B. It is not necessary to take photographs of injuries if they are described in detail in the physician's notes.

C. The patient should be offered prophylaxis for pregnancy.

D. A bimanual exam should be avoided to prevent further trauma to the patient.

E. The police should begin questioning the patient during the exam so as to get the most accurate details.

12. You are examining a female athlete with amenorrhea. Which of the following is true?

A. Physical activity alone can induce amenorrhea.

B. Initial treatment is usually oral estrogens.

C. In athletes who have been amenorrheic for more than 12 months, assessment of bone mineral density should be considered.

D. A pregnancy test is not necessary.

E. After administration of progesterone (10 mg for 5 to 10 days) in a female with hypothalamic pituitary axis suppression, withdrawal bleeding is the expected finding.

13. Which of the following is true regarding labial adhesions in the prepubescent years?

A. Adhesions are usually symptomatic.

B. Urinary incontinence can occur.

C. The etiology of adhesions is usually sexual abuse.

D. In a child without symptoms and with minimal adhesion, surgical correction is usually appropriate.

E. Adhesions may resolve spontaneously in puberty due to increased estrogen production.

14. Which of the following is not a typical response to estrogen in the female newborn?

A. Breast enlargement

B. Vaginal bleeding that lasts more than 2 months

C. Thickened hymen

D. Whitish vaginal discharge

E. Fused labia minora

15. Which of the following is true regarding fibrocystic breast disease?

A. Women with fibrocystic breast disease and atypical lobular hyperplasia who are younger than 45 years old are only slightly more likely to get breast cancer.

B. Atypical lobular hyperplasia is a potentially malignant finding.

C. Oral contraceptives are contraindicated in women with fibrocystic breast disease.

D. Most fibrocystic breast disease is malignant.

E. If a cyst aspiration is performed in the office and the cyst disappears completely with clear non-bloody fluid, the fluid should still be saved for microscopic analysis.

16. Which of the following would be an effective treatment for gonorrhea?

A. Amoxicillin 400 mg—single oral dose

B. Ceftriaxone (Rocephin) 125 mg—single intramuscular dose

C. Metronidazole (Flagyl) 500 mg—single oral dose

D. Tetracycline 500 mg four times per day for 7 days

E. Azithromycin (Zithromax) 1 g—single oral dose

17. Which of the following is a true statement regarding oral contraception?

A. Rifampin, phenobarbital, phenytoin, and certain antibiotics can significantly increase the serum concentration of estrogen.

B. The concentration of estrogen can fluctuate by as much as 120% if other medications are taken with the pill.

C. Up to one-fourth of women taking oral contraceptive pills may experience a delay in resuming ovulation after cessation of the pill.

D. Patients who have been taking the pill for more than 5 years should be advised to wait 4 to 6 months before attempting to conceive.

E. Women who smoke but who are not at increased risk of premature heart disease may safely use the pill into their 50s.

18. The subtypes of human papillomavirus (HPV) that most correlate with cervical dysplasia are:

A. 6 and 11

B. 6, 11, and 18

C. 31 and 33

D. 33 and 35

E. 16 and 18

19. Which of the following is true with regard to possible colposcopic findings?

A. Dysplastic epithelium will generally turn a lush red color with the application of acetic acid.

B. Normal epithelium does not stain well with Lugol's solution.

C. Squamous metaplasia is an abnormal finding.

D. Endocervical columnar cells can commonly appear white after an application of acetic acid.

E. Corkscrew vessels are a normal finding.

20. You see a 40-year-old patient presenting with heavy, prolonged periods. She is afebrile, and her vital signs are stable. On physical exam, you find her uterus is enlarged. Her pregnancy test is negative, and her hemoglobin level is 10.5. A pelvic US confirms multiple fibroids. Medical treatment options at this time include:

A. Leuprolide acetate

B. Medroxyprogesterone acetate

C. Testosterone transdermal patch

D. Conjugated estrogen

E. Acetaminophen therapy

21. The previous patient tries oral contraceptives but is not satisfied with the result. She would like to discuss uterine artery embolization. In considering if she is a good candidate, you need to consider which factor:
A. Age
B. Anemia
C. Number of fibroids
D. The presence of pedunculated fibroids
E. Iodine allergy

22. A 25-year-old woman presents complaining of an increased number of periods. She brings in a calendar indicating the following dates as the first days of her last four periods: April 2, April 21, May 11, and May 30. Her bleeding pattern is defined as:
A. Menorrhagia
B. Metrorrhagia
C. Polymenorrhea
D. Amenorrhea
E. Oligomenorrhea

23. A 24-year-old woman G1P1001 on oral contraceptives (OCPs) presents with heavier, prolonged bleeding with her last menstrual cycle. Her OCP contains 35 μg of ethinyl estradiol. She is sexually active with two new partners in the past year. She recently started taking loratadine (Claritin) for allergic rhinitis. The most likely cause of her menorrhagia is:
A. Accumulated estrogenic effect of her oral contraceptive pill
B. Drug–drug interaction
C. Pituitary adenoma
D. Pelvic inflammatory disease
E. Anovulation

24. A 45-year-old G3P2012 woman with a history of a tubal ligation 10 years ago presents to you complaining of increased vaginal bleeding. Her periods in the past were every 25 to 28 days and lasted 4 or 5 days. Now she is bleeding every 14 to 35 days and her bleeding is heavier, lasting 7 to 10 days. What is the most accurate descriptive term for her bleeding, and what is the most likely cause?
A. Menometrorrhagia: anovulation
B. Menometrorrhagia: hyperplasia
C. Metrorrhagia: endometrial cancer
D. Menorrhagia: endometrial cancer
E. Menorrhagia: hyperplasia

25. A 48-year-old G0P0 woman presents to the emergency room complaining of heavy vaginal bleeding and dizziness. She has no other significant past medical history. She has increased bleeding with menstruation the past few months. She is afebrile, pulse 100, and blood pressure 110/70 in the recumbent position. When standing, her pulse is 120 and blood pressure 98/60. Her exam is unremarkable except that she has a large amount of blood in the vaginal vault. She has a negative pregnancy test and a hemoglobin of 9 mg/dL. Your initial treatment includes:
A. High doses of nonsteroidal anti-inflammatory agents
B. Conjugated estrogen (Premarin)
C. Blood transfusion—2 units of packed red blood cells
D. Medroxyprogesterone (Depo-Provara)
E. A high-dose combination oral contraceptive pill

26. A 37-year-old woman G0P0 presents to your office complaining of heavy bleeding with her last period and recent intermenstrual bleeding. Your initial evaluation should include an evaluation for which of the following?
A. Hyperprolactinemia
B. Hypothyroidism
C. Pelvic inflammatory disease (PID)
D. Endometrial hyperplasia
E. Pregnancy

27. A 16-year-old G0P0 girl presents to your office complaining of prolonged periods. She reports menarche 4 months ago. Since then she has had three periods, each lasting 10 to 14 days, with heavy bleeding the first 5 or 6 days. She has never been sexually active. Your evaluation should include:
A. Pelvic ultrasound
B. Bleeding time
C. Endometrial biopsy
D. 17-Hydroxyprogesterone level
E. Cervical cultures

28. A 47-year-old female presents for brief consultation. She believes that she is going through "the change" and would like to be tested for menopause. She notes that her last menstrual period was 2 months ago. She has not experienced hot flashes but notes fatigue and some difficulty concentrating. Her past medical history is unremarkable. She has one sexual partner, her husband. Based on her current symptoms, you provide a provisional diagnosis, order additional testing, and ask her to return for a complete physical examination. Which of the following describes your provisional diagnosis and plan?
A. Stress-induced oligomenorrhea; no laboratory studies
B. Perimenopause; UCG, CBC, and thyroid-stimulating hormone (TSH)
C. Depression; Beck's depression inventory at next visit
D. Hypothyroidism; TSH
E. Menopause; UCG, FSH, estrogen, and progesterone

29. A 57-year-old woman presents with a complaint of vaginal irritation. Which of the following findings on microscopic examination of her vaginal secretions would be indicative of a diagnosis other than vaginal atrophy?
A. pH 6.0
B. Clue cells
C. The absence of lactobacilli
D. Many white blood cells
E. Many bacteria

30. A 52-year-old female presents for her annual examination. She recently read an article on vaginal cancer in a women's magazine and would like to know more about her risk for the disease and the disease itself. Her past medical history is significant for total abdominal hysterectomy 10 years ago. She has no current complaints. Which of the following statements provides her with correct information?
A. She is at decreased risk for vaginal cancer because it is most commonly seen in women younger than the age of 50.
B. Since she has had a hysterectomy, she need not be concerned about vaginal cancer.

C. She is at high risk for clear cell adenocarcinoma because of her hysterectomy.

D. Common symptoms of vaginal cancer include vaginal bleeding, vaginal irritation, and painful urination.

E. Common symptoms of vaginal cancer include abdominal distension and weight loss.

31. A 56-year-old postmenopausal woman comes to your office complaining of a 1-year history of recurrent irritation in what she describes as her pubic area. She reports itchiness, and sometimes a blood-tinged discharge. The patient has tried metronidazole (Flagyl) suppository per vagina and topical cream over her labia, with little relief of her discomfort. Recently, the patient feels a pea-sized lump on her labia, and this is why she has come to see you. What is the most likely diagnosis?

A. Bartholin cyst

B. Cystic adenosis

C. Squamous cell carcinoma of the vulva

D. Bartholin gland carcinoma

E. Sebaceous cyst

32. A 40-year-old woman calls your office at the end of a busy day complaining to your receptionist of a very heavy "period" with clots that came 1 week early. Her husband has been using condoms but occasionally forgets. She has cramping and some nausea. She has had two normal children. There is no chest pain, pelvic pain (apart from cramping), flank pain, nor dysuria. There are no bleeding tendencies in the family. You relay the message for her to come right in and you squeeze her between your scheduled patients. The most appropriate encounter in the office would be:

A. Your staff takes vital signs. She appears normal, so you give her reassurance, advising her to return if her cramps or bleeding worsen.

B. You insist on doing a pelvic examination, even though she protests being examined while bleeding.

C. You order a serum beta human chorionic gonadotropin (BHCG) because your office is out of urine testers. The results will come back tomorrow.

D. You send her for a pelvic ultrasound, which may not be done until tomorrow.

E. You do an immediate endometrial biopsy while she is in the office.

33. A 14-year-old girl presents to your office complaining of pain in her left breast for 3 months. She says she feels "something" in her breast and is worried. She began menstruating at age 12, has a 28-day cycle, and finished her last period 5 days prior to her visit. She denies any change in size of the breast mass during her cycle or any exacerbating or ameliorating factors. Her family history is negative for breast cancer. On exam, you palpate two small 1-cm round rubbery masses in the right lower quadrant of her left breast. The masses are tender and noncompressible; otherwise, the exam is benign. No nodes are palpated in either axilla. The most likely diagnosis is:

A. Cyst

B. Fibroadenoma

C. Carcinoma of the breast

D. Fibrocystic change

E. Abscess

34. A 43-year-old female is scheduled for total abdominal hysterectomy with bilateral salpingoophorectomy. The indication for her surgery is pelvic pain due to chronic pelvic inflammatory disease. Which of the following hormone replacement therapy options would initially be best for this patient in the postoperative period:

A. Conjugated estrogen (Premarin) 0.625 mg PO daily

B. Conjugated estrogen (Premarin) 0.3 mg and medroxyprogesterone acetate (Provera) 5 mg PO daily

C. Conjugated estrogen (Premarin) 0.625 mg and medroxyprogesterone acetate (Provera) 5 mg PO daily

D. Transdermal estradiol—17B (Climara) 0.1 mg patch twice weekly

E. Transdermal estradiol—17B (Climara) 0.05 mg patch twice weekly and medroxyprogesterone acetate (Provera) 5 mg PO daily

35. Which of the following is a side effect of hormone replacement therapy?

A. Weight loss

B. Insomnia

C. Diarrhea

D. Hirsuitism

E. Nausea

36. Which of the following conditions constitute a relative contraindication for the use of hormone replacement therapy?

A. Leukemia

B. Acne

C. Congestive heart failure

D. Melanoma

E. Down's syndrome

37. Compared to estrogen therapy, raloxifene (Evista) is more likely to cause which of the following?

A. Hot flashes

B. Migraine headaches

C. Cough

D. Nausea

E. Arthritis

38. What is the major advantage of raloxifene (Evista) over estrogen?

A. Better control of atrophic vaginitis

B. Better control of hot flashes

C. Fewer endometrial changes

D. Fewer thromboembolic events

E. Better lipid effects

39. A 28-year-old woman presents to your office complaining of irregular periods every 2 to 4 months for the past 8 months. She reports menarche at age 15. She started on an oral contraceptive pill at the age of 17. She had a regular period up until 9 months ago. She stopped taking the oral contraceptive pill 9 months ago. On exam, she has normal vital signs. Her exam is unremarkable except for obesity and mild facial hair that she reports she has had "for as long as I can remember." This patient most likely has an anovulatory pattern of bleeding secondary to:

A. Obesity

B. Polycystic ovarian syndrome (Stein–Leventhal syndrome)

C. Prolonged oral contraceptive use
D. Turner syndrome
E. Perimenopause

40. A 41-year-old nonsmoking woman presents to your office with heavy bleeding. After a complete evaluation, you determine she has dysfunctional uterine bleeding. What would be your first treatment choice?
A. Dilation and curettage
B. Oral contraceptive pill
C. Endometrial ablation
D. Hysterectomy
E. Hospitalization for transfusion

41. A 27-year-old P5G5005 woman presents to the office with a history and exam consistent with dysfunctional uterine bleeding of 2 years' duration. She had an onset of menses at age 9. She has used oral contraceptives for a total of 5 years since age 15. Her height is 68 inches and her weight is 260 lbs. She is a smoker. She also has a history of diabetes type 2 and HTN. You decide to proceed with an evaluation of her endometrium with an endometrial biopsy. Which of the following is associated with an increased risk of endometrial cancer in this woman?
A. Smoking status
B. OCP use
C. Parity
D. Age
E. Early onset of menses

42. A 55-year-old woman presents with vaginal spotting. Her last period was 14 months ago. Her history and exam are otherwise unremarkable. She refuses an endometrial biopsy but agrees to have a transvaginal ultrasound to evaluate her endometrial stripe. The following result would be reassuring:
A. Anything less than 3 cm
B. Anything less than 2.5 cm
C. Anything less than 1 cm
D. Anything less than 8 mm
E. Anything less than 3 mm

43. A female patient presents her completed basal body temperature chart to you following 1 month of strict measurements taken first thing in the morning using a basal body temperature thermometer. Day 1 is the first day of her menstrual period. Her chart is shown in Table 4.1. Which day has the highest likelihood of achieving conception with coitus?
A. Day 13
B. Day 14
C. Day 15
D. Day 16
E. Day 17

44. A couple in your office has not achieved pregnancy after several months of basal body temperature charting and ovulation predictor testing. They have used a home ovulation predictor kit for 2 months, which detects luteinizing hormone in the urine before ovulation occurs. See Table 4.2. They have intercourse as directed, and the husband's sperm is normal. What could be the cause of her infertility based on the following results?

Table 4.1 Basal body temperature chart

Cycle Day No.	Temperature Recording on Morning Awakening (°F)	Coitus: ✓ If Yes
1 (menses)	97.6	
2 (menses)	97.6	
3 (menses)	97.8	
4 (menses)	97.7	
5	97.5	
6	97.5	✓
7	97.6	
8	97.8	✓
9	97.9	
10	97.6	
11	97.7	
12	97.5	
13	97.6	
14	97.6	✓
15	97.4	✓
16	98.7	✓
17	98.6	✓
18	98.6	✓
19	98.7	
20	98.6	✓
21	98.5	
22	98.5	
23	98.6	
24	98.6	
25	98.6	✓
26	98.5	
27	98.7	
28	98.6	✓
29	98.2	
30	98.0	

Table 4.2 Results of home ovulation predictor kit for 2 months

Month 1	Strip positive on days 5 and 16
Month 2	Strip positive almost everyday

A. Submucosal fibroids
B. Hypothyroidism
C. Asherman syndrome
D. Polycystic ovarian syndrome
E. Endometriosis

45. After performing a Papanicolaou test, the pathologist report lists "atypical glands of undetermined significance," abbreviated AGUS. Which statement is correct?
A. A more significant underlying abnormality may be associated with AGUS than with ASCUS (atypical squamous cells of undetermined significance).
B. AGUS is seen more frequently than ASCUS.
C. Endometrial biopsy is never warranted in the initial evaluation of AGUS.
D. The subclassification of AGUS that favors a reactive process is common and requires no follow-up.
E. Glandular abnormalities are very distinct on colposcopic examination.

46. When adding an androgen to estrogen–progesterone hormone replacement therapy (HRT), which is true?
A. The risk of coronary artery disease will increase significantly.
B. Moderate hirsutism will occur in more than half the female patients on this regiment.
C. The combination of HRT and an androgen will result in increased bone mass.
D. There have been no studies indicating improved sexual function with the addition of androgens.
E. Hepatotoxicity is not a concern with the addition of androgens, especially at high doses.

47. What study is best for evaluating a patient for an endometrial polyp?
A. Pelvic ultrasound
B. Hysteroscopy
C. MRI
D. Laparoscopy
E. Endometrial biopsy

48. After a woman has had three consecutive, satisfactory, normal Pap smears she can consider having a Pap smear less frequently. All women having risk factors should continue to have their Pap smears yearly. These risk factors include:
A. Age younger than 25
B. Few lifetime sexual partners
C. Substance abuse
D. Nulliparity
E. High socioeconomic status

49. Koilocytosis is a term used to describe squamous cells on a Pap smear displaying cytoplasmic vacuolization and nuclear abnormalities. Koilocytosis is used to describe cellular changes associated with the following diagnosis:
A. Atypical squamous cells of uncertain significance (ASCUS)
B. Low-grade squamous intraepithelial lesion (LGSIL)
C. High-grade squamous intraepithelial lesion (HGSIL)
D. Atypical glands of uncertain significance (AGUS)
E. Carcinoma in situ (CIS)

50. Some Pap smears demonstrating low-grade intraepithelial lesions (LGSIL) will spontaneously regress to normal without any treatment. The percentage of all LGSIL Pap smears that will eventually revert to normal is approximately:
A. 5%
B. 20%
C. 40%
D. 60%
E. 80%

51. A 24-year-old recent immigrant from Trinidad comes to your office complaining of lesions on her vulva for the past week. She admits to unprotected sex with a new boyfriend. On exam, the patient has four painless, sharply demarcated ulcers with a beefy red friable base of granular tissue on opposite sides of her vulva, in a "kissing" fashion. Your differential diagnosis is granuloma inguinale, also known as donovanosis. Which of the following statements about granuloma inguinale is true?
A. Co-infection of syphilis and donovanosis is uncommon.
B. The diagnosis is easily made on culture.
C. This disease is endemic in temperate regions.
D. Untreated donovanosis can progress to cause elephantiasis.
E. It is rare for significant tissue destruction to occur before patients seek treatment.

52. A 17-year-old sexually active woman presents for her annual Pap smear and renewal of oral contraceptives. A screening culture for chlamydia and gonorrhea is collected at the same time. She denies any vaginal discharge or irritation. The culture is positive for chlamydia. According to the Centers for Disease Control and Prevention (CDC), which of the following is an accepted regimen for treatment of chlamydia infection?
A. Doxycycline (Vibramycin) 100 mg PO bid for 7 days
B. Penicillin 250 mg PO qid for 7 days
C. Azithromycin (Zithromax) 500 mg PO bid for 7 days
D. A single dose of ceftriaxone (Rocephin) 125 mg IM
E. Because she is asymptomatic, no treatment is necessary.

53. An 18-year-old unmarried sexually active female presents for evaluation of mucopurulent vaginal discharge. Culture subsequently identifies *Neisseria gonorrhea* as the cause. Which of the following includes the most appropriate measures in this patient's management?
A. A single dose of ceftriaxone (Rocephin) 125 mg IM and azithromycin (Zithromax) 1 g, testing and treatment of all sexual partners, emphasis of condom use, testing for HIV should be offered, resumption of sexual activity 24 hours after her antibiotics are finished
B. A single dose of ceftriaxone (Rocephin) 125 mg IM and azithromycin (Zithromax) 1 g, testing and treatment of all sexual partners, emphasis of condom use, testing for HIV should

be offered, resumption of sexual activity after both partners have been treated and symptoms have regressed

C. A single dose of azithromycin (Zithromax) 1 g, testing and treatment of all sexual partners, emphasis of condom use, testing for HIV should be offered, resumption of sexual activity after both partners have been treated and symptoms have regressed

D. A single dose of ceftriaxone (Rocephin) 125 mg IM and azithromycin (Zithromax) 1 g, testing and treatment of all sexual partners, emphasis of condom use, resumption of sexual activity after both partners have been treated and symptoms have regressed

E. A single dose of azithromycin (Zithromax) 1 g, testing and treatment of all sexual partners, emphasis of condom use, resumption of sexual activity after both partners have been treated and symptoms have regressed

54. A 23-year-old woman presents with chief complaint of a yellowish green malodorous vaginal discharge. Speculum exam is performed and the cervix is noted to be slightly red and irritated. A probe for gonorrhea and chlamydia is collected as well as wet prep and KOH. The wet prep is significant for *Trichomonas vaginalis*. Which of the following is most appropriate?
A. Initiate treatment with clindamycin (Cleocin).
B. Initiate treatment with metronidazole (Flagyl).
C. There is no need for treatment of her sexual partner.
D. She will need follow-up wet prep in 2 weeks.
E. Sexual contact should be avoided until 48 hours after initiation of therapy.

55. Which of the following are risk factors for ectopic pregnancy?
A. Previous abdominal surgery
B. Previous pelvic inflammatory disease
C. Previous ectopic pregnancy
D. Endometriosis
E. All of the above

56. Menopause is defined as the end of the last menstrual period. The following statement is true regarding menopause:
A. The mean age for the start of menopause is 45.5 years.
B. Vasomotor and psychologic symptoms are caused by decreased estrogen levels.
C. Menopause is a physiologic event and its timing may be determined genetically.
D. Progestins have little effect on vasomotor symptoms.
E. Vaginal changes occur 1 or 2 years after the onset of menopause.

57. Breast pain or mastalgia is most common in women aged 30 to 50 years. The following statement is true regarding breast pain:
A. Thirty percent of women develop breast pain in their lifetime.
B. Cyclical breast pain may be caused by costochondritis.
C. Cyclical breast pain often affects the upper outer quadrants and may refer to the medial aspects of the upper arm.
D. There is strong evidence of the effect of evening primrose oil for treating breast pain.
E. Mastalgia is usually associated with malignancy.

58. Which of the following places the patient at risk for endometrial hyperplasia?
A. Early menopause
B. Low BMI

C. Long-term OCP use
D. Multiparity
E. Polycystic ovarian syndrome

59. You perform an endometrial biopsy on a 48-year-old perimenopausal woman. Which of the following choices correctly pairs the pathologist's report with your treatment recommendations?
A. Cystic hyperplasia—continuous estrogen therapy
B. Simple hyperplasia—dilatation and curettage
C. Complex hyperplasia without atypia—radiation therapy
D. Complex hyperplasia with atypia—radiation therapy
E. Endometrial carcinoma—chemotherapy

60. Which of the following patients have an increased risk of endometrial cancer?
A. Women with regular menstrual cycles
B. Women younger than age 40
C. Multiparous women
D. Hypothyroid women
E. Women taking tamoxifen (Nolvadex)

61. A 25-year-old woman presents to the office complaining of a "very large lump" near her vagina. The most common vulvar mass is:
A. Lipoma
B. Dermatofibroma
C. Bartholin's gland cyst
D. Sebaceous cyst
E. Ganglion cyst

62. A 43-year-old female presents with complaints of changes in her menstrual pattern. She notes that her past three periods have been very light with spotting for 1 or 2 days. Which of the following options represents a correct first response to her concern?
A. Order a TSH level
B. Order a prolactin level
C. Perform an endometrial biopsy right away
D. Prescribe HRT
E. Order a urine pregnancy test

63. A 47-year-old obese diabetic female calls with complaint of four heavy long periods in a row. She had this problem in the past and received a prescription that corrected the problem. She is requesting a prescription for that medication. Which of the following would be your next course of action?
A. Order medroxyprogesterone acetate
B. Check an FSH level
C. Perform a Pap smear
D. Check a TSH and prolactin level
E. Endometrial biopsy

64. A 45-year-old woman presents with complaints of difficulty sleeping, irritability, memory difficulty, and occasional hot flushes. She has skipped one or two menses this year. Which of the following medications would be appropriate to treat her symptoms of perimenopause?
A. L-Thyroxine
B. Alprazolam (Xanax)
C. 5 mg medroxyprogesterone acetate daily

D. Progesterone-only oral contraceptive pills

E. Combination oral contraceptive pills

65. While performing a sports physical on a 13-year-old girl, you note that she has just started breast development (Tanner 2). There is no pubic hair development yet (Tanner 1). Although she is not concerned, her mother is anxious to know when her daughter will start menstruating. You tell her:

A. She should start her menses within the year because 13 is the average age for menarche.

B. The patient should already be menstruating and an evaluation for the delay is necessary.

C. Not to worry, primary amenorrhea occurs only if menarche is not achieved by 18 years of age.

D. Without pubic hair development, there may be an insensitivity to gonadotropins.

E. Within 2 years of breast development, most girls will start menstruating.

66. A 21-year-old college student calls the office in the morning crying. She states that while having intercourse the night before, the condom broke and she is very afraid of pregnancy. You offer her emergency contraception. Which is correct?

A. Emergency contraception must be taken within 24 hours to be effective.

B. Any oral contraceptive can be used to provide pregnancy protection.

C. Prescribing an antiemetic is important with high-dose estrogen use.

D. Both estrogen and progesterone must be taken to stop ovulation.

E. Mifepristone (RU 486) is likely to cause immediate bleeding.

67. A 35-year-old woman, whose child you delivered last year, forgets her oral contraceptive pills while going out of town for a 3-day "honeymoon." When she returns, she calls 2 days later to say that she and her husband had intercourse during the week. She asks if there is anything that can be done to prevent pregnancy? Options for her include:

A. A single dose of 50 mg of RU 486 (Mifepristone)

B. Ovral two tablets followed in 12 hours by two tablets

C. A Copper T intrauterine device (IUD) placed in the office

D. A and C

E. A, B, and C

68. A 22-year-old woman comes to you to discuss contraception. She has been using condoms for the past 6 months and she would like to try oral contraceptives. She has heard some information about "the pill" but would like your expert opinion. Which of the following statements is correct about oral contraceptives?

A. Personal history of DVT is a relative contraindication to oral contraceptive use.

B. Oral contraceptives are not indicated for the treatment of acne.

C. Combination oral contraceptives should never be used by a breast-feeding woman.

D. Oral contraceptives improve cycle control for women with polycystic ovarian syndrome.

E. Menorrhagia is usually exacerbated by oral contraceptives.

69. Oral contraceptives are an effective means of contraception. In addition, oral contraceptives improve many conditions that are not fertility related. In which of these patients is hormonal contraception contraindicated?

A. A woman whose maternal grandmother had postmenopausal breast cancer

B. A woman who has active liver disease from chronic hepatitis C

C. A 40-year-old woman who has never had any children

D. A woman with type 2 diabetes mellitus whose mother had coronary artery disease

E. A 25-year-old woman with a previous history of chlamydia PID

70. A 28-year-old G2P2 woman comes to your office to discuss contraception. She delivered her second baby vaginally 3 months ago. Approximately 2 weeks after delivery, she received depo-medroxyprogesterone acetate (Depo-Provera) 150 mg intramuscularly. She has been dissatisfied with this method because of frequent spotting. She took oral contraceptives as a teenager but does not remember much about their use. In counseling her, you review the side effects of oral contraceptives. Which of the following is true?

A. Breakthrough bleeding is the most common reason for women to discontinue oral contraceptives.

B. Weight gain of 5 lbs or more per year is common for women on oral contraceptives.

C. Heavy, prolonged menstrual periods (menorrhagia) are common during the first 3 months of oral contraceptive use, but menses return to baseline after several cycles.

D. Women who start on oral contraceptives should return for a blood pressure check after 3 months of use so that significant hypotension can be diagnosed and treated.

E. Heavy, prolonged menstrual periods (menorrhagia) are common throughout the duration of use of oral contraceptives.

71. A 24-year-old G1P1 woman presents to your office for re-evaluation. You delivered her first child vaginally 6 months ago and she has been breast-feeding since then. She started combination oral contraceptives following her 6-week postpartum visit with you. She had some occasional spotting initially, then had a full menses approximately 1 week ago. She has noticed that her breast milk supply was abundant initially, but over the past month, her milk supply has decreased. She resumed work 2 months ago and rarely pumps her breasts while separated from her infant. Her weight dropped initially after delivery but has now stabilized to approximately 5 pounds above her pre-pregnancy weight. Which of the following should you recommend?

A. The diminishing breast milk supply is not likely due to the oral contraceptives.

B. We must draw labs to evaluate this patient's symptoms.

C. The patient's weight loss is a common side effect of initiating oral contraceptives.

D. The patient is likely to have irregular menstrual cycles while on oral contraceptives.

E. Intermenstrual bleeding is a not a common side effect of oral contraceptives and she should notify you immediately if this occurs.

72. You started a 25-year-old nullipara woman on oral contraceptives 2 months ago. She complains of mild nausea and intermenstrual spotting during the first month of use. She has had no leg pain or swelling, no chest pain, and no persistent headaches. She is otherwise happy with this form of contraception and says that she is using it as directed. Her blood pressure is not significantly different from when you last saw her. Which of the following is true regarding the side effects of oral contraceptives?

A. Lower progestational activity is associated with less breakthrough bleeding.

B. Hypercoagulability, which is rare, is due to the progestational activity.

C. Nausea is associated with the estrogenic activity of the pill.

D. Decreased libido is due to the estrogenic affects of OCPs.

E. Telangectasias may be due to the progesterone effects.

73. A 38-year-old G4P4 woman wishes to discuss contraception. She is in excellent health except that she smokes 10 to 15 cigarettes per day. She is well informed about the advantages and disadvantages of many methods of contraception and she would like to try oral contraceptives. Which of the following is true regarding oral contraceptive pill use in women her age?

A. The dose of estrogen is directly related to the risk of intermenstrual bleeding in women older than the age of 35.

B. The risk of mortality from myocardial infarction exceeds the risk of mortality from stroke in women who use oral contraceptives.

C. Women between the ages of 35 and 39 who smoke and take oral contraceptives are at 10 times the risk of death compared to women of this age who take oral contraceptives but do not smoke.

D. For women aged 35 to 39, the absolute risk of death due to oral contraceptives in a smoker is less than the risk of death due to pregnancy.

E. Pills that contain 50 μg or more of estrogen are associated with a lower risk of thromboembolic disease, especially in women older than the age of 35.

74. A 30-year-old G1P1 woman presents for her annual well woman exam. She has been taking oral contraceptives on and off for the past 12 years. She hears about oral contraceptives in the news periodically and has several questions about them. Her last Pap smear was 13 months ago. She had one abnormal Pap smear approximately 5 years ago, but all her Pap smears have been normal since then. Women who take oral contraceptives:

A. Are 5 to 8 times as likely to develop breast cancer as women who do not

B. Are less likely to develop ovarian cancer than those who do not

C. Are more likely to develop PID than women who use depo-medroxyprogesterone acetate (DMPA or Depo-Provera) for contraception

D. Are more likely to develop cervical cancer than those who do not; this is why women should not get their pills refilled if their last Pap smear was more than 12 months previously

E. Are at lower risk of developing a chlamydia cervicitis compared to women who use other forms of contraception

75. Benefits of oral contraceptives include:

A. Reduction in rheumatoid arthritis development

B. Decreased ectopic pregnancy

C. Improved libido

D. A and B

E. A, B, and C

76. A 16-year-old patient is considering starting sexual activity. She has heard a lot about "the pill" and she would like your advice on oral contraceptives. Oral contraceptives have which of the following effects?

A. Increase the likelihood of PID

B. Prevent pregnancy about 90% of the time

C. Protect against unintended pregnancy about 7 days after initiation

D. Do not affect volume of menstrual flow

E. Increase the incidence of ovarian cysts

77. Which of the following is true about the effectiveness of oral contraceptives?

A. Oral contraceptives are less effective at preventing pregnancy than condoms with spermicide when each method is used correctly.

B. "Actual use" effectiveness is higher than "theoretical use" in pregnancy prevention.

C. Effectiveness is not diminished if the pills are taken at different times of day.

D. Skipping pills twice a week is not associated with a significant decrease in efficacy.

E. Theoretical use of oral contraceptives is comparable to female sterilization (tubal ligation).

78. You are rounding on a 17-year-old G1P1 patient you delivered yesterday. You are discussing contraception options with her and she asks you about "the shot" that several of her friends have received. Regarding DMPA (Depo-Provera), you tell her:

A. In actual use, DMPA is less effective than oral contraceptives at preventing pregnancy.

B. It is associated with a return to normal fertility 3 months (12 weeks) after the last injection.

C. Amenorrhea is the most common side effect after 12 months of use.

D. Breakthrough bleeding is uncommon during early use. If noted, it should be investigated further (e.g., endometrial biopsy).

E. It is more likely to cause severe headaches than are oral contraceptives.

79. A 25-year-old G1P1 patient comes in to discuss contraception. Menarche was at age 12 and her menses have always been regular and relatively light. She has a distant history of chlamydia infection with her first pregnancy 5 years ago. She is recently married and would like to have a second child in the near future. She is concerned about her family history of premature coronary disease because her father had a myocardial infarction (MI) at age 40. She is personally in good health and does not smoke. She has seen advertisements for Depo-Provera and wonders if it is the right contraceptive for her. Women who use Depo-Provera:

A. Are at increased risk of MI and stroke compared with nonusers

B. Discontinue use most frequently for persistent abnormalities of their menstrual cycle

C. Have an increased risk of PID compared with women who use other contraceptives

D. May gain weight initially, but infrequently have persistent weight gain associated with its use longer than 12 months

E. Have a lower risk of later osteoporosis because of the increase in bone density associated with its use

80. A 32-year-old G2P2 woman comes in for her postpartum visit. She was undecided about a contraceptive method at the time she left the hospital. She is in excellent health and does not smoke. Menarche was at age 13. Her menses have been regular with moderate flow except during her pregnancies and periods of lactation. She is pretty sure that she is finished with childbearing but her husband would like her to get pregnant one more time, to "try for a boy." Which of the following is a true feature of a copper intrauterine device (Cu-IUD)?

A. It is not readily reversible and fertility rates after removal are decreased compared to age-matched controls not using an IUD.

B. It does not allow for sexual spontaneity because it is only effective at certain times during the menstrual cycle.

C. It is not very cost-effective because it is much more expensive than other methods and needs to be replaced yearly.

D. It is contraindicated in women with dysmenorrhea and menorrhagia.

E. The Paragard-T IUD (Cu T 380A) can remain in place for up to 20 years.

81. The IUD is contraindicated in women who:

A. Have an active cervical infection or PID

B. Have irregular menstrual cycles

C. Have a history of chlamydia

D. Are in the first 3 months postpartum and are breast-feeding

E. Both A and C are correct

82. Which of the following statements about barrier methods of contraception are correct?

A. They include condoms, diaphragm, and cervical caps.

B. All barrier methods are effective in preventing STDs.

C. They increase the likelihood of PID compared with the IUD.

D. They have the same contraindications as the hormonal forms of contraception.

E. The use of spermicide in conjunction with the barrier decreases the effectiveness.

83. A 17-year-old G2P1011 woman presents to your office reporting condom breakage the last time she had intercourse. A friend urged her to come to discuss the "morning after pill" with you. The following is true about emergency contraception:

A. It is effective when used within 96 hours of unprotected intercourse.

B. It includes high-dose oral contraceptive pills.

C. It is not approved by the U.S. Food and Drug Administration.

D. It should only be used within the first 5 days of the patient's last menstrual period.

E. It would be appropriate for a woman who is less than 6 weeks (42 days) past her last menstrual period.

84. Which of the following statements about emergency contraception is correct?

A. These methods do not require a negative pregnancy test prior to use.

B. These methods can be used by patients who are up to 7 weeks (49 days) past their last menstrual cycle.

C. This is not a form of abortion since it prevents ovulation.

D. There are very few reported effects from high-dose oral contraceptive pills.

E. The effectiveness of emergency contraception decreases each day from the time of unprotected intercourse.

85. You saw a 22-year-old G0P0 patient in the office last week for her annual well woman exam. Her Pap smear comes back with low-grade squamous intraepithelial lesion (LGSIL). This diagnosis on a Pap smear:

A. Is sensitive but not specific for CIN 1 on histology

B. Is specific but not sensitive for CIN 2 on histology

C. Encompasses CIN 1 and HPV changes

D. Is a true cancer precursor

E. Is an indication for a loop electrical excision procedure (LEEP) procedure

86. A 22-year-old G0P0 patient comes to your office for annual well woman exam and Pap smear. She has had annual Pap smears since the age of 18 and all of them have been normal. She has been sexually active with one male partner since the age of 20. She has no history of sexually transmitted diseases. Which of the following statements are true?

A. Pap smears should be repeated annually for all patients.

B. Pap smears are sensitive but not specific for the detection of HGSIL.

C. Pap smears are an effective screening test for the detection of endometrial carcinoma.

D. Pap smears should be initiated within 3 years of the age of first sexual activity or age 21, which ever is younger.

E. Because of their increased sensitivity, liquid-based cytology (such as ThinPrep Pap smears) is the recommended screening test for all women.

87. While counseling a 36-year-old G2P2 woman on contraception, she wants to know more about IUDs. You think she may be a candidate for a progesterone-containing IUD such as Progestasert or Mirena. Advantages over a copper IUD include:

A. May be left in place longer for more years of contraception

B. Will prevent more pregnancies

C. Decreased risk of ectopic pregnancy

D. Improved menorrhagia

E. Less likely to be spontaneously expelled

88. A 45-year-old woman presents to your office complaining of irregular periods over the past 4 months. Her exam is unremarkable. Her FSH = 25 and her TSH = 1.85. Which of the following statements about perimenopause is correct?

A. Perimenopausal bleeding changes occur after menopause.

B. Anovulation becomes more prevalent during this time.

C. She will no longer need birth control.

D. Her estrogen levels have declined.

E. There is no correlation between the age when her mother experienced menopause and when she will.

89. A 43-year-old woman presents to your office complaining of irregular, heavy periods over the past 9 months. After a thorough investigation, you determine her irregular bleeding is secondary to anovulation during perimenopause. You discuss her options for treatment and she decides she would like to try an oral contraceptive. For which of the following conditions would you encourage her to use oral contraceptives over other forms of treatment:

A. Fibroids

B. Hypertension

C. Hypercholesterolemia

D. Tobacco use

E. Coronary artery disease

90. A 48-year-old woman presents to your office for her yearly well woman exam. She has noticed a lengthening in her menstrual cycle and an occasional skipped period. She complains of increased fatigue recently. On further questioning, she states she has noticed that she has had difficulty sleeping recently. But her major complaint is the intermittent hot flashes. Her labs include an FSH = 30 and a TSH = 1.24. If this patient declines estrogen hormone replacement therapy, which treatment option is best to reduce her hot flashes?

A. Dress in cooler clothing

B. Venlafaxine (Effexor)

C. Thyroid hormone replacement

D. Clonidine

E. Dong quai

91. A 42-year-old woman presents to your office complaining of new-onset menometrorrhagia. After your initial evaluation, you decide to proceed with an endometrial biopsy. This procedure could help in identifying:

A. Endometrial cancer

B. Endometrial polyps

C. Endometrial hyperplasia

D. All of the above

E. A and C

92. You receive the endometrial biopsy report back from a 45-year-old woman with irregular spotting and it shows simple hyperplasia without evidence of atypia. Treatment should include:

A. Dilatation and curettage

B. High-dose oral contraceptives ×3 months

C. Methoxyprogesterone ×14 days

D. Hysterectomy

E. Endometrial ablation

93. A 48-year-old woman presents to your office with abnormal vaginal bleeding. You complete an endometrial biopsy as part of the workup and the report returns showing complex hyperplasia with atypia. You explain to the patient that her risk of developing uterine cancer if she does not receive treatment is:

A. Not increased

B. 5%

C. 30%

D. 90%

E. Not determinable without more information

94. A 60-year-old woman G3P3003 presents complaining of vaginal spotting over the past 2 days. She has no significant past medical history. She is not on any medications. She is sexually active with her long-term male partner. She had a normal Pap smear in the past 4 months. On her exam, she has mild vulvar and vaginal atrophy but is otherwise unremarkable. You tell her that:

A. She likely has endometrial cancer.

B. Her bleeding is from her vaginal atrophy and reassure her.

C. She needs a referral for a hysterectomy.

D. She needs further evaluation with a transvaginal ultrasound and/or an endometrial biopsy.

E. A and D

95. A 25-year-old woman presents to your office complaining of vaginal spotting and moderate lower abdominal pain. She reports a positive home pregnancy test. She is G4P1021. She reports a previous first trimester miscarriage and a second trimester abortion. She has had nine lifetime sexual partners. She has a history of herpes but reports no active lesions. She also reports she is a smoker and occasionally smokes marijuana. You are concerned about an ectopic pregnancy because of her multiple risk factors. These include:

A. Drug use

B. Previous miscarriage

C. Previous abortion

D. Age

E. Smoking status

96. After confirming the previous patient's pregnancy and performing a complete evaluation, you are uncertain of the cause of the bleeding. An ultrasound is performed but is inconclusive. You decide to pursue with close follow-up in the office and a serial number of quantitative BHCG tests performed every 48 hours. Which of the following sequences would increase your suspicion of an ectopic pregnancy?

A. 675; 950; 1,050

B. 50,000; 70,000; 80,000

C. 920; 1,845; 3,600

D. 56; 100; 345

E. 540; 350; 158

97. A 46-year-old woman presents to your office. During the review of systems, she admits that her desire for sex has diminished. She is interested in sildenifil (Viagra) to "spice up" her relationship with her husband. You tell her that the most common cause of decreased libido in perimenopausal women is:

A. Diminishing testosterone levels

B. Circulatory decrease leading to vaginal dryness

C. Depression and anxiety

D. Declining estrogen production

E. Lifestyle factors that interfere with intimacy

98. A 19-year-old female presents to your office complaining of crampy, lower abdominal pain beginning with the onset of her menses every month and lasting for 2 or 3 days. She denies any pain between menses. She reports radiation of the pain to her lower back and upper thighs, along with accompanying nausea, fatigue, and headache. She states this has been present for several years but has been getting progressively worse. She denies history of sexually transmitted disease or trauma. Physical exam is unremarkable. The most likely diagnosis is:

A. Premenstrual syndrome

B. Primary dysmenorrhea

C. Secondary dysmenorrhea

D. Endometriosis

E. Uterine fibroids

99. What tests are appropriate to further evaluate this patient?

A. CBC and erythrocyte sedimentation rate (ESR)

B. Pelvic ultrasound

C. Cervical smear, GC, and chlamydia testing

D. A, B, and C

E. A and C

100. A concerned mother brings her 15-year-old daughter to your office because she has never had a period. The daughter is very self-conscious and says that she is just a late bloomer. After establishing rapport with the patient, you proceed with history and physical. The patient denies any history of sexual activity, sexually transmitted diseases, or monthly symptoms of bloating, breast tenderness, or abdominal cramping. Physical exam reveals a normal uterus and female genitalia, minimal breast development, and no visible axillary and pubic hair. The most likely cause of this patient's primary amenorrhea is:

A. Imperforate hymen
B. Hypothalamic failure
C. Hypothyroidism
D. Testicular feminization
E. Prolactinoma

101. Which of the following are commonly associated with the above disorder?

A. Anorexia nervosa
B. Substance abuse
C. Grave's disease
D. A and B
E. All of the above

102. Treatment should include:

A. No treatment is required in a patient this young
B. Discovering and treating the underlying cause
C. Bromocriptine
D. Surgical treatment
E. OCPs

103. A 39-year-old G2P1001, with a last menstrual period 6 weeks earlier, presents with spotting for 2 days. She is without pain and has normal vital signs and an unremarkable exam with a small, retroverted uterus and a closed cervical os. Her urine qualitative test for BHCG is positive and a transvaginal ultrasound reveals nothing in the uterus or adnexa. The appropriate next step might include:

A. Serum progesterone
B. Laparoscopy
C. Quantitative BHCG
D. A and C
E. All of the above

104. Barrier methods of contraception include condoms, diaphragms, cervical caps, and spermicidal jellies. Which pair correctly identifies the method of contraception with the pros or cons:

A. Polyurethane condom: less breakage
B. Spermicidal jelly (nonoxynol 9): increased risk of STDs
C. Diaphragm: decreased bacterial colonization of the vagina
D. Cervical cap: improved efficacy in parous women
E. Vaginal sponge: must be replaced for each intercourse

105. Condoms are most likely to prevent which sexually transmitted disease?

A. Trichomonas
B. Human papillomavirus
C. Syphilis
D. Herpes simplex virus
E. Chancroid

106. A 16-year-old G1P0 patient at $14\frac{2}{7}$ weeks gestation presents for her initial prenatal visit. She has been sexually active for $1\frac{1}{2}$ years and has not used contraception except for occasional condom use. She has had two different sexual partners (lifetime) and has been with her current partner for the past 5 months. She has never had a Pap smear. As part of her prenatal care, you perform a Pap smear and a probe for gonorrhea and chlamydia. Her Pap smear comes back with LGSIL. Regarding this patient:

A. When confirmed by biopsy, her abnormality is likely to regress 70% of the time.
B. Her lesion is likely to progress to invasive cancer because of immunosuppression in pregnancy.
C. If the Pap smear is repeated and is normal, follow-up with annual Pap smears is recommended.
D. Because she is pregnant, you should repeat a Pap smear at her next appointment (4 weeks) to rule out a false positive.
E. Colposcopy cannot be performed during pregnancy.

107. A 25-year-old G1 P0010 patient presents for a well woman exam. Her last Pap smear was 5 years ago at the time of her elective abortion. She recalls being told that it was "not completely normal" but is unsure of the diagnosis. She does remember being told that she needed "some other test" done but was unable to schedule it because of financial issues. She is now working full-time and has health insurance through her employer and would like to be checked. She used to smoke one-half to one pack of cigarettes per day but stopped 6 months ago. Her cervix appears grossly normal. Because of her history, you do a ThinPrep Pap smear (liquid-based cytology), which reveals HGSIL. Which of the following is true about HGSIL?

A. It is seen more frequently on Pap smears than is LGSIL.
B. When confirmed with colposcopy, HGSIL will proceed to invasive cervical cancer approximately 30% of the time.
C. HGSIL encompasses the histologic terms CIN 2 and CIN 3 but not carcinoma in situ (CIS).
D. Treatment options for biopsy-confirmed HGSIL include a "wait and watch" approach.
E. Treatment with cryotherapy is as effective as and less invasive than treatment with LEEP.

108. A 17-year-old G0P0 patient presents for a well woman exam. Two months ago, she became sexually active for the first time and her friends urged her to come in for a Pap smear. She has had one partner and has used condoms with spermicide with every act of intercourse. Her Pap smear returns with Atypical Squamous Cells of Undetermined Significance (ASCUS). Which of the following statements are true regarding ASCUS?

A. ASCUS should encompass no more than 5% of the cytologic diagnoses at most institutions.
B. ASCUS can be classified as favors reactive or favors dysplasia, or can be unclassified.
C. ASCUS is a cancer precursor and should be managed with immediate cryotherapy or LEEP.
D. A and B
E. None of the above

109. A 34-year-old G1P1 woman comes in for well woman exam. She has had multiple normal Pap smears in the past with her most recent one having been 1 year prior to your appointment with her. Her examination is unremarkable. Her Pap smear comes back with Atypical Squamous Cells of Undetermined Significance (ASCUS). Follow up of ASCUS on a Pap smear can be appropriately managed by which of the following methods below

A. Colposcopy with directed biopsy

B. Repeating Pap smear every 4 to 6 months until 3 consecutive normal Pap smears at which time referring the patient back for annual screening

C. Repeating Pap smear every 4 to 6 months until 3 consecutive abnormal Pap smears at which time refer the patient for colposcopy

D. A and B

E. A and C

110. A 45-year-old G3P3003 woman comes in for well woman exam. She has been feeling well and has no complaints. Her menstrual cycles are regular and she has had no intermenstrual bleeding. She is monogamous with her husband of 20 years. Her last Pap smear was 5 years ago at her post-partum check up. She had a bilateral tubal ligation following the birth of her third child (who had been unplanned). Her cervix appears normal and the remainder of her exam is normal. Her Pap smear comes back showing AGUS. Appropriate workup for a woman of this age with a Pap smear with AGUS includes:

A. Repeating Pap smear in 4 to 6 months, and if that one is abnormal, scheduling a colposcopy

B. Treatment with metronidazole or clindamycin vaginal cream, then repeating Pap smear

C. Endometrial biopsy and colposcopy with directed biopsy and endocervical curettage

D. Repeating Pap smear in 12 months because AGUS is less likely to be associated with preinvasive or invasive disease than ASCUS

E. Hysteroscopy with or without endometrial biopsy

111. A 68-year-old G3P2013 patient presents for routine health care. She has only become your patient recently after hypertension was diagnosed during an emergency room visit for a severe headache. Prior to that she had not been to a doctor for approximately 35 years since her last children (a set of twins) were born. After several visits for her hypertension, you convince her to come in for a well woman exam. Her exam is unremarkable except for contact bleeding while taking the Pap smear sample. Her Pap smear comes back with a diagnosis of cervical cancer. Cervical cancer diagnosed on a Pap smear:

A. Is rarely a true-positive diagnosis

B. Can be a false-positive diagnosis in the setting of a chlamydial infection

C. Is most closely correlated with HPV serotypes 16, 18, 31, or 33

D. Is equivalent to the histologic term CIS

E. Is rarely associated with inflammation

112. A 38-year-old female presents to you asking for her ovaries to be removed because her mother died at age 39 and her sister died at age 41 from ovarian cancer. Which approach may be appropriate for this patient?

A. You test her for the BRCA-1 and BRCA-2 gene

B. You refer her for prophylactic oophorectomy

C. You screen her with the CA-125 serum marker

D. You screen her with transvaginal ultrasonography

E. All of the above

113. Regarding mammography for the detection of breast cancer:

A. Annual screening should begin at age 40 for the general population.

B. Women with the BRCA mutation should begin annual mammography at age 35.

C. Ten percent to 15% of all breast cancers are not detected by mammogram.

D. A and C

E. All of the above

114. A 48-year-old female with stress incontinence has failed a decent trial of Kegel's exercises (pelvic floor rehabilitation). Other nonsurgical method(s) you may offer her is/are:

A. Vaginal weights

B. Pessary

C. Topic estrogen therapy

D. A and C

E. All of the above

115. A 57-year-old female presents with the complaint of leaking urine. Steps to take in the initial evaluation and management of urinary incontinence may be all of the following *except*:

A. Teaching the patient pelvic floor muscle exercises

B. Starting the patient on estrogen replacement therapy

C. Obtaining a patient record of her urinary output, voiding and incontinence frequency, and fluid intake

D. Obtaining a urinalysis and urine culture

E. Obtaining a post void residual urine

116. A 17-year-old female presents at your office for a cervical smear and pelvic exam. She is sexually active with one partner and denies any current or past sexually transmitted diseases. She has no history of abnormal Pap smears. She does report a clear, odorless vaginal discharge. She is currently taking low-dose oral contraceptives. Examination of the labia and vagina is unremarkable. On cervical exam, you see a rough, red epithelium covering most of the surface of the cervix, with smooth epithelium only at the very rim. Based on the history and clinical exam, your diagnosis is:

A. Diethylstilbesterol (DES) adenosis

B. Cervical condyloma

C. Chronic cervicitis

D. Cervical ectropion

E. Giant cervical erosion

117. Which of the following statements is *true* about cervical polyps:

A. Patients with symptomatic polyps should be reassured that there is no need for removal because these are benign growths, and symptoms will improve with time.

B. Benign polyps can be friable, leading to spotting after intercourse or tampon use.

C. They cannot be removed in the office setting.

D. Removal usually requires local anesthesia to ensure patient comfort.

118. You are making rounds in the hospital on one of your patients who delivered the night before. She is a 24-year-old G1P1 who is married, monogamous, smokes half a pack of cigarettes a day, but with an otherwise unremarkable medical history. She is recovering well from delivery and is preparing for discharge. In your discussion of contraception, she asks about the T380A copper IUD. She reports that she wants to discontinue use of the pill because of issues with moodiness and difficulty remembering to take it. She definitely does not want to become pregnant for at least 5 years, but she does plan on having other children in the future. She is concerned about the efficacy of the IUD, as well as its effects on her future fertility. You tell her:

A. The IUD is very effective, but she is likely to have problems with fertility after removal.

B. Evidence from the United States indicates that the IUD is effective in preventing pregnancy, but there is little long-term and international data on its efficacy.

C. The IUD is as effective as tubal ligation and its effects are almost immediately reversible upon removal.

D. The IUD is very effective, but she will have to wait 6 months postpartum to have it inserted, until her uterus returns to its prepregnancy size.

E. The T 380A copper IUD is a very effective form of birth control, but the patient will have to have it changed each year to maintain this high degree of efficacy.

119. Your patient's sister told her that copper IUDs give women genital infections. You tell your patient the following about IUDs:

A. In low-risk women, the IUD is only associated with increased infection within the first few weeks after insertion.

B. The copper IUD can lead to lighter, less crampy menstrual cycles.

C. A change in the amount or character of cervical mucous may occur with IUD use and is suggestive of infection.

D. The only contraindication to placing an IUD is if a woman has an active sexually transmitted disease.

120. After discussing the contraception issue with her husband, your patient decides that she would prefer using an injectable progestin (Depo-Provera) instead of the IUD. The patient is concerned about weight gain with this method of contraception. You tell her:

A. There is no evidence that women gain weight on this drug.

B. Women do gain weight on this drug due to a slowing of the metabolism. Patients who take this drug should take additional measures to increase their metabolic rate to counter this effect.

C. Women do gain weight on this drug, but it is all due to water retention. Decreasing salt in the diet can lessen this effect.

D. Women do gain weight on this drug due to an increase in appetite. If patients are aware of this effect beforehand, and try to maintain their prior eating patterns, this effect can be moderated.

E. Women do gain weight on this drug, but it is only 2 or 3 pounds and plateaus after the first year.

121. A 19-year-old white female presents to your office for her annual physical. She is sexually active and uses condoms on a regular basis with her current boyfriend. She relates to you that last month she noticed several blisters in the groin area that were painful. The blisters erupted after several days and the lesions became dry and scaly. Which test will be most helpful in confirming the diagnosis in this patient?

A. Tzank prep

B. HSV titre

C. RPR

D. Viral culture

E. Cervical cultures

122. A 48-year-old female patient presents to discuss her perimenopausal symptoms. She has been having hot flashes, night sweats, and mood disturbances. She is very bothered by these symptoms and would like some medication to provide relief, but she has read several recent articles about the dangers of hormone replacement therapy. You tell her:

A. Hormone replacement therapy is no longer recommended due to the risks outweighing the benefits.

B. Combination therapy (0.625 mg estrogen and 2.5 mg progesterone) is associated with an increased risk in breast cancer with any use.

C. Combination therapy (0.625 mg estrogen and 2.5 mg progesterone) is associated with a one-third reduction in colorectal cancer risk after 5 years of use.

D. There is currently no safe alternative to combination therapy to treat these symptoms.

E. None of the above

123. As you delve more into the patient's history, you find that she had a partial hysterectomy 5 years ago, with one ovary left behind. Knowing this, you explain to the patient that she is a candidate for estrogen-only therapy. You tell her that estrogen-only therapy:

A. Carries the same risks and benefits as the combination therapy

B. Does not carry any of the risks of combination therapy

C. Will help protect her from osteoporotic changes

D. Is no longer deemed appropriate due to the increased risk of breast cancer

E. None of the above

124. A 19-year-old co-ed presents to the health clinic on campus complaining of diffuse abdominal pain for the past several days. She states that she had a fever of 101°F, dyspareunea, nausea, and several episodes of vomiting. On exam, her external genitalia appear normal, as does her cervix. However, she has findings of cervical motion tenderness, adnexal tenderness, and lower abdominal tenderness. At this point, you have a high clinical index of suspicion for which disease process?

A. Appendicitis

B. Cervicitis

C. Pelvic inflammatory disease

D. Cholecystitis

E. Ovarian cyst

125. After discussing the possible diagnosis and treatment plan with the previous patient, you screen for pregnancy. The BHCG comes back as positive. What would be appropriate therapy for this patient?

A. Outpatient therapy: ofloxacin (Floxin) 400 mg bid and metronidazole (Flagyl) 500 mg bid

B. Outpatient therapy: ceftriaxone (Rocephin) 250 mg IM and doxycycline (Vibramycin) 100 mg bid

C. Inpatient therapy: clindamycin (Cleocin) 900 mg IV q8hrs and gentamicin (Garamycin) loading dose (2 mg/kg) followed by a maintenance dose (1.5 mg/kg) q8hrs

D. Inpatient therapy: cefoxitin (Mefoxin) 2 g IV q6hrs and doxycycline (Vibramycin) 100 mg IV q12hrs

E. Inpatient therapy: clindamycin (Cleocin) 900 mg IV q8hrs and ciprofloxacin (Cipro) 500 mg q12hrs

126. While taking an oral contraceptive pill, a patient complains of a myriad of side effects. Of the list below, which is an estrogen-mediated side effect?

A. Breakthrough bleeding
B. Mood labiality
C. Vascular headache
D. Weight gain
E. Hirsuitism

127. A couple presents to your office for family planning counseling. They have been trying to get pregnant for the past 2 years without success. While taking her history, it is revealed that she has had worsening dysmenorrhea over the past 3 years. Prior to that, she had pain-free cycles. If endometriosis is the working diagnosis, what would be the next step for this patient?

A. Watchful waiting
B. Trial of leuprolide (Lupron)
C. Referral to OB/GYN for possible exploratory laparoscopy
D. Trial of high-dose NSAIDs
E. Trial of continuous oral contraception

128. A 28-year-old woman presents to your office complaining of left lower quadrant abdominal pain. She denies fever, chills, nausea, vomiting, dyspareunia, or vaginal discharge. During the pelvic exam, there was no cervical motion tenderness but positive for left adnexal fullness and tenderness. After a negative serum HCG, the patient was sent for an ultrasound that revealed a 5-cm complex cyst of the left ovary and no fluid in the cul-de-sac. What would your next step be?

A. Refer to OB/GYN for surgical evaluation
B. Pursue other etiologies of pelvic pain
C. Repeat ultrasound in several weeks
D. Pain management with NSAIDS
E. Both C and D

129. Which of the following medications is a frequent cause of galactorrhea?

A. Ibuprofen (Advil)
B. Levothyroxine (synthroid)
C. Enalapril (Vasotec)
D. Metaclopramide (Reglan)

Answer Key

1.	B	43.	C	85.	C	127.	C
2.	D	44.	D	86.	D	128.	E
3.	C	45.	A	87.	D	129.	D
4.	C	46.	C	88.	B		
5.	C	47.	B	89.	A		
6.	E	48.	C	90.	B		
7.	E	49.	B	91.	E		
8.	A	50.	D	92.	C		
9.	D	51.	D	93.	C		
10.	C	52.	A	94.	D		
11.	C	53.	B	95.	E		
12.	C	54.	B	96.	A		
13.	E	55.	E	97.	E		
14.	B	56.	C	98.	B		
15.	B	57.	C	99.	C		
16.	B	58.	E	100.	B		
17.	C	59.	B	101.	D		
18.	E	60.	E	102.	B		
19.	D	61.	C	103.	D		
20.	B	62.	E	104.	B		
21.	D	63.	E	105.	A		
22.	C	64.	E	106.	A		
23.	D	65.	E	107.	B		
24.	A	66.	C	108.	C		
25.	B	67.	D	109.	D		
26.	E	68.	D	110.	C		
27.	B	69.	B	111.	C		
28.	B	70.	A	112.	E		
29.	B	71.	A	113.	D		
30.	D	72.	C	114.	E		
31.	C	73.	D	115.	A		
32.	B	74.	B	116.	D		
33.	B	75.	D	117.	A		
34.	D	76.	C	118.	C		
35.	E	77.	E	119.	D		
36.	C	78.	C	120.	D		
37.	A	79.	B	121.	B		
38.	C	80.	D	122.	C		
39.	B	81.	A	123.	C		
40.	B	82.	A	124.	C		
41.	E	83.	B	125.	C		
42.	E	84.	E	126.	C		

Gynecology Answers

1. B

Infertility is the inability of a couple to conceive despite one full year of unprotected intercourse. The most common cause of infertility is male factors, including primary testicular disease (30% to 40%), disorders of sperm transport (10% to 20%), and hypothalamic pituitary disease (1% or 2%). Ovulatory dysfunction is the second most common cause of infertility (18%). Tubal and peritoneal factors make up the third most common factor in infertility (22%), with pelvic inflammatory disease and subclinical pelvic chlamydia infections as major contributors. Infertile women may also have endometriosis at a high prevalence rate. Unexplained factors make up about 28% of infertility causes. These couples may benefit from empiric therapy of ovulatory stimulation with clomiphene citrate and/or intrauterine insemination. The cervical factor is considered the midcycle interaction of spermatozoa and cervical mucus, and it is not as common in infertility as the factors listed previously. The uterine factor is generally associated with recurrent pregnancy loss and is not generally considered a cause of infertility. However, myomas may cause infertility if they are located near the uterotubal junction or are large enough to distort the anatomy of the fallopian tube and ovary. A complete sexual history is essential in assessing infertility at the initial visit.

2. D

The most common cause of male infertility is varicocele, which is a dilatation of the pampiniform plexus of the scrotal veins. Vericoceles are 10 times more likely to occur on the left than on the right, likely related to the fact that the left testicular vein drains into the left renal vein. Varicoceles are present in about 15% of the normal population, and they are estimated to be present in 25% to 40% of men with male factor infertility. They are thought to influence semen quality by increasing testicular temperature, likely causing progressive impairment of spermatogenesis. Varicoceles can be repaired in a number of ways, including retroperitoneal ligation of the internal spermatic vein, laparoscopic retroperitoneal ligation, inguinal ligation, and transfemoral vein embolization by interventional radiology. The most common complications are hydrocele formation, reccurrence of the varicocele, and testicular infarction or atrophy. The other listed causes also cause male infertility but not as commonly as varicocele.

3. C

Coarctation of the aorta is the most common cardiovascular anomaly in patients with Turner's syndrome. Evaluation of heart, kidneys, and ovaries is warranted after establishing the diagnosis of Turner's syndrome because both congenital heart defects and renal malformations occur in 30% of girls with Turner's syndrome. Coarctation of the aorta, ventricular septal defect, horseshoe kidneys, and unilateral renal agenesis have all been reported. The karyotype observed in Turner's syndrome is 45, XO. Up to 30% of girls with Turner's syndrome have normal pubertal development but less than 5% menstruate spontaneously. Very rarely, pregnancies in Turner patients have been reported. Female patients with a karyotype of XO have decreased height, with a final height between 55 and 58 inches (141 to 146 cm). Some of the common somatic features of Turner's syndrome are low nuchal hairline, webbed neck, small mandible, prominent ears, high arched palate, broad chest with widely spaced nipples, and more than 50% will have cubitus valgus, an elbow deformity that increases the carrying angle of the arm.

4. C

Typically, menses occur every 21 to 35 days and volume is usually less than 60 cc. Repeated blood loss of greater than 80 cc can lead to anemia. The normal bleeding duration is 4 to 6 days. Abnormal uterine bleeding can be either anatomic or, more likely, dysfunctional (DUB). Anatomic causes include trauma, infection such as cervicitis and salpingitis, carcinomas, polyps, uterine fibroids, and adenomyosis. More than 75% of DUB is due to anovulation. Causes of anovulation include thyroid abnormalities, both hypothyroidism and hyperthyroidism, adrenal disease, polycystic ovarian syndrome, endometriosis, premature menopause, medication, stress, and nutritional abnormalities such as morbid obesity, malabsorption, or anorexia nervosa. The degree of endometrial growth and thus shedding is related to the degree of estrogen exposure. Moreover, long-term exposure to unopposed estrogen can lead to endometrial hyperplasia and abnormal uterine bleeding. In females older than 40 years of age with abnormal bleeding, carcinoma is the most important consideration, but it is not the most common cause. The most common cause of uterine bleeding in postmenopausal women is atrophy of the vaginal mucosa or endometrium. During the course of a workup for DUB, an endometrial biopsy must be done. If hyperplasia is discovered, the patient must have further evaluation including dilation and curettage. Uterine bleeding in a premenarchal girl is only rarely due to neoplasm; more common causes are foreign body, vulvovaginitis, and urologic factors.

5. C

Several studies now show an increased incidence of preterm birth in women with bacterial vaginosis. In addition, bacterial vaginosis can complicate pregnancy by increasing the risk of a low–birth-weight infant, chorioamnionitis, amniotic fluid infection, and postpartum endometritis. Vaginosis is associated with the presence of fetal fibronectin, which in turn is associated with preterm delivery and infection. Bacterial vaginosis is a polymicrobial infection in which there is an overgrowth of anaerobic bacteria. *Gardnerella vaginalis* is only one of the many organisms involved and may not always be present in bacterial vaginosis. This overgrowth is characterized by a malodorous, grayish vaginal discharge with a pH generally greater than 4.5, but usually there is not external irritation of the vulva. Clue cells are a common microscopic finding and need to be at least 20% of the epithelial cells seen on the wet prep. Clue cells are epithelial cells "peppered" with adherent coccobacilli. The microorganisms causing bacterial vaginosis can be found in the upper genital tract and are associated with some cases of acute salpingitis.

6. E

The absolute contradictions to the use of oral contraceptives include thrombophlebitis or thromboembolic disorders, cerebral vascular or coronary artery disease, breast or other estrogen-dependent neoplasms, undiagnosed genital bleeding, cholestatic jaundice, and hepatic tumors. A history of heavy smoking (greater than 15 cigarettes per day) in a woman older than 35 years is an absolute contraindication. These recommendations were based on older, higher dose pills. However, there have been no new studies to challenge these contraindications. The product insert clearly states that women with these conditions may not receive oral contraceptives. Among the relative contraindications are hypertension, surgeries that require a period of immobilization, major injury to the lower extremity, migraines, tobacco use, diabetes mellitus, sickle cell disease, major depression, gallbladder disease, hepatitis, and age older than 40 years if there is an additional risk such as for coronary artery disease. These prescribing recommendations for oral contraceptives are applicable to all delivery systems of hormonal contraception (i.e., transdermal patches and vaginal rings).

7. E

Up to 20% of the female population is colonized with yeast and is asymptomatic. Although cultures will identify these women as carrying a yeast species, they do not necessarily require therapy. Many of the over-the-counter medications for yeast are used inappropriately, either for normal discharge or for infections other than yeast. A physician should evaluate all women experiencing symptomatic discharge for the first time. About 90% of yeast infections are caused by *Candida albicans*. Evaluation of a patient with suspected yeast infection should include a speculum exam, vaginal pH, microscopic exam of discharge, a whiff test, and possibly fungal cultures. If the exam is not consistent with yeast infection, then cultures for chlamydia, gonorrhea, and trichomonas may aid in identifying the cause of the abnormal vaginal discharge. Although rare, there is resistance of antifungals to *C. albicans*. Recurrent candidiasis should be evaluated by fungal cultures and the investigation of possible systemic causes, such as HIV or diabetes mellitus. If resistance is present to topical treatment, then a 14-day course of oral azole therapy or the use of a broader spectrum topical antifungal is indicated. The treatment can be followed by a 6-month maintenance regimen with topical suppositories.

8. A

The medroxyprogesterone acetate (Depo-Provera) intramuscular injection is a form of birth control given by injection every 12 weeks. It is an excellent means of contraception, with a failure rate of only 0.3%. However, like any nonbarrier method of contraception, there is no protection against sexually transmitted diseases. Patients must be cautioned about potential side effects. These include menstrual irregularities such as spotting, amenorrhea, and weight changes, with the average gain being 5 lbs. Also noted are dizziness, headache, depression, bloating, acne, and edema. Current U.S. Food and Drug Administration (FDA) black box warnings recommend against the use of medroxyprogesterone acetate for long-term contraception. This recommendation is due to bone loss that has been demonstrated with increased use.

9. D

The laboratory evaluation for patients presenting with hirsutism varies depending on the presentation. However, because the cause of hirsutism is androgenic effects on the pilosebaceous unit, the workup always begins with androgen levels. Generally, patients should have a serum testosterone level and a DHEAS level. This measures increased androgen production from the ovary and adrenal gland, respectively. Hyperprolactinemia and late-onset congenital adrenal hyperplasia are both rare causes but may be evaluated with prolactin and 17-hydroxyprogesterone levels. Polycystic ovarian syndrome (PCOS), also called Stein–Leventhal syndrome, is the most common cause of excessive androgen production. Although traditionally the diagnosis is made with an LH-to-FSH ratio greater than 3:1, not all women with PCOS have this lab abnormality. Because it is now thought to be on the continuum of the metabolic syndrome, fasting glucose, insulin, and triglyceride levels may be more important in diagnosing the disorder. Ovarian tumors will produce testosterone levels greater than 200 mg/dL. Adrenal tumors cause DHEAS levels to climb above 700 mg/dL. If these levels are obtained, further evaluation with CT scan would be indicated. An overnight dexamethasone suppression test should be performed if Cushing's disease is suspected, although Cushing's disease is a very rare cause of hirsutism.

10. C

Urinary tract infection is a potential complication of pessary use. Severe complications of pessary use are infrequent. However, patients must be advised that potential complications may include vaginitis, vaginal discharge, ulceration, and bleeding. If used improperly by being left in place too long, they may cause abscess, erosion into the rectum or bladder, and possibly fistula formation. Use of topical estrogen in postmenopausal women who are not on hormone replacement therapy can prevent device erosion through atrophic vaginal mucosa. Douching is not recommended, but the device should be cleaned at a minimum of once per week with soap and water. Pessary devices may be preferred to reconstructive surgery in woman who plan to become pregnant because vaginal delivery may damage or reverse the surgical repair and require reoperation following delivery.

11. C

Although the risk of pregnancy is low after a rape (about 1%), a patient should be offered pregnancy prophylaxis. This is usually effective if given within 72 hours of exposure. There are many combinations of emergency contraception that are effective. Forcible rape is a fast growing crime in the United States. Rape victims often feel powerless and have problems returning to family life, jobs, and other previously comforting situations. The fact that rape may produce a post-traumatic syndrome should be considered, and all patients should be offered comprehensive psychologic therapy. If a victim has been abused previously, she may have a more dramatic and severe reaction than a first-time victim. It is essential to take photographs of injuries whenever possible, preferably by a photographer from the police department. A pelvic exam with palpation of the vaginal mucosa is essential because visual inspection can fail to detect small lacerations. With adult patients, only a physician and female nurse should be present in the room. If the patient is a child, the parent should also be present.

12. C

The "female athlete triad" consists of amenorrhea, osteoporosis, and eating disorders. Initial treatment revolves around reducing physical stress. It is necessary for these patients to decrease training and improve eating habits. Menstrual abnormalities can occur in some form or severity in up to two-thirds of female athletes. The abnormalities can include primary amenorrhea, which is the absence of menarche by age 16 in a female with or without secondary sexual characteristics, and secondary amenorrhea, which is the absence of menses for three consecutive cycles or more in a previously menstruating woman. Contributory factors may include low body weight and body fat, eating disorder, thyroid abnormality, exogenous hormone use such as testosterone, and hypothalamic–pituitary axis suppression from physical and/or emotional stress. Physical activity alone does not induce amenorrhea in the absence of an eating disorder. Evaluation should include a thorough dietary and exercise history along with a physical exam focusing on sexual characteristics and the pelvis. Further evaluation should include a pregnancy test, thyroid-stimulating hormone level, prolactin level, progesterone challenge, and possibly an estradiol level. Low follicle-stimulating hormone and luteinizing hormone levels can suggest hypothalamic–pituitary axis suppression. A bone mineral density test should be considered in any woman without menses for more than 12 months.

13. E

Labial adhesions are common in prepubescent females. They are seen most commonly in children younger than 2 years old. The etiology is not clear, but it may be due to abrasion secondary to diaper rash or harsh soaps. Rarely, sexual abuse may be the cause. Most adhesions are insignificant and asymptomatic. When treatment is indicated, external estrogen cream applied daily for 2 or 3 weeks is effective in 90% of girls with adhesions. For most cases, surgery is not required. If urinary retention or frequent urinary tract infections exist, surgical division of the labia may be considered. Most cases resolve spontaneously with the onset of puberty and a natural increase in estrogen.

14. B

From birth and for a few weeks after, a newborn girl responds to maternal estrogen. Breast enlargement may occur but is temporary and should subside by the second week as the hormones are cleared from the newborn's system. The breasts should not be squeezed or massaged because this could result in an infection under the skin.

In addition to the enlargement, there may be some discharge from the nipples. This too is common and should be of no concern, disappearing within 2 weeks. The discharge is called witch's milk.

Both the external and the internal genitalia may be affected. The uterus may enlarge and newborn girls may initially have prominent labia and a thickened hymen as a result of the estrogen exposure. They sometimes also experience a type of vaginal discharge called pseudomenstruation due to the withdrawal of the maternal hormones. The discharge is white and occasionally tinged with blood. This condition is common and should not last beyond the first week of life. New mothers should always be warned about these effects in order to prevent unnecessary anxiety.

15. B

Fibrocystic breast disease is common and most changes are benign. However, there are some diagnoses, such as atypical lobular hyperplasia, diffuse papillomatosis with atypia, and atypical epithelial hyperplasia, that are premalignant in nature. If a woman has a history of atypia and has a family history of breast cancer, her risk is about 20% for developing breast cancer in the next 15 to 20 years. Treatments suggested to reduce pain associated with fibrocystic breast disease include nonsteroidal anti-inflammatory drugs, acetaminophen, oral contraceptives, tamoxifen, danazol, bromocryptine, decrease in the amount of nicotine and caffeine intake, evening primrose oil, breast supports, and topical heat application. Cysts can be aspirated for both treatment and diagnosis. The fluid can be discarded on the conditions of normal mammography, complete resolution of the mass with aspiration, and clear fluid. If the mass remains or the fluid is bloody, further evaluation is needed.

16. B

There are multiple drug regimens that are appropriate for gonorrhea. One dose of ceftriaxone intramuscularly will treat gonorrhea. It is important to remember that there is often a concomitant infection with *Chlamydia trachomatis* for which doxycycline 100 mg taken twice a day for 7 days or a single 1-g dose of azithromycin can be used. Gonorrhea is often asymptomatic in women until tubal scarring or pelvic inflammatory disease is present.

17. C

Fertility may return immediately upon cessation of the oral contraceptive pill. In the past, most family physicians recommended that patients wait two or three cycles before attempting to conceive because the dating of pregnancies was difficult without a regular menstrual pattern. Now, with accurate early ultrasound, a woman can attempt to conceive immediately. Liver enzyme-inducing medications, such as phenytoin, carbamazepine, phenobarbital, rifampin, tetracycline, and penicillin, may reduce the effectiveness of the pill. In fact, they may reduce the estrogen concentration by 30% to 50%. Although one-fourth of women will experience a delay in return to normal ovulatory cycles after stopping the pill, most women will ovulate immediately. In women who are nonsmokers and are not at a high risk for premature cardiovascular disease, it is safe to continue a low-estrogen contraceptive pill into perimenopause. However, oral contraceptives are contraindicated in women older than 35 years who smoke.

18. E

The finding of HPV DNA in the genital system of a female corresponds with cervical dysplasia. In the United States, HPV is the most common sexually transmitted disease. Some of the HPV subtypes are associated with visible warts, whereas some are associated with dysplasia. Subtypes 6 and 11 typically have a low malignant potential. The subtypes 31, 33, and 35 have an intermediate potential for dysplasia. The subtypes 16 and 18 have the greatest oncogenic potential and are associated with flat condylomatous lesions. Several tests are now available for HPV subtyping, which can be done from the Pap smear sample or a cervical biopsy. See Figure 4-1.

19. D

Following the application of acetic acid or Lugol's solution, dysplastic epithelium will turn whiter or lighter compared to the surrounding normal tissue. The degree of this change often correlates with the degree of the dysplasia. Lugol's solution is readily taken up by normal squamous epithelium because of the large glycogen stores. Abnormal squamous epithelium will have a larger nucleus to cell ratio with decreased glycogen and thus decreased staining

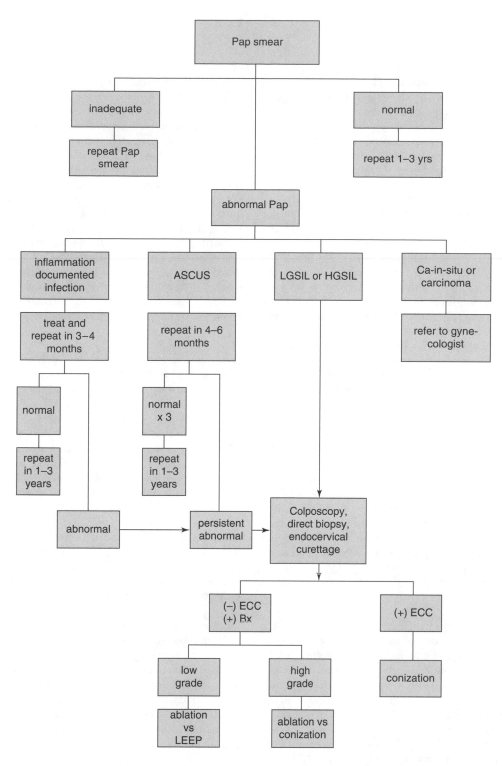

Figure 4-1. *Algorithm for the management of an abnormal pap smear.*

with Lugol's solution. Squamous metaplasia is a normal process, occurring around the transformation zone. It can also be seen in areas of previous cervicitis or regions with reparative changes. Endocervical cells, which are columnar, can appear slightly "whiter" than the surrounding epithelium with the application of acetic acid. If there is any suspicion regarding the staining, a biopsy is warranted. The vascular pattern abnormalities include punctations, mosaicism, and corkscrew vessels. These changes can be suggestive of moderate to severe dysplasia, or even invasive carcinoma.

20. B

Medroxyprogesterone acetate can greatly reduce blood loss and is an excellent treatment for a variety of gynecologic conditions that result in menorrhagia and iron deficiency anemia. There is evidence that women who use injectable progesterone have lower hysterectomy rates for uterine fibroids than other women. Gonadotropin-releasing hormone agonist administration can greatly reduce the volume of a patient's fibroids. Unfortunately, this effect is temporary and, as a result, this treatment is largely reserved for preoperative therapy to facilitate the removal of the uterus or fibroid. Treatment with nonsteroidal anti-inflammatory drugs (NSAIDs) or oral contraceptives may be effective in decreasing abnormal uterine bleeding. Oral contraceptives may reduce the perceived amount of blood loss. Despite this, they can occasionally stimulate the growth of the fibroids causing other bulk-induced symptoms such as pelvic discomfort to increase. Testosterone and estrogen are not appropriate treatment options.

21. D

Women wanting to avoid hysterectomy now have the option of uterine fibroid embolization (UFE). This procedure involves an interventional radiologist injecting tiny polyvinyl alcohol particles into the uterine arteries. Since the hypervascular fibroids have no collateral vascular supply, they undergo ischemic necrosis. Women with pedunculated, submucosal, or subserosal fibroids are not considered ideal candidates for this procedure. In addition, since the effects of UFE on future fertility are not well-known, the procedure is generally not done on women desiring future fertility. UFE is also generally not performed on postmenopausal women. Menorrhagia is improved in over 90% of women undergoing UAE.

22. C

The normal menstrual cycle is generally 21 to 35 days in length, with a menstrual flow lasting 2 to 7 days and a total menstrual blood loss of 20 to 60 mL. Common terminology when discussing vaginal bleeding presentations includes menorrhagia (heavier uterine bleeding during periods), metrorrhagia (uterine bleeding with unpredictable intervals), menometrorrhagia (heavier uterine bleeding with unpredictable intervals), hypermenorrhea (heavier uterine bleeding at a predictable yet abnormal interval), polymenorrhea (uterine bleeding at abnormally short intervals), and oligomenorrhea (abnormally light or infrequent uterine bleeding).

23. D

PID in its classic form presents with fever, pelvic discomfort, cervical motion tenderness, and adnexal tenderness. However, many patients present with atypical symptoms and can present without having any symptoms. PID can cause menorrhagia or metrorrhagia, so the patient presenting with abnormal vaginal bleeding should be fully evaluated for PID. Pituitary disease is more likely to present as amenorrhea than vaginal bleeding. Oral contraceptives can cause irregular spotting, but because of the atrophic changes they cause in the endometrium, they rarely cause heavy bleeding. Loratadine (Claritin) has no interaction with OCPs.

24. A

Abnormal vaginal bleeding is a common problem in the perimenopausal period. Up to 90% of women have a change in their bleeding pattern prior to total cessation of menstruation. The most common physiologic cause of menstrual changes is anovulation. Menometrorrhagia best describes this patient's bleeding pattern since she is bleeding irregularly and heavier than her normal period. While the most likely cause is anovulation, the patient should have further evaluation to rule out hyperplasia or endometrial cancer as a cause.

25. B

Conjugated equine estrogen (Premarin) has traditionally been used to treat an acute episode of heavy uterine bleeding because it can be administered intravenously, resulting in quick action, and will stop most uterine bleeding no matter what the cause within 24 to 48 hours. The dose commonly used is 25 mg of conjugated estrogen IV every 4 hours. Progestins are not helpful acutely but should be added to the estrogen regimen once the bleeding has stopped. An alternative treatment is the use of an injectable GnRH agonist, such as Lupron (leuprolide). It is thought that the mechanism of action is an estrogen surge, and this approach has the added benefit of amenorrhea after the initial event. In either case, the control lasts only for a few weeks, and further treatment is based on the etiology of the bleeding. NSAIDs, medroxyprogesterone (Provera), and oral contraceptives are useful for chronic menorrhagia but do not work quickly enough in a woman with severe uterine bleeding. In addition, nausea limits using high doses of estrogen orally, but lower doses can be used in a patient with acute bleeding who is hemodynamically stable. Although this patient has signs of hypovolemia and anemia, neither is severe enough to warrant an emergency transfusion.

26. E

Hyperprolactinemia is more likely to present as amenorrhea rather than vaginal bleeding. The initial evaluation of any patient presenting with vaginal bleeding should include an evaluation for pregnancy, especially because one of the first warning signs of ectopic pregnancy is vaginal bleeding. Even after a miscarriage, there may be resolving levels of beta-human gonadotropin that would confirm a pregnancy. A patient with hypothyroidism may experience changes in her menstrual cycle, including amenorrhea, oligomenorrhea, polymenorrhea, or menorrhagia. PID and endometrial hyperplasia can cause menorrhagia or metrorrhagia.

27. B

Since this patient just began her menses, subtle bleeding disorders may manifest for the first time. Formation of a platelet plug is the first step of homeostasis during menstruation. Patients having disorders interfering with the normal platelet plug formation can experience menorrhagia. Bleeding can be particularly severe at menarche, due to the dominant estrogen stimulation causing increased vascularity. The two most common disorders are von Willebrand's disease and thrombocytopenia. Von Willebrand's disease is the most common congenital cause of hypermenorrhea and can be diagnosed by an abnormal bleeding time, abnormal platelet function, and decreased factor VIII activity. Thrombocytopenia is usually due to autoimmune destruction, bone marrow suppression, or platelet consumption. The other options are not indicated in this patient because of her age, no risk factors for STDs, and presentation.

28. B

Menopause is a retrospective diagnosis made 1 year after cessation of menses for women in the age range of 45 to 55 years. No routine tests are done to diagnose menopause, although FSH and LH may be useful for the patient who is very young or is taking oral contraceptives. For 5 to 7 years preceding menopause, women may experience symptoms of menopause and may be said to be in "perimenopause." This patient reports two such symptoms: fatigue and concentration problems. With only 2 months of amenorrhea, she cannot be diagnosed with menopause. Since she has not been diagnosed with menopause, pregnancy must be ruled out. Although stress may cause amenorrhea, other causes for her symptoms, such as anemia and hypothyroidism, must be investigated.

29. B

Vaginal atrophy can occur with any estrogen deficiency state. Thus, women in menopause, lactating and postpartum women, as well as those taking progesterone-only or low-dose oral contraceptives may experience vaginal atrophy. Low estrogen states lead to thinning of the vaginal tissue with decreased glycogen-rich secretions. Decreased glycogen production decreases normal flora (lactobacilli) and vaginal pH rises. A pH level above 4.5 with bacteria, white blood cells, and red blood cells on microscopy are characteristic findings for vaginal atrophy. In contrast, clue cells are characteristic of bacterial vaginosis.

30. D

Vaginal cancer is a rare genital cancer, occurring most often between the ages of 50 and 70 years. One type of cancer, clear cell adenocarcinoma, occurs decades earlier in women whose mothers took diethylstilbestrol (DES). DES was given to pregnant women between 1945 and 1970 in an attempt to prevent miscarriage. Other women at increased risk for vaginal cancer include those with a history of cervical cancer, cervical precancerous conditions, HPV infection, or uterine prolapse. Symptoms of vaginal cancer may include: bleeding or discharge not related to menstrual periods, difficult or painful urination, dyspareunia, pelvic pain, constipation, or a palpable mass. Weight loss and abdominal distension are more commonly associated with ovarian cancer.

31. C

Vulvar cancer is a rare malignancy that accounts for less than 1% of all cancers in women. It encompasses 5% of all genital cancers and occurs less often than endometrial, ovarian, and cervical cancer. It is overwhelmingly squamous in origin, but melanoma, Paget's disease, adenoma, and basal cell carcinomas also occur. It affects women in the postmenopausal age group and often presents with a long history of local vulvar irritation, pruritis, bleeding, and discharge. Sometimes, pruritis is the only complaint, causing delay in diagnosis. Early lesions may appear as chronic dermatitis that develops into a lump, ulceration, or cauliflower-like growth. Bartholin cyst is a swelling of the Bartholin's gland deep in the posterior portion of the labia minora that occurs in young women. The cyst is most often associated with a pressure sensation and/or dyspareunia. If the cyst becomes infected, it may be painful. Cystic adenosis is a submucosal cyst of the vagina, not labia. They are often asymptomatic and are remnants of the mullerian duct. Bartholin gland carcinoma is an extremely rare form of vulvar cancer that often metastasizes early due to the rich lymphatic supply. Sebaceous cysts are benign, discrete, white cysts originating from the pilosebaceous unit that are generally asymptomatic unless they rupture or become infected.

32. B

Acute, heavy bleeding requires close observation and accurate diagnosis. The source should be determined by thorough exam. It is important to consider ectopic pregnancy, degenerating fibroids, spontaneous abortion, and trauma. An ultrasound, BHCG, reassurance, and eventual endometrial biopsy in this 40-year-old may ensue, but the first step is a good pelvic examination.

33. B

The most common adolescent breast disorder is breast mass, the majority of which are fibroadenomas or benign cysts. Most fibroadenomas are benign, mobile, well-defined rubbery-feeling masses. Multiple fibroadenomas occur in 10% to 20% of patients. Fibroadenomas tend not to vary in size during the menstrual cycle, often distinguishing them from cysts. Cystosarcoma phylloides is a rare variant of a fibroadenoma, distinguished by having a more cellular stroma. It is typically larger than a fibroadenoma and can rarely be malignant. In one biopsy series of adolescent breast masses, 71% were found to be fibroadenomas, 11% were abscesses, and 2% were cystosarcoma phylloides. Breast cysts vary in size over the course of a menstrual cycle, so a patient should be re-examined 2 weeks after the initial examination. Persistence of the mass or its enlargement over three menstrual cycles is an indication for surgical consultation. Aspiration can be attempted under local anesthesia, often resulting in curative drainage if it proves to be a cyst. If no fluid is obtained, an excisional biopsy is indicated. When multiple small masses are palpable, associated with pain or tenderness and varying with the stage of the menstrual cycle, they are most often fibrocystic lesions. Prolonged use of combination oral contraceptives of low progesterone potency may be beneficial in reducing the frequency of fibrocystic changes. Using combination oral contraceptives with a lower estrogen dose (20 μg) may lessen OCP-associated breast pain. A biopsy is rarely indicated with this presentation. Carcinoma of the breast in the adolescent is rare. The efficacy and possible sequelae of mammography in managing adolescent breast masses are unknown. The dense breast tissue of the adolescent obstructs the visualization of a palpable mass; thus, mammography is not advised for this age group. Ultrasonography is useful in distinguishing cystic from solid masses.

34. D

Severe menopausal symptoms often begin within days following surgical menopause. Patients usually require higher levels of estrogen replacement therapy for symptomatic control. Appropriate starting doses of estrogen for this patient include conjugated estrogens (Premarin) 1.25 mg daily, oral estradiol—17B (Estrace) 4 mg daily, or transdermal estradiol—17B (Climara) 0.1 mg twice weekly. Combined therapy with progesterone is indicated for prevention of endometrial hyperplasia in patients who have an intact uterus, prophylaxis against osteoporosis, or for treatment of breast tenderness related to estrogen use.

35. E

Hormone replacement therapy (HRT) is an effective treatment for menopausal hot flashes, but it is not without side effects. Despite continuous therapy with estrogen and progesterone, many women continue to have vaginal bleeding. Additional problems include weight gain, nausea, abdominal pain, depression, headaches, and breast tenderness. Hirsutism can be seen if androgens are added to HRT.

36. C

Absolute contraindications to the use of HRT include the presence of an estrogen-related cancer, undiagnosed abnormal vaginal bleeding, liver disease, active thromboembolic disorders, pregnancy, and prior complications of HRT. Relative contraindications include risk for thromboembolic disorders, gallstones, the presence of conditions aggravated by fluid retention, active endometriosis, uterine fibroids, acute intermittent porphyria, and previous breast cancer. Since congestive heart failure may be worsened by fluid retention, it is a relative contraindication for HRT.

37. A

Raloxifene (Evista) is a selective estrogen receptor modulator (SERM), which acts as both an estrogen agonist and an antagonist. Other medications in this class are tamoxifen (Nolvadex) and clomiphene (Clomid). Raloxifene has prospectively proven beneficial effects on bone and reduces the risk of breast cancer. It also improves lipid profiles. However, because of the antagonist effects, it may exacerbate menopausal symptoms, such as hot flashes and atrophic vaginitis.

38. C

As a SERM, raloxifene (Evista) acts on target tissues to produce some effects that are similar to estrogen and others that are distinctly different. Like estrogen, raloxifene can cause thromboembolic events, improve serum lipids, and increase bone density. Unlike estrogen, typical side effects include hot flashes and atrophic vaginitis. A major advantage of raloxifene over estrogen is the lack of proliferative effect on the endometrium, which in turn reduces the risk of endometrial adenocarcinoma.

39. B

This patient's history and exam is most consistent with polycystic ovarian syndrome (or Stein–Leventhal syndrome). Making the diagnosis of PCOS involves the evaluation of clinical features, endocrine abnormalities, and the exclusion of other etiologies. Women with PCOS can present with oligomenorrhea or dysfunctional uterine bleeding from prolonged anovulation. In addition, these women can have hirsutism, acne, and central obesity. Hormonally they can have increased testosterone activity, elevated luteinizing hormone concentration with a normal FSH level, and hyperinsulinemia due to insulin resistance. In fact, this disorder is related to the metabolic syndrome (e.g., truncal obesity can increase one's risk of developing either disease). PCOS usually has its onset during puberty, and so these women will usually report a long history of irregular periods. This patient had years of regular periods because she was taking an oral contraceptive pill. The length of time she has been on oral contraceptives should not affect her subsequent ovulatory pattern.

40. B

Dilation and curettage (D&C) is a useful test in evaluating the cause of vaginal bleeding but is not effective as the sole treatment for menorrhagia. It provides a blind sampling of the endometrium and is useful in patients with cervical stenosis or other anatomic factors preventing an adequate endometrial biopsy in the office. OCPs provide an option for treatment of both the acute episode of bleeding and future episodes of bleeding, as well as prevention of long-term health problems from anovulation. OCPs are effective in treating dysfunctional uterine bleeding no matter what the pattern of bleeding. Patients who are unable to tolerate hormonal management can consider endometrial ablation. The techniques of electrocautery, laser, cryoablation, or thermoablation all result in destruction of the endometrial lining. Women who undergo hysterectomies may have the option of an abdominal or vaginal hysterectomy. Women who undergo vaginal hysterectomies have fewer complications and shorter hospital stays. The size of the uterus at the time of surgery determines if this approach is possible because the surgeon must be able to remove the uterus completely through a vaginal incision. See Figure 4-2.

41. E

The main factor that increases a woman's risk of endometrial cancer is chronic, unopposed estrogen exposure. Higher parity, smoking, and the use of oral contraceptives decrease the amount of estrogen and therefore the risk of endometrial cancer. Factors associated with an increased risk of endometrial cancer include early menarche, obesity, and chronic anovulation. Diabetes is associated with endometrial cancer, probably because of its link to obesity. The risk of endometrial cancer increases after the age of 35 years.

42. E

The results of a transvaginal ultrasound evaluation of a patient's endometrial stripe need to be interpreted based on whether a patient is pre- or postmenopausal. For all women, the thicker the endometrial stripe, the more likely the patient has an endometrial abnormality. There are some conflicting results regarding the exact cutoff point for an abnormal endometrial stripe, but postmenopausal patients with an endometrial stripe greater than 4 or 5 mm should have a biopsy for histologic diagnosis.

43. C

The basal body temperature (BBT) chart is a take-home test couples can use to help determine when ovulation has occurred in order to properly time intercourse. The follicular phase is characterized by temperature between 97°F and 98°F, and the luteal phase generally has a temperature greater than 98°F. Temperature rise corresponds to the thermogenic properties of progesterone on the central nervous system, which rises with the LH surge. Ovulation probably occurs the day before the first temperature elevation, and it may be marked by a slight drop in temperature. The most likely time for conception, based on a single artificial insemination, is the day before the temperature rise. On day 16, the temperature jumps from a cycle low of 97.4°F on day 15 to a high of 98.7°F. Hence, day 15 is the optimal day for achieving conception based on temperature. The BBT is most helpful when there is a clear temperature jump, as in this patient. When the BBT does not change or has no clear pattern, there may be an anovulatory pattern, and other diagnostic tests should be pursued.

44. D

Persistently elevated LH levels or evidence of two "ovulations" are seen in months 1 and 2. POS can cause aberrant LH pulses throughout the menstrual cycle as in this patient. In patients taking clomiphene citrate, there may also be two LH surges, seen in month 1. The first surge is due to the clomiphene effect and the second surge is the "true" LH surge. However, this patient is not taking clomiphene citrate. Submucosal fibroids may impair fertility but will not cause changes in LH levels. Hypothyroidism is also a cause for infertility but is screened with thyroid function tests, not an ovulation predictor kit. Endometriosis and Asherman syndrome (uterine synechiae) can also cause infertility by mechanically blocking ovum and sperm passage and egg implantation. None of these would produce increased levels of LH.

45. A

Although a rare lesion, AGUS is associated with a significant abnormality in 20% to 50% of patients, making evaluation of all AGUS Paps essential. All patients should undergo colposcopy and endocervical curettage. If the patient is older than 35 years or has

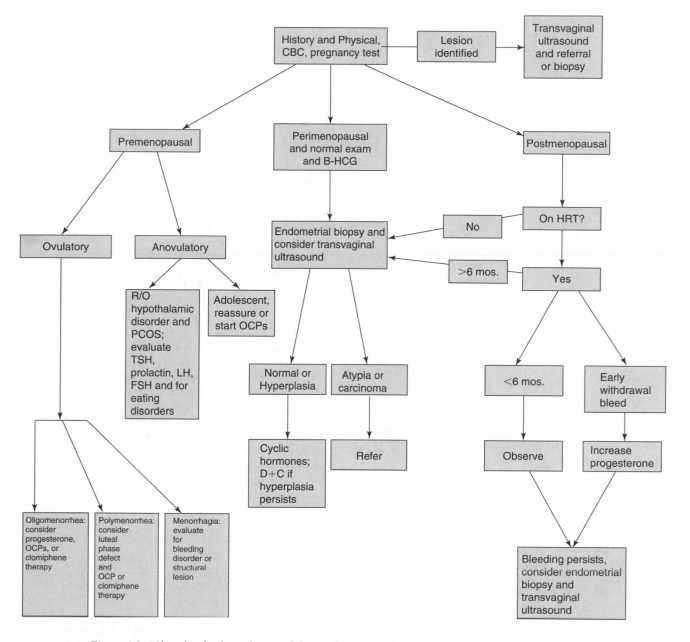

Figure 4-2. *Algorithm for the evaluation of abnormal vaginal bleeding.*

abnormal bleeding, an endometrial biopsy is also warranted. After the initial evaluation, management depends on the subclassification of the AGUS Pap. When the subclassification favors a reactive process or is unqualified and the colposcopy is negative, the patient may undergo repeat Pap smears every 4 to 6 months until four consecutive negative results are obtained, at which point the patient can return to routine screening. If any subsequent Pap reads as AGUS, a cone biopsy of the cervix should be considered. If the AGUS reading is subclassified as favoring neoplasia, the patient similarly undergoes colposcopy and ECC. However, even if the results are negative, a cone biopsy is warranted because of the high rate of adenocarcinoma in this group. If the colposcopy or ECC is positive, the patient can go straight to surgery for definitive treatment with hysterectomy. Glandular changes are notoriously difficult to see on colposcopy and can be easily missed, especially if a squamous lesion coexists.

46. C

Before menopause, the ovaries produce androgens. Subsequently, the adrenal gland secretes androgens but at much lower level. A significant benefit from adding androgens to HRT is increased bone mass. A small number of studies indicate improved sexual dysfunction with testosterone/estrogen combinations. Possible side effects include mild hirsuitism, occurring in less than 25% of women on androgen combination; abnormal liver function tests with high doses of androgen; and a small effect on lipid profile. Although there is a concern over increased risk of coronary artery disease with long-term use of androgen, there is no clear-cut evidence for this.

47. B

Hysteroscopes allow the physician to directly visualize the endometrial lining. This direct exploration of the uterus is useful in identifying structural abnormalities such as fibroids and endometrial polyps. The other study that is useful in evaluating a patient for an endometrial polyp is a sonohysterogram. Sonohysterography (SHG) involves performing a transvaginal ultrasound following installation of saline into the uterus. The study is most useful for differentiating focal from diffuse endometrial abnormalities. SHG done after an abnormal vaginal ultrasound can help guide the decision of doing a hysteroscopy to evaluate a focal abnormality versus performing an endometrial biopsy or D&C for a diffuse endometrial abnormality.

48. C

Age itself is not a risk factor for an abnormal Pap smear result. However, the risk of cervical cancer increases if the patient had sexual intercourse or contracted HPV at an early age. Risk factors include multiple sexual partners, multiparity, tobacco and/or alcohol abuse, low socioeconomic status, and history of sexually transmitted diseases (including HPV).

49. B

Koilocytosis is used to describe cellular changes associated with HPV infection. Lesions classified as either koilocytosis or mild dysplasia progress to high-grade intraepithelial lesions at similar but low rates. Both of these lesions are categorized as LGSIL in the Bethesda system for reporting Pap smear results. A traditional Pap smear has a sensitivity of 50% to 60% and a specificity of approximately 90% of cellular abnormality. Liquid-based cervical cytologic smears, trade name ThinPrep, improve the adequacy of the sample and lead to increased diagnosis of low-grade lesions. A study in 2001 found this method (ThinPrep) to be cost-effective in reducing the rates of cervical cancer.

50. D

More than 1 million women are diagnosed with LGSIL each year. The natural history of LGSIL is that 85% to 95% of patients will not progress to a more advanced lesion and 60% will actually revert to a normal Pap smear. While there is a low rate of progression, due to the risk of a woman being lost to follow-up and the common occurrence of colposcopy being indicated in follow-up cytology, it is recommended that all patients with LGSIL undergo colposcopy. If the colposcopy is satisfactory and there is no presence of CIN 2 or 3, the patient can be managed with repeat cytologic testing at 6 and 12 months or HPV testing at 12 months with referral to colposcopy if either is positive. CIN 2 or 3 should be treated with ablation or excision. Up to 15% of women with an LGSIL on Pap smear actually have a higher grade lesion when tissue biopsy is performed (1).

51. D

Donovanosis is rare in the United States but is common in tropical zones such as India, the Caribbean, Brazil, South Africa, and Australia. With the influx of immigrants from these regions, this disease may increase in incidence. Donovanosis is caused by *Calymmatobacterium granulomatis*, which is very difficult to culture. Diagnosis is usually made by a smear that demonstrates the typical cytoplasmic inclusions, called Donovan bodies. Because it is not usually painful, significant tissue destruction can occur prior to diagnosis. The destruction is local and can cause phimosis and paraphimosis in men. Both men and women can develop subcutaneous inguinal granulomas called pseudobuboes and eventual lymphatic destruction leading to elephantiasis of the legs and genitalia. Coinfection of syphilis and donovanosis is common. The CDC recommends treatment with trimethroprim-sulfamethoxazole or doxycycline. Other antibiotics that can be used include ciprofloxacin and erythromycin.

52. A

The recommended treatments are doxycycline 100 mg orally twice a day for 7 days or azithromycine 1 g orally in a single dose. Alternative regimens include erythromycin, ofloxacin, or levofloxacin. Treatment is required even in asymptomatic patients. The highest prevalence of chlamydia in the United States is among sexually active adolescents, with estimates as high as 20%. A majority of teens are asymptomatic, but mucopurulent discharge, a cervix that bleeds easily, and dysuria should prompt investigation. Because this infection is often asymptomatic and can lead to serious consequences such as PID and infertility, universal screening of all sexually active women younger than 25 years is recommended. The diagnosis of chlamydia is usually made using nucleic acid amplification test, which can screen for both chlamydia and gonorrhea. The sensitivity and specificity for chlamydia are 85% and 94% to 99.5%, respectively.

53. B

Neisseria gonorrhea may be treated with any number of antibiotic regimens as outline by the CDC. Ceftriaxone and azithromycin are but one treatment option. Note that the azithromycin is for treatment of chlamydia, which shows a high rate of coinfection with gonorrhea. All sexual partners within 60 days of the onset of her symptoms should be tested and treated for infection. Testing for HIV should be offered and the patient should be counseled regarding the ability of condoms to protect her against HIV, gonorrhea, chlamydia, and other sexually transmitted diseases. Partners should not resume sexual activity until both have been treated and no longer have any symptoms of disease, which is likely to be much longer than 24 hours.

54. B

Trichomonas vaginalis is diagnosed using microscopic examination of vaginal secretions in the office. Treatment is with metronidazole given as either a single 2-g dose or a short course of 500 mg PO bid for 7 days. Sexual partners should be treated. There is no need for follow-up examination unless the patient's symptoms worsen or fail to resolve. Sexual contact should be avoided until treatment has been completed and both partners are asymptomatic.

55. E

Patients may have one or more of these as risk factors for ectopic pregnancy. In addition to these factors, previous pelvic and tubal surgery, previous ectopic pregnancy, infertility treatments, uterine abnormalities, tobacco abuse, and DES exposure are also associated with ectopic pregnancy. Reported rates of ectopic pregnancy range from 0.5% to 2% of all pregnancies. Patients often present with adnexal pain and vaginal spotting early in pregnancy. Rarely, patients present in full-blown hemorrhagic shock from ruptured ectopic pregnancy. Diagnosis depends on careful physical exam focused on the pelvis, determination of pregnancy, and ultrasound evaluation. BHCG levels less than 1500 mIU/ml and progesterone levels less than 25 ng/mL are also associated with ectopic pregnancy. Treatment depends on the gestational age. If diagnosed early, medical therapy with methotrexate may spare the patient surgery. After 8 weeks, surgery is required to evacuate the ectopic pregnancy.

56. C

Menopause is often diagnosed retrospectively when a woman has not had a menstrual period in 12 months. Although the mean age for the start of menopause is 50 years, menopausal symptoms often begin in the perimenopausal years. Perimenopause is considered to begin if a woman older than 40 years has signs of menopause, such as vaginal dryness and hot flashes. Decreased estrogen levels cause urogenital symptoms, but the exact etiology of vasomotor and psychologic effects related to menopause remains unclear. There is good evidence from randomized prospective trials that progestins reduce vasomotor symptoms.

57. C

Mastalgia is extremely common, affecting 70% of women. Breast pain can be differentiated into cyclical or noncyclical mastalgia. Cyclical pain is thought to be due to hormone changes but no physiologic explanations have been proven. It is usually bilateral and spontaneously resolves within 3 or 4 months of onset in 20% to 30% of women. However, it can relapse and remit, causing up to 60% of women to develop recurrent symptoms 2 years after treatment. Noncyclical pain may be caused by true breast pain or chest wall pain located over the costal cartilages. The cause of mastalgia is multifactorial and many treatment options have been utilized, including better fitting bras and application of topical heat. Medications used to treat breast pain include NSAIDs, evening primrose oil, hormones, and even tamoxifen. The overall evidence is poor regarding outcome of treatment, however.

58. E

Endometrial hyperplasia, abnormal thickening of the uterine lining, can lead to endometrial cancer if left untreated. Risk factors for endometrial hyperplasia include chronic anovulation, polycystic ovarian syndrome, obesity, unopposed exogenous estrogen use, tamoxifen use, diabetes mellitus, nulliparity, late menopause, and hypertension. OCP use can actually decrease the risk of endometrial cancer by 50%.

59. B

Treatment of endometrial hyperplasia is based on the pathologic diagnosis. *Simple* or *cystic hyperplasia* has a low risk of malignancy. Treatment can include observation, D&C, and hormonal endometrial shedding induced with either progesterone alone or cyclic estrogen and progesterone. *Complex (adenomatous) hyperplasia without atypia* carries a slightly increased risk of malignancy. This can be treated as above except that estrogen should not be used. *Complex hyperplasia with atypia* progresses to malignancy in about 25% of cases. Treatment is generally with total abdominal hysterectomy and bilateral salpingoophorectomy (TAH-BSO). Patients who are poor surgical candidates or who desire fertility may be treated with high-dose progesterone and regular endometrial surveillance. *Endometrial carcinoma* is treated with TAH-BSO plus adjuvant radiation.

60. E

Although the peak age for endometrial cancer is 60 years, most physicians agree that women who are 40 years of age or older are at increased risk. Other risk factors include diabetes, use of tamoxifen, irregular menstrual cycles, and the presence of atypical glandular cells (AGUS) on a Pap smear. Use of OCPs, cigarette smoking, and multiparity are considered protective factors. See Table 4.3.

Table 4.3 Risk factors for endometrial cancer

Risk Factor	Relative Risk
Nulliparity	2–3
Late menopause	2–4
Diabetes mellitus	2–8
Tamoxifen use	2–3

Obesity
  21–50 lbs overweight
  50 lbs overweight
	3
	10

Unopposed estrogen therapy	4–8

61. C

The Bartholin's gland cyst is the most common mass found in the vulvar region. This cyst develops if the Bartholin's gland duct becomes obstructed. The Bartholin's gland provides lubrication and is situated near the vaginal opening at approximately 5 and 7 o'clock just inside of the labia minora. If the duct is obstructed, the gland fills with mucus and can grow very large. Patients are symptomatic because of pain or superinfection. Treatment requires incision and drainage. However, a simple incision and drainage results in a very high recurrence rate, and the definitive treatment requires the re-establishment of an epithelial tract. This is done by the placement of a Word catheter or marsupialization. It is very rare that total excision of the gland is needed. Because the Bartholin gland begins to involute after the age of 30 years, cysts are rare in older women. Lipomas and sebaceous cysts can occur but are rare.

62. E

Menstrual patterns vary widely during the perimenopause. For the perimenopausal patient with absent or decreased menses, the first step in evaluation is to rule out pregnancy. An endometrial biopsy is indicated for patients with menometrorrhagia in this age group because this is the usual bleeding pattern associated with endometrial cancer. Other causes of menstrual irregularity include thyroid disorders and prolactin secreting tumors.

63. E

This patient has several risk factors for endometrial cancer: age older than 40 years, obesity, and diabetes. Other risk factors include being Caucasian, nulliparity, hypertension, and family history. Endometrial carcinoma is the most common pelvic cancer in women but has an excellent prognosis. Menorrhagia in this patient requires evaluation with endometrial sampling prior to hormonal therapy. A younger patient could be treated with medroxyprogesterone acetate or combination oral contraceptives without first taking a biopsy of the endometrium.

64. E

Patients may complain of classic menopausal symptoms for years before the cessation of menses. Symptoms are treatable with a combination of estrogen and progesterone. Traditional combination oral contraceptive pills provide these hormones in dosages high enough to prevent pregnancy. Women in perimenopause have a high rate of unintended pregnancy, over 50%, second only to teenagers. Despite recent data on HRT, perimenopause and acute menopausal symptoms may still be treated with hormone therapy.

65. E

Primary amenorrhea is usually considered to be absence of menses by the age of 16 years. In the United States, girls have been achieving menarche increasingly earlier for unknown reasons. The average age of menarche is 12.8 years but can range from 8 to 16 years. Primary amenorrhea can occur because of hypothalamic, pituitary, gonadal, or anatomic abnormalities. In this patient, thelarche (breast development) is apparent, which indicates normal hypothalamic, pituitary, and ovarian function resulting in estrogen production. Pubic hair development follows thelarche within 1 year. Menarche follows thelarche by 2 years on average, so it would be safe to tell the mother that menses can be expected when the patient is 15 years old. See Table 4.4.

66. C

Hormonal emergency contraception was officially recognized by the FDA in 1997, using a combination of 100 μg of ethinyl estradiol and 1 mg of levonorgestrel taken within 72 hours of unprotected intercourse and repeated in 12 hours. This method is currently available either as a prepackaged prescription marketed as the "Preven Emergency Contraceptive Kit" or by combining several pills of Ovral, Lo/Ovral, Levelen, Nordette, Alesse, and others. The main side effect of this method is nausea and vomiting, which can be alleviated by prescribing an antiemetic. Both high-dose estrogen and high-dose progesterone alone will prevent pregnancy, but the progesterone-only method appears to have fewer side effects associated with it. It consists of 0.75 mg levonorgestrel given within 72 hours and repeated in 12 hours. It is available as a prepacked prescription under the name "Plan B."

Mifepristone is an antiprogesterone usually associated with abortion but is also effective as emergency contraception. A common side effect is delayed menses.

67. D

This is a common scenario with the unprotected intercourse occurring several days prior. Unfortunately, although the Ovral dose is appropriate for emergency contraception, it is past the 72-hour limit for effectiveness. Both the mifepristone and the IUD can be utilized up to 5 days after the unintended intercourse and still provide emergency contraception. This patient is an ideal candidate for the IUD because she is multipara and is presumably in a monogamous relationship. The IUD has a very high success rate and has the added benefit of providing contraception for 10 years if the woman chooses to leave it in place. The limiting factor for mifepristone is availability.

68. D

Concerns about estrogen causing a decrease in the breast milk supply through decreasing prolactin levels are only a relevant during the first several weeks while breast-feeding is being established. Once the milk supply is well established, which may take 6 weeks, combination pills could be used instead of a progestin-only pill. The failure rate of progestin-only pills is nearly four times as high as combination contraceptives. All the other statements are false. Indications for combination contraceptive use include cycle regulation, menorrhagia, and mild to moderate acne.

69. B

Oral contraceptives are contraindicated in patients who have active liver disease, whatever the cause. The other patients are all candidates. OCPs have not been shown to increase the risk of breast cancer. Although the risk of thromboembolic complications increases, women over age 35, especially nonsmokers, may use OCPs. Although OCPs may impair glucose tolerance, their use is

Table 4.4 Tanner stages of sexual maturity

Stage	Boys	Girls
1	Childlike penis No enlargement of testicles No pubic hair	No breast development No pubic hair
2	Penis unchanged Scrotum and testicles enlarge Small amount of fine long pubic hair	Breast buds Small amount of fine, long pubic hair
3	Penis elongates Continued growth of testicles and scrotum Coarse and curly pubic hair	Breasts enlarge, areolas enlarge Pubic hair coarse and curly
4	Penis increased in diameter Darkening of scrotum Adult hair texture over pubic area	Continued breast growth Adult hair texture over pubic area
5	Adult penis, scrotum Pubic hair extends to thighs	Adult breast contours Pubic hair extends to thighs

not an absolute contraindication in women with diabetes. In fact, there is a high incidence of maternal and infant morbidity associated with unintended pregnancies in women with uncontrolled diabetes. As for the patient with a history of PID, OCPs reduce the likelihood of salpingitis. The etiology of this effect is not fully understood but may be due to thickened cervical mucus preventing pathogenic bacteria from ascending into the upper genital tract, decreased menstrual blood (which acts as a culture medium), less dilated cervical canal, and decreased uterine contractions.

70. A

Breakthrough bleeding or spotting between menses is common during initiation of oral contraception and is the most common reason for women to discontinue OCPs. Intermenstrual bleeding can occur in 10% to 20% of women initially and persists in 5% of women. Management of this side effect can be accomplished by switching to a pill with higher estrogen activity if it occurs early in the cycle or higher progestational activity if it occurs after the 14th day. Weight gain can occur on OCPs but the same number of women may lose weight. Initially, if weight is gained, it is most likely due to water retention. Estrogen can cause fat deposition on the hips after many months of use. Either way, weight gain does not continue and will respond to diet and exercise. The estrogen component can increase blood pressure, and current recommendations are to recheck blood pressure in 3 months. Menses usually becomes lighter with hormonal contraception and, in fact, amenorrhea can occur.

71. A

The diminishing of the breast milk supply can occur due to OCPs, but it is unlikely to be related to OCPs in this patient. It is more likely due to her return to work and decreased stimulation to the nipples. Lab work would be unlikely to provide any information. However, any postpartum woman with excessive fatigue, cardiac symptoms, or goiter should be evaluated for thyroid dysfunction, which can occur transiently in 6% of women after delivery. This patient's weight loss is unlikely due to any hormonal contraceptive. Although she can expect regular menses, breakthrough bleeding or spotting between menses is common during initiation of oral contraception.

72. C

Nausea correlates with the estrogenic activity of the pill. Intolerable nausea or vomiting can be improved by switching to a pill that has a relatively lower estrogenic activity. Low progesterone activity is associated with late-cycle spotting. Estrogen is responsible for the increased risk of thrombosis and telangectasias. However, decreased libido is due to the reduction in natural testosterone (androgenic effect).

73. D

Smoking and advanced age are risk factors for thrombotic complications of OCPs, but physicians frequently overestimate this risk if the patient is a light smoker who smokes less than 20 cigarettes per day. Although increased for women who smoke, the true magnitude of the risk is still low. For example, the risk of death for women aged 35 to 39 years is 4 per 100,000 women-years for OCP users who do not smoke and 13 per 100,000 women-years for OCP users who smoke. The risk of death from pregnancy is 19 per 100,000 women-years for women in this age

range. While the relative risk is increased, the absolute risk is still small. The risk of stroke exceeds the risk of myocardial infarction (MI) in women of any age who smoke and use OCPs. Pills with 50 μg or more of estrogen are not currently used because thromboembolic risk increases with higher doses of estrogen and lower doses of estrogen have been shown to be effective contraceptives. If the patient is a heavy smoker, smoking 20 or more cigarettes per day, then the risks outweigh the benefits and the patient should not be on OCPs.

74. B

One of the benefits of OCPs is a decreased risk of ovarian cancer, and another is decreased risk of endometrial cancer. With long-term use, the reduction of ovarian cancer is 80% and the reduction of endometrial cancer is 50%. There is a very small increase in the relative risk of breast cancer in OCP users, but the absolute risk is very low. It should be noted that the breast cancers that are found are usually found at an earlier stage and confined to the breast. Although health professionals often tie the Pap smear to refilling OCPs, there is no evidence that OCPs increase the risk of cervical cancer. Women who use OCPs have 10% to 70% less risk of PID than nonusers but the risk of chlamydia cervicitis is somewhat increased.

75. D

OCPs have many benefits, including the reduction of other medical problems. These include osteoporosis, endometriosis, and rheumatoid arthritis. Overall, OCP use reduces the hospitalization rate for women. Because of the anovulation, it is an excellent method to reduce ectopic pregnancy. In addition, it reduces the risk of PID, which is a leading cause of ectopic pregnancy. One of its drawbacks is the reduction of libido that can occur. The cause may be related to the reduction in testosterone production in women on OCPs. Other women may feel more sexual enjoyment because the fear of pregnancy is reduced.

76. C

Teens are good candidates for OCPs because the medical and social risks of pregnancy are great. Teens need special education regarding OCPs because there are many circulating misconceptions. OCPs need to be used on a daily basis to prevent unintended pregnancy. Teens may not understand the importance of daily use. They may also stop contraception for minor side effects such as the nausea or spotting. Discussing the side effects thoroughly will improve compliance. The pill will not provide pregnancy protection immediately. Protection usually starts 7 days from the initiation of OCPs, and only if the pills were started in the first half of the cycle. Most clinicians will recommend a barrier method for the first month in order to be certain that pregnancy will not occur. Barrier methods include condoms, diaphragm, and spermicides. The other statements are true of OCPs.

77. E

The lowest expected pregnancy rate is 0.1 per 100 women-years for OCPs and 0.2 to 0.5 per 100 women-years for tubal ligation. Most women do not have perfect (theoretical) use and the actual use effectiveness is 4 to 5 pregnancies per 100 women. Without any contraception, 85% of women will become pregnant in any given year. Skipping pills or taking them at different times of day are examples of actual use and are both causes of decreased effectiveness. Other methods that have similar effectiveness include depomedroxyprogesterone acetate (Depo-Provera) and intrauterine devices with the added advantage that theoretical and actual use are similar. The theoretical effectiveness of barrier methods is 2 to 3 pregnancies per 100 women-years.

78. C

Amenorrhea is the most common side effect of DMPA, with over 80% of women becoming amenorrheic after 5 years of use. Other side effects include irregular or breakthrough bleeding, which occurs in 50% of women in early use. A benefit of DMPA is that the perfect use and typical use are the same and result in only 0.3% pregnancy use per year. The rate for typical use of oral contraceptive pills is 4% to 5%. The average length to return to fertility is 5 to 8 months after DMPA, but it can take 1 year. The estrogenic component of OCPs is associated with vascular headaches and therefore DMPA is unlikely to contribute to migraines. In addition, women with seizure disorder can experience a reduction in seizure frequency.

79. B

Fifty percent of women will have breakthrough bleeding during the early months on DMPA. Irregular and unpredictable menses are the most common reason women discontinue DMPA use. Women should be counseled about this common side effect prior to initiation. Because DMPA does not contain estrogen, it does not increase the risk of MI, stroke, or other thromboembolic diseases. DMPA may be associated with bone loss and may put long-term users at increased risk for osteoporosis. This risk is further increased if the patient is a smoker. Women gain an average of 3 to 5 lbs per year on an ongoing basis while using DMPA, with the mean being 13.8 lbs after 4 years of use.

80. D

Menorrhagia and dysmenorrhea are relative contraindications to copper IUD use. Both of these conditions can be worsened by copper IUD use, although the cramping and heavy flow tend to subside after the first several cycles. One benefit of the copper IUD is that it is nonhormonal, and women who have not tolerated other hormonal methods of contraception can usually use this one successfully. Contraception occurs because both tubal and uterine transport of sperm are diminished. The IUD also alters the endometrial lining and the copper component may be toxic to the sperm as well. Contrary to popular belief, the copper IUD prevents fertilization. Women who have copper allergy or Wilson's disease may not use the copper IUD.

81. A

Active cervical infections and PID are two absolute contraindications to use of an IUD. Other absolute contraindications are anatomic uterine abnormalities, recurrent PID, and pregnancy. If the copper IUD is used, then copper allergy is also a contraindication. Women with a past history of chlamydia or risk factors for sexually transmitted diseases should be cautioned prior to the placement of an IUD, but it is not an absolute contraindication. Women should be counseled carefully about the risks of PID with an IUD in place and advised on using condoms for protection. Other precautions include HIV disease, nulliparity, abnormal vaginal bleeding of unknown etiology, and previous problems with IUDs.

82. A

Unlike hormonal methods of contraception, the only contraindications to barrier methods are latex allergy and inability to use the products correctly. Male condoms are usually made of latex but are also made of polyurethane and lambskin; however, lambskin does not offer protection from STDs and there is still not enough clinical experience with polyurethane to know if it will protect from infections. The diaphragm requires a fitting from a physician and some women may be unable to learn proper insertion technique. It will not offer effective STD protection and may increase the rate of urinary tract infections. A major benefit is that it may be placed up to 6 hours before intercourse, thereby improving spontaneity. The cervical cap also requires a prescription and is more difficult to place than a diaphragm. It has some of the same side effects and precautions as a diaphragm, but its main advantage is that spermicidal jelly does not need to be reapplied for repeat intercourse. It may be left in place for up to 48 hours.

83. B

Oral contraceptive pills are the most common form of emergency contraception. Other forms include inserting an IUD, high-dose estrogen regimens, and high-dose progesterone. Effectiveness diminishes with increasing time from intercourse. It should not be taken more than 72 hours after unprotected intercourse. The patient should be sure that she is not already pregnant prior to use and she should have a negative urine HCG. Women who are 42 days past the first day of the last menstrual period have a high likelihood of being pregnant. Women should be counseled about not relying on this form of contraception, and if appropriate, they should be counseled on other methods.

84. E

Emergency contraception in the form of oral contraceptive pills needs to be used within 72 hours of unprotected intercourse. The patient should be sure that she is not already pregnant prior to use and she should have a negative urine HCG. Women who are 42 days past the first day of the last menstrual period have a high likelihood of being pregnant. When educating women, let them know that the sooner the pills are taken after unintended sexual intercourse, the more effective they are at preventing pregnancy. The prevention rate is 75% to 88% of pregnancies. Because of the high-dose estrogen in combination OCPs, nausea is a very common side effect.

85. C

The Bethesda system does not differentiate between HPV changes and CIN 1. LGSIL on Pap correlates well with HPV changes or CIN 1 seen on histology at the time of biopsy. The Bethesda system was initially developed in 1988 and modified in 1991 as a means to better correlate cytology with pathology and to provide a more consistent way to report abnormalities. The report will contain comments about the specimen's adequacy; a category of abnormality such as normal, benign cellular changes, squamous, or glandular cell abnormalities; and a description of the abnormality, such as reactive or dysplastic. Overall sensitivity of the Pap smear is higher than 80% and false negatives are usually due to sampling error by the physician or screening error by the technician. Sensitivity improves with higher grade lesions. LGSIL, including CIN 1, has a high rate of regression back to normal and does not necessarily constitute a cancer precursor. LEEP is not indicated in this patient. See Table 4.5.

Table 4.5 Bethesda system

Adequacy of specimen
Satisfactory for evaluation
Satisfactory for evaluation but limited by (SBLB): no endocervical cell, inadequate history provided
Unsatisfactory for evaluation, specify reason

Descriptive diagnosis
Within normal limits
Benign cellular changes (BCC)
Infection: Trichomonas vaginalis, Candida, Coccobacili c/w shift in vaginal flora, Actinomycese species, HSV
Inflammatory changes, except cellular changes of HPV infections
Epithelial cell abnormalities
Squamous cell
ASCUS: borderline changes more reactive than definitive
LSIL: borderline changes including HPV, mild dysplasia, CIN 1
HSIL: moderate dysplasia or CIN 2 severe dysplasia or CIN 3, and CIS, +/− HPV changes
Squamous cell carcinoma: cancer or invasive
Glandular cell
Endometrial cells, cytological benign in a post menopausal woman—endometrial hyperplasia or cancer
AGCUS (atypical glandular cells of undetermined significance): borderline cells between reactive changes to premalignant/malignant process
ACIS: adenocarcinoma in situ
Adenocarcinoma: endocervical suggesting adenocarcinoma or ACIS, endometrial suggesting possible endometrial cancer, extrauterine that could be from vagina, ovary, tube, or metastatic
Other malignant neoplasms: small cell carcinoma, melanoma, lymphoma, sarcoma, etc.
Hormonal evaluation (vaginal smears only): hormonal pattern compatible or incompatible with age and history
Hormonal pattern incompatible with age and history: specify
Hormonal evaluation not possible due to: specify

---

86. D

The U.S. Task Force on Preventive Services and the American Academy of Family Physicians recommend that cervical cancer screening be performed on all women within 3 years of initial sexual activity or age 21, whichever comes first. If a patient has had three consecutive normal Pap smears and is low risk, she may be screened on a 2- or 3-year interval. However, annual screening is recommended for women with high risk factors for cervical cancer, which are considered sex prior to age of 20 years, two or more sexual partners in her lifetime, having a male partner who has had multiple partners, a history of a Pap smear abnormality, or immunosuppression. Pap smears are not effective in detecting the presence of endometrial abnormality, but they are very sensitive and specific for high-grade cervical lesions. The liquid cytologic Paps do increase sensitivity, but they do so by finding more low-grade lesions. This technology is not cost-effective for low-risk women (2).

87. D

There are currently two FDA-approved progesterone-containing IUDs on the market. The Progestasert (Alza Pharmaceuticals)

releases progesterone over the course of 1 year. The Mirena (Berlex Laboratories) contains levonorgestrel and is left in place for 5 years. Contraception occurs, as with a copper IUD, because uterine and tubal motility is decreased. In addition, the progesterone will cause anovulation, thicken cervical mucus, and alter the endometrium. For this reason, it is beneficial in women who have heavy periods or who would like an IUD but do not wish to have dysmenorrhea. The contraceptive rate is similar for both types of IUDs. The risk of ectopic pregnancy is increased with the Progestasert for unknown reasons. The rate of ectopic pregnancy with the T Cu-380A is 0.25 per 1,000 women-years, compared to Progestasert's rate of 4 or 5 per 1,000 women-years.

88. B

There is a correlation between when mothers and daughters experience menopause. Women during the perimenopausal years actually have higher levels of estrogen, probably due to the ovarian follicular response to elevating levels of FSH. Only 10% of women cease menstruating abruptly. Most women will experience several years of increasing anovulation leading up to menopause.

Since ovulation still does occur, it is necessary to consider the possible need for birth control.

89. A

The use of oral contraceptives until menopause has been found to be safe in women with no risk factors for cardiovascular disease. Since hypertension, hypercholesterolemia, and smoking are all risk factors for cardiovascular disease, oral contraceptives should be avoided in women having these conditions. If menorrhagia has been a problem due to fibroids, an oral contraceptive may be helpful in reducing the amount of bleeding. It will not alter the size of the fibroids but may make her symptoms better.

90. B

Hot flashes are characterized by a sudden reddening of the skin followed by an intense feeling of heat and sometimes conclude with profuse perspiration. They occur most frequently at night and can interfere with sleep. Ten percent to 25% of women will begin to have hot flashes perimenopausally. The hot flash is believed to originate in the hypothalamus. Many remedies have been tried, and the most effective treatment is estrogen replacement or phytoestrogen supplementation. Other nonhormonal treatments are also under investigation. Currently, the serotonin reuptake inhibitor class (SSRI) has the greatest evidence for altering hot flashes. Several studies show a 50% to 75% reduction in the perception of hot flashes. Wearing cooler clothing does not alter hot flashes. Thyroid replacement would not only be ineffective for this patient but also be dangerous because her TSH demonstrates appropriate thyroid function. Clonidine has been used in the past because it reduces vascular reactivity. However, several trials show no improvement over placebo, and nausea, depression, fatigue, and headaches limit its tolerability. Dong qui is a Chinese herb that is prescribed for menopause, but it has no proven effect on hot flashes.

91. E

The endometrial biopsy provides an adequate method of sampling the endometrial lining to identify histologic abnormalities. It is used to identify diffuse problems of the endometrium, such as hyperplasia. There is always a risk of sampling error since it is done blindly. This is increased if the lesion is discrete. If a patient with a high pretest probability of an abnormality has a negative biopsy, further evaluation should be pursued. Since the endometrial polyp is a discrete lesion, it is best identified either by pelvic ultrasound, especially sonohysterography, or by hysteroscopy.

92. C

Endometrial hyperplasia is an overgrowth of the glandular epithelium of the endometrial lining. This usually occurs when a patient is exposed to unopposed estrogen, either iatrogenically or because of anovulation. Most patients without atypia will respond to progestin therapy. If the patient is receiving estrogen therapy and she has a uterus, progesterone must be added, either continuously or cyclically. If the hyperplasia is due to anovulation, such as occurs during perimenopause, a combined estrogen–progesterone supplement will help prevent further endometrial changes.

93. C

The risk of endometrial hyperplasia progression is related to the presence and severity of atypia. Overall, the rate of progression for complex hyperplasia with atypia is about 30%. Therefore, patients having complex hyperplasia with atypia should have a hysterectomy due to the high incidence of subsequent endometrial cancer. Progestin therapy can be used to treat endometrial hyperplasia without atypia, but it is less effective for those patients displaying atypia. Progestin therapy can be used in patients who refuse hysterectomy due to fertility concerns.

94. D

She needs further evaluation with a transvaginal ultrasound and/or an endometrial biopsy. Endometrial cancer most often presents as postmenopausal bleeding in the sixth and seventh decades, although only 10% of patients with postmenopausal bleeding when investigated will have endometrial cancer. Uterine cancer is the fourth most common cancer in women. Risk factors for endometrial cancer include nulliparity, late menopause (after age 52 years), obesity, diabetes, unopposed estrogen therapy, tamoxifen, and a history of atypical endometrial hyperplasia.

95. E

The patient does have multiple risk factors for ectopic pregnancy, including her history of herpes, multiple sexual partners, and cigarette smoking. Factors associated with high risk for ectopic pregnancy include fallopian tube surgery, tubal sterilization, previous ectopic pregnancy, DES exposure in utero, IUD use, and documented tubal pathology. Factors associated with a moderately increased risk include technology-assisted pregnancies, previous genital infections, and multiple sexual partners. Prior abdominal or pelvic surgery, cigarette smoking, vaginal douching, and early age at first intercourse are also associated with a slight increase in risk. Smoking may confer risk through ciliary dysfunction in the fallopian tubes, similar to the ciliary dysfunction in the respiratory system. It is important to remember that more than 50% of women presenting with an ectopic pregnancy do not give a history of any risk factors.

96. A

BHCG is produced by the trophoblastic cells of the developing embryo. In a normal intrauterine pregnancy, BHCG doubling time ranges from 1.5 days in early pregnancy to 3.5 days at 7 weeks gestation. Both ectopic pregnancies and abnormal intrauterine pregnancies (IUPs) have impaired HCG production with prolonged doubling times. Thus, serial quantitative measurements of BHCG concentrations can be helpful in distinguishing normal IUPs from abnormal IUPs and ectopics. Serial measurements are performed at 48-hour intervals. Pregnancies that demonstrate a greater than 66% increase in 48 hours likely represent ectopics or IUPs that are likely to abort. A consistently declining BHCG level generally indicates a nonviable pregnancy. Nearly all ectopic pregnancies are associated with a BHCG level of less than 50,000 mIU/mL, so a level above 50,000 can help to exclude the diagnosis of ectopic pregnancy. High-frequency transvaginal scanners are capable of reliably detecting an IUP when BHCG levels range from 1,000 to 2,000 mIU/mL (approximately 5 weeks gestation). Therefore, repeating an ultrasound when the BHCG level reaches this range is often helpful.

97. E

Disorders of desire are common, although physicians often do not elicit them. Multiple factors are involved, but lifestyle, relationships, and the level of intimacy and comfort are clearly the most important factors in a woman's desire. Depression can play a role in decreased libido, but it causes only a small fraction of the problem. No study has ever shown hormone levels to be directly related to libido, and survey studies of postmenopausal women demonstrate that sexual functioning is mainly dependent on a patient's physical well-being and on her relationship's health. Estrogen is involved in the health of the vaginal mucosa and the surrounding tissues. There is benefit in local estrogen if the sexual problem is related to vaginal or vulvar atrophy causing dysperunia. Testosterone has long been touted as a cure for libido. It is involved in the female sexual response, but no long-term studies have evaluated its effectiveness or safety if given as a supplement. This is an area that has not received the proper scientific attention and much research needs to be done.

98. B
Dysmenorrhea or painful menstruation can be classified as primary or secondary, with primary being defined as painful menses in the absence of pelvic disease and secondary being the occurrence of painful menstruation caused by pelvic disease. Patients with primary dysmenorrhea report a history of intermittent, cramping, lower abdominal pain, which is usually most intense on the first day of menses and may last up to 3 days. Accompanying symptoms may include headache, back pain, upper thigh pain, vomiting, nausea, diarrhea, and asthma exacerbation. All are mediated by prostaglandin release from the degenerating endometrium. Secondary dysmenorrhea has its onset after 20 years of age, with pain lasting for 5 to 7 days, and is usually without the accompanying symptoms described in the question. Premenstrual syndrome is a cluster of affective, cognitive, and physical symptoms that occurs before the onset of menses.

99. C
History and physical are the key elements in diagnosing primary dysmenorrhea. A cervical smear and GC/chlamydia test should be performed on all patients presenting with dysmenorrhea. A CBC and ESR would be appropriate to help detect chronic, underlying infection or inflammation if secondary dysmenorrhea was suspected. Pelvic ultrasound is appropriate only in patients who have abnormal findings on pelvic exam or who have not responded to therapy for primary dysmenorrhea. Because dysmenorrhea is associated with ovulatory cycles, it does not present with menarche but only later, as eggs are released on a consistent basis. Treatment is usually aimed at blocking prostaglandin, which is the cause of the dysmenorrhea, with prescription-strength NSAIDs.

100. B
The most common cause of primary amenorrhea with absent breast development and normal pelvic exam is hypothalamic dysfunction. This may indeed be a cause for "late blooming." Also to be considered is gonadal failure due to either Turner's syndrome or a primary ovarian disease. A patient with an imperforate hymen would likely have normal breast development and complain of monthly symptoms associated with menstruation. In addition, she would have abdominal pain due to the hematocolpos. A patient with a thyroid disorder would likely have normal breast development and may report symptoms associated with hypo- or hyperthyroidism. A patient with testicular feminization would have abnormal findings on pelvic exam, such as absence of all pubic and axillary hair and a short, blind vagina. Prolactinoma is a rare cause of delayed maturation and menses. A serum prolactin level should be drawn to evaluate this possibility.

101. D
Grave's disease and other primary thyroid disorders do not cause hypothalamic failure. However, many other disorders are associated with hypothalamic failure. Causes include constitutional delay ("late bloomer"), anorexia nervosa, protein malnutrition, extreme sports training, substance abuse, and GnRH absence. Hypothalamic failure should always be suspected as the cause of primary amenorrhea if a girl of 14 or 15 years of age does not develop breast tissue. A simple examination or ultrasound can determine if the internal organs are intact. If they are, the delay is almost certainly due to a hypothalamic disorder. Less commonly, the pituitary gland may also be involved as with Sheehan syndrome (pituitary destruction following shock), panhypopituitarianism, isolated gonadotropin deficiency (LH and FSH), and hemosiderosis usually occurring due to thalassemia major.

102. B
Primary amenorrhea occurs in girls who are 14 years old and have had no menses as well as no secondary sexual characteristic development or in girls who are 16 years old and have had no menses. Treatment involves identifying and addressing the underlying cause. Breast development or thelarchy occurs 2 years before menarche, which is why workup can begin at 14 years if a girl has no secondary sexual characteristics, such as breast development or pubic or axillary hair. A physician can evaluate secondary sexual characteristics even prior to a full pelvic exam. Simple blood work consisting of thyroid-stimulating hormone and prolactin levels, along with a pregnancy test, can be performed. In addition, the patient's lifestyle should be evaluated for exercise, eating habits, emotional stress, and drugs of abuse. Medications should also be reviewed. All these areas may prove to be the cause of the amenorrhea and are amenable to treatment.

103. D
While visualizing an intrauterine pregnancy virtually rules out an ectopic pregnancy, the finding of free fluid or an adnexal mass is highly suggestive of the diagnosis; a pelvic ultrasound may not be able to visualize either an early intrauterine or ectopic pregnancy. The most important information at this point is the quantitative BHCG level. Once above 1,800 mIU/mL IRP (International Reference Preparation), the "zone of discrimination," a gestational sac should be visualized on transvaginal sonogram. Below this level, a repeat BHCG can be done in 48 hours and should demonstrate a rise of at least 66% if the pregnancy is viable. A failure to rise 66% in 48 hours suggests the possibility of a nonviable or ectopic pregnancy. With a normally rising BHCG, a repeat ultrasound can be obtained once the BHCG is above 1,800 mIU/mL IRP. A BHCG above 1,800 mIU/mL IRP with an empty uterus on ultrasound suggests ectopic pregnancy. A single serum progesterone level may also be useful. A level above 25 ng/mL suggests a viable pregnancy, whereas a single level below 5 ng/mL suggests a nonviable or ectopic pregnancy. Early diagnosis of ectopic pregnancy is important because it results in decreased mortality and preserved fertility. Management of ectopic pregnancy is most commonly via laparoscopic surgery, but in early cases it might include medical management with methotrexate or expectant management if the BHCG is very low and falling. Dilation and curettage is used in some cases to distinguish between ectopic pregnancy and miscarriage.

104. B
Barrier methods are excellent choices for contraception but have lower rates of efficacy than hormonal or surgical methods. Some of the decrease in efficacy occurs because they are user dependent and require patient skill and commitment. Although nonoxynol 9 was

initially thought to provide superior protection from sexually transmitted diseases, including HIV and gonorrhea, the incidence of vaginal irritation and mucosal breakdown is now well documented. This breakdown is actually associated with an increased risk of contracting HIV, and current recommendations are to avoid condoms with nonoxynol 9. Efficacy rates for pregnancy prevention with use of spermicide alone range from 5% to 50%, making it a poor contraceptive choice. Polyurethane condoms are indicated for men and women with latex allergy. They appear equally effective at preventing pregnancy as regular condoms, but they are very expensive and have a higher rate of breakage (approximately 8%). The diaphragm is associated with increased rates of *Escherichia coli* colonization, which is cause for the increase in urinary tract infection rates in women users. The cervical cap becomes less effective with parity. One of the benefits of the female sponge is that it can be used for repeated intercourse. Currently off the market, it is due to return with a new manufacturer. Concerns are being raised about the presence of nonoxynol 9 in the sponge and whether the prolonged contact with vaginal mucosa can increase the risk of HIV.

105. A

Condoms are effective at preventing those STDs that are spread by fluids and mucosal surfaces. These infections include gonorrhea, chlamydia, HIV, and trichomonas. Because the condom does not cover all of the pubic skin, STDs such as HPV, syphilis, herpes simplex virus (HSV), chancroid, lice, and crabs may still be transmitted. It is important to advise your patients that condoms do not prevent all STDs.

106. A

Abnormal Pap smears occur in 5% of pregnancies. Most of the Paps are reported as LGSIL or ASCUS. Invasive cancer is very rare in pregnancy, with an incidence ranging from 0.4% to 0.012%. Despite the relative immunosuppression of pregnancy, the majority of cases of LGSIL (and even HGSIL) will regress spontaneously in the postpartum period. Approximately 20% of patients will have persistent CIN 1 changes and only 10% will progress to HGSIL. Therefore, LGSIL is not considered a true cancer precursor. Pap smear abnormalities need to be confirmed by colposcopy with directed biopsy prior to treatment. Because cytology can be false negative up to 50% of the time, colposcopy is indicated, even in pregnant patients. Colposcopy should be done early in pregnancy. Biopsies can be performed, but bleeding will be more significant than in nonpregnant women. Endocervical curettage is not done in pregnancy.

107. B

Roughly one-third of biopsy-proven HGSIL will proceed to invasive cervical cancer and HGSIL is considered a true cancer precursor. Because of this, observation or treatment with cryotherapy is inadequate. These patients should be referred for a LEEP. In most populations, there should be fewer cases of HGSIL than LGSIL reported on Pap smears. LGSIL is equivalent to the histologic term CIN 1 and HPV changes, whereas HGSIL encompasses CIN 2, CIN 3, and CIS.

108. C

Pap smears are screening tests and, therefore, abnormalities need to be confirmed by a diagnostic test such as colposcopy with directed biopsy prior to treatment. Although cervical cancer can occasionally present as ASCUS on Pap smear, most women with ASCUS on their Pap smears do not have cervical cancer. Multiple infections including those from HPV or chlamydia can cause ASCUS Pap smears. HPV typing is an effective method of triaging Pap smears with ASCUS. Patients with ASCUS with high-risk virus serotypes should be evaluated with colposcopy, whereas those patients with low-risk virus serotypes can have Pap smear surveillance. If the Pap smear returns to normal, the patient may be returned to annual screening.

109. D

This is an inappropriate way to manage patients with ASCUS. Most algorithms recommend repeat Pap smears every 4 to 6 months, but if any of the repeat Paps are abnormal the patient should be referred for colposcopy. Newer technology allows patients to be tested for the presence of not only HPV but also the subtype. This newer triage method can allow patients with oncogenic subtypes to undergo immediate colposcopy and allow patients with low-risk subtypes to continue receiving Pap smear observation. Studies now prove that empiric metronidazole does not "improve" a Pap smear or clarify triage. In addition, if a diagnosed infection is present, then treatment and re-Pap are appropriate. At that time, if the results are abnormal, colposcopy is appropriate. Acceptable methods for the management of ASCUS include all of the other choices, although recent data suggest that reflex HPV testing may be the most cost-effective.

110. C

AGUS is associated with a high probability of finding a high-grade lesion or even preinvasive and invasive cancer. In 20% to 50% of cases, a significant lesion is found on colposcopy and biopsy. ASCUS is associated with a significant lesion only 5% to 15% of the time. AGUS smears can represent an abnormality from the endometrium, endocervix, or ectocervix. Immediate colposcopy with biopsy, endocervical curettage, and endometrial biopsy (depending on age) is indicated. If the source of the AGUS is not found, a cone biopsy of the cervix is warranted. Studies show that doctors tend to overmanage ASCUS but do not employ an aggressive enough approach to AGUS.

111. C

Cervical cancer rates have dramatically decreased in the United States and other developed countries due to screening and precancer treatment. Cervical cancer continues to kill many women in developing countries, and it is still the second leading cancer diagnosis worldwide in women. We now know that cervical cancer is associated with high-risk HPV serotypes such as 16, 18, 31, and 33. Also associated with cervical cancer are smoking, low socioeconomic status, other sexually transmitted diseases, and more than two lifetime sexual partners. The diagnosis of cervical cancer in the United States occurs most frequently in women who have not been adequately screened with Pap smears, such as indigent women, African Americans, Hispanics, and women older than the age of 65. Sixty percent of women with invasive cervical cancer have not had a Pap smear in the past 5 years. Although sensitivity is limited, usually by obscuring inflammation, specificity of the Pap smear for cervical cancer is excellent and the patient should be managed aggressively. False-negative rates are between 10% and 15%, but false positives are unlikely. CIS is still a premalignant histologic diagnosis because the cellular abnormality has not crossed the basal membrane.

112. E

Seventy-five percent of women with ovarian cancer are diagnosed at an advanced stage, with a 5-year survival of less than 30%.

These sobering statistics make early detection crucial to survival. Unfortunately, a standard screening protocol has not yet been defined for patients with a strong family history suggesting genetic predisposition to developing ovarian cancer. Women with BRCA-1 and BRCA-2 mutations have a 40% to 60% chance of developing cancer in their lifetime, and women with a high incidence of ovarian cancer in their family should be tested for this mutation. Those who are positive can elect for prophylactic oophorectomy. If these women choose to delay this procedure, screening with both CA-125 and transvaginal ultrasonography becomes important. The screening intervals have not been determined. These tests have proved inadequate in sensitivity, specificity, and positive predictive value for early detection in the general population; thus, they are not recommended for widespread screening.

113. D

The American Cancer Society also recommends clinical breast examination every 3 years starting at age 20, then yearly when the patient turns 40. Monthly self breast exam should also begin at age 20. Women with a family history of BRCA gene mutation should begin annual mammography screening between ages 25 and 35. Patients with a palpable breast mass not detected by mammogram should be evaluated thoroughly with ultrasound and needle biopsy.

114. E

The object of Kegel's pelvic muscle exercises is to rehabilitate or strengthen the pelvic floor muscles and improve resting urethral tone. This can better be achieved through the use of biofeedback devices such as vaginal weights or pelvic floor electrical stimulating devices. Unfortunately, electrical stimulation devices are not commonly covered by third-party provider insurance. Occlusive devices such as pessaries, urethral plugs, and urethral stents prevent loss of urine, but plugs and stents are not widely accepted by patients. Estrogen replacement can cause thickening of the urethral mucosa, and pseudoephedrine, an alpha-adrenergic drug, can increase resting urethral tone. If these methods fail, standard surgical procedures, such as retropubic urethropexies or suburethral slings, or minimally invasive procedures, such as the tension free vaginal tape (minimally invasive suburethral sling) or periurethral injections of collagen or carbon-coated beads, are good options.

115. A

Pelvic floor muscle exercises are specific for stress incontinence and are not recommended unless full evaluation suggests that is the cause. Estrogen replacement therapy, however, is useful in the management of overactive bladder as well as stress incontinence, and it may be started empirically. The 24-hour record is essential to assessing triggers such as caffeine and severity of the incontinence. Urinary tract infection is the most common, easily treatable cause of urge incontinence, and it must be ruled out in every case. A post-void residual urine, obtained by catheterization after the patient urinates, can be useful to diagnose overflow incontinence, hematuria, chronic urinary tract infections, and kidney or metabolic abnormalities.

116. D

Cervical ectropion is a nonpathologic finding that appears as a red velvety, well-demarcated area on the ectocervix. It is commonly seen in teenagers, pregnant women, and women taking oral contraceptives. Ectropion is often accompanied by an increased clear cervical discharge due to the exposed, mucous-producing, glandular epithelium. It can sometimes be confused with chronic cervicitis, but the latter would appear more reddened, with denuded epithelium, and be accompanied by a mucopurulent discharge. DES adenosis is a developmental birth defect seen in women who were exposed to DES in utero and is characterized by glandular tissue on the cervix and vaginal walls. This can undergo malignant transformation. Since DES was prescribed between 1940 and 1970, this patient, who is 17 years old in 2002, would not have been exposed.

117. A

Although the majority of cervical polyps are benign, carcinomatous change (most often adenocarcinoma or squamous cell carcinoma) has been reported to occur in 1.7% of cases. Suspicion should be heightened in patients with polyps that present with bleeding or increased vaginal discharge. All polyps that are removed should be sent for pathology to detect these rare cancers. Most cervical polyps can be removed in the office with no local anesthesia since there is little or no pain associated with removal. Some patients report mild cramping, which is best treated with NSAIDs. Benign polyps may be friable, leading to spotting after intercourse or tampon use. Particularly large or friable polyps can be considered for removal in the operating room due to concerns about excessive bleeding. Polyps as large as 17 × 10 × 5 cm have been reported, but the majority are less than 5 cm in length.

118. C

The IUD is one of the most effective forms of birth control on the market, equaling or exceeding the success rate of tubal ligation. It has been used for many years as the primary form of birth control throughout the world, although is used by less than 1% of women in the United States due to negative perceptions on the part of physicians and patients. These perceptions are held over from the 1970s when several forms of IUDs (i.e., the Dalcon shield), which are no longer in use, were associated with elevated rates of PID. The copper IUD is approved for 10 years of continuous use and can be inserted immediately postpartum, although expulsion rates are lower if insertion is delayed until 6 to 8 weeks postpartum. There are no indications that IUDs are associated with infertility, and return of fertility has been documented within hours of removal.

119. D

Any woman with multiple sexual partners, endometritis, purulent cervicitis, or sexually transmitted disease within the 3 months prior is at increased risk of infection due to her exposures and is not a good candidate for IUD placement at that time. The copper IUD alters sperm motility as well as ovum and sperm interaction by causing an inflammatory response in the endometrium. The increase in tubal and uterine fluids can lead to a change in the amount and character of cervical mucous but should not be reported as mucopurulent or foul smelling. The IUD itself does not cause PID, and it is not associated with an increased risk of infection outside the first few weeks of insertion.

120. D

Depo-Provera users gain an average of 5.4 lbs after 1 year of use, 8.1 lbs after 2 years of use, and 13.8 lbs after 4 years of use. Although progesterones can cause some fluid retention, the primary etiology is likely an increased appetite. The most important thing for patients to realize is that the weight gain is avoidable if they maintain the eating habits they had before starting the medication. There is no evidence that use of injectable progesterone slows the metabolism, although a decrease in glucose tolerance has been observed, necessitating close observation of diabetic patients receiving this therapy.

121. B

This is a typical scenario for HSV 2. Over 50 million Americans have HSV 2. Clinical diagnosis is difficult and does not distinguish between HSV 1 and HSV 2, which is important for prognosis. A viral culture is the gold standard, but the ability to obtain viral particles diminishes rapidly as the lesion heals. In this patient, there would not be any virus to culture. Likewise, cytology, in the form of Pap smears or Tzank preps, is nonspecific and unlikely to be positive once healing starts. New-generation serology enzyme-linked immunosorbent assay tests can detect HSV 2 antibodies with a sensitivity of 80% to 98%, but false negatives can occur, especially early in the initial infection. Specificity is 96%. If confirmation is needed, an immunoblot assay can be performed. It is important to counsel patients that condoms do not protect against certain STDs, such as HSV and HPV. With HSV 2, the initial outbreak is usually worse than subsequent outbreaks. HSV 1 can occur in the genital mucosa but has a much lower likelihood of reoccurring than HSV 2. Many patients describe a prodromal period before the eruption of vesicles that includes itching and pain. When evaluating this patient, an HSV antibody and serologic screen for syphilis should be obtained because HSV and syphilis can coexist in approximately 5% of lesions. Approximately 20% of Americans are positive for HSV 2, and more than 60% are positive for HSV 1.

122. C

Both the Heart and Estrogen/Progestin Replacement Study and the Women's Health Initiative (WHI) provided substantive evidence that the risks of combination HRT are greater than previously thought. The additional risk to an individual woman is still small for each disease state, as can be seen by showing the increase per 10,000 women for each disease state:

- An additional 8 cases of invasive breast cancer per 10,000 women
- An additional 7 heart attacks per 10,000 women
- An additional 18 blood clots per 10,000 women
- An additional 8 pulmonary emboli per 10,000 women

These studies also showed benefits of combination therapy to include a 34% reduction in hip fractures, a 37% reduction in colorectal cancer, and a 24% reduction in total fractures. There was no difference in the mortality rates between the treated and non-treated groups. These results were seen after 5 years of therapy, making it impossible to comment on the effects of shorter term combination therapy. Combination therapy may still be a very appropriate short-term therapy for women with perimenopausal symptoms. The important message is that we must educate our patients about the risks and benefits and allow them to make an educated decision based on their values and comorbidities.

123. C

The studies mentioned previously apply only to combination therapy. WHI does have an estrogen-only arm, which did not show the statistically significant negative outcomes evident in the combination therapy arm. The jury is still out on whether patients in the estrogen-only category may be able to reap the benefits of estrogen without the adverse affects seen with combination therapy greater

than 5 years. It is well documented that estrogen helps to protect against postmenopausal bone loss.

124. C

The other answers need to be considered as possible causes, but none of them match the history to indicate PID. Cervicitis would usually include a friable cervix and mucopurulent discharge. PID is the result of an ascending bacterial infection. The most common causative agents are *Neisseria gonorrhea* and *Chlamydial trachomatis*. Retrograde menstruation is thought to play a role in the ascension of infection. Serious sequelae include infertility, tubo-ovarian abscess, and later higher risk of ectopic pregnancy.

125. C

The patient must be evaluated for ectopic pregnancy immediately. The next step would be to admit the patient for parenteral treatment secondary to high risk of maternal and fetal morbidity. The choice of antibiotics can be narrowed to what is safe in pregnancy. Tetracyclines, which include doxycycline, and quinolones are contraindicated due to teratogenicity. The tetracycline family causes fetal bone and tooth abnormalities and maternal liver toxicity that is different from fatty liver of pregnancy. Although the quinolones have not been definitely proven to be teratogenic, there is concern over cartilaginous formation in fetuses exposed.

126. C

Nausea, breast tenderness, and vascular headaches are all estrogen-mediated side effects. Acne, weight gain, and hirsuitism are androgen related. Breakthrough bleeding can be linked to the ratio of estrogen-to-progesterone. Early cycle breakthrough bleeding usually requires more estrogen, whereas late cycle breakthrough bleeding requires more progesterone.

127. C

Endometriosis can be seen in 20% to 75% of women who are part of an infertile couple. The true incidence of endometriosis is not known because it requires surgery to diagnose. It is estimated that 20% of women with pelvic pain have endometriosis. In this situation, the couple has been trying to conceive for an extended period of time. A full evaluation of all causes of infertility should be performed, after which laparoscopic surgical excision or laser ablation is the treatment for endometriosis and infertility. Although a trial of OCP or Lupron may treat the pain, these would not improve rates of conception. Medication may help establish a presumptive diagnosis, but in a couple attempting to conceive, surgical evaluation and treatment is necessary.

128. E

Functional ovarian cysts are a normal occurrence during the menstrual cycle. Usually growing between 2 and 3 cm, the follicular cyst forms during the first half of the cycle and regresses upon ovulation. The corpus luteum cyst then takes over and can persist past the typical 2-week luteal phase. The above functional cyst has likely had some bleeding into it, which gives it the appearance of complex cyst. The cyst should be evaluated with serial ultrasound. If the cyst persists beyond 9 weeks, surgical evaluation should be sought to rule out ovarian cancer.

129. D

Many common medications can be associated with galactorrhea. A patient must be questioned carefully about use of prescription, over-the-counter, and recreational drugs to ascertain whether this may be the etiology of his or her galactorrhea. Common medications that can cause galactorrhea include phenothiazines, estrogen, alpha methyldopa, metoclopramide, TCAs, SSRIs, opiates, and cimetidine. The etiology of galactorrhea has a large differential diagnosis. Most galactorrhea is idiopathic, but medications can cause 20% of cases. Physiologic milk production can occur due to pregnancy, adolescent hormone fluctuations, or breast stimulation. Irritation of the breast or chest wall from ill-fitting undergarments, herpes zoster, or even burns can incite galactorrhea. Neoplasia, most commonly intracranial, should also be considered in the etiology. Systemic illnesses such as hypothyroidism, renal failure, and Cushing's disease are rare but possible causes.

References

1. Wright TC Jr, Cox JT, Massad LS, Twiggs LB, Wilkinson EJ; for the 2001 ASCCP-sponsored consensus conference. 2001 Consensus Guidelines for the Management of Women with Cervical Cytological Abnormalities. *JAMA.* 2002;287: 2120–2129.

2. U.S. Preventive Services Task Force. Screening for cervical cancer: Recommendations and rationale. *Am Fam Physician.* 2003;67(8):1759–1766.

Chapter 5

Psychiatry Questions

1. Regarding U.S. Preventive Services Task Force (USPSTF) recommendations for depression screening in primary care, which is true?

A. The USPSTF recommends routine screening of adults based on fair evidence that it improves outcomes and outweighs risks.

B. The Zung self-assessment depression scale is the best screening device.

C. Positive screening using the Beck depression inventory does not need to be followed by a standard diagnostic interview.

D. Screening for depression is not recommended.

2. The use of benzodiazepines in pregnancy is associated with which of the following?

A. Ebstein's abnormality

B. Failure to thrive

C. Development of attention deficit hyperactivity disorder (ADHD) in child

D. Increased risk of oral clefts

E. Spina bifida

3. The highest rate of illicit drug use is found among individuals of the ages:

A. 16 to 20

B. 21 to 29

C. 30 to 39

D. 51 to 60

E. 61 and older

4. A 34-year-old woman presents with complaints of disturbed sleep due to nightmares, intermittent abdominal pain, rectal pain, diarrhea, dyspareunia, myofascial pain, occasional paresthesias in the hands, occasional panic attacks, and an avoidance of driving 3 months after being in a car crash in which her daughter (a passenger) was killed. Given her most likely diagnosis, which of the following statements is false?

A. Mental status exam is likely to reveal alexithymia (inability to verbalize or identify feeling states), as well as withdrawal and social isolation.

B. Mental status exam is likely to reveal amnesia for various aspects of the traumatic event.

C. Abdominal pain is likely due to a previously overlooked physical internal trauma.

D. This patient is likely to exhibit self-harming behaviors or aggressive behaviors when stressed.

E. Further examination is likely to reveal comorbid psychiatric disorders.

5. A 52-year-old white female is seen in your office after referral from a local ER, for a long history of complaints including multiple burning sensations and excruciating pain in the right foot as well as in the genitals and rectum, and diffuse low back pain. She insists that these symptoms, as well as her GI distress, spastic bladder, and pain with weight bearing, are due to a parasitic infestation. Your medical student notes the presence of "la belle indifference," in that the patient has become unemployed and nearly bedridden yet had to be urged to see a physician by her family. Which of the following is the most likely diagnosis?

A. Schistosomiasis

B. Systemic lupus erythematosis

C. Progressive supranuclear palsy

D. Somatization disorder

E. Multiple sclerosis

6. A true statement concerning competence is:

A. Competence is a medical concept.

B. Refusal of a medically indicated procedure is evidence of incompetence.

C. The presence of psychiatric symptoms is evidence that the patient is incompetent.

D. Competence is a legal concept.

E. Physicians, because of their superior medical knowledge, are the final arbiters of competence.

7. A 45-year-old typist has had symptoms of carpal tunnel unresponsive to conservative therapy. In follow-up to her carpal tunnel release, she describes diffuse burning pain of her limb, hyperesthesia, hyperhidrosis, weakness, and periodic blanching of her limb. You suggest which of the following?

A. That such pain is common following carpal tunnel surgery

B. A trial of a nonsteroidal anti-inflammatory agent

C. Immobilization of the limb

D. Waiting for 3 months and then reassessment

E. A trial of an oral corticosteroid and sympathetic blockade

8. A 22-year-old female patient has had severe, recurrent depression, associated with multiple suicide attempts. She has been stabilized for the past 3 months on sertraline. She tells you she is pregnant. You tell her:

A. Stop your sertraline because of the risk of fetal malformations.

B. Stop the sertraline because of the risk of premature delivery.

C. Add a mood stabilizer, such as lithium.

D. Continue sertraline and carefully monitor for depression.

E. Substitute St. John's Wort for sertraline.

9. True statements concerning the PLISSIT model of sexual counseling includes all of the following *except*:

A. P stands for permission: giving the patient validation and permission to discuss his or her problem.

B. LI stand for limited information concerning sexual health.

C. SS stand for sexual satisfaction: assessing the patient's current satisfaction with his or her sexual role and function.

D. IT stand for intensive therapy: providing therapy for the patient's difficulty.

10. Risk factors for developing alcohol withdrawal include which of the following?

A. Alcohol consumption for less than 1 year

B. Female gender

C. Tremors and anxiety appearing within 8 hours of cessation

D. Absence of other acute medical problems

E. Age younger than 40 years

11. Separation anxiety would be suggested by all of the following symptoms *except*:

A. School avoidance

B. Refusal to go to sleep without the presence of an attachment figure

C. Temper tantrums when parents leave for an evening out

D. Fear that child will be separated from a parent by a kidnapping or accident

E. Running away from a parent at a mall

12. A 76-year-old is hospitalized for pneumonia. The patient has fluctuating levels of attention, changes in awareness, and marked disturbance of the sleep–wake cycle. You initially recommend which of the following?

A. Haldol regularly until symptoms abate

B. Respirdal regularly until symptoms abate

C. Valium to prevent the patient's injury

D. A family member or sitter to regularly sit with the patient

E. Isolation in a quiet, dark room

13. You have successfully treated and maintained a 34-year-old male with major depression and no other health problems on 40 mg of fluoxetine qid for 6 months. He now presents complaining of persistent anorgasmia, which has become a significant problem in his new relationship. All of the following would be possible ways of treating this *except*:

A. Decrease the dose of fluoxetine by 10 to 20 mg a day

B. Prescribe sildenefil (Viagra)

C. Prescribe bupropion in addition to fluoxetine

D. Switch the patient to bupropion only

E. Add mirtazapine in addition to fluoxetine

14. The drug of choice for panic disorder is:

A. Clomipramine

B. Alprazolam

C. Clonazepam

D. Busipirone (Buspar)

E. Any selective serotonin reuptake inhibitor (SSRI)

15. You manage medications for a psychiatrically stable 28 year-old patient with bipolar disorder on lithium 600 mg bid. Besides this patient's regular preventive care, you should be monitoring:

A. CBC, serum creatinine, thyroid-stimulating hormone (TSH), and ECG every 3 months, serum lithium as needed

B. CBC, serum lithium, and serum creatinine every 6 months

C. CBC, serum creatinine, serum lithium, and TSH every 6 months

D. CBC, serum creatinine every 6 months, ECG and TSH every year

E. TSH, serum creatinine, and serum lithium every 6 months

16. A 21-year-old female complains of the inability to have intercourse with her boyfriend due to pain when he attempts penetration. She reports adequate desire and lubrication. A pelvic examination is difficult because the patient complains of discomfort with insertion of the speculum and an examining finger due to spasm of the muscles of the outer vagina. The hymenal ring is not intact. This woman has:

A. Vaginismus

B. Sexual aversion disorder

C. Inhibited female orgasm

D. Hypoactive sexual desire

E. Dyspareunia

17. You are treating a 35-year-old white female with major depression. When taking sertraline (Zoloft) in the past she has experienced sexual dysfunction. Which one of the following antidepressants would be the best alternative?

A. Paroxetine (Paxil)

B. Bupropion (Wellbutrin)

C. Sertraline (Zoloft)

D. Fluoxetine (Prozac)

E. Citalopram (Celexa)

18. A 27-year-old woman comes to your office with the complaint of a creeping, crawling sensation of the legs interfering with sleep. Your management might include all of the following *except*:

A. Evaluation of renal function

B. Evaluation of iron levels

C. EMG

D. Assessment of whether the woman is pregnant

E. Starting her on an SSRI

19. The patient in question 18 has an appropriate evaluation and all testing is normal; you prescribe which of the following?

A. Clonazepam

B. Levo-dopa/carbiodopa (Sinemet)

C. Oxycodone

D. Triazolam

E. Folic acid

20. The least understood phase of the sexual response cycle, which is also likely responsible for the majority of lifetime sexual problems, is the:

A. Refractory stage

B. Desire stage

C. Orgasm stage

D. Arousal stage

E. Plateau stage

21. A 32-year-old married female with a history of Bipolar I disorder, without psychotic features, currently euthymic, presents with her husband to discuss family planning. She does not have a history of dangerous or suicidal behaviors, or drug use while mentally ill. She is currently maintained on 600 mg of lithium bid. Which of the following is true regarding the management of bipolar disorder in pregnancy?

A. Since the need for mood stabilizers greatly decreases during pregnancy, she may consider discontinuing the medication.

B. She should definitely continue the lithium in the first trimester due to the high-risk of relapse during pregnancy.

C. Should she decide to continue the lithium during the first trimester, it should be given in smaller divided doses to avoid high peak plasma levels.

D. The risk of relapse decreases in the postpartum period.

E. She should switch to valproate.

22. A child is most at risk for abuse if he:

A. Was born prematurely

B. Lives in a poor family

C. Is African American

D. Lives in a home where there is partner abuse

E. Lives in a home where alcohol is used regularly

23. A 45-year-old woman with a history of depression reports having symptoms of the flu and increasing irritability. She even reports having slapped her husband during an argument. She states that this type of action is very uncharacteristic of her. This event took place after she discontinued a medication. Which of the following medications might she have been taking?

A. Amitriptyline

B. Bupropion

C. Phenelzine

D. Paroxetine

E. Nefazodone

24. A 65-year-old presents at the urging of his wife, who complains about her husband's snoring. Which of the following is true?

A. Ninety percent of men habitually snore by age 65.

B. Empiric treatment with a short-acting benzodiazepine is indicated.

C. If a sleep study were performed, a respiratory disturbance index of 5 would support the diagnosis of sleep apnea syndrome.

D. A change in shirt collar size would suggest a diagnosis of sleep apnea syndrome.

E. A history of sudden weakness associated with emotional outbursts would suggest sleep apnea.

25. A 19-year-old female is brought into your office by her parents. They are concerned because their daughter has been going out 1 to 3 Saturday nights a month for the past 3 months and drinks 8 to 12 beers plus 1 to 3 shots each night. When talking with the family, which is the most appropriate term to use in describing their daughter's drinking behavior?

A. Substance misuse

B. Substance abuse

C. Substance dependence

D. Alcoholism

E. Normal teenage binge drinking

26. Before you enter a clinic room to see your next patient, a 14 year-old girl, you read the nurse's note that says the mother thinks the patient is depressed. After visiting with the two of them for a few minutes, you request a private interview with the girl. During the visit, she minimizes her mother's concerns, states her mother is always nagging her, attempts to convince you that her 12 hours of sleep each day is normal, and suggests it would help a lot if you could get her mother off her back. When you talk with the mother, she appears quite distressed and feels the problems with her daughter are urgent. She is afraid her daughter will attempt suicide, and wants you to run some tests to see how depressed her daughter actually is. Which of the following is likely to be true about this situation?

A. It is important to spend most of your time with the patient in order to support her autonomy and status as a patient in her own right.

B. Spend equal amounts of time with both the patient and her mother, and then jointly in order to facilitate a conversation between the two of them to clarify the situation.

C. You should run a blood screen to test for illicit drugs.

D. One or both of them probably need to be referred for a psychiatric evaluation.

27. Jared Smith, a 14-year-old white male, is brought to see you by his mother, a single parent with two other children. Mrs. Smith states that her son was physically abused by his biologic father, but the abuse ended 5 years ago when she divorced him and moved back to town to be near her family. Since that time, she has periodically had trouble with him. Jared is sassy and at times disrespectful. The teachers in his junior high school last year reported that he tended to project an anti-authority attitude, particularly to female teachers. Jared has reportedly run away from home on two occasions. He has spent the night in a youth center once. Recently, he has been in trouble for truancy, vandalism, and initiating fights at school. Mrs. Smith was encouraged by the school counselor to have Jared see a doctor in order to have a complete physical and maybe even a drug screen. Mrs. Smith thinks he might have ADHD or a learning disability. The most likely DSM-IV diagnosis is:

A. Oppositional defiant disorder

B. Attention deficit hyperactivity disorder

C. Unipolar manic disorder

D. Conduct disorder

E. Antisocial personality disorder

28. A 78-year-old woman has relatively well-controlled hypertension, periodic headaches, relatively benign osteoarthritis, and a history of depression. She has been on sertraline (Zoloft), 50 mg per day, for 2 years. During clinic visits her affect is normal and she is not tearful. Her short- and long-term memory are intact. She scores 29 or 30 on the mini-mental status exam (MMSE). However, she regularly brings up and wants to talk about a number of issues from her past, most of which seem disconnected from the reasons for her clinic visits. What is the most likely explanation for her behavior?

A. She is showing early signs of developing Alzheimer's dementia.

B. She is engaged in the "life review" developmental task that is typical of the elderly.

C. Her depression is not well controlled.

D. She is engaging in attention-seeking behavior.

E. She is suffering from dissociative identity disorder.

29. A 6-year-old white male is brought to your office because of problems at school. His teachers report that he has difficulty remaining seated, often squirms in his seat, and is easily distracted. He has difficulty completing tasks and sustaining attention. He talks excessively and often blurts out answers to questions before they have been completed. He also has trouble playing quietly. He has behaved in this manner for at least 6 months and is falling behind the other students academically. His physical examination is normal and there is no evidence of tics or psychosis. What is the most appropriate next step?

A. Start methylphenidate (Ritalin)
B. Order an EEG
C. Refer to a psychiatrist
D. Check T4 and TSH levels
E. Schedule him for an assessment including written feedback from teachers

30. Which of the following is true regarding partner abuse?

A. Anxiolytic medications are an important first-line approach to treating battered women.
B. The successful treatment of alcoholism in a battering husband is likely to prevent further episodes of battering.
C. The incidence of underlying mental illness (DSM-IV Axis 1 disorders) is no different in batterers than in the general population.
D. The natural history of domestic violence is generally unpredictable.

31. The pharmacotherapy of attention-deficit disorder is described by which of the following statements?

A. Antidepressants such as desipramine are generally considered first-line medications for this disorder.
B. Appetite and long-term growth suppression may occur in children on medication for this disorder.
C. In most cases, medication alone provides adequate management for this disorder.
D. Administration of dextroamphetamine does not usually induce behavioral stimulation in children.
E. It is important to ensure that children take "drug holidays" on weekends and in the summer.

32. Which of the following symptoms is not consistent with panic attacks?

A. Diaphoresis
B. Numbness
C. Chest pain
D. Dizziness
E. Hallucinations

33. A 39-year-old female was repeatedly raped by a group of three gang members 2 weeks previous to seeing you. Her symptoms included flashbacks; recurrent distressing dreams; physiologic reactivity to internal or external cues that resemble the rape; feelings of detachment from others; restricted range of affect; efforts to avoid thoughts, feelings, or conversations associated with the rape; sleep disturbance; hypervigilance; and exaggerated startle response. Which of the following is the most appropriate diagnosis?

A. Anxiety disorder not otherwise specified
B. Post-traumatic stress disorder (PTSD)
C. Major depressive disorder
D. Acute stress disorder
E. Obsessive–compulsive disorder

34. "Atypical" depression includes all of the following features *except*:

A. Leaden paralysis
B. Panic attacks
C. Long-standing pattern of interpersonal rejection
D. Hypersomnia
E. Anorexia

35. The most effective treatment for a patient with "atypical" depression, as in the previous question, is:

A. Sedative–hypnotic agents
B. Mirtazapine
C. Hypnosis
D. Bupropion
E. MAOIs

36. John Smith is in your office to establish care. He is complaining of irritability, difficulty getting to sleep, difficulty concentrating, and excessive worry. These symptoms have been consistent over the past 8 months. The most appropriate diagnosis for Mr. Smith is:

A. Major depressive disorder with anxiety
B. Anxiety disorder with depression
C. Generalized anxiety disorder
D. Mood disorder not otherwise specified
E. Obsessive–compulsive personality disorder

37. Your patient, Jane McGiveren, is concerned about losing her job because of tardiness. She would like you to put her on an antidepressant because she is having a difficult time getting to bed and a difficult time getting up in the morning. You investigate Ms. McGiveren's symptoms more and find out that her sleep disturbance has to do with her inability to relax once she gets into bed. She tells you she has some minor "quirks" and that it takes her about an hour and a half to settle down at night because she repeatedly has to check to make sure she locked the door, shut off the oven, and organized her children's school supplies. She states that she knows that her behavior is out of control but if she does not go through this routine she would never be able to go to sleep. A similar situation occurs in the morning with her checking that the stove is off, confirming that the front door is locked, and spending quite a bit of time retracing her driving route to make sure she did not run anyone over. The most appropriate diagnosis for Jane is:

A. Generalized anxiety disorder
B. Obsessive–compulsive personality disorder
C. Panic disorder
D. Obsessive–compulsive disorder
E. Delusional disorder

38. The first-line agent for individuals who suffer from panic disorder is:

A. Benzodiazepines
B. SSRIs
C. MAO inhibitors
D. Tricyclics
E. Beta-blockers

39. The current treatment of choice for individuals with specific phobias, such as fear of spiders, elevators, airplanes, or blood, is:

A. Benzodiazepines
B. Cognitive behavioral therapy

C. Systematic desensitization

D. SSRI

E. Biofeedback

40. Which of the following would not be a treatment of choice for an individual suffering from anxiety with depression?

A. Buspirone (Buspar)

B. Paroxetine (Paxil)

C. Sertraline (Zoloft)

D. Citalopram (Celexa)

E. Bupropion (Welbutrin)

41. The most effective approach to the reduction of symptoms in post-traumatic stress disorder is:

A. SSRIs

B. Systematic desensitization

C. Benzodiazepines

D. Aggressive treatment of acute distress disorder

E. Progressive muscle relaxation

42. Which of the following would be the most appropriate short-term adjunctive therapy for an SSRI for panic disorder?

A. Beta-blocker

B. Bupropion

C. Benzodiazepine

D. Amitriptyline

E. Desensitization therapy

43. A 58-year-old patient presents with complaints of frequent headaches and fatigue. She reports that she has been experiencing increasing difficulty for the past 6 weeks since her husband died suddenly of an acute myocardial infarction. He was 67 and had seemed to be in good health. The patient reports that she frequently has some difficulty sleeping, and when she does sleep, she dreams of her husband. She has been crying, has not been interested in being around other people, has had trouble concentrating since she returned to work several weeks after the funeral, and has felt irritable in situations in which she would typically have been patient. Her appetite is fine most of the time. She is not suicidal. The patient states she is troubled by thoughts of guilt; she feels she should have made him go to his doctor for a checkup. The most appropriate diagnosis would be:

A. Bereavement

B. Adjustment reaction with depressed mood

C. Somatization disorder

D. Major depressive episode

E. Dysthymia

44. In the previous case, your initial treatment recommendations should include which of the following:

A. An SSRI to help with her organic symptoms

B. A referral to psychotherapy to help her get on with life

C. Discouraging the patient from being angry since this may contribute to the development of depression

D. Ventilation of feelings and encouragement to talk about positive experiences with the loved one

45. A 45-year-old executive presents at your office and is complaining about his inability to carry out his job. He was recently promoted and his new job requires him to travel and present in front of 40 to 50 individuals in meetings. He has sent his partner to the past two meetings because of fear of getting in front of a group that large. The patient reports no additional symptoms of anxiety. An appropriate treatment for him would be:

A. Alprazolam 0.5 mg bid

B. Lorazepam 0.5 mg tid

C. Paroxetine 20 mg qid

D. Propranolol 40 mg prn

E. Biofeedback

46. Characteristics that distinguish seasonal affective disorder (SAD) from major depressive disorder are increased appetite and weight gain, and:

A. Lesser impact on self-esteem

B. An increased likelihood of cyclothymic periods

C. Psychomotor retardation rather than agitation

D. An increased suicidal potential

E. Mania

47. In the assessment and management of acute alcohol withdrawal, which of the following is not a red flag suggesting the need for inpatient medical management of the condition?

A. A history of severe withdrawal symptoms such as seizures

B. Pregnancy

C. Unwillingness to follow treatment plan or follow-up with providers

D. Hypomagnesemia

E. A concomitant well-controlled seizure disorder

48. Postpartum depression is more likely when:

A. The mother is older than 40 years of age.

B. The baby's father is not supportive.

C. The baby is born prematurely.

D. This is the first child.

E. The baby is of the "wrong" gender.

49. Which of the following is required in order to make the diagnosis of Bipolar II disorder?

A. One or more major depressive episodes

B. One or more manic episodes

C. Persistent delusions

D. Onset in middle age

E. At least one manic episode

50. A woman in an abusive relationship is most at risk of being killed by her abuser when she:

A. Attempts to leave the relationship

B. Gets pregnant

C. Becomes employed outside the home

D. Tries to stand up to her abuser

E. Reports the violence to her family physician

51. A 24-year-old white female has had a depressed mood on most days for several years. She has low self-esteem, low energy, and difficulty making decisions. There is no evidence of psychosis or mania. There is no weight change or sleep disturbance. This presentation is most consistent with a diagnosis of:

A. Cyclothymic disorder

B. Dysthymic disorder

C. Anxiety disorder

D. Borderline personality disorder

E. Major depressive episode

52. In the assessment of a depressed patient, which of the following is not considered important in determining lethality of a plan to commit suicide?

A. Whether the person has a specific plan and the means to carry it out

B. Whether or not there is a history of suicidal behavior

C. The presence of hallucinations commanding the person to commit suicide

D. Socioeconomic status

E. The presence of progressive psychomotor retardation

53. Appropriate advice regarding sleep hygiene or sleep habits includes which of the following?

A. If you cannot get to sleep in 45 minutes, stay quietly in bed until sleep comes.

B. Perform vigorous exercise immediately prior to lights out.

C. Take 2 ounces of alcohol prior to bed. May repeat once if not sleepy.

D. Engage in behavioral relaxation techniques as needed.

E. Use over-the-counter sleep aids for insomnia.

54. Which one of the following is required in order to make the diagnosis of Bipolar I disorder?

A. One or more manic episodes

B. Persistent delusions

C. Onset in middle age

D. At least one depressive episode

E. Behaviors such as checking

55. Which of the following is the most commonly used illicit drug?

A. Cocaine

B. LSD

C. Marijuana

D. Methamphetamine

E. Heroin

56. A 35-year-old male is admitted to the hospital for pancreatitis. He admits to excessive drinking over the past 5 years and understands that it is a problem for his family. This patient has considered quitting alcohol in the past and thinks that now might be a good time to do so. He is in which stage in the readiness for change?

A. Denial

B. Precontemplation

C. Contemplation

D. Preparation

E. Action

57. The most appropriate intervention for this patient's alcohol use would be:

A. Confront the patient with the facts about the morbidity and mortality associated with pancreatitis.

B. Talk with the patient about formulating a plan for stopping.

C. Hold a family meeting and confront the patient.

D. Encourage inpatient treatment.

E. Reinforce his thinking about quitting by exploring the pros and cons.

58. All of the following are risk factors for developing PTSD following a traumatic event *except*:

A. Female gender

B. Prior divorce

C. Low level of education

D. Concomitant substance abuse

E. Previous history of depression

59. Using the stages for readiness for change, helping the patient formulate a plan to stop his or her alcohol use is most appropriate during which stage?

A. Precontemplation

B. Contemplation

C. Preparation

D. Action

E. Follow-up

60. Which of the following is not a short-term effect of marijuana use?

A. Increased heart rate, anxiety

B. Trouble with concentration and problem solving

C. Distorted perception

D. Seizure

E. Loss of coordination

61. A 7-year-old is brought into your office because he is driving his parents wild. He will not do anything they tell him and is always running around and on the go. They are convinced that he has ADHD and desire that you put him on Ritalin. What would be the most appropriate first step here?

A. Start with Ritalin 5 mg PO bid and follow up in 3 weeks.

B. Refer the parents to a parenting class.

C. Speak to the child's teacher.

D. Refer the child to a child psychologist.

E. Tell the family that his behavior is normal, and they should not be so worried.

62. Regarding the use of antidepressants in pregnancy, which of the following is true?

A. Tricyclic antidepressants (TCAs) can be used safely throughout pregnancy.

B. Fluoxetine (Prozac) can be harmful in the first trimester.

C. TCAs are associated with behavioral effects in offspring.

D. Other SSRIs (besides fluoxetine) have not been studied as much but probably share the risk of harm in the first trimester.

E. Venlafaxine (Effexor), bupropion (Welbutrin), and serzone (Nefazadone) are safer than TCAs.

63. The illicit drug most commonly found to cause visits to the emergency department is:

A. Methamphetamine

B. Heroin

C. Marijuana

D. Cocaine

E. Opium

64. Which of the following is not true regarding divorce?

A. After divorce, men's standard of living increases while women's decreases.

B. Elementary-age children fair better than other aged children when parents divorce.

C. Women older than 30 years who divorce are less likely than their divorced male counterparts to remarry.

D. Neither joint nor sole custody has been shown to be clearly superior to the other in the effect on children's long-term well-being.

E. Older women cope better than older men in the postdivorce period.

65. An antidepressant medication that might be activating for a patient whose depression is partially manifested in depressed mood, marked fatigue, and lethargy is which of the following?

A. Nortriptyline

B. Sertraline

C. Nefazodone

D. Venlafaxine

E. Buspirone

66. The cardiac effects of antipsychotics include:

A. Prolonged QT but not QTc

B. SVT

C. Decreased contractility

D. Elevated CPK-MB

E. Prolonged QTc and Torsades de Pointes

67. Which of the following statements is true regarding the treatment of PTSD?

A. The use of SSRIs is associated with the lowest rate of relapse among all forms of treatment.

B. Psychoanalysis is more effective than hypnosis.

C. The use of a polypharmacologic approach is associated with better outcomes.

D. Support groups are useless in treating PTSD.

E. Of the nonpharmacologic treatments of PTSD, cognitive–behavioral techniques, including exposure therapy, have the most empirical support.

68. A 74-year-old nursing home patient with Parkinson's disease and dementia is found delirious, febrile, diaphoretic, and unable to respond coherently. The neurologic exam is difficult and reveals lead pipe rigidity but no clear focal change. The only recent medication changes were made by the consulting neurologist, who noted worsening cognitive and behavioral changes over stable Parkinson's. He discontinued amantadine and started olanzapine at a low dose. Of the following, you would be most likely to find:

A. Elevated troponin I

B. Lacunar infarct of the basal ganglia on MRI

C. Subdural hemotoma on CT scan

D. Elevated serum CPK

E. Prompt recovery with physosstigmine administration

69. The differential diagnosis for the previous patient includes all of the following except:

A. Lethal catatonia

B. Central pontine myelinosis

C. Serotonin syndrome

D. Encephalitis or other infectious syndrome (i.e., urosepsis)

E. CVA

70. Which of the following is correct concerning sleep changes with aging?

A. Increased rapid eye movement (REM) sleep

B. Decreased sleep efficiency

C. Decreased nocturnal awakenings

D. Decreased time from lights out to sleep (sleep latency)

E. Delayed sleep phase (later to bed, later to rise)

71. Melancholic depression includes all of the following features except:

A. More common after age 50

B. Better response to psychotherapy than medications

C. Significant weight loss

D. Diurnal variation in mood symptoms

E. Profoundly depressed mood and anhedonia

72. Which of the following has been found to buffer the stress of children whose parents divorce?

A. A positive relationship with both parents

B. A positive relationship with one parent

C. No positive relationship with either parent

D. 50–50 joint custody of the children

E. None of the above

73. A diagnosis of major depressive disorder is suggested over that of adjustment disorder by which of the following?

A. Symptoms of anxiety and depression 4 months after divorce or loss of spouse

B. Suicidality

C. Concomitant substance abuse

D. Feelings of hopelessness and worthlessness

E. Panic attacks

74. Which of the following is not a possible result of valproic acid therapy?

A. Hyperammonemia

B. Life-threatening pancreatitis

C. Transient alopecia

D. Development of the polycystic ovarian syndrome

E. Hypothyroidism

75. Which of the following statements is true regarding the diagnosis of a major depressive episode?

A. There is virtually always a clear precipitating factor.

B. Symptoms must present for 2 weeks, with a clear change in baseline status.

C. Both a depressed mood and diminished interest in pleasurable activities are required.

D. The individual is more likely to evidence psychomotor agitation than psychomotor retardation.

E. Difficulty getting to sleep is a common complaint.

76. Which of the following is true of the use of mood stabilizers in pregnancy?

A. Lithium is not associated with the development of Ebstein's abnormality.

B. Lithium may be associated with a perinatal syndrome of cyanosis and hypotonicity.

C. Valproic acid and carbemazepine are associated with an increased risk of Ebstein's abnormality.

D. Lithium is characterized as a pregnancy category X drug.

77. A man in his mid-50s is having difficulty with maintaining erections. He has experienced transient difficulties with impotence before. He acknowledges this has been during stressful periods of his life, and that he is currently under stress in his job. The physical exam is unremarkable and the patient is otherwise healthy. The most appropriate step to take is to:

A. Prescribe Viagra on a prn basis.

B. Order blood work, including testosterone level.

C. Make a referral to a sex therapist for conjoint therapy.

D. Encourage the man to use relaxation strategies to deal with underlying stress.

E. Refer him to a urologist for an evaluation.

78. All of the following are features of generalized anxiety disorder *except*:

A. Excessive anxiety or worry, which is difficult to control, occurring more days than not for at least 6 months

B. Associated with at least three of the following: difficulty breathing, irritability, mind going blank, muscle tension, and sleep disturbance

C. May present as a feeling of "lump in the throat"

D. Is rarely associated with other psychiatric illnesses such as major depression and alcoholism

E. Has a lifetime prevalence of 5% and is more common in females

79. Which of the following statements is false regarding panic disorder?

A. Panic attacks are associated with sweating, trembling, and shaking.

B. Panic attacks reach their peak within 10 minutes.

C. They commonly present as chest pain or a choking sensation.

D. Patients are indifferent to the thought of continued attacks.

E. Panic attacks can occur unexpectedly.

80. You are treating a 28-year-old female who is complaining of an inability to reach orgasm. What is the most appropriate first step in working with this patient?

A. Review patient medications

B. Check TSH, testosterone, and estrogen levels

C. Refer to sex therapy

D. Take a detailed sexual history

E. Screen for depression

81. In providing supportive psychotherapy to patients, which of the following techniques are most likely to be emphasized?

A. Confrontation and clarification

B. Interpretation and empathic validation

C. Clarification and affirmation

D. Affirmation and empathic validation

E. Interpretation and encouragement to elaborate

82. Which of the following statements is true regarding delirium tremens (DTs):

A. DTs is considered the first stage of alcohol withdrawal.

B. It does not follow a "sundowning" phenomenon.

C. It never begins less than 4 days after cessation of drinking.

D. Unlike other psychoses, insight into hallucinations is retained.

E. Adequate early identification and early treatment intervention of alcohol withdrawal can prevent the development of DTs.

83. Regarding depression and pregnancy, which of the following is false?

A. Decisions to continue or initiate pharmacologic therapy should be made on an individual risk–benefit basis.

B. Patients with histories of severe and recurrent depression are at moderate risk for relapse during pregnancy and in the postpartum period, and a prophylactic antidepressant should be considered.

C. The incidence of depression in all women is greater during pregnancy than in the postpartum period.

D. Women who develop postpartum blues may be managed with interpersonal or supportive therapy.

E. When major depression emerges during pregnancy or postpartum, medication should be strongly considered.

84. The medical or "organic" differential diagnosis of depression (secondary depression) includes all of the following *except*:

A. Cushing's disease

B. Subcortical CVA

C. Parkinson's disease

D. Folate deficiencies

E. Vitamin E deficiency

85. All of the following are helpful interventions in preventing delirium in hospitalized older patients *except*:

A. Initiating cognitively stimulating activities three times daily, such as word games or discussion of current events

B. Relaxation tapes, music, and massage to manage insomnia

C. Nighttime diazepam for regulating sleeping patterns

D. Early recognition and management of dehydration

E. Early mobilization activities

86. Which of the following methods of counseling is most useful in helping the ambivalent patient to change a given behavior?

A. Operant conditioning

B. Reverse psychology

C. Unconditional positive regard

D. Decision balance techniques (helping the patient weigh the pros and cons of a behavioral change)

E. Threatening dismissal of patient

87. Children and adolescents from divorced families are more likely to be at a greater risk for all of the following *except*:

A. Suicide

B. Homosexuality

C. Future divorce

D. Poor school performance

E. Substance abuse

88. Motivational counseling is recommended and supported by empirical evidence as treatment for all of the following *except*:

A. Gambling

B. Obesity

C. Homosexuality

D. Spousal abuse

E. High-risk sexual behaviors

89. A 41-year-old male patient with bipolar disorder (stable), a 30 year history of type 1 diabetes, and essential hypertension presents complaining of worsening erectile dysfunction (ED). Potential likely causes of this gentleman's ED include all of the following *except*:

A. Psychogenic

B. Atherosclerosis

C. Diabetic neuropathy

D. Medication induced

E. Prostate disease

90. The previous patient may have multiple contributing causes of ED, but he notifies you he has stopped taking his antihypertensive medication because this seemed to be the major culprit to him. Reviewing his chart, you see he has failed several ACE inhibitors (ACE-I) and angiotensin receptor blockers (ARBs). With further inquiry, he admits to stopping them because of sexual dysfunction. Assuming you would like to maintain this patient on at least a small dose of ACE-I, other options for treating his ED would include all of the following *except*:

A. Regular exercise

B. Relaxation techniques

C. Viagra

D. Substitute valproic acid for lithium

E. Add high-dose fluoxetine

91. You have a depressed patient with osteoarthritis who has recently had a GI bleed despite the continued use of a COX-II inhibitor. His current medication regimen includes high-dose

bupropion (Wellbutrin) daily. Which of the following would be inappropriate for pain control?

A. Acetaminophen

B. Gabapentin

C. Tramodol

D. Vicodin

E. Amitryptiline

92. Which of the following has been found to be an effective and simple screening tool for assessing problems with alcohol abuse?

A. Blood alcohol level

B. CAGE method

C. SASSI assessment

D. Asking patient how many drinks he or she has on average

E. Asking the patient's family how much he or she drinks on average

93. Lithium is contraindicated in which of these general medical conditions?

A. COPD

B. Psoriasis

C. Hypertension

D. Down's syndrome

E. Cystic fibrosis

94. Which of the following is false regarding the differences between men and women with depression?

A. Women attempt suicide more frequently but are not as successful.

B. Atypical symptoms are experienced more often in women.

C. Depression is more prevalent in men.

D. Women usually have more association of thyroid disease and migraine headaches.

E. Women more often experience guilt.

Chapter 5

Answer Key

1. A	**43.** A	**85.** C
2. D	**44.** D	**86.** D
3. A	**45.** D	**87.** B
4. C	**46.** C	**88.** C
5. D	**47.** D	**89.** E
6. D	**48.** B	**90.** E
7. E	**49.** A	**91.** C
8. D	**50.** A	**92.** B
9. C	**51.** B	**93.** B
10. C	**52.** E	**94.** C
11. E	**53.** D	
12. D	**54.** A	
13. B	**55.** C	
14. E	**56.** C	
15. E	**57.** E	
16. A	**58.** D	
17. B	**59.** C	
18. C	**60.** D	
19. B	**61.** C	
20. B	**62.** A	
21. C	**63.** D	
22. D	**64.** B	
23. D	**65.** B	
24. D	**66.** E	
25. A	**67.** E	
26. A	**68.** D	
27. D	**69.** C	
28. B	**70.** B	
29. E	**71.** B	
30. C	**72.** B	
31. D	**73.** D	
32. E	**74.** E	
33. D	**75.** B	
34. E	**76.** B	
35. E	**77.** D	
36. C	**78.** D	
37. D	**79.** D	
38. B	**80.** D	
39. C	**81.** D	
40. E	**82.** E	
41. D	**83.** C	
42. C	**84.** E	

Psychiatry Answers

1. A

The USPSTF gave a B rating for recommending routine screening for depression in adults and concluded there was insufficient data to make a recommendation for children. In addition, there is no evidence to suggest that any one rating scale is more useful than others, and shorter ones may be just as effective and more efficient. All positive screenings should be followed by a full diagnostic interview to assess via DSM-IV criterion.

2. D

Benzodiazepines have been associated with the development of oral clefts. Additionally, the use of benzodiazepines perinatally is associated with hypotonia, apnea, hypothermia, and feeding difficulties.

3. A

The highest rates of illicit drug use are found among individuals ages 16 to 20 (35.6%).

4. C

This patient most likely has post-traumatic stress disorder (PTSD). The most likely cause of the abdominal pain and other non-PTSD symptoms (paresthesias, dyspareunia) is concomitant somatization disorder, which has an extremely high comorbidity with PTSD. It may be present in the subsyndromal form, whereas this patient has a "textbook" diagnosis.

The essentials of a PTSD diagnosis include exposure to or witnessing a serious trauma, symptoms of re-experiencing the event, symptoms of increased arousal, emotional numbing, avoidance of stimuli associated with the trauma, and symptoms that last longer than 1 month and cause significant distress or impairment.

5. D

La belle indifference refers to a relative lack of concern about apparently severe and disabling symptoms. Although frequently mentioned in the literature as a feature of conversion disorder, la belle indifference is not pathognomonic for somatization or conversion disorder. The diagnosis relies on lack of support for other physical diagnoses as well as the presence of at least two GI complaints, four pain complaints, one sexual symptom, and one pseudoneurologic complaint. However, some studies have shown that there is a high prevalence of subsyndromal somatization (where not all the criteria are met) in the primary care population. The differential diagnosis for la belle indifference includes hemineglect, frontal lobe injury, multiple sclerosis, and other neurologic syndromes. Multiple sclerosis would be the most likely disease in the differential and should be ruled out.

Somatization disorder often involves multiple symptoms from several possible organ systems. Despite multiple subjective complaints, there are few, if any, objective findings. Evaluation

may also be confounded by coexisting mental illness. However, a physician needs to consider the possibility of organic diseases, such as systemic lupus erythematosis, that involve several organ systems and may present with multiple symptoms.

6. D

Competence is a legal, not medical, concept. Hence, the courts have the final say in judging an individual competent or not. The presence of psychiatric symptoms or cognitive impairment is not, in and of itself, an indicator of incompetence. Neither is refusal of a "medically indicated" procedure. It is important to remember that a patient may be able to answer questions and make decisions in some aspect of his or her life but not in others (e.g., competent to participate in treatment decisions but not to handle complicated financial decisions).

7. E

This patient has symptoms suggestive of reflex sympathetic dystrophy, a medical emergency warranting aggressive treatment. Reflex sympathetic dystrophy presents following injury or postoperatively with symptoms and signs of autonomic dysregulation, sensory and motor abnormalities, trophic symptoms (e.g., muscle atrophy, altered hair growth), and psychologic symptoms. Judicious physical therapy, sympathetic blockade, systemic corticosteroids, and psychologic interventions are effective. Referral is usually warranted given the severe morbidity of this condition.

8. D

This patient has a very high risk of depression relapse because of her short duration of current treatment and multiple severe depressive episodes. The risk of severe depression certainly outweighs the unproven risk of a selective serotonin reuptake inhibitor (SSRI) to which she is responding. There is no convincing evidence that the SSRIs are associated with an increased risk of fetal malformations or premature delivery. Lithium would be inappropriate during pregnancy, and the best evidence suggests St. John's Wort is ineffective in patients with major depression and safety in pregnancy has not been established.

9. C

The PLISSIT model of sexual counseling is a useful framework for addressing sexual issues. The P stands for permission: giving the patient validation and permission to discuss his or her problem; LI stand for limited information concerning sexual health; SS stand for specific suggestions regarding the concern; and IT stand for intensive therapy: providing therapy for the patient's difficulty.

10. C

Risk factors for alcohol withdrawal include age older than 40 years, male gender, daily consumption greater than one-fifth of liquor, excessive drinking for greater than 10 years, tremors and anxiety within 8 hours of cessation, and the presence of an acute medical problem.

11. E

Separation anxiety is characterized by excessive fear in the face of separation from the presence of a significant figure such as a parent or guardian. Children will often have unrealistic concerns about horrible events such as kidnapping and would be unlikely to run away from a parent at a mall. Such individuals will often throw tantrums when parents leave. They may refuse to go to school, or even sleep in the absence of their parents. Somatic symptoms are common. Prior to age 8 months, infants have not established a concept of normalcy. Typically between 8 and 14 months, children develop familiarity with parents and home environment and when removed from either may exhibit signs of fear and feel threatened by change in the environment. Separation anxiety usually resolves around the age of 2 years. Resolution requires development of safety and trust in non-parental individuals and environmental exposure outside the home.

12. D

This patient has delirium, an acute medical and psychiatric emergency. Treatment of delirium should be aimed at uncovering the underlying causes, such as infection, hypoglycemia, medication side effects, withdrawal, fecal impaction, hypoxia, pain, or central nervous system abnormalities. Diagnosis and treatment of the underlying problem should take precedence. Involving family members can be helpful. While overstimulation may be harmful, sensory isolation is likely to exacerbate this patient's problem. Medications, such as the typical and atypical neuroleptics, can be helpful but are secondary to correcting the cause of delirium.

13. B

The SSRIs all are capable of delaying orgasm and can cause anorgasmia as well as decreased arousal. Occasionally, the patient's body will adjust to the drug, and this side effect will decrease or disappear. Effective treatments include lowering the dose of SSRI, adding bupropion or switching to bupropion, and adding mirtazapine. Mirtazapine is unique among the antidepressants in that it possesses antagonistic properties at the 5-HT3 receptor sites. Increased activation of 5-HT3 receptors by SSRIs is thought to result in most of the side effects from the SSRIs. Although sildenefil might be helpful in obtaining an erection, it is not likely to benefit this gentleman in achieving orgasm.

14. E

The SSRIs all possess antipanic properties, and most have been shown to effectively treat panic disorder and panic symptoms, with few side effects. Most patients will respond to a dose of sertraline as low as 50 mg qid. Effective doses are often between 50 and 200 mg/day. SSRIs are safe, well tolerated, and are not addictive. Using PRN benzodiazepines as a rescue medicine is appropriate in the initiation of therapy, and in some cases for continued management, but SSRIs are the more definitive therapy. Venlafaxine may be as effective but may require a long withdrawal schedule if the patient wants to discontinue the drug due to the possibility of withdrawal symptoms. Special caution should be paid to use of SSRIs in child and adolescent patients.

15. E

It is not necessary to monitor a CBC with lithium treatment because the hematopoeitic effects are limited to benign leukocytosis.

Hypothyroidism is a more common and more serious adverse effect of lithium. ECGs only need to be followed as needed in patients with symptoms of cardiac arrhythmia or failure, older patients (older than 40 years), and patients with known cardiac disease. Because of potential nephrotoxicity, especially with long-term use, renal function should be closely monitored.

16. A

The woman would not have sexual desire or lubrication if she was suffering from sexual aversion disorder, inhibited female orgasm, or dyspareunia. There is insufficient information to determine how well functioning she is in the orgasm phase. Vaginismus is the condition in which the vaginal introitus closes so tightly that penetration is impossible. This involuntary spasm of the muscles surrounding the vaginal entrance occurs whenever an attempt is made to introduce an object into the vaginal orifice. Dyspareunia is defined as the occurrence of pain during sexual intercourse.

17. B

Some studies estimate that SSRIs affect sexual functioning in more than one-half of those who take them. SSRIs can affect any of the stages of the sexual response cycle (desire, arousal, orgasm). Most often, the impact includes diminished desire, arousal, and anorgasmia in women and diminished desire, impotence, and delayed ejaculation in men. It is important to ask about sexual functioning when assessing a patient for depression and other mood disorders because diminished sexual functioning is a common symptom. Doing so also helps to later distinguish this primary symptom from the secondary effects of the antidepressant. Bupropion is relatively free from sexual side effects.

18. C

The patient has symptoms strongly suggestive of restless legs syndrome. Although frequently idiopathic, this condition is associated with iron deficiency, pregnancy, and renal failure. A CPK and EMG are not indicated. SSRIs can be effective in some patients. Symptoms of itching, pulling, and an inability to remain still are common. Symptoms are typically worse in the evening hours while resting.

19. B

The patient has restless legs syndrome (RLS). Although RLS may respond to benzodiazepines or opioid analgesics, contemporary first-line management leans toward dopaminergic agents including carbidopa or levodopa, pramipexole (Mirapex), and pergolide mesylate (Permax). RLS sometimes responds to iron replacement even when iron studies are sometimes normal. Folic acid deficiency is not commonly associated with RLS. SSRIs are becoming common agents associated with RLS.

20. B

Masters and Johnson outlined three stages of the sexual response cycle and described them as being analogous in men and women. They included the arousal, orgasm, and refractory periods. Subsequent researchers conceptualized and investigated a fourth stage preceding the other three: desire. Increasingly, it is thought that it is necessary to identify the primary biologic and psychosocial root of the problem, and most frequently it is in the desire phase.

21. C

Pregnant women usually need a higher dose of lithium than before pregnancy. Lithium doses should be cut in half during labor to avoid toxic levels related to fluid loss. In general, the natural course of bipolar disorder is not known during pregnancy, but the postpartum period is known to be a time of high risk for relapse; up to 50% will relapse if not treated with a mood stabilizer before or immediately after delivery. In general, the decision to continue prophylactic drug therapy should be made on a risk–benefit basis with the patient adequately informed and involved. Consultation with a psychiatrist can be beneficial in assessing the individual risk. In general, a person without a history of psychosis or dangerous behaviors such as drug use or suicide attempts while manic or depressed may be able to go without drug therapy. Also important are the patient's history of relapse off medication and social support. Patients with chronic and severe mental illness should usually be co-managed with a psychiatric consultant.

22. D

Although poverty (a major stressor) and the disinhibitory effect of alcohol abuse increase the likelihood of abuse, partner abuse in the home is the strongest predictor of potential child abuse. Depending on the study, it has been estimated that 16% to 40% of women are abused during pregnancy (endangering the fetus). Similarly, 35% to 70% of men who batter their partner also abuse their children. Child abuse comes in many forms, including physical, mental, and sexual abuse. Signs of physical abuse include cigarette burns, unexplainable fractures, and unexplained bruises and are potentially easier to identify than behavioral patterns. Behaviors that suggest possible abuse include aggressive behavior, "fear of home," runaway behavior in adolescents, withdrawn behavior, and self-destructive behavior. Physicians need to be alert for both physical and behavioral traits and in some states are required to report both abuse and suspicion of abuse to the appropriate protective agencies.

23. D

Patients taking SSRIs and who discontinue abruptly may be at risk for serotonin withdrawal syndrome. This syndrome can be described with the acronym FLUSH:

Flu-like symptoms including myalgia, loose stools, and nausea
Lightheadedness and dizziness
Uneasiness and restlessnesss
Sleep and sensory disturbances
Headache

It is recommended that patients taper off slowly. Physicians should recommend that patients decrease the daily dose by approximately 25% per week. Among the SSRIs, this is most true for paroxetine (Paxil), then citalopram (Celexa) and sertraline (Zoloft), and then fluoxetine (Prozac), which has a very long half-life due to a metabolite.

24. D

Obstructive sleep apnea (OSA) is common and can be challenging to diagnose as patients age because approximately 50% of men and 40% of women at age 65 habitually snore. A history of functional compromise, daytime sleepiness, obesity, or secondary findings (e.g., retrognathia, a "bull neck," or cor pulmonale) on the physical examination might support the diagnosis. Increasing collar size has been linked with the presence of sleep apnea. A sleep study is often warranted to evaluate for OSA. The respiratory disturbance index (RDI) counts the frequency of apneas and hypopneas each hour; an RDI greater than 20 is suggestive of OSA; an

RDI of 5, unless associated with prolonged apneic periods or other physical signs, is not supportive. Treatment with a benzodiazepine would be contraindicated, until a clearer diagnosis is made, because it would aggravate OSA.

25. A

Use the following when categorizing substance abuse:

- Substance misuse: this applies to individuals who occasionally will use an illegal or legal substance to excess.
- Substance abuse: a maladaptive pattern of substance use occurring within a 12-month period that causes impairment in social or occupational functioning (job) legal, and interpersonal problems.
- Substance dependence: a maladaptive pattern of substance use occurring within a 12-month period, leading to significant impairment or distress and characterized by either tolerance (need for markedly increased amounts of the substance or marked diminished effect with continued use of the same amount of substance) or withdrawal (even if withdrawal does not happen because the patient uses a substance to relieve or avoid withdrawal symptoms).

26. A

Negotiating visits with adolescents can be tricky. It is important to foster their sense of growing autonomy, privacy, and being a patient in their own right. On the other hand, it is important to remember that adolescent development is a process during which parents remain important in adolescents' lives. Parents can provide important background information that the teenager may be unaware of or minimizes. Parents may have concerns that teenagers flatly deny. Barring abusive situations or cases involving emancipated minors, a history should include a balance from both parents and the adolescent. A drug screen could be a part of the workup if a parent presents credible grounds for concern. It is advisable to negotiate the decision to obtain the screen in order to obtain the teenager's cooperation and consent, however.

27. D

Conduct disorder is characterized by aggression to people or animals, destruction of property, deceitfulness or theft, and serious violations of rules. It is considered a more serious problem than oppositional defiant disorder, which is characterized by an argumentative, defiant, blaming, angry, vindictive, annoying, or spiteful attitude and behavior. There is not enough information in this question to determine whether or not a mood disorder is present. A personality disorder is defined by the DSM-IV as an enduring pattern of inner experience and behavior that differs markedly from the expectations of the individual's culture, is pervasive and inflexible, has an onset in adolescence or early adulthood, is stable over time, and leads to distress or impairment. Personality disorders are thought to be maladaptive perceptions and responses to the actions of others and stressful life events. Each personality disorder is categorized into one of three clusters based on the behavioral characteristics.

28. B

We continue to develop psychosocially throughout our life spans. Elderly people are typically engaged in the struggle of what Erik Erikson terms ego integrity versus ego despair. Part of this is a normative process of "life review"—reviewing the elements of the past to determine whether or not life has been worth living, whether or not it has had meaning. Arriving at a positive conclusion allows us to maintain or develop a sense of integrity about our lives. This reminiscing should not be considered attention-seeking. Nor should it be considered a sign of dementia (confabulating and living in the past because the short-term memory is fading), especially since she scores well on the MMSE. This patient's depression seems well controlled based on her affect and lack of organic symptoms of depression. Dissociative identity disorder is a fairly rare condition that people experience in the aftermath of serious trauma (e.g., child sexual or physical abuse).

29. E

On the surface, it may seem clear that this child has ADHD. However, the differential diagnosis for these symptoms includes mood disorders, learning disabilities, family dysfunction, and classroom environmental issues. Therefore, a thorough assessment is the best next step. Children who are having difficulty learning, are distressed by a troubled home situation, or are anxious or depressed may act out behaviorally. Although medication, including Ritalin, may be a helpful part of eventual treatment, it is very important to assess the child carefully in order to determine if he really does have ADHD. There also may be comorbid conditions that need attention. ADHD is reported in approximately 3% to 5% of school-age children. It may also persist into adulthood.

30. C

The history of domestic violence is fairly predictable in that a cycle has been identified, with tension-building, acute battering, and honeymoon phases. When women present with symptoms associated with or directly caused by domestic violence, anxiolytic and other psychiatric medications may be helpful at some point. But it is very important to address the other psychosocial issue before offering medication. Alcohol or other substance abuse treatment for batterers has not been shown to significantly reduce abuse because it does not effectively address the underlying power and control issues or the batterer's emotional dependency. It is tempting to think of batterers as psychiatrically different than the rest of the population, but this is not the case. The incidence of mood, anxiety, and other disorders has not been found to be different.

31. D

Stimulant medication, such as methylphenidate, and nonstimulant medications, such as atomoxetine, are first-line choices. Appetite changes can result from the nausea caused by stimulant medication. But studies have shown that children on stimulant medication catch up to the average growth rates in the long term. For mild cases, behavioral intervention and psychoeducation are usually sufficient interventions. For moderate and severe cases, medication and psychoeducation and behavioral changes are necessary. The stimulant medications generally have an effect that improves behavioral and emotional regulation. Depending on behavioral performance, some parents choose to withhold medications on weekends and at other non-performance-oriented times to allow the child a break from the side effects of stimulant medication. Some children require continuous daily medication for successful treatment.

32. E

The essential feature of a panic attack is a discrete period of intense fear or discomfort that is accompanied by at least 4 of 13 cognitive or somatic symptoms. Hallucinations are not among the typical symptoms. A few typical symptoms include heart palpitations, sweating, shortness of breath, chest discomfort, nausea, dizziness, and parasthesias. Patients may experience a feeling of impending doom or detachment from oneself (depersonalization). Situations may trigger panic attacks; however, some occur unexpectedly without situational context.

33. D

According to the DSM-IV criteria, traumatic experiences resulting in these symptoms are to be diagnosed as a stress disorder. Post-traumatic stress disorder is used for symptoms that last more than 1 month, whereas acute stress disorder symptoms are the same but the duration is less than 1 month.

34. E

Atypical depression is commonly associated with hyperphagia, a reversed diurnal variation in mood, as opposed to classic depression (worse in afternoon or evening, rather than morning), somatization, and mood lability. It is more common in females and usually has an earlier age of onset than classic depression.

35. E

MAOIs are considered the treatment of choice if not contraindicated by other factors, but antipsychotics and imipramine, as well as other TCAs, may also be effective.

36. C

Individuals with excessive worry, more days than not, for a period of more than 6 months have generalized anxiety disorder if they also have three or more of the following symptoms: restlessness, easily fatigued, difficulty concentrating, irritability, muscle tension, or sleep disturbance. John does not exhibit the necessary symptoms for a major depressive disorder, such as depressed mood or anhedonia.

37. D

The most appropriate answer here is obsessive–compulsive disorder (OCD). OCD and obsessive–compulsive personality disorder (OCPD) are differentiated in that OCD is manifested by obsession and compulsions, whereas OCPD involves a pervasive pattern of preoccupation with orderliness, perfectionism, and control. Most individuals with OCD are aware their behaviors are irrational. In OCPD, their behaviors are consistent with their personality and therefore their behaviors usually only irritate those around them.

38. B

Although benzodiazepines might be appropriate to manage the symptoms of panic disorder, because of their side effects authorities now favor SSRIs as first-line therapy. If the symptoms are severe, benzodiazepines are an appropriate addition to the SSRI. The beta-blockers are effective for performance anxiety but are less effective for panic attacks.

39. C

The current treatment of choice for specific phobia is systematic desensitization. This treatment focuses on helping the person manage his or her anxiety while being progressively introduced to the panic-producing agent. Benzodiazepines and SSRIs may help manage some of the symptoms but are not seen as curative. Cognitive–behavioral therapy and biofeedback may also be helpful, but exposure to the anxiety-producing agent has been found to be more effective.

40. E

Buspirone, paroxetine, sertraline, and citalopram have been found to be effective in the treatment of anxiety with depression. Although bupropion is effective as an aid to smoking cessation and for depression, it has relatively little anxiolytic effects.

41. D

Although all of the above can be effectively used in the treatment of PTSD, the most effective treatment is to avoid the condition altogether by aggressively treating the individual after the traumatic event occurs.

42. C

A benzodiazepine, such as clonazepam, is the best short-term medication for the initial treatment of panic disorder because of its long-acting mechanism of action. This will greatly decrease the potential for abuse. It is also important to explain and contract with the patient when using any benzodiazepines that the treatment is for a short time and is being used only until the SSRI is in full effect. The other medications are either ineffective or have an unfavorable side effect profile (amitriptyline). Cognitive–behavioral therapy, not desensitization therapy, might be an effective counterpart to medication.

43. A

Whenever a patient presents with these types of symptoms following the death of a close family member, bereavement is the appropriate diagnosis. Even though this is an "adjustment reaction with depressed mood," it is considered a normal reaction to a traumatic loss. A diagnosis of major depression is not given until symptoms have been present for at least 2 months. Other symptoms not related to grief can help distinguish between the two. These include guilt not related to the circumstances around the death, thoughts of death other than those pertaining to a wish to have died with or instead of the deceased, marked psychomotor retardation, prolonged and marked functional impairment, and hallucinations not related to the deceased. This patient does not meet the criteria for diagnosis of somatization disorder. Dysthymia is only diagnosed if the depressive symptoms have been present for at least 2 years without a 2-month period of remission. This patient might be at risk for prolonged bereavement or major depressive disorder given the sudden nature of her husband's death; close follow-up would be warranted.

44. D

Since this patient's reaction is normal in these circumstances, grief counseling support is likely the most beneficial initial intervention. An SSRI would take 3 to 6 weeks to be effective. By that time, her symptoms may well have diminished. Also, both medication and a referral to therapy may pathologize this normal reaction. A short-acting medication to help her sleep may be useful. Anger is a normal part of the grief process; expressing it does not contribute to the development of depression.

45. D

The current treatment of choice for simple stage fright is a single dose of a beta-adrenergic receptor blocker prior to the performance. The other psychoactive agents here could be appropriate if there were other symptoms of anxiety. Biofeedback and psychotherapy might also be appropriate but would take longer to work and are sometimes not needed. It is important to attempt a

trial of medication to confirm that adverse side effects do not occur prior to actual use for "stage fright."

46. C

Seasonal affective disorder (SAD) is a depression variant associated with lack of exposure to light that occurs in northern climates during winter. Exposure to bright light, as delivered by a light box, can be helpful in addition to the more common therapies for major depressive disorder. Symptoms are the "hibernation" type, including lethargy, increased appetite, and weight gain. SAD is more common in women, but it does affect both sexes. Although possible in children and teenagers, it is less common under the age of 20 years. Risk of occurrence decreases with age. SAD is more common among inhabitants of northern geographic latitudes.

47. D

Hypomagnesemia in and of itself is not necessarily an indication for inpatient management of alcohol withdrawal. Ninety percent of all cases of alcohol withdrawal do not progress past stage 1, and serum magnesium levels routinely drop in these patients but usually return to normal without replacement. Other red flags include uncontrollable or dangerous behavior, previously failed outpatient detoxification, longer term and more severe alcohol use, and other concomitant medical illnesses that may limit the patient's physiologic reserve capacity.

48. B

Social support is one of the most important predictors of postnatal adjustment. The relationship between the mother and her partner is a key element of this support network and strongly impacts the mother's perception of her future well-being, safety, security, and hopefulness. All other things being equal, and if they have never had a prior episode of depression, women tend to be less susceptible to mood disorders as they age. This may be because of the role of life experiences, maturation, and coping skills development.

49. A

Bipolar disorders in general have their onset in the second or third decade of life. By definition, Bipolar II disorder includes recurrent major depressive episodes with hypomanic (not manic) episodes. Although people with bipolar disorder may experience transient delusions, hallucinations, and other perceptual problems, these are not persistent in nature.

50. A

Often the primary and most common psychologic factors underlying the reason why partners (chiefly men) become batterers pertain to emotional dependency and need for control. Any change in circumstances that threatens the relationship increases the likelihood of an escalation of tension and subsequent violence. All of these options potentially fit into that category. However, the time when intimate partners are most likely to be killed is when they attempt to leave the relationship.

51. B

Dysthymia is defined if depressed mood has been present for most days for at least 2 years without a 2-month period of remission. The diagnosis of major depression requires additional clinical features. Exclusion of normal bereavement, drug abuse, and manic episodes is required. Fatigue, self-reproach, poor concentration, and thoughts of death (not limited to suicide) are common.

52. E

A history of suicidal behavior and the presence of a specific plan are important indicators of lethality. Psychiatric disturbances, such as hallucinations, and major stressors, such as economic instability or poverty, make an already dangerous situation more unstable. On the other hand, psychomotor retardation often deprives the person of the energy needed to develop and act on a plan. Physicians need to be cautious, then, in treating the severely depressed and suicidal patient. It is possible for the patient to improve enough that he or she may still be depressed and also regain the energy needed to develop and act on a suicide plan. Careful follow-up is necessary.

53. D

Appropriate sleep hygiene or sleep habits are very important, even for the treatment of primary sleep disorders. Avoidance of caffeine, smoking, stimulants, and medications known to interfere with sleep is prudent. Alcohol and over-the-counter sleep aids may actually disrupt the sleep cycle, impair function, and have carry-over to the next day. Cognitive–behavioral techniques, relaxation therapy, and other behavioral interventions (such as scheduling worry time prior to bed) have been proven effective. If the patient cannot go to sleep within 15 minutes, he should get up and engage in some quiet activity.

54. A

Bipolar disorders in general have their onset in the second or third decade of life. By definition, Bipolar I disorder includes at least one manic episode. Although people with bipolar disorder may experience transient delusions, hallucinations, and other perceptual problems, these are not persistent in nature. Many people with bipolar disorder have or will have one or more depressive episodes, but this criterion is not required to make the initial diagnosis. Checking is usually associated with obsessive–compulsive disorder.

55. C

Marijuana is the most frequently used illegal drug in the United States. Nearly 69 million Americans older than the age of 12 years have tried marijuana at least once and 20 million are regular users. About 10 million had used the drug in the last month. Among teens 12 to 17 years old, the average age of first trying marijuana was 14 years. A yearly survey of students in grades 8 through 12 shows that 23% of 8th-graders have tried marijuana at least once, and by 10th grade 21% are "current" users (i.e., used within the past month). Among 12th-graders, nearly 50% have tried marijuana or hash at least once, and about 24% were current users. Other researchers have found that use of marijuana and other drugs usually peaks in the late teens and early twenties, then declines in later years.

56. C

Because the patient understands he has a problem and is considering quitting, he is in the contemplation stage. The stages are as follows:

- Precontemplation: has not considered that there is a problem with the substance
- Contemplation: has wondered whether or not she should stop using the substance
- Preparation: is beginning to formulate a plan to stop using
- Action: has begun making behavioral or situational changes
- Follow-up: continued implementation or alteration of plan, despite possible setbacks

57. E

During the contemplation stage, it is important to solidify the patient's decision to quit by exploring the costs and benefits of quitting. Although family meetings can be helpful in working with these patients, usually this is done when the patient is in the precontemplation stage in which he or she does not see the alcohol as a problem. Talking about the negative health outcomes might be helpful with some patients; however, these can be seen as threats and put the physician and patient in adversarial positions. Inpatient treatment might be an appropriate treatment for the patient, but that step would occur in the preparation or action stage.

58. D

The largest risk factor for PTSD is lack of functional social support. A family history of anxiety disorders and prolonged early separation from parents are additional risk factors. Alcohol and drug dependence are associated with exposure to adverse and traumatic events, but epidemiologic studies have shown that they are not risk factors for developing PTSD.

59. C

It is during the preparation stage that a plan should be formulated to stop the alcohol use. During the precontemplation stage, the patient does not acknowledge drinking as a problem. During the contemplation state, the patient may be considering stopping. During the action phase, the patient will have already put into practice behavioral changes that were identified in the preparation stage. In the follow-up stage, the focus is on continuing to work on the plan.

60. D

The short-term effects of marijuana use are all of the above except seizure. Other signs and symptoms that often occur after marijuana use include the following: The person may seem dizzy and have trouble walking; seem silly and giggly for no reason; have very red, bloodshot eyes; and have a difficult time remembering things that just happened. When the early effects fade, over a few hours, the user can become very sleepy.

61. C

In order to make the diagnosis of ADHD, it is necessary to have impairment due to the condition in two or more settings (school and home). Since you only have symptoms in one setting, the diagnosis of ADHD would be premature. Therefore, speaking to the child's teacher will help with the diagnosis. A referral to a therapist could be appropriate once you have a better understanding of the problem. Parenting classes may be beneficial, but it is important to rule out ADHD before using this referral. Parents will often feel blamed if they are referred for parenting classes. If this is an appropriate referral, great care should be used in presenting this option.

62. A

TCAs and fluoxetine have been well studied in pregnancy, do not increase the risk of structural or behavioral teratogenesis, and do not clearly cause any perinatal syndromes. The other SSRIs are not as well studied but do not appear to increase the rate of teratogenesis. Serotonin–norepinephrine reuptake inhibitors and other newer antidepressants have not been well studied in this regard. MAOIs have not been thoroughly studied, but current data suggest they are problematic and should not be used in pregnancy. Any drug use in pregnancy should involve a careful discussion with the patient and weighing the benefits and harms of treatment.

63. D

Drug-related emergency department visits included an estimated 131 cocaine mentions per 100,000 population, 55 heroin mentions, 73 marijuana mentions, and 35 for stimulant mentions per 100,000 population. Together, these four drugs accounted for 35% of all drug mentions in DAWN-reportable ED visits in 2004.

64. B

Divorce is disruptive for the entire family. Particularly at risk are elementary-aged children. Neither joint nor sole custody arrangements have been shown to be associated with better outcomes for the children. After divorce, women are often economically challenged, whereas men's standard of living often increases. Women older than age 30 are less likely to remarry. Older women cope better than older men after divorce.

Elementary-age children tend to fare worse after divorce than children of other ages. Divorce clearly affects the whole family, and although there is no clearly superior method of custody, a respectful relationship between parents focused on the children's best interests will help ensure most favorable outcomes.

65. B

Nortriptyline, nefazodone (Serzone), and venlafaxine (Effexor) all tend to be somewhat sedating and have a calming effect. A patient experiencing lethargy and fatigue might benefit more from an activating or stimulating antidepressant such as sertraline (Zoloft).

66. E

The antipsychotic agents may prolong the QTc and lead to Torsades de Pointes, a serious and potentially life-threatening arrhythmia. The older tricyclic antidepressants also may prolong the QT interval, whereas the newest agents (such as the SSRIs) are relatively devoid of cardiac problems.

67. E

Several studies show that cognitive–behavioral techniques have lower rates of relapse than pharmacologic treatments for PTSD. However, CBT requires more active participation than drug treatment and is less generalizable. There are no good empirical data to support psychoanalysis over hypnosis. Polypharmacologic approaches are often used but lack evidenced-based support. Support groups are generally considered beneficial, especially in the case of rape victims.

68. D

This patient has the neuroleptic malignant syndrome (NMS), which usually occurs during the period of initiation of an antipsychotic medication (including atypical antipsychotics), as well as with discontinuation of antiparkinsonian agents. In addition, this patient has an organic brain disorder, which further predisposes to NMS. CPK levels are ubiquitously elevated (usually between 2,000 and 15,000 v/L) in patients with NMS. Treatment is withdrawal of olanzapine, re-initiation of amantadine, and supportive therapy to correct temperature dysregulation. Benzodiazepines, dopaminergic agonists, and dantrolene may be used, and the latter two agents have been shown to reduce mortality. ECT is a controversial treatment.

69. C

All of the noted conditions could potentially present in a similar fashion except serotonin syndrome, which is characterized by abdominal pain, diarrhea, sweating, fever, tachycardia, elevated blood pressure, altered mental state, myoclonus, and even death.

70. B

Predictable changes in sleep occur in healthy elders. These include slightly decreased total sleep time, decreased deep and REM sleep, longer sleep latency, increased nocturnal awakenings, and advanced sleep phase (earlier to bed, earlier to rise).

71. B

Melancholic depression is specified by either the presence of a marked and pervasive anhedonia or a loss of pleasurable response to pleasurable stimulus of any sort, as well as three of the following: mood worse in morning, early morning awakening, marked psychomotor retardation or agitation, significant anorexia or weight loss, excessive or inappropriate guilt, or distinctly different subjective feel of the depressed mood by the subject. The significance of differentiating patients with melancholic depression is controversial, but it is thought to be a more severe form of depression and may warrant referral to a psychiatrist and more aggressive treatment, especially if initial treatment response is not optimal. TCAs may be more effective than SSRIs for this type of depression.

72. B

It has been suggested that a positive relationship with one parent can act as a buffer against the stress and disruption resulting from the divorce process, whereas a close bond to both or neither parent does not appear to act as a buffer. It is possible that a close bond to one parent, as opposed to both parents, decreases the likelihood of loyalty conflicts, which lowers the likelihood of feelings of anxiety about potentially alienating one parent by being forced to take sides.

73. D

The other options are nonspecific or suggest another diagnosis. Differentiating a major depressive episode from that of grief or bereavement can sometimes be difficult. There are a number of overlapping symptoms, and it is not unusual for some people to meet the criteria for depression, especially in the acute stages of grief. Grief and bereavement may evolve into a depressive disorder. Symptoms from grief and bereavement usually start to resolve after several months. Uncomplicated grief usually resolves with supportive or grief counseling or no intervention. Differentiating between major depression and normal grief is important because patients with major depression are at greater risk for suicide. People with a history of a depressive disorder are at a higher risk of relapse following a significant loss.

The shared symptoms of grief include sadness, tearfulness, decreased appetite, sleep disturbances, and decreased interest in activities. Mood fluctuations are more common in grief ("waves" of grief with remission in between), versus a more persistent depressed mood with major depression. In normal grief, shame and guilt are usually limited to not having done enough for the deceased while alive, or survivor guilt. Guilt and shame in a depressive disorder are often described as feelings of worthlessness or of being a bad person. Hopelessness and anhedonia that persist after the acute period of grief are more suggestive of a depressive disorder.

74. E

Valproic acid most commonly causes weight gain, tremor, alopecia, and gastrointestinal disturbance. The transient alopecia can be treated with selenium and zinc in some patients. There have been some reports of abnormal thyroid studies in patients on valproic acid, but their clinical significance is not clear. Hyperammonemia usually is limited and does usually require stopping the drug.

75. B

According to the DSM-IV, to be diagnosed with a major depressive episode, a patient must have experienced symptoms for at least 2 weeks. These symptoms must include anhedonia *or* dysphoria, along with four others, including disturbance of sleep, appetite, concentration, energy, self-esteem, hopefulness, or psychomotor activity. In depression, the latter is most likely to be psychomotor retardation (whereas anxiety is likely to be marked by psychomotor agitation). Depression can have its onset with or without an identifiable stressor. Early morning awakening is a common complaint with depression, not difficulty initiating sleep.

76. B

Traditionally, lithium has been thought to be associated with a 10-fold increase in Ebstein's abnormality with exposure in the first trimester. More recently, a well-designed study did not find this association, but further confirmation is probably warranted. Lithium is currently classified as a class D drug for use in pregnancy (positive evidence of human fetal risk, but the risks may be acceptable in a serious disease or life-threatening circumstance). Valproic acid and carbemazepine are associated with a 10-fold increase in neural tube defects with first-trimester exposure, and they are also associated with oral clefts. No behavioral teratogenicity has been confirmed with any of these agents. Daily folate supplementation with 1 mg folate can reduce the risk of anticonvulsant-associated neural tube defects.

77. D

It is very unlikely for an otherwise healthy male whose sexual functioning has been normal to have a low testosterone level. Although a referral for Viagra may eventually be needed, the most appropriate approach would be to address the stress issues and re-evaluate. Premature prescription of Viagra can make a man inappropriately psychologically dependent on the medication.

78. D

Generalized anxiety disorder (GAD) is associated with excessive worry or anxiety and a host of somatic symptoms. It is more common in women than men. GAD is highly comorbid with many psychiatric illnesses, such as major depression in 62% and alcoholism in 37%. A sensation of a "lump in throat" is common with panic attacks as well.

79. D

The diagnosis of panic disorder requires both the occurrence of unexpected panic attacks and that this be followed by at least 1 month of at least one of the following: persistent worry about having more attacks, worry about the implications of the attack, or a significant change in behavior related to the attacks. Panic attacks are often associated with sweating, trembling, and shaking, and they can mimic choking or a heart attack.

80. D

Although all of the above might be appropriate in working up this individual's problem, taking the sexual history is the first step. Through the sexual history, the physician can determine whether this is a primary or secondary sexual dysfunction. The sexual history can also be useful to rule out any technique problems with the couple. Often, the inability to reach orgasm can be due to inadequate foreplay and stimulation.

81. D

The goal of supportive psychotherapy is to help the patient adapt to stresses while providing affirmation and validation. The therapist hopes to strengthen defenses to facilitate the patient's adaptive capacity to handle the stresses of daily living. This goal often involves restoring a patient to a previous level of functioning that has been compromised by a crisis. The therapist may help the patient view reality more accurately and anticipate the consequences of the patient's actions and thereby improve his or her judgments. At the other end of this spectrum are interventions such as clarification, confrontation, interpretation, and more insight-oriented techniques.

82. E

Delirium tremens is considered the third and most severe stage of alcohol withdrawal. Patients can develop DTs as early as 24 hours and as late as 10 days after the cessation of drinking. Withdrawal of ethanol causes a functional decrease in the inhibitory effects of the neurotransmitter GABA. The withdrawal of the GABA effects leads to a marked elevation of sympathetic activity and catecholamine release. The symptoms of DTs include mental confusion, tremor, sensory hyperacuity, visual hallucinations (e.g., bugs and snakes), autonomic hyperactivity, diaphoresis, dehydration, electrolyte disturbances (hypokalemia and hypomagnesemia), seizures, and cardiovascular abnormalities. Patients typically experience significant "sundowning" or worsening symptoms with the onset of darkness and loss of visual cues to reality. Loss of insight into the hallucinosis of alcohol withdrawal defines the difference between DTs and stage 2 hallucinosis. Such hallucinations may cause panic and violent or aggressive behaviors. Mortality may be as high as 35% if untreated, but early recognition and treatment reduces this to 5%. Comorbid medical conditions including infection and hepatitis may increase the risk for DTs.

83. C

The incidence of depression is about the same in pregnant and nonpregnant women. However, the incidence of depression is significantly increased during the postpartum period. Although many women experience postpartum blues, and can often be managed with supportive therapy alone, patients who meet criteria for major depressive disorder should be treated aggressively. Current evidence suggests depression can be managed with medications during pregnancy and the postpartum period with little risks to the developing fetus or neonate. The best evidence supports the use of the SSRIs. Nonetheless, a careful discussion of risks and benefits of pharmacologic therapy should be initiated.

84. E

Vitamin E deficiency is not associated with depression. Some studies have implicated both folate and B12 deficiencies as being associated with depression. Other medical conditions that may contribute to depression include Cushing's disease, Addison's disease, hypothyroidism, hepatitis, HIV, anemia, and cancer. It is important to identify and treat depression early because it may play a direct role in patient compliance with medical treatment.

85. C

Risk factors for the development of delirium in elderly hospitalized patients include cognitive impairment, sleep deprivation, immobility, visual impairment, hearing impairment, and dehydration. Research has shown that developing protocols for treating target risk factors can reduce the number and duration of delirious episodes in hospitalized older patients. Benzodiazepines can exacerbate delirium and should be avoided. Nighttime benzodiazepines have a tendency to cause anterograde amnesia, worsening of existing memory impairment, insomnia, and confusion.

86. D

The decision balance technique has been shown to be most useful in counseling patients in the contemplation and preparation stages of behavioral change. This technique has the patient list the pros and cons of changing and keeping a behavior. For example, the patient might list for smoking cessation that a factor in favor of continuing smoking is the ability to relax; a con is that it costs a lot. A pro to quit smoking might be improved stamina and a con might be the risk of being teased by friends who continue to smoke.

87. B

There is no demonstrated relationship between sexual preference and history of divorce in the family. However, children of divorced parents have a greater chance of substance abuse, depression, poor school performance, and future divorce.

88. C

Although motivational counseling is an effective behavioral intervention for problems ranging from compulsive gambling to risky sexual behavior, there is no evidence that it is effective in changing sexual orientation. Moreover, intervention to change sexual orientation is not warranted.

89. E

All of these problems are linked to ED, but prostatic disease is less likely in a younger male, whereas atherosclerosis, psychogenic, neuropathic, and medication-induced problems would be more common, especially in this patient with long-standing type 1 diabetes mellitus.

90. E

Because this patient has diabetes, the use of an ACE-I or ARB is preferred because of their favorable effect on morbidity and possibly mortality. Relaxation and couples therapy may help with contributing psychologic factors. Valproic acid tends to interfere less than lithium with erectile dysfunction in males.

Because of probable organic contributors to ED, silandefil (Viagra) would be reasonable if coronary artery disease was unlikely to be present. Of course, stressing the importance of good diabetic control and the role of diabetes in ED is important. Fluoxetine and other SSRIs are commonly associated with sexual dysfunction. Even if this patient was depressed, other options would be better.

91. C

Tramodol has been shown to cause seizures in some patients on antidepressant medications. Because of bupropion's association with seizures, this combination would be inadvisable.

92. B

The CAGE method has been found to be an effective initial screening tool to identify problem drinking. This method involves four questions:

> Have you ever felt that you ought to *cut* down on your substance usage?
> Have you ever been *annoyed* by people criticizing your substance use?
> Have you ever felt *guilty* or bad about your substance use?
> Have you ever had to use the substance first thing in the morning to get your day going, steady your nerves, or to treat a hangover (*eye opener*)?

One positive response indicates high risk for alcohol abuse and further evaluation is indicated. The SASSI is a more in-depth assessment device and would be an appropriate evaluation if the CAGE is positive. Because of denial and minimization, asking the patient how much he or she drinks is not a good measure of true consumption. Asking the patient's family about alcohol consumption might be an appropriate assessment; however, many family members minimize and deny the extent of the patient's alcohol consumption.

93. B

Lithium can aggravate a number of medical conditions and interact with a number of commonly prescribed medications. Antihypertensives should be switched to nonthiazide diuretics or nondiuretic therapy because these drugs can elevate lithium levels. Lithium may cause exacerbation of psoriasis and acne, or other dermatologic reactions, early in the course of therapy. Although this is not an absolute contraindication, other treatments may be a better choice.

94. C

Depression is more prevalent in women than men. Moreover, women typically attempt suicide more frequently but tend to use less lethal means. Atypical symptoms are more common in women, who also tend to experience more guilt than men. Thyroid disease and migraine are also more common comorbidities.

Chapter 6

Surgery Questions

1. A 36-year-old data entry clerk presents to your office complaining of tingling and pain in the right thumb and wrist, worse by the end of the day. Occasionally, she is awakened at night from the pain. Phalen's, Tinel's, and median nerve compression tests are positive. The hand and wrist appear otherwise normal, with full range of motion, good perfusion, and no focal signs of inflammation or trauma. Which of the following treatment modalities would be your first choice in alleviating pain in this patient?
A. Steroid and lidocaine injection into the carpal tunnel
B. Wrist splinting in neutral or slight extension
C. Trigger point injection
D. Surgical release of the transverse carpal ligament
E. Iontophoresis therapy

2. The following positive physical examination finding is helpful in diagnosing rotator cuff disease:
A. Drop arm test
B. "Popeye muscle"
C. Adson's maneuver
D. Sulcus test
E. Spurling's test

3. A 20-year-old man with a history of epileptic seizure presents to the emergency room complaining of left shoulder pain following a grand mal seizure. He presents holding his left arm adducted and rotated inward. Which radiologic study is the most important for this patient's diagnosis?
A. True AP view
B. Transcapular lateral view
C. Axillary lateral view
D. Scapular Y view
E. Serendipity view

4. Which of the following diseases is associated with frozen shoulder (adhesive capsulitis)?
A. Diabetes mellitus
B. Osteoarthritis
C. Hypertension
D. Pregnancy
E. Gout

5. A 45-year-old woman presents to the emergency room when you are on call. She complains of epigastric pain, radiating to the back. She also has nausea and vomiting. She states that she has had similar symptoms for many years but has never felt this bad. She does not use tobacco or alcohol. You suspect obstruction of the common bile duct because the patient is jaundiced. The optimal diagnostic study is:

A. Ultrasound evaluation
B. Computerized tomography (CT) scan of the abdomen
C. Plain abdominal films, flat and upright
D. HIDA scan
E. Endoscopic retrograde cholangiopancreatography

6. A teenage boy is brought in by his mother to see you for 1 day of abdominal pain in the right lower quadrant, nausea, and anorexia. He appears unwell and states that even the car ride to the office was painful for him. The best method of diagnosis for his condition is:
A. CT scan
B. History and physical exam
C. Ultrasound
D. Barium enema
E. Complete blood count

7. On a routine physical exam, you think you feel a pulsatile mass in the abdomen of a 65-year-old woman. She has no abdominal complaints. You are concerned about an abdominal aortic aneurysm (AAA). Which of the following is correct?
A. Women's risk of AAA is three times higher than that for men.
B. Aneurysm diameters of 6 cm or more are at the greatest risk of rupture.
C. Physical exam is not accurate in diagnosing aneurysms.
D. An aneurysm is defined as a dilation of 100% or greater from the baseline diameter.
E. Aortic aneurysms are most commonly suprarenal.

8. Which of the following statements about hemorrhoids is correct?
A. A palpable rectal mass is usually associated with internal hemorrhoids.
B. Internal hemorrhoids, although not usually painful, become so with prolapse.
C. In patients with thrombosed external hemorrhoids, removing the largest portion of the clot will hasten recovery.
D. Hemorrhoids are associated with age older than 50 years, pregnancy, and portal hypertension.
E. Treatment of hemorrhoids includes a low-residue diet.

9. Which. of the following statements about colorectal cancer is true?
A. Villous adenomatous polyps have only a 5% chance of becoming malignant.
B. The average time from development of a polyp to malignant transformation is 5 years.

217

C. One-half of all colon cancers occur in the transverse colon.

D. Risk factors for colon cancer include Lynch syndrome, inflammatory bowel disease, and familial adenomatous polyposis syndrome.

E. Presenting with hematochezia has a worse prognosis than presenting with constipation.

10. A 25-year-old man is seen in the emergency room complaining of pain in his scrotum. The presence of pyuria is most associated with:

A. Varicocele

B. Acute orchitis

C. Testicular torsion

D. Epididymitis

E. Testicular cancer

11. A major advantage of cryotherapy is:

A. Its use in deeper lesions, such as dermatofibroma

B. The preservation of skin pigment in visible areas

C. Minimal to no scarring that results from treatment

D. That it is painless

E. It can be used in areas with hair growth

12. In treating recurrent ingrown toenails (onychocryptosis), which is true?

A. At the time of the nail removal, nerve block is necessary on the ingrown side only.

B. Epinephrine in the anesthetic will be very helpful in reducing bleeding after toenail removal.

C. The toebox should fit snugly to provide support for the affected foot.

D. Phenol can only be used for total nail ablation.

E. A periosteal elevator will reduce injury to the nail bed during toenail removal.

13. The best tool for evaluating benign prostatic hypertrophy (BPH) is:

A. Rectal exam

B. Prostate-specific antigen (PSA) level

C. History

D. Urodynamics

E. Urinalysis

14. Which of the following statements concerning tonsils and adenoids is correct?

A. The immune function of tonsils and adenoids diminishes in the third decade of life.

B. Children have a higher risk of postoperative bleeding after a tonsillectomy or adenoidectomy.

C. Asymmetric enlargement of the tonsils is a common finding.

D. Tonsillar and adenoid hypertrophy is the most common cause of obstructive sleep apnea in children.

E. CT scan is the best tool to evaluate hypertrophy.

15. Otitis media with effusion is common in both children and adults. Which of the following conditions can lead to otitis media with effusion?

A. Eustachian tube dysfunction

B. Hearing loss

C. Poor development of the mastoid air cells

D. Cholesteatoma

E. Tympanostomy tube placement

16. A 63-year-old man, previously healthy, presents to your office with 2 days of left abdominal pain and intermittent diarrhea. He has been taking soups and juices at home. On exam, he is afebrile. He does have left lower quadrant guarding but no peritoneal signs. The best course of action at this time would be:

A. Immediate endoscopic confirmation of the diagnosis, with admission for intravenous antibiotics after the procedure

B. CT scan of the abdomen with IV and oral contrast, and if it reveals no complicated disease, the patent can be sent home with an oral quinolone and metronidazole

C. Arrange for a double contrast barium enema and treat with sulfamethoxazole-trimethoprim as an outpatient

D. Refer the patient to a registered dietician for counseling on a high-fiber diet with follow-up in your office in a week

E. Make the patient NPO, in anticipation of surgery

17. A 68-year-old man presents to the office with a complaint of progressive blurry vision and inability to read the newspaper "for a while now." He has hypertension and smokes. You are able to do a fundoscopic exam and see multiple small round yellow to white lesions consistent with drusen lateral to the optic disc. See Figure 6-1. The most likely diagnosis is:

A. Diabetic retinopathy

B. Glaucoma

C. Cataracts

D. Retinal detachment

E. Macular degeneration

18. When performing a "cover test" on a 4-year-old girl, you notice that the left eye moves laterally when the right eye is covered. The most serious consequence of this disorder is:

A. Strabismus

B. Cataracts

C. Nystagmus

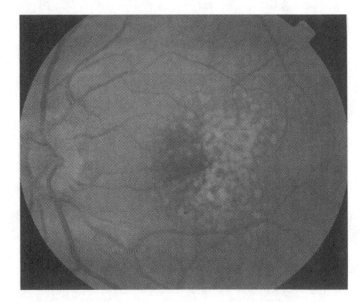

Figure 6-1.

D. Amblyopia

E. Leukocoria

19. A 78-year-old woman complains of itchy eyelids, with morning crusting for several months. Which of the following is the most likely diagnosis?

A. Chalazion

B. Allergic conjunctivitis

C. Blepharitis

D. Eczema

E. Viral infection

20. When patients present with suspected conjunctivitis, immediate referral to an ophthalmologist is warranted if:

A. There is bilateral itching

B. Mucopurulent discharge is present

C. The patient also has chlamydia

D. There is photophobia

E. The conjunctivitis is bilateral

21. On a routine urinalysis, a 50-year-old man is noted to have microscopic hematuria. He is asymptomatic and cannot recall if he ever had hematuria previously. After taking a history, you decide to further evaluate this finding. Which factor increases the likelihood that there is a serious underlying abnormality?

A. Acetaminophen use for chronic low back pain

B. A high number of squamous cells on microscopic examination of the urine

C. Recent vigorous exercise

D. Stress incontinence

E. Cigarette smoking

22. When a 35-year-old man presents to the emergency room with right flank colicky pain, you suspect nephrolithiasis. The imaging modality with the highest specificity and sensitivity is:

A. Intravenous pyelogram

B. Noncontrast CT scan

C. Abdominal radiograph

D. Ultrasound

E. Nuclear scan

23. A 60-year-old man has symptoms of prostate enlargement. If he also has mild hypertension, a good choice for initial therapy is:

A. Tamsulosin (Flomax)

B. Oxybutynin (Ditropan)

C. Terazosin (Hytrin)

D. Finasteride (Proscar)

E. Tolterodine (Detrol)

24. A 58-year-old man complains of painful legs. His physical exam reveals a loss of hair over the lower shins and dystrophic nails. An ankle brachial index is 0.80. The best course of action would be:

A. Prescription for exercise and smoking cessation

B. MRI of the lumbar spine

C. Ice and NSAID therapy

D. Duplex scan of the lower extremity veins

E. Arteriography of the lower extremities

25. You are examining a patient. During the fundoscopic exam, you notice increased cupping, but the patient denies any symptoms. The most likely diagnosis is:

A. Primary angle-closure glaucoma

B. Retinal detachment

C. Hypertensive retinopathy

D. Primary open-angle glaucoma

E. Diabetic retinopathy

26. An 85-year-old woman from a nursing home is brought by ambulance to the emergency room for vomiting. The patient complains of abdominal pain but has appropriate vital signs and normal mentation. The exam reveals a distended abdomen with an old lower abdominal midline scar. An x-ray reveals dilated loops of bowel and air in the rectum. The most appropriate next step in treatment is:

A. Rectal tube decompression and intravenous antibiotics

B. Nasogastric tube placement and intravenous isotonic saline infusion

C. Rectal suppository of promethazine (Phenergan) and oral ice chips afterwards

D. Narcotic analgesics and intravenous antibiotics

E. CT scan with contrast via nasogastric tube

27. Which of these patients will require tetanus prophylaxis?

A. A 24-year-old man with a cooking knife laceration to his finger; his last tetanus immunization was 8 years ago.

B. A 9-year-old girl with a stellate laceration from broken glass; her last tetanus immunization was 4 years ago.

C. A 45-year-old woman with a cut on her leg from a metal table corner; her last tetanus immunization was 9 years ago.

D. A 35-year-old man with a mild second-degree campfire burn to his arm; his last tetanus immunization was 4 years ago.

E. A 40-year-old man with a crushing hammer blow to his finger; his last tetanus immunization was 6 years ago.

28. Keratoacanthomas (KAs) should be biopsied because they are often indistinguishable from (see Figure 6-2):

A. Dematofibromas

B. Amelanotic melanomas

C. Squamous cell carcinomas

D. Angiokeratomas

E. Basal cell carcinomas

29. When undergoing a cystoscopy, which patient should get antibiotic prophylaxis?

A. A 53-year-old woman with mitral valve prolapse with regurgitation

B. A 70-year-old man with a pacemaker

C. A 35-year-old woman who had a ventricular sepal defect closed as a child

D. A 45-year-old man with a flow murmur

E. A 40-year-old woman with a secundum atrial septal defect

30. A 35-year-old man presents for a pre-employment physical. His only complaint is of a heavy feeling in this groin. On exam, there is a palpable but small bulge at the top of the scrotum that increases with Valsalva maneuver. The most likely diagnosis is:

A. Direct inguinal hernia

B. Varicocele

C. Indirect inguinal hernia

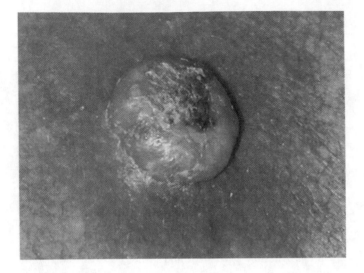

Figure 6-2. Keratocanthoma.

D. Hydrocele

E. Femoral hernia

31. The main risk factor for the development of a pterygium is:

A. Ultraviolet light exposure

B. Tobacco abuse

C. Chlamydial infection

D. Tear duct obstruction

E. Exposure to allergens

32. You suspect that a patient with unexplained gastrointestinal bleeding has a Meckel's diverticulum. The best diagnostic study would be:

A. CT scan

B. Abdominal flat and upright x-ray

C. Technicium-99m pertechnetate scan

D. Tagged RBC scan

E. Upper GI series with small bowel followthrough

33. After examining a man in the emergency room for colicky left flank pain, a CT scan demonstrates a distal ureteral stone that is 4 mm in diameter and no hydronephrosis. The best course of action is:

A. Urology evaluation for urgent extracorporeal shockwave lithotripsy

B. Preparation for placement of percutaneous nephrostomy tube

C. Admission for intravenous antibiotics

D. Preparation for ureteroscopy and stone retrieval

E. Ambulatory management with urine straining

34. After performing a flourescein test on a boy hit with a football, you notice a small area on the right eye that fluoresces green under the blue light. Assuming that the remainder of the full eye exam is normal, the best treatment for this is:

A. Topical analgesic drops

B. Topical antibiotic drops

C. Patching of the eye

D. Topical steroid drops

E. Contact lens use

35. A serious consequence of repeated concussions is the second impact syndrome. This is defined as:

A. Prolonged confusion lasting more than 1 week

B. Neck strain or "whiplash"

C. Loss of consciousness

D. Uncoordinated movement

E. Progressive cerebral edema

36. Which test is currently indicated to screen patients for lung cancer?

A. Sputum cytology

B. No screening is indicated

C. CT scan

D. Chest x-ray

E. Spirometry

37. Which of these skin lesions is not associated with a possible underlying systemic malignancy?

A. Generalized pruritis

B. Seborrheic keratosis

C. Acanthosis nigricans

D. Melasma or chloasma

E. Palmar–plantar keratoderma

38. In men with prostate cancer, all the treatment options have risks and side effects. Which treatment and risk pair is incorrect?

A. Radical nerve-sparing (suprapubic) prostatectomy: erectile dysfunction

B. Observation: metastasis

C. Radiotherapy: diarrhea

D. Radical nerve-sparing (suprapubic) prostatectomy: urinary urgency

E. Radiotherapy: erectile dysfunction

39. A man complains of a "lump" on his upper back. He states it has been slowly enlarging for many years but has never bothered him. On exam, it is compressible with a visible central punctum, and there is no erythema. You are able to express some white foul-smelling material from the lesion. You advise him:

A. It can be removed intact to prevent rupture into the surrounding dermis.

B. It should be biopsied via fine needle aspirate.

C. The lesion can be treated with cryotherapy.

D. The lesion is likely infected and should be treated with antibiotics prior to any removal.

E. Steroid injection into the area will reduce its size.

40. Keratosis pilaris is associated with which condition?

A. Varicella infection

B. Asthma

C. Vitiligo

D. Acne vulgaris

E. Type 2 diabetes mellitus

41. A pale lesion seen on the back of the patient has a "stuck on" appearance. There are multiple lesions like this over the entire back. This lesion is most likely a:

A. Skin tag

B. Seborrheic keratosis

C. Nevus sebaceous

D. Urticaria

E. Psoriasis

42. Actinic keratoses are seen frequently in elderly patients. What can these lesions become and what is the treatment of choice?

A. Basal cell carcinoma; excisional biopsy

B. Malignant melanoma; cryotherapy

C. Squamous cell carcinoma; cryotherapy

D. Malignant melanoma; wide excision

E. Squamous cell carcinoma; punch biopsy

43. Risk factors for the development of a squamous cell carcinoma (SCC) include which one of the following?

A. Previous burn injury

B. Female gender

C. Dark complexion

D. Family history of SCC

E. Younger age

44. Basal cell carcinomas (BCCs) may be treated with cryotherapy if:

A. There is a recurrence and re-excision would be cosmetically unacceptable.

B. The lesion occurs on the cheek.

C. The lesion is a sclerosing BCC.

D. The lesion occurs in the nasolabial fold.

E. The lesion is 2 cm in diameter.

45. A 15-year-old boy shows you his "cool" mole, which has a ring of pale skin around it, during a well checkup. You proceed to do a thorough check for:

A. Malignant melanoma

B. Alopecia areata

C. Basal cell carcinoma

D. Junctional nevi

E. Foreign body reaction

46. In African American patients, malignant melanomas most commonly occur on which body part?

A. Upper back

B. Lower legs

C. Lower arms

D. Forehead

E. Foot sole

47. Prognosis of malignant melanoma is most dependent on:

A. Diameter of the lesion

B. Location of the lesion

C. Amount of pigment in the lesion

D. The presence of bleeding or crusting

E. Depth of the lesion

48. An elderly woman presents to you with a pink scaling rash on her right areola. She has recently changed the detergent that she uses to wash her bras and attributes the rash to irritation. Other than the skin changes, the breast exam is normal. If the rash does not resolve with topical corticosteroid cream, the next step is:

A. Antibiotic treatment

B. Mammography

C. Antifungal cream

D. Vitamin D treatment

E. PUVA treatment

49. A mother asks about treatment for her 10-year-old daughter's atopic dermatitis. Appropriate treatment options include:

A. Radioallergosorbent testing (RAST)

B. Antibiotic treatment

C. HEPA filter use

D. Topical antihistamines

E. Ammonium lactate lotion

50. Guttate psoriasis most often presents after:

A. Severe sunburn

B. Group A beta-hemolytic streptococcal pharyngitis

C. Staphylococcal impetigo

D. Drug allergy

E. Herpes zoster outbreak

51. The Koebner phenomenon is defined as:

A. Lichenification of frequently rubbed skin

B. Thinning of the skin in response to corticosteroid use

C. Urticarial lesions in response to stroking the skin

D. Enlargement of the nose in rosacea

E. Lesion formation at the site of trauma

52. Junctional nevi are differentiated from dermal nevi in all but which of the following ways?

A. Junctional nevi are often lighter in color.

B. Dermal nevi are papular.

C. Dermal nevi occur most often on the face.

D. Junctional nevi are intraepidermal.

E. Dermal nevi often contain a terminal hair.

53. After examining a newborn infant, you note that over the lumbar region and buttocks there is a dark brown plaque with sharply demarcated border. It looks as if the infant were wearing a "bathing trunk." In counseling the parents, you tell them that:

A. Although unsightly, the lesion is of cosmetic importance only.

B. The lesion is relatively common.

C. No new lesions can develop.

D. Excision is mandatory but can be delayed until the patient is an adult.

E. This type of lesion can be associated with meningeal involvement.

54. A 16-year-old female is brought to your office complaining of mid-back pain for 2 months. She denies any history of trauma, radicular symptoms, fever, weight loss, or nocturnal pain. Her BMI is 23, she has regular menses, and she reports no other chronic medical problems. She is a competitive water skier who noticed the onset of these symptoms coincident with the beginning of her skiing season this year. Exam is significant for a moderate thoracic kyphosis, with no tenderness to palpation or localized deformity of the spine. Films of the thoracic spine reveal anterior wedging greater than 5% in three consecutive vertebral bodies. This patient's diagnosis is:

A. Juvenile, postural round back

B. Spondylolisthesis

C. Scheuermann's disease

D. Osteoporosis

E. Malignancy

55. You measure her kyphotic curve and find it to be 65%. The most appropriate treatment at this point would be:

A. Overhead arm extensions

B. Upper trunk and postural exercises

C. Surgical correction with posterolateral fusion

D. TLSO bracing

E. None of the above

56. Concerning seborrheic keratosis, which is true?

A. They are most commonly seen on the lower extremities.

B. They do not require treatment.

C. They are often seen in adults younger than age 50 years.

D. Liquid nitrogen is not appropriate for treatment.

E. The tendency to develop seborrheic keratoses is not inherited.

57. Which statement is incorrect regarding the management of basal cell carcinoma?

A. For large tumors with well-defined borders, excisional surgery is the preferred method of treatment.

B. Moh's surgery is necessary for BCCs on the cheek in order to be assured of cure.

C. Cryotherapy may be used for superficial BCCs with well-defined margins.

D. Because the dermis of the shoulder and back is thick, it is best to avoid curettage in these areas.

E. Radiation therapy may be used for areas where a good cosmetic result is an important consideration.

58. A 30-year-old male presents with a scaling red eruption over the entire scalp. You suspect seborrheic dermatitis and treat appropriately. Despite care, his skin condition does not improve. You order some blood work, including:

A. HIV

B. Antinuclear antibody

C. Lipid profile

D. Rheumatoid factor

E. Liver function tests

59. A 28-year-old woman presents to your office complaining of a lump under her axilla that is painful and swollen. She recalls frequent "blackheads" and multiple large pores in the same area. You recommend:

A. Surgery as soon as possible

B. Topical antibiotics

C. Oral anti-inflammatories

D. Oral antibiotics with good tissue penetration

E. Cold compresses with domboro's solution

60. A 25-year-old man presents to your office requesting a "mole check." He has noticed several moles on his back and extremities. He states that his father had several suspicious moles removed from his back but does not know if any were cancerous. Which characteristic would make you suspicious for dysplastic nevi?

A. Irregular borders that can fade into the surrounding normal skin

B. Smaller than 6 cm

C. Present at birth or developed within the first few weeks of life

D. Occur most frequently on the thighs

E. Uniform in color

61. A 35-year-old African American woman complains during a routine exam about an "unsightly" scar. It is at the location of her appendectomy site and is a dome-shaped linear lesion that is significantly wider than the original incision. You tell her:

A. These lesions can be treated best with intralesional corticosteroids after a healing period of several months.

B. Caucasian patients are more likely to develop these lesions.

C. These lesions can expand in size for decades.

D. Surgical excision often provides the best cosmetic appearance.

E. The head and neck are often spared from developing these lesions.

62. In order to reduce the pain and burning associated with injecting local anesthesia, the family physician may:

A. Warm the lidocaine to body temperature

B. Mix the lidocaine with sodium bicarbonate to raise the pH

C. Spray the skin with ethyl chloride

D. Inject into the subcutaneous tissue rather than the dermis

E. All of these techniques may be employed

63. A 55-year-old woman complains of right shoulder pain. The pain is increased at night when she tries to lie on the right side and also when she tries to reach overhead. In order to differentiate between impingement and rotator cuff tear, you:

A. Test for the Neer sign, forcibly flexing the shoulder overhead to reproduce pain

B. Order AP and axillary radiographs of the shoulder

C. Perform a subacromial bursal injection

D. Test for the Hawkins sign, forcibly internally rotating the humerus while the arm is in flexion to reproduce pain

E. Palpate for pain over the greater tuberosity

64. A 25-year-old obese woman complains of numbness and tingling of the little and ring finger in her left hand. She states that the symptoms are worse when she raises her hands. The elevated arm stress test (EAST) is positive on the left. The most likely diagnosis is:

A. Thoracic outlet syndrome

B. Carpal tunnel syndrome

C. Impingement syndrome

D. Chronic shoulder subluxation

E. Ulnar artery thrombophlebitis

65. You are asked to evaluate a 78-year-old male patient who has no family physician for a right total knee arthroplasty. His activity has been limited by knee pain, but he still climbs his staircase and mows his lawn. He has been trying to lose weight to improve his osteoarthritis and has managed to lose 20 lbs in the past 6 months but remains at 240 lbs. His last cardiac stress test was less than 2 years ago when his left knee joint was replaced. Factors that will increase this patient's risk of postoperative complications include:

A. His advanced age

B. His obesity

C. Recent weight loss

D. His functional capacity

E. His unknown cardiac status

66. While working at a local urgent care center, several patients present with animal bites and exposures. In order to judiciously use resources, which patient requires immediate rabies prophylaxis?

A. A 23-year-old male bitten by the neighbor's dog after he tried to feed it treats

B. A 7-year-old girl scratched by a friend's cat after picking it up

C. A 40-year-old man sprayed by a skunk while out hiking in the woods

D. A 30-year-old woman bitten by a hare while working in the garden

E. A 17-year-old boy bitten by a fox while out hunting with his dog

67. A 45-year-old man complains of seeing "dust." Taking a further history confirms that he is complaining of floaters. During the exam, you review possible etiologies that include:

A. Migraine headache

B. Keratitis

C. Myopia

D. Strabismus

E. Corneal abrasion

68. A 14-year-old girl with type 1 diabetes mellitus controlled via insulin pump is seen in one of the urgent visit slots in your office because of periorbital swelling in the right eye. The most likely organism in this patient is:

A. *Mucormycosis* sp.

B. *Haemophilus influenza*

C. *Aspergillosis* sp.

D. *Moraxella catarhalis*

E. *Streptococcus pneumoniae*

69. When examining a patient with a red eye, uveitis may be differentiated from keratitis by:

A. Decreased visual acuity

B. Ciliary flush

C. Photophobia

D. Periorbital pain

E. Constricted pupil

70. A 45-year-old man returns from a golfing vacation to report that he has a painful right elbow. On examination, the right medial epicondyle is tender to palpation and the patient has increased pain with wrist flexion. The best course of action is:

A. Refrain from golfing for suspected golfer's elbow

B. Refer to orthopaedics for this unusual presentation

C. Recommend surgery for radial tunnel decompression

D. Obtain x-rays for suspected radial head fracture

E. Splint the elbow for triceps tendonitis

71. After lifting her 4-year-old girl by the arms, a mother reports that her daughter began to cry and would not use her right arm. She is keeping the arm close to her side in a pronated position. The most effective treatment for this orthopaedic disorder is:

A. Splinting and/or casting depending on the length of time the radius was subluxed

B. Referral to orthopaedics for evaluation and possible surgical repair

C. X-ray evaluation prior to any manipulation

D. Limitation of activities that require reaching overhead

E. Rapid reduction by supinating the forearm

72. You see a 35-year-old man who fell onto his outstretched hand while playing basketball and dislocated his left elbow. You treat

him with reduction and splinting. The most common long-term complication of this injury is:

A. Motor weakness of the forearm

B. Olecranon bursitis

C. Ulnar nerve palsy

D. Limited extension

E. Medial epicondylar pain

73. A 28-year-old man presents to the office complaining of a painful right index finger. While working on his deck, a splinter punctured that same finger and the next day he noted swelling and pain. On exam, there is erythema and swelling of the pad extending to but not crossing the distal interphalangeal joint (DIP), but you see no pus. You decide to treat him with:

A. Nail removal to allow the infection to drain with subsequent daily soaking

B. Acyclovir for presumed herpetic whitlow, which should never be drained

C. Dorsal midaxial incision with packing removal in 2 or 3 days

D. Intramuscular cephalexin (Rocephin) and recheck in 2 days

E. Central volar incision with closure in 1 or 2 days to avoid future disability

74. Lateral femoral cutaneous nerve syndrome occurs most often in:

A. Type 2 diabetic patients

B. Elderly women after hip fracture

C. Patients with motor weakness of the hip abductors

D. Obese patients

E. Patients with lumbar disk herniation

75. Which of the following is correct regarding avascular necrosis of the femoral head?

A. It is associated with sharp pain with rapid onset.

B. It is associated with chronic inflammatory conditions.

C. CT scan with contrast is the diagnostic study of choice.

D. It is more common in older patients.

E. Early surgical reconstruction is the treatment of choice.

76. A 70-year-old male presents to your office complaining of left upper arm pain after falling off his back porch. He states he broke his fall by catching the railing with his left arm. He has noticed pain and weakness with movement, especially abduction of the shoulder. What is the most likely diagnosis?

A. Adhesive capsulitis

B. Rotator cuff tear

C. Posterior shoulder dislocation

D. Epicondylitis

E. Acromioclavicular sprain

77. A 50-year-old man who's only past medical history is hypothyroidism presents to the office complaining of painful shoulder with an increasing feeling of stiffness. On exam, he has decreased range of active and passive movement. What is the most likely diagnosis:

A. Osteoarthritis

B. Impingement syndrome

C. Adhesive capsulitis

D. Anterior shoulder dislocation

E. Rotator cuff tear

78. A 45-year-old female presents to the emergency room complaining of right shoulder pain. She states she slipped on a wet floor at home and fell onto her outstretched hand. She denies loss of consciousness, headache, or hand, hip, or leg pain. After your exam, you are sure there is a posterior shoulder dislocation. Which of the following would be a confirmatory x-ray?

A. True AP view
B. Oblique
C. Axillary view
D. Lateral
E. None of the above

79. A 25-year-old male reports to your office complaining of low back pain and right leg numbness. He reports acute onset of symptoms after lifting a heavy box. Physical exam reveals numbness of his lateral thigh and anterior shin along with weakness in dorsiflexion of his right great toe. The remainder of the physical is unremarkable and history reveals no other reported deficits or symptoms. What nerve root(s) is affected by his injury?

A. L3
B. L4
C. L5
D. L4 and L5
E. L3 and L4

80. What is the next best step for this injury?

A. Radiographs of the thoracic and lumbar spine to evaluate for bony injury
B. Bed rest for 1 or 2 weeks
C. Immediate surgery
D. Muscle relaxants, NSAIDs, and cold packs, followed by physical therapy
E. Back bracing until symptoms subside

81. A 52-year-old female patient presents to your office complaining of neck pain and occipital headaches. She denies any history of trauma. She states these symptoms have been gradual in onset over the past few years, with increasing frequency in the past 2 months. She denies any visual symptoms or jaw claudication. Exam reveals restricted lateral flexion and rotation of the neck, as well as weakness of deltoids bilaterally. Plain films reveal osteophytes and narrowed disc spaces, indicative of degenerative changes. What is the most likely diagnosis?

A. Brachial plexus neuropathy
B. Cervical spondylosis
C. Neck strain
D. Migraine with neurologic deficit
E. Temporal arteritis

82. What is the appropriate treatment for this condition?

A. Physical therapy
B. NSAIDs and muscle relaxants
C. Operative treatment, if symptoms are severe
D. Cervical collar
E. C or D

83. A 49-year-old white male presents to clinic with rectal bleeding for 2 weeks. The patient states that the bleeding usually occurs after a bowel movement. The patient denies pain. He also admits to itching near the anal region. The patient denies history of weight loss, other changes in bowel habits, and personal or family history of colon cancer. On exam, the patient is guiac positive with

internal hemorrhoids located in the anterior and posterior regions. What is the most appropriate management?

A. Consult a surgeon for hemorrhoidectomy
B. Treatment with Anusol, a stool softener, and avoidance of specific dietary components
C. Schedule flexible sigmoidoscopy and a double contrast enema
D. A and C
E. B and C

84. You perform a lipoma excision from a patient's forearm. The incision is linear. When deciding on the best closure and suture, you choose:

A. 3–0 silk subcutaneously, 4–0 nylon interrupted for the skin
B. 4–0 nylon mattress sutures for the skin
C. 4–0 chromic gut interrupted sutures for the skin
D. 3–0 nylon subcutaneously, 4–0 polypropylene (Prolene) intracuticularly
E. 3–0 polyglactic acid (Vicryl) subcutaneously, 4–0 nylon interrupted for the skin

85. Subungual hematoma evacuation requires:

A. A perforation of 1 or 2 mm to prevent reclosure
B. Complete digital block
C. Partial nail removal
D. Hematoma involvement of more than 50% of the nail
E. Antibiotic use after evacuation

86. When performing an incision and drainage of an abscess on the buttocks:

A. A small linear incision is used to minimize scaring.
B. Once drained, the cavity should be closed in two layers.
C. A field block with lidocaine with epinephrine will provide adequate anesthesia.
D. Antibiotics should be prescribed for all patients after drainage.
E. Cryogenic anesthetics do not provide adequate anesthesia.

87. You are rounding on a 63-year-old man from your practice who has undergone a colon resection for bleeding diverticuli 2 days ago. He does complain of pain at the incision site but is pleased with the patient-controlled anesthesia. On reviewing his vital signs, you note a fever to 101°F. Which of these is the most likely cause of fever at 48 hours post-op?

A. Deep venous thrombosis
B. Wound infection
C. Inflammation
D. Intra-abdominal abscess
E. Atelectasis

88. You are consulted by a surgeon to follow a 72-year-old man with type 2 diabetes mellitus during the postoperative period following a colon resection. After reviewing his preoperative records, you start him on insulin, aware that hyperglycemia is involved in:

A. Postoperative myocardial infarction
B. Wound infection
C. Pressure ulcers
D. Hypertension
E. Oligouria

89. While you are working at a local urgent care center, a 15-year-old male presents after burning himself at a barbecue. His burns involve his anterior left arm and half his left chest. He is in pain and you diagnose superficial partial-thickness burns. You quickly calculate the percentage of his body affected as:

A. 16.5%

B. 20%

C. 9%

D. 13.5%

E. less than 5%

90. When counseling a 45-year-old man who desires a vasectomy, you tell him the most common complication of the procedure is a sperm granuloma, which is associated with an increased risk of:

A. Reanastomosis

B. Epididymitis

C. Anti-sperm antibodies

D. Infection

E. Hematoma

91. While playing football, a 17-year-old student was hit on the right neck and shoulder area. He developed sharp burning shoulder pain that radiated down the arm. His arm also felt limp and lifeless. Which of the following statements regarding "burners" are true?

A. Burners by definition are transient and resolve spontaneously.

B. Patients with recurrent burners may have an associated increased risk of disc herniation.

C. He may return to play when he has complete resolution of pain and neurologic symptoms, and full range of motion of his cervical spine.

D. A and C

E. All of the above

92. The most specific physical exam maneuver or finding for anterior cruciate ligament (ACL) tear is:

A. Hemarthrosis

B. Anterior drawer sign

C. McMurray sign

D. Lachman maneuver

E. Apprehension test

93. While trying to catch a baseball, a 28-year-old male complains of sudden onset of knee pain. The pain subsided somewhat and he continued to play. Two or 3 days later, he developed knee swelling. He also complained of locking and pain with squatting. You suspect a meniscal tear. Which of the following is correct?

A. Young patients tend to present more frequently with an effusion or hemarthrosis than older patients.

B. Most meniscal tears are peripheral and do not heal well.

C. Patients with degenerative tears tend to be younger, athletic patients.

D. History and clinical exam is not sufficient to diagnose meniscal damage; an MRI is required.

E. Aggressive treatment with surgical debridement should be delayed as long as possible.

94. Which of the following has a causal relationship with cataracts?

A. Hypertension

B. Smoking

C. Hypothyroidism

D. UV-A exposure

E. Asthma

95. Which of the following is contraindicated in the treatment of seasonal allergic conjunctivitis?

A. Normal saline or liquid tear drops

B. Wearing occlusive glasses and being in an air-conditioned setting

C. Topical corticosteroids

D. Histamine antagonists

E. Mast cell stabilizers

96. A homeless male was found in an alley after a snowstorm. His core body temperature was 92°F and he was shivering, confused, incoherent, tachycardic, and tachypneic. Which of the following methods of rewarming is appropriate for this patient?

A. Passive rewarming by moving him to a warm environment and covering him with blankets

B. Active external rewarming with exogenous heat sources such as heated blankets, hot packs, or heat lamps

C. Active core rewarming using heated humidified air or intravenous fluid

D. Active core rewarming via peritoneal dialysis or hemodialysis

E. Active core rewarming using gastric or colonic irrigation

97. A 32-year-old male slammed his index finger into a car door about an hour ago. His finger is throbbing and the nail is a purplish color. Which of the following is true?

A. Risk of distal phalanx fracture with this mechanism of injury is rare; thus, radiographs are performed only in select cases.

B. The patient requires immediate subungual decompression with cautery or heated paper clip.

C. With simple subungual hematomas, splints should be placed for 2 or 3 weeks.

D. Subungual hematoma involving greater than 25% of the nail is likely to have nail bed laceration.

E. Prophylactic antibiotics with penicillins or first-generation cephalosporins should be given.

98. Which of the following statements regarding bites are true?

A. Human bites cause more serious infections than cat or dog bites.

B. Signs of infection are evident within 12 hours in cat bites and within 24 hours in dog bites.

C. Wounds should be left open if they are clinically infected wounds, puncture wounds, or wounds older than 24 hours.

D. If a confined animal observed for 10 days remains healthy, a bite victim does not need rabies prophylaxis.

E. All of the above

99. Which suture material is most useful for epidermal skin closure?

A. Cat gut

B. Polyglactic acid (Vicryl)

C. Monofilament nylon (Maxon)

D. Polyglycolic acid (Dexon)

E. Chromic

100. Regarding genu valgum and genu varum, which of the following is true?

A. Physiologic genu valgum (knock-knees) is not a normal variation in children.

B. Blount disease is a rare pathologic form of genu valgum (knock-knees)

C. Physiologic genu varum (bowlegs) is a normal variation in children younger than age 2 years.

D. Rickets is not a consideration with either condition.

E. Obese children are at less risk for Blount disease.

101. The incidence of sepsis, renal failure, and overall mortality in burned children is considerably higher if fluid resuscitation is delayed more than ____ hour(s) from thermal injury.

A. 1

B. 2

C. 4

D. 6

E. 12

102. Which statement is correct regarding incision and drainage?

A. Both carbuncles and furuncles should be incised and drained.

B. Incision and drainage is not indicated when the lesion becomes fluctuant and boggy.

C. The incision should be closed after 1 or 2 days of active drainage for better cosmesis.

D. Packing is contraindicated because it will trap bacteria in the wound.

E. Antibiotics such as first-generation cephalosporins or penicillins are always used after drainage.

103. Which of the following is true about Osgood–Schlatter disease:

A. It is a repetitive stress injury to the patellar tendon just inferior to the patella.

B. Virtually no patients grow out of this condition.

C. It is more common in females.

D. Treatment includes relative rest, strengthening, and stretching regimens.

E. Patients with Osgood–Schlatter disease are at greater risk of developing arthritis.

104. A 28-year-old woman complains that "every time I pick up my child, I get a sharp pain in my wrist." On physical exam, there is local tenderness at the tip of the radial styloid, positive Finkelstein's test, and pain aggravated by resisting thumb extension and abduction. What is the most likely diagnosis?

A. Carpal tunnel syndrome

B. Gamekeeper's thumb

C. Dorsal ganglion cyst

D. Carpometacarpal osteoarthritis

E. De Quervain's tenosynovitis

105. A 17-year-old skier seeks evaluation for pain and swelling in the thumb following a fall on the slopes 3 days prior. He has trouble flexing his thumb, and you find local swelling and tenderness along the ulnar side of the metacarpal (MP) joint. He has diminished strength on pinching the thumb and first finger together. What is your treatment of choice for this acute injury?

A. Immobilization with thumb spica splint

B. Local corticosteroid injection

C. Phonophoresis with hydrocortisone gel

D. Arthrodesis or reattachment of the distal torn ligament

E. Ice over the MP joint

106. A machinist presents to your office complaining of 2 weeks' duration of a painful index finger, which feels "locked up." He complains that when he uses scissors or fingernail clippers, he gets a sharp pain at the base of the finger on the palmar side. You find tenderness at the metacarpophalangeal (MCP) head of the finger, locking at the proximal interphalangeal (PIP) joint, and pain on passive extension of the finger. The symptoms have occurred for the past $1\frac{1}{2}$ months. He denies any inciting event leading to these symptoms. What is the diagnosis?

A. Tendon cyst

B. Trigger finger

C. Dupuytren contracture

D. Mallet finger

E. Osteoarthritis

107. A 57-year-old Caucasian woman presents to your office complaining that she cannot open her hands all the way, with one hand worse than the other. She has noted gradual contracture of her fourth and fifth fingers over the past 5 years. She denies pain, and she states that she is able to perform activities of daily living. You diagnose Dupuytren contracture because of the gradual progression of the disease, mild puckering of the skin over the fourth and fifth flexor tendons in the palm, mild fixed flexion contracture of the affected fingers, and painless palmar nodules and thickening. She has no active signs of tenosynovitis. What is the therapy of choice in her present condition?

A. Prompt surgical release to resolve the contracture before it is beyond surgical means of repair

B. Corticosteroid injection to the affected tendons to decrease inflammation in the flexor tendons to prevent fibrosis

C. Heated massage and stretching exercises to delay worsening fibrosis of the flexor tendons

D. Observation only

E. Long-term oral steroid use to halt the progression of the disease

108. Which of the following conditions is *not* associated with an increased risk of epistaxis (nose bleeds)?

A. Humid conditions

B. Septal deviation

C. Pregnancy

D. Sinusitis

E. Renal failure

109. A 35-year-old male reports to your acute clinic with an active nosebleed. The bleed appears to be coming from the anterior portion of the nasal septum and is stopped by direct pressure. It is not described as brisk, but it appears to continue once the pressure is released. Initial management includes:

A. Having the patient lie back and relax

B. Applying 1:1,000 epinephrine to the vestibule with a cotton ball

C. Having the patient hold pressure, checking every 1 or 2 minutes for persistence or cessation of bleeding

D. Cauterizing the bleeding site with a silver nitrate stick

E. C and D

110. Which of the following is true regarding overuse syndromes?

A. Overuse syndromes are rarely seen in family medicine offices.

B. Fibromyalgia is considered an overuse syndrome.

C. Sports participation can prevent overuse injury.

D. These syndromes are rarely seen in younger patients.

E. Patellar tendonitis is considered an overuse syndrome.

111. Which of these factors is included in the development of overuse syndromes?
A. Ergonomic factors, including temperature and vibration
B. Comfortable postures in the workplace
C. Psychosocial factors do not play a role
D. Relaxed pace work environment
E. Obesity

112. Popliteal cysts are commonly associated with:
A. Rheumatoid arthritis
B. Medial gastrocnemius strain
C. Degenerative meniscal tears
D. A and C
E. All of the above

113. The following finding on physical exam is suggestive of patellofemoral pain syndrome:
A. Patellae point away from each other
B. Tenderness present at the inferior pole of the patella
C. Patella moves laterally upon full extension
D. Bowlegs (genu varus) when standing
E. Q angle less than 25 degrees

114. While swinging a baseball bat during a game, a patient hears a pop in her knee and develops severe pain. Her leg becomes locked in a partially flexed position and the knee now looks deformed. On exam, manipulation of the patella produced significant anxiety. Range of motion was quite limited and an effusion was noted. Lachman and McMurray's tests were negative, and no pain or laxity was elicited upon valgus strain. Medial joint line tenderness was absent. The patient likely has:
A. Anterior cruciate ligament tear and should receive aspiration of the joint, knee immobilization, and possible ACL reconstruction
B. Medial collateral ligament tear and should receive rest, ice, compression, elevation (RICE); crutches; NSAIDs; and a hinged brace for 6 weeks to 3 months with strengthening exercises
C. Medial meniscal tear and should receive RICE, analgesics, and surgical debridement
D. Patellofemoral instability and requires compressive dressing, protective splinting in extension, joint aspiration, analgesics, and ice for 24 to 48 hours, then immobilization, modified weight bearing and isometric exercises of the quadriceps
E. Patellofemoral pain syndrome and requires a program of strengthening and flexibility of the quadriceps and hamstrings, NSAIDs, and a knee sleeve

115. A patient with osteochondritis dissecans will show which finding on radiograph?
A. Osteonecrotic fragment fractures from the articular surface of the femoral condyle
B. Fracture of the femur just proximal to the knee joint
C. Abnormal positioning of the patella onto the trochlea
D. Signs of osteopenia in the bone shaft
E. Narrowing of the joint space

116. A 30-year-old healthy woman who has decided to train for a marathon comes to you for advice on proper hydration. You recommend the following:
A. 15 oz. of water consumed every 20 minutes of exercise

B. 12 oz. of a sport drink containing 8% carbohydrate every 20 minutes of exercise
C. 20 oz. of a sport drink containing 8% carbohydrate every 60 minutes of exercise
D. 12 oz. of a sport drink containing 12% carbohydrate every 15 minutes of exercise
E. Drink whenever she feels thirsty

117. A 35-year-old female complains of increased nervousness and heart palpitations. Physical examination reveals a resting heart rate of 113 beats per minute and an enlarged thyroid gland is palpable and exophthalmos. You suspect Grave's disease. What is the next step to confirm your diagnosis?
A. Obtain an electrocardiogram
B. Order thyroid ultrasound
C. Order TSH, T3, and T4 levels
D. Order a fine needle aspiration of the gland
E. No further workup is necessary

118. Which of the following athletes would require further evaluation prior to being cleared to play on his or her pre-participation physical examination?
A. A 12-year-old female soccer player with a history of exercise-induced asthma well-controlled on montelukast (Singulair) and albuterol MDI
B. A 16-year-old female gymnast with asymptomatic mitral valve prolapse (MVP)
C. A 14-year-old male HIV-positive tennis player with no apparent manifestations of AIDS
D. A 17-year-old male cross country runner with a history of a stress fracture last season that is now healed
E. A 15-year-old healthy male football player whose 25-year-old cousin recently collapsed and died

119. A 35-year-old woman complains of right upper quadrant pain for the past 3 days. This pain is worsened by eating, and today she has had nausea and vomiting. Physical examination: temperature, 100.6°F heart rate, 103; weight, 237 lbs. She appears uncomfortable; on abdominal palpation she has a positive Murphy's sign. Laboratory examination demonstrates elevated WBCs but otherwise is normal. Ultrasound of the gallbladder demonstrates the presence of stones in the gallbladder and fluid around the gallbladder. What is your diagnosis?
A. Pancreatitis
B. Cholelithasis
C. Choledocholithasis
D. Cholangiitis
E. Cholecystitis

120. A 7-year-old boy complains of pain bilaterally in the posterior heel. He is an avid soccer player and the pain typically occurs after he finishes practice or a game. Examination reveals tenderness at the junction of the Achilles tendon and the calcaneus. What is your diagnosis?
A. Sever disease
B. Achilles tendonitis
C. Gastrocnemius strain
D. Plantar fasciitis
E. Morton's neuroma

Chapter 6

Answer Key

1. C	43. A	85. A
2. A	44. B	86. C
3. C	45. A	87. C
4. A	46. E	88. B
5. E	47. E	89. C
6. B	48. B	90. A
7. B	49. E	91. D
8. D	50. B	92. D
9. D	51. E	93. A
10. D	52. A	94. B
11. C	53. E	95. C
12. E	54. C	96. A
13. C	55. D	97. B
14. D	56. B	98. E
15. A	57. B	99. C
16. B	58. A	100. C
17. E	59. D	101. B
18. D	60. A	102. A
19. C	61. C	103. D
20. D	62. E	104. E
21. E	63. C	105. A
22. B	64. A	106. B
23. C	65. B	107. C
24. A	66. E	108. A
25. D	67. C	109. E
26. B	68. E	110. E
27. E	69. E	111. A
28. C	70. A	112. D
29. A	71. E	113. C
30. C	72. D	114. D
31. A	73. C	115. A
32. C	74. D	116. B
33. E	75. B	117. C
34. B	76. B	118. E
35. E	77. C	119. E
36. B	78. C	120. A
37. D	79. C	
38. D	80. D	
39. A	81. B	
40. B	82. E	
41. B	83. E	
42. C	84. E	

Chapter 6

Surgery Answers

1. C

A trigger point is defined as the presence of discrete focal tenderness located in a palpable taut band of skeletal muscle, which produces both referred regional pain and a local twitch response. This patient had no signs of local inflammation. In the absence of a definable trigger point, dry needling or lidocaine injection is unnecessary. Local application of steroid and/or lidocaine, either by direct injection into the carpal tunnel space or by iontophoresis, may significantly alleviate the pain from soft tissue inflammation in carpal tunnel syndrome. Iontophoresis is the use of electric impulses from a low-voltage current to drive topical corticosteroids into soft tissue structures. Wrist splinting is a noninvasive, cost-effective treatment to relieve compression of the median nerve, but it requires a great deal of patient compliance. Surgery is not the first step in this patient's management but should be considered if all other treatment modalities fail.

2. A

The drop arm test is helpful in diagnosing rotator cuff disease, with the patient unable to oppose even gentle downward force on the affected arm held in 90° abduction. Failure is primarily due to weakness in the supraspinatus muscle, one of the four ("SITS") rotator cuff muscles: supraspinatus, infraspinatus, teres minor, and subscapularis. The "Popeye muscle" is a bulge associated with proximal biceps tendon rupture. Adson's maneuver tests for thoracic outlet syndrome, where the radial pulse is lost with shoulder extension and ipsilateral head rotation while holding the breath. The sulcus test indicates glenohumeral instability, where downward traction on the adducted arm results in dimpling of the skin distal to the acromion. Spurling's test is associated with cervical spine pathology, resulting in ipsilateral pain from lateral head flexion and rotation with compression.

3. C

The patient probably has a posterior shoulder dislocation based on the seizure history and his presentation of shoulder pain with an adducted and internally rotated arm. The first three views listed in the question (true AP, transcapular, and axillary lateral) should all be obtained for shoulder traumas. The axillary lateral view, however, is important to confirm the diagnosis of glenohumeral dislocation, especially posterior type.

4. A

Secondary adhesive capsulitis is associated with many conditions. Diabetes, myocardial infarction, stroke, thyroid disease, and rheumatoid arthritis are all linked to frozen shoulder. However, the mechanisms are unclear, whether it is due to trauma, autoimmune reaction, inflammatory conditions, or a combination of these. Although the diagnosis of adhesive capsulitis is usually made clinically, arthrography is the imaging test of choice to document decreased joint volume if the diagnosis is unclear. It is an invasive test but can definitively demonstrate loss of joint volume.

5. E

Endoscopic retrograde cholangiopancreatography (ERCP) is the gold standard in diagnosing choledocolithiasis. It has the added benefit of being therapeutic because sphincterotomy and removal of impacted stones is possible. If biliary pancreatitis is present, early ERCP may reduce morbidity and mortality. The complications of ERCP are pancreatitis, infection, biliary duct perforation, and hemorrhage. Ultrasound is an excellent choice for gallstones in the gallbladder and has a high sensitivity for acute cholecystitis. However, up to half of biliary duct stones are missed, likely due to abdominal gas. Also, small stones (less than 2 mm) are easily missed on ultrasound. CT scan can be helpful in determining if there is evidence of pancreatitis. High-resolution CT scans that provide three-dimensional images of the biliary duct may be comparable to ERCP but do not offer therapeutic options. Abdominal films are unlikely to be helpful, although there may be a sentinel loop of duodenum seen in acute pancreatitis. A HIDA scan uses technetium-labeled iminodiacetic acid that is injected intravenously. Because it is excreted by the liver into the bile, the gallbladder and ducts should be seen within 30 to 45 minutes of administration. Nonvisualization of the gallbladder is usually due to obstruction of the cystic duct. Repeating the scan 4 hours after initial administration will reduce the false-positive rate for gallbladder nonvisualization. Ninety-five percent of common bile duct stones originate in the gallbladder. The complications are acute pancreatitis and cholangitis. The classic presentation of cholangitis, called Charcot's triad, consists of chills, pain, and jaundice. If there is hypotension and altered mental status as well, the presentation is called Reynold's pentad and is indicative of ascending cholangitis and sepsis. Pancreatitis may be difficult to differentiate from cholangitis in that symptoms are similar. However, enzyme levels, particularly lipase and amylase, are higher in pancreatitis.

6. B

Despite all the diagnostic tests available to the clinician, acute appendicitis is diagnosed at the bedside. Because time is essential in preventing rupture of the appendix, radiologic studies are done only when the diagnosis is in question. Almost 100% of patients will have abdominal pain and anorexia. However, only 50% of patients have the classic symptoms of periumbilical pain migrating to McBurney's point along with anorexia and nausea. The most common findings on exam in appendicitis are right lower quadrant tenderness, fever, guarding, and peritoneal signs, including Psoas sign, Obturator sign, and Rovsing's sign. CT scans, specifically appendiceal CTs, are both sensitive and specific for acute appendicitis if the diagnosis is in question. It requires gastrografin contrast given as an enema. The CT can identify periappendiceal inflammation. However, it requires time, is costly, and exposes patients to radiation. Ultrasound provides information without exposing patients to radiation, which makes it a good choice for women. It can evaluate other pelvic causes of pain as well as evaluate the appendix. The diagnosis of appendicitis is more likely if compression with the probe over McBurney's point causes tenderness or the appendix is noncompressible. There are multiple conditions that may mimic appendicitis on an ultrasound, namely Meckel's diverticulum, diverticulitis, endometriosis, and pelvic inflammatory disease. Barium enema is no longer used in the diagnosis of appendicitis due to the advent of CT and ultrasound. The component of the CBC that may be helpful is the white count, which is elevated in 80% of patients with appendicitis. There is almost always a neutrophilia and elevated band count, even with a normal WBC. However, this is a very nonspecific test.

7. B

Physical exam is very helpful in diagnosing asymptomatic abdominal aortic aneurysms. Three-fourths of all aneurysms are found incidentally, and physical exam has a sensitivity of 30% to 76%, increasing as the diameter increases. Specificity is poor, however, and a negative finding does not rule out an aneurysm. Factors that can make the physical diagnosis difficult are obesity, inability to lie down, ascites, lumbar lordosis, and aortic tortuosity. Women have a much higher risk of AAA rupture. Because the infrarenal diameter is, on average, 3 mm smaller than in men, they also rupture at a smaller diameter. Women are also screened less often for aneurysm. Rupture is the greatest risk of an aneurysm because it carries 75% to 90% mortality. The risk of rupture rises exponentially after 6 cm, smaller in women. Elective repair has a mortality of 3% to 5% and is now often performed at 5 cm. Aneurysms are defined as dilations of vessels 1.5 times the baseline diameter. Most AAAs are infrarenal and the diagnosis of an aneurysm can be made by comparing the infrarenal to suprarenal diameter. There is evidence that in a screened population of 65-year-old patients, if the ultrasound is negative, the chance of developing an aneurysm on a repeat screen is less than 1%. AAAs are found in 5% to 8% of people older than the age of 60 years, 10 times as often in men. After the age of 85 years, women's risk increases to a third of that of men. Several studies have advocated a single ultrasound screening for men 60 to 80 years old. Risk factors for AAA are smoking, hypertension, peripheral vascular disease, and a first-degree relative with the condition.

8. D

Hemorrhoids are found in almost one-half of all 50-year-olds and are increased in pregnant women and those with portal hypertension. Other risk factors include diets that are high in fat, diets low in fiber, employment that requires prolonged standing or sitting, and any condition that requires straining at defecation. Palpable rectal masses are usually external hemorrhoids. In order for an internal hemorrhoid to be felt, it must prolapse out of the rectum and remain prolapsed. Internal hemorrhoids are usually not associated with pain. Even prolapsed internal hemorrhoids do not hurt. However, if the prolapsed internal hemorrhoid becomes edematous or thrombosed, the sphincter may go into spasm. Most hemorrhoids are composed of complex venous channels and any remaining clot will cause reaccumulation of thromboses. Treatment of hemorrhoids involves increasing fiber and bulk in a diet. Also indicated are increased water intake, avoiding prolonged sitting or standing, and sitz baths. Most hemorrhoids will respond to these interventions. However, about 10% of hemorrhoids require surgical intervention. Mild internal hemorrhoids can be treated in the office with band ligation, which has been shown to have the best long-term outcome. Because of discomfort and rare complications, some practitioners are using infrared coagulation for treatment. Prolapsed internal hemorrhoids, as well as mixed internal and external hemorrhoids, may require surgical excision.

9. D

Hematochezia has a much better prognosis than other symptoms because it is associated with cancers in the descending colon. Ninety percent of rectosigmoid cancers present at a Dukes stage A. If the bleeding is maroon colored, it is likely an ascending colon cancer, which presents at a Duke B or higher 75% of the time. Any other symptoms, such as constipation or iron deficiency anemia, almost always represent a cancer at a Dukes stage C. Polyps found on endoscopy are either hyperplastic, which have no malignant potential, or adenomatous. Tubular adenomas are pedunculated and have a 4% chance of becoming malignant. Villous adenomas are broad based and tend to be larger; these have a 20% chance of malignant change. Of course, tubulovillous adenomas are intermediate in both appearance and malignant potential. The time from polyp to cancer is indeed 10 to 15 years but decreases as it moves distal. The shortest time for transformation is in the rectosigmoid region. Although only one-third of polyps occur in the proximal colon, fully half of all cancers arise in the ascending and transverse colon. There are many risk factors for colon cancer, although 75% occur without identifiable risk factors. Lynch syndrome is also called hereditary nonpolyposis colon cancer and is associated with other adenomatous cancers, such as uterine, breast, and stomach. Inflammatory bowel disease increases the risk of colon cancer, with increasing risk for each year of disease. Familial adenomatous polyposis syndrome results in an almost 100% chance of colon cancer by age 40. It is an autosomal dominant syndrome and results in the formation of hundreds of polyps in the colon.

10. D

Epididymitis is most associated with pyuria; in fact, the absence of pyuria will call the diagnosis into question. Presentation is usually gradual onset of pain with dysuria. Diagnosis can be made with exam and culture. It is the most common cause of scrotal pain and swelling in young men. Etiologies in young men are usually STDs, namely *Neisseria gonorrhea* and *Chlamydia trachomatis*. Varicoceles are dilated blood vessels in the pampiniform plexus and are a common cause of infertility, accounting for 30% of cases. Patients usually complain of a mass above the left testis that can be accentuated by the Valsalva maneuver into a "bag of worms." Acute orchitis presents with sudden pain and an enlarged, tender testis. Urinalysis may reveal hematuria. The etiology is usually pyogenic bacteria or viruses. Treatment is aimed at the primary cause and includes rest and elevation of the scrotum. Testicular torsion is an emergency that presents with acute pain, nausea, and vomiting. The scrotum may be edematous and red. The testis is tender and retracted upward. Urinalysis is usually normal, and if the diagnosis is in question, nuclear scanning or duplex ultrasound can determine blood flow. Testicular cancer rarely presents with pain, but it is possible if a hematoma forms as a result of minor trauma or the cancer bleeds into the enclosed space of the tunica albuginea. It is a cancer of young men, the average age being 35 years old. On exam, there is a nontender mass, which will be intratesticular on ultrasound. There may be associated findings such as gynecomastia, pulmonary metastasis, and elevated tumor markers, namely alpha-fetoprotein and human chorionic gonadotropin. See Table 6.1.

Table 6.1 Differential diagnosis of acute scrotal pain

Testicular torsion
Epididymitis
Torsion of appendix testis or appendix epididymis
Incarcerated inguinal hernia
Testicular tumor
Idiopathic scrotal edema
Acute hydrocele
Henoch–schonlein purpura
Spermatocele
Varicocele

11. C

Cryotherapy is an easily learned and safe method for family practitioners to treat a large number of different lesions. Some of the greatest advantages are ease of mastery, safety of the treatment, and minimal or no scarring. Cryotherapy has some limitations, namely that it does not allow pathology to be sent. Cosmetically, it can destroy hair follicles and decrease skin pigment, thereby limiting its use in patients with darker skin. It is not effective for certain deep lesions, such as dermatofibromas, malignancies other than superficial basal cell carcinoma, and vascular lesions. Although local anesthesia is not needed and the freezing is associated with anesthesia, there is burning on both the initial freeze and the thaw, which may not be tolerated by some, especially children.

12. E

Ingrown toenails are extremely common. The definitive treatment is partial or total toenail removal. Although instruments such as scissors and hemostats can be used to lift the nail up, a small periosteal elevator is the least likely to injure the nail bed. When performing a nail removal, a digital nerve ring block is necessary to provide full anesthesia, even if only the medial or lateral portion of the nail is being removed. Because the toe is a terminal appendage with limited collateral blood supply, epinephrine should not be used due to the risk of tissue ischemia. Other body regions where epinephrine is contraindicated include fingers, earlobes, the nose, the penis, and other vascularly compromised areas. Epinephrine is poorly absorbed in mucus membranes and is of little benefit in those areas. Predisposing conditions leading to ingrown toenails include tightly fitting shoes, fungal infections (especially after successful treatment with oral antifungals), toe injuries, structural abnormalities, repeated impact on the toenail such as running, and improper trimming of toenails. Phenol can be used to ablate the nail bed but is also successful in providing partial ablation. The cotton applicator soaked in phenol is used to cauterize the nail bed and nail matrix area for about 3 minutes, and then it is neutralized with isopropyl alcohol.

13. C

Benign prostatic hypertrophy is very common, with more than 90% of octogenarian men affected. By the age of 50 years, almost one-fourth of men have decreased flow. The history is the most important method for assessing the presence and severity of BPH. There is controversy surrounding the rectal as an assessment tool because the size felt on exam does not correlate with symptoms. However, if there is enlargement on exam, the likelihood of BPH is five times higher. The PSA level increases with age, prostatitis, and prostate cancer. It is neither sensitive nor specific enough to evaluate BPH. Urodynamic evaluation is not warranted routinely unless the diagnosis is uncertain or the symptoms are severe. Urinalysis may help in differentiating the irritative symptoms of BPH, such as urgency or frequency from a urinary tract infection. Most of the symptoms of BPH can be attributed to hypertrophy of the transition zone that surrounds the urethra. This process is testosterone dependent. The most common symptoms of BPH include decreased stream force, hesitancy, incomplete emptying, straining, dribbling, nocturia, frequency, urge incontinence, and dysuria.

14. D

Although obesity is strongly associated with adult obstructive sleep apnea syndrome (OSAS), it is rare in children. When children have OSAS, it is almost always due to hypertrophy of the lymphoid tissue in the upper airways. The tonsils and adenoids are part of Waldeyer's ring and their removal is one of the most common procedures performed in the United States. The immune function of tonsils and adenoids is most active from 3 to 10 years of age, although adenoids begin to diminish in size by age 6. Their removal does not seem to have a significant impact on immunologic function. There are multiple indications for the removal of tonsils, including recurrent tonsillitis of greater than six episodes per year or greater than three episodes for more than 2 years, chronic tonsillitis resistant to treatment; peritonsillar abscess; OSAS or persistent snoring: and speech abnormalities. Adenoids are removed for hypertrophy associated with chronic or recurrent acute otitis media; OSAS, craniofacial abnormalities such as the so-called "adenoid facies"; dental occlusion abnormalities; and speech abnormalities. The procedure is safe, with hemorrhage the most significant complication, with rates of only 0.5% to 2%. Bleeding is most common in teens and adults. Asymmetrical enlargement of the tonsil is never a normal finding and should prompt referral to an ENT for possible malignancy. Besides history, the best tool to assess hypertrophy is fiber-optic nasopharyngoscopy.

15. A

Eustachian tube (ET) dysfunction is a leading cause of otitis media with effusion, both acute and chronic. ET dysfunction leads to reflux and bacteria insufflation into the middle ear. If the middle ear is improperly ventilated, the cells undergo a metaplasia from squamous cells to columnar and goblet cells, which produce fluid, an effect that is reversible once ventilation is re-established. Otitis media can lead to hearing loss in about 70% of children with effusions that persist for more than 3 months. Any child with a persistent effusion over 3 months should undergo hearing evaluation and possible tympanostomy tube placement. The mastoid air cells are fully developed by the age of 5 years, but chronic otitis media can limit the aeration of the cells. Acquired cholesteatomas arise when squamous cells from the external ear invade the middle ear, mastoid process, and the canal wall. These benign squamous epithelial lesions can invade surrounding tissue because they produce strong lytic enzymes.

16. B

This presentation is highly suggestive of diverticulitis, albeit a mild case. Diverticular disease is extremely common, with up to 50% of

Americans older than 70 years being affected. If diverticulitis is suspected, an outpatient CT with oral and IV contrast should be scheduled as soon as possible. This is to ensure that there is no free air, no abscess, and no other organ involvement. If a CT is unavailable, a well-appearing patient may undergo an upright abdominal film to evaluate for free air. Those patients with no peritoneal sign and the ability to take liquids can be treated at home with bowel rest, oral rehydration, and broad-spectrum antibiotics, such as amoxicillin clavulanate or quinolone-metronidazole combination. These will cover the offending organisms, namely anaerobes and gram-negative rods, particularly *Bacteroides fragilis* and *Escherichia coli*. Sulfamethoxazole-trimethoprim may be used, but in combination with metronidazole. Endoscopy and barium enema are no longer recommended because the increased pressure of the study may cause a perforation in acutely inflamed tissue. With barium, there is the added risk of spilling into the peritoneum and causing a severe peritonitis. Although fiber therapy is helpful in decreasing the intraluminal pressure, this should be tried after the acute diverticulitis has resolved. Surgery is rarely indicated in patients with a first attack, especially if it is mild. If the attack is recurrent, or does not respond to intravenous fluids and antibiotics, then surgical evaluation is warranted. Of course, if any of the complications of diverticulitis—namely phlegmon, abscesses, perforation, fistula formation, or stricture and obstruction—are present, then surgical evaluation is immediate.

17. E
Macular degeneration is the most common cause of visual loss in the elderly. It is a progressive disease that destroys the macula, the area of central vision on the retina. There are two basic types, exudative and, more commonly, nonexudative. Both cause visual loss, but exudative macular degeneration is most likely to result in severe changes. The nonexudative type causes visual loss through the deposition of drusen, which is calcified extracellular material, and atrophy of the retina. The exudative type occurs when abnormal vessels grow into the subretinal space, causing distortion of the macula. There is limited treatment with laser, but only for select patients with the exudative type. Patients can be taught to develop peripheral vision, since that remains intact, and are able to use magnifying aids. Prevention is important; dietary intake of the antioxidants lutein and zeaxanthin, both carotinoids, should be encouraged. Smoking cessation, control of blood pressure, and lipid management may all help reduce the incidence of macular degeneration. Diabetic retinopathy is a major cause of vision loss in middle-aged patients with diabetes. Patients may complain of blurry vision, but they will also complain of floaters and poor night vision. Diagnosis is through fundoscopic exam. Glaucoma causes peripheral vision loss and may otherwise be silent. Patients who are older, African American, or have a family history should be screened for this disease. Cataract causes visual loss by opacification of the lens. A fundoscopic exam will be difficult due to the opacification, and diagnosis is via slit lamp. Finally, retinal detachment is usually sudden and accompanied by flashing lights. It may be precipitated by trauma or diabetic retinopathy.

18. D
Family physicians are often the first line in detecting early visual problems in children. The cover test reveals strabismus, which is the most common cause of amblyopia. Strabismus occurs when the two eyes do not work as a single unit. The affected eye may deviate out, in, up, or down, and sometimes only intermittently. The deviation may be very subtle. Strabismus may occur because

of refractive errors, poor extraoccular muscle development, or nerve palsies. Amblyopia is permanent and uncorrectable reduction in the visual acuity not caused by any eye or neurologic abnormality. Other causes of amblyopia are refractive errors and deprivation, which can be caused by any obstruction to vision, such as cataracts, ptosis, or hemangiomas. Cataracts may be congenital and are detected when a red reflex is absent. Leukocoria is a white light pupillary light reflex. Besides cataracts, vitreous opacities, hyphema, and retinal diseases such as retinoblastoma all cause leukocoria. Nystagmus is a sign of neurologic abnormality.

19. C
Blepharitis is inflammation at the lid margin, and it has multiple causes. It is one of the most common eye complaints, resulting in itching, crusting, tearing, and burning. Diagnosis is by examination, but treatment is aimed at the underlying etiology. All patients should practice good eye hygiene with daily warm compress soaks and eyelid scrubs. Chalazion is an obstruction of a meibomian gland under the tarsal plate. These may present acutely as an infection or chronically as a nontender lump on the upper eyelid. A similar problem is a hordeolum or stye, which is a blockage and infection of a more superficial gland along the eyelash line called the glands of Zeiss. When acne rosacea affects the eye, it is called ocular rosacea. Treatment of the rosacea elsewhere and good eyelid hygiene are the appropriate treatment. Sometimes oral antibiotics are necessary to control the rosacea. Seborrheic dermatitis is an allergy to a ubiquitous skin fungus called *Pityosporum ovale*. Patients will often have dandruff and scaling in areas with increased sebum, such as eyelids, nasolabial folds, and eyebrows. Treatment is by local reduction of the fungus with lid hygiene. Bacterial infections may be chronic and require topical antibiotic ointment or ophthalmic drops. If the infection does not resolve, lid cultures may be taken to direct therapy with oral antibiotics.

20. D
Photophobia is not found with any of the common and more benign causes of red eye. It is indicative of a problem other than conjunctivitis, such as iritis, uveitis, glaucoma, or cellulitis. Other indications for immediate referral are pain, visual changes, suspected ocular herpes, and uncertain diagnosis. Conjunctivitis is the most common cause of red eye. Bilateral itching is highly suggestive of allergic conjunctivitis, especially if the patient has other signs of atopy. Treatment is with a topical or systemic antihistamine medication. Other topical treatments that may work are nonsteroidal anti-inflammatory agents or mast cell stabilizers. Mucopurulent discharge is indicative of bacterial or chlamydial infection. Cervical lymphadnopathy is absent in acute bacterial conjunctivitis, but it is often present in chlamydial infections. Bacterial etiologies differ for children and adults. *Streptococcus pneumoniae* and *Haemophilus influenzae* are most common in children, whereas *Staphylococcus aureus* and *Streptococcal* species are most often seen in adults. Gram-negative organisms such as *Escherichia coli* and *Pseudomonas* are rare, but they do occur in adults. The best treatment is with a broad-spectrum topical antibiotic with activity against both gram-positive and gram-negative organisms, such as erythromycin. *Chlamydia trachomatis* infections are important because the trachomal form is responsible for the most common cause of preventable blindness in the world. It is endemic in Africa, Asia, and the Middle East but rare in the United States. The type of chlamydial conjunctival infection seen most often in the United States is the inclusion type, which is sexually transmitted both to adults and to newborns during birth.

An evaluation for genital infection is warranted if chlamydial conjunctivitis is found. Treatment is with the same antibiotics used to treat genital chlamydia, such as doxycycline, erythromycin, and azithromycin, but for a longer course. Most conjunctivitis is bilateral or becomes so with autoinoculation.

21. E
The finding of incidental microscopic hematuria remains a controversial clinical problem. There are several causes of hematuria that do not require a full evaluation, including exercise, recent trauma, infection, sexual activity, and viral infections. When patients have three or more red blood cells (RBCs) per high-powered field in at least two of three clean catch urine samples, there should be further evaluation. Risk factors that increase the likelihood that there is a serious urologic problem include smoking, age older than 40 years, nonsteroidal anti-inflammatory drug (NSAID) abuse, exposure to certain chemicals and dyes, pelvic radiation, chronic urinary tract infection, and previous gross hematuria. If there is accompanying proteinuria, red cell cast, or renal insufficiency, the hematuria is likely due to renal disease, such as glomerular nephropathy, infection, tumor, interstitial nephritis, papillary necrosis, or vascular disease. Otherwise, the focus is on the lower urinary tract, which is evaluated with radiologic study of the upper tract with CT scan or intravenous pyelogram and cystoscopy of the bladder. Most lower urinary tract disease consists of stones, infections, cystitis, bladder tumor, stricture, BPH, coagulopathy, and trauma. See Table 6.2.

Table 6.2 Causes of hematuria

Type	Cause
Glomerular hematuria	IgA nephropathy (Berger's disease) Mesangioproliferative glomerulonephritis Focal segmental proliferative glomerulonephritis
Nonglomerular hematuria	Exercise Bladder tumors Renal artery embolism/thrombosis Arteriovenous fistula Renal vein thrombosis Stones Urinary tract infections Renal cell carcinoma Papillary necrosis (consider in diabetics, blacks, and analgesic abusers) Injury Ureteral carcinoma Menstrual contamination Interstitial cystitis Extracorporeal shock-wave lithotripsy
Medications	Anticoagulants and analgesics

22. B
Nephrolithiasis occurs in about 3% of the population. Risk factors include male sex, previous calculi, and white ethnicity. There are many options for evaluating suspected nephrolithiasis, but noncontrast helical CT scan is fast becoming the imaging of choice. It is fast and does not require contrast, which is safer in people with compromised renal function. Although it is more expensive than intravenous pyelography, it provides more information and may diagnose other causes of the flank or abdominal pain. Intravenous pyelogram was previously considered the gold standard in imaging, but it required bowel preparation and proper hydration in order to obtain the most accurate results. Abdominal x-rays are helpful only if the stone is radiolucent, such as a calcium oxalate or calcium phosphate stones. Ultrasound is quick and safe, but it cannot detect ureteral stones. It is very helpful in assessing hydronephrosis. There are currently no nuclear scans that are helpful in the diagnosis of nephrolithiasis.

23. C
There are two broad groups of medications for BPH, the alpha-1 blockers and 5-alpha reductase inhibitors. Among the alpha-1 blockers, terazosin and doxazosin (Cardura) both improve urinary flow as well as reduce blood pressure. Although tamulosin belongs to this group, it is highly selective for the alpha-1A receptor and thus has minimal to no cardiac effects. Finasteride is a 5-alpha reductase inhibitor, which inhibits the conversion of testosterone to the more active hormone, dihydrotestosterone. It has no effect on blood pressure. Both oxybutynin and tolterodine are useful in urge incontinence and work through anticholinergic pathways.

24. A
This patient has both symptoms and signs of peripheral arterial disease. The pain is called claudication and occurs in the calf, thigh, or buttocks depending on the level of arterial involvement. The pain occurs with exertion and should resolve with rest. His exam is also consistent with arterial disease. The skin may be cool and hairless. The nails are often thick and dependent rubor may be present. The ankle brachial index (ABI) is the ratio of the systolic blood pressure of the dorsalis pedis or posterial tibial artery over the systolic pressure of the brachial artery. Normally, this is 1.0 or higher. Anything less than 0.95 is abnormal. Most patients with intermittent claudication have a ratio of 0.5 to 0.8. An ABI less than 0.5 is consistent with severe ischemic disease and rest pain. The first step in treatment for intermittent claudication is lifestyle management, especially tobacco cessation and the start of an exercise program. Antiplatelet medications such as aspirin, ticlopidine (Ticlid), and clopidogrel (Plavix) also have a proven role in treatment. The MRI is helpful if there is a suspicion of spinal stenosis causing pseudo-claudication or lumbar disc disease. Ice and NSAIDS may be used for muscular strain. The duplex scan is used for the evaluation of possible deep vein thrombosis. Arteriography is not indicated for mild intermittent claudication. It is useful only if surgical intervention is anticipated in patients unresponsive to lifestyle and medical management.

25. D
Primary open-angle glaucoma is one of the leading causes of blindness in the world. It is most common in the elderly, African Americans, those with a family history, patients with hypertension or diabetes, and patients with myopia. Screening is important because patients remain asymptomatic. Since central vision usually

234   Chapter 6

remains intact bur peripheral vision is lost, most patients do not complain of visual changes until late in the disease process. Screening is achieved via measurement of intraoccular pressure, but optic nerve damage can be seen when characteristic cupping occurs. Primary angle-closure glaucoma comprises only about 10% of glaucoma and occurs more frequently in people of Asian descent, women, and patients with hyperopia. Cupping is not normally seen. Treatment is aimed at reducing intraocular pressure by reducing the amount of fluid the eye produces, increasing absorption, or improving fluid drainage. Retinal detachment is separation of the sensory retina from the underlying retinal pigment epithelium. Patients usually present acutely with the sensation of flashing lights or floaters. Patients continue to have good vision except for minor field defects unless the fovea detaches. Hypertensive retinopathy and diabetic retinopathy are due to the vascular changes that each disease causes. Patients will be known to have the disorder, although the retinopathy may be present at initial diagnosis. Hallmarks of diabetic retinopathy are microaneurysms, hemorrhages, cotton–wool spots, retinal edema, exudates, and neovascularization. Hypertensive retinopathy is marked by arteriovenous nicking, retinal hemorrhages, macular edema, and cotton–wool spots.

26.   B

This patient has a small bowel obstruction, but because of air in the rectum, it may be presumed to be a partial one. Both her presentation and her physical exam are typical of obstruction. Postoperative adhesions are the most frequent cause of obstruction, followed by tumors and hernias. Lower abdominal and pelvic surgery further increases the risk of later obstruction, perhaps because bowel in the lower quadrants has looser mesenteric fixation. These patients should have immediate saline resuscitation since most are not only fluid depleted but also have electrolyte disturbances. The nasogastric tube is essential in providing upper intestinal decompression and limiting the vomiting, which can lead to aspiration. Also indicated may be antibiotics for gram-negative and anaerobic bacteria because of the possibility of translocation. Nearly 60% to 80% of patients with partial obstructions can be successfully treated without surgery. However, this requires frequent re-evaluation and immediate surgical referral for any deterioration. Rectal tubes do not decompress the obstruction and may lead to erosions and perforations. Antiemetic medications will not be helpful in this situation because the nausea is due to obstruction and not a central process. Although abdominal pain is present, most patients will have resolution of pain with decompression. CT scan is a very important modality if the picture is ambiguous, there is a history of intra-abdominal malignancy, there is no previous surgery, or an abscess is suspected as the cause of obstruction. Even then, oral contrast is not advised due to the risk of aspiration.

27.   E

Tetanus occurs when *Clostridium tetani*, an anaerobic bacteria, releases exotoxins. Tetanus is a serious problem worldwide and can have a mortality rate approaching 50%. In the United States, tetanus affects patients older than the age of 65 half of the time, likely because of waning immunity. It is most likely to cause death in infants and the elderly. Clean minor wounds, such as cuts, are the least likely to become infected with *C. tetani*. Wounds that cause devitalization, such as avulsion injuries, crush injuries, burns, and frostbite, and wounds that are deep, such as puncture wounds, are most likely to become infected. Because *C. tetani* lives

in the soil and is a colonizer in 10% of adult colons, wounds that are contaminated with soil, feces, or saliva are also likely to become infected. Tetanus prophylaxis is recommended in a variety of wounds. Immunity depends on the basic series of three vaccines. If patients are uncertain of their series or are known to have less than three vaccines, then tetanus immunoglobulin (TIG) is indicated in addition to Td in wounds other than clean minor ones. For patients with the basic series and a Td within 5 years, no Td is needed for any type of wound. If the last dose was between 5 and 10 years ago, then a dose of Td is indicated for all wounds other than clean minor wounds. If the interval since the last vaccine was more than 10 years ago, any type of wound requires a dose of Td.

28.   C

Keratoacanthomas are solitary lesions that may mimic invasive squamous cell carcinomas. They are flesh-colored domes with a central keratin plug. Because they often appear on the face and grow rapidly, they are commonly brought to the attention of the family physician. Although KAs are squamous cell tumors, most will resolve spontaneously over a period of months to years, albeit with scarring, and are not associated with malignant potential. A biopsy is warranted to rule out invasive squamous cell carcinoma. Dermatofibromas are also dome shaped, but they are dermal lesions and will dimple inward if squeezed. Amelanotic melanomas are rare and not usually mistaken for a classic KA. Angiokeratomas are small vascular lesions, most commonly found around the genitalia. Basal cell carcinomas have a characteristic pearly appearance and grow slowly as opposed to KAs, which grow rapidly.

29.   A

Invasive procedures cause transient bacteremia. Normally, this is cleared rapidly by the body, but certain cardiac abnormalities predispose patients to endocarditis. Patients with high risk of endocarditis include those with prosthetic valves (including animal valves), those with previous endocarditis, and those with cyanotic congenital heart defects. Patients with moderate risk include those with mitral valve prolapse with regurgitation, hypertrophic cardiomyopathy, congenital heart defects, and valve dysfunction. Both high- and moderate-risk patients require prophylaxis. This is given as amoxicillin: 2 g given 1 hour before the procedure. If the gastrointestinal or urogenital system is involved, then 2 g of ampicilllin is given intravenously along with gentamicin at the time of the procedure and ampicillin is given again 6 hours later. There are many situations in which prophylaxis is not indicated. Patients with isolated secundum atrial septal defect, septal defects repaired more than 6 months previously, CABG, pacemakers, defibrillators, mitral valve prolapse without regurgitation, and functional murmurs do not require routine prophylaxis.

30.   C

Groin hernias are among the most common surgical problem seen by family physicians. Many patients are asymptomatic or have only a mild heaviness in the groin. Indirect inguinal hernias are the most common type found in both men and women. These herniations occur through the potential space of the inguinal canal and lateral to the inferior epigastric artery. Because there is a congential component, up to 20% of patients will have a bilateral inguinal hernia. Direct inguinal hernias come through acquired defects in the abdominal wall, medial to the inferior epigastric artery. Often, it is difficult to differentiate between the two types of inguinal hernia except at the time of repair. Femoral hernias are rare but occur most often in elderly women, likely due to increased intra-abdominal pressure and pelvic floor relaxation. Varicoceles are dilated and tortuous veins in the pampiniform plexus and spermatic vein. Usually asymptomatic, it is often described as a "bag of worms." A hydrocele can also be felt as a scrotal swelling but it is due to fluid in the tunica vaginalis.

31. A

A pterygium is an overgrowth of hyalanized bulbar conjunctiva that crosses the limbus (the sclerocorneal junction). It is most strongly associated with chronic sunlight exposure and distance from the equator. Although usually asymptomatic, pterygia are often brought to a family physician's attention by patients who do not like the cosmetic appearance or find the lesion to be red and inflamed. It is important to follow these lesions because with continued growth, they can block vision, cause astigmatism, or even obstruct ocular motion. Pterygia are notoriously difficult to treat because the recurrence rate is very high, ranging from 40% to 75%. After surgical excision, the lesion tends to regrow even more rapidly. Newer techniques to reduce recurrence include chemotherapeutic agents, radiation, and conjuctival graphs. A similar lesion to a pterygium is a pinguecula, which is also a conjunctival lesion. It does not cross the limbus and often has a yellow appearance due to elastin degeneration. Ultraviolet light exposure is associated with cataract formation as well, and the patient should be instructed in the use of wide-brimmed hats and appropriate sunglasses.

32. C

Meckel's diverticulum is the most common congenital abnormality of the gastrointestinal tract. Although it occurs in 2% of the population, only 5% to 25% of patients with a Meckel's diverticulum will have complications. The diverticulum can mimic almost any GI problem, and it should be considered in any patient with unexplained abnormal pain, nausea, vomiting, and bleeding. Most complications occur because of ectopic mucosa; this occurs in more than half of all diverticula. The most common ectopic tissue by far is gastric mucosa, followed distantly by pancreatic mucosa. The acid production of the ectopic gastric mucosa is the cause of most of the complications. Diagnosis is difficult because the diverticulum is small, does not readily fill with contrast, and is located in the middle of the small bowel. Because bleeding is only intermittent and small, a tagged RBC scan is of little use, but technetium-99m pertechnetate accumulates in gastric tissue, illuminating the ectopic mucosa. The sensitivity and specificity are high in children but fall to only 62% and 9%, respectively, in adults. The use of pentagastrin, cimetidine, and glucagon may help increase the accuracy of the scan. If the patient had no bleeding but Meckel's was suspected for other reasons, an ultrasound examination may be beneficial.

33. E

The main determinants in the passage of stones are size and location. Stones that are less than 4 mm will usually pass in 1 or 2 weeks and most require no intervention other than pain control. Even stones that are 5 mm can pass, but they are less likely to do so. If the stone is greater than 5 mm, then a urologist should be consulted. The more distal the stone, the more likely it is to pass. A 4-mm stone in the distal ureter has a 75% chance of passing spontaneously. For stones that do not pass in 2 weeks, stones greater than 5 mm, or stones that are causing complications, there are several options for treatment. Extracorporeal shockwave lithotripsy is appropriate for renal stones less than 2 cm and ureteral stones less than 1 cm. It is avoided in women of child-bearing age because of possible effects on the ovaries and it still requires the passage of stone fragments. Percutaneous nephrostomy tube and retrograde ureteral stent placement are temporizing methods for those patients with hydronephrosis from stone obstruction. Antibiotics are advised whenever the patient has concomitant infection, especially with staghorn calculi. Ureteroscopy is invasive but provides definitive treatment. It usually requires postoperative stent placement and can lead to ureteral stricture.

34. B

Corneal abrasions are the most common traumatic eye injury, occurring twice as often among boys. Patients will usually recall an injury with subsequent pain. Luckily, these injuries heal very rapidly because the corneal epithelium regenerates easily. Although patching was once considered the best treatment option, multiple prospective controlled trials now disprove its benefit. It may, in fact, increase the risk of infection, and in infants it may cause amblyopia. Management is with topical antibiotics to reduce the risk of infection, which is increased until the protective epithelium of the cornea regenerates. The most common organisms to secondarily infect corneal abrasions are pseudomonal species and *Staphylococcus aureus*. Topical analgesics and steroids have no role in the treatment of corneal abrasions and may increase the risk of complications. Sterile contact lenses have been used in adults as a bandage, but their use has not been investigated in children.

35. E

The second impact syndrome is the most dreaded consequence of repeated concussions. It occurs when a concussion is sustained prior to recovery from the previous concussion. It results in sudden and progressive brain edema that can result in death. A concussion is an axonal shear injury that, depending on the severity, can cause a variety of symptoms. There are three grading scales widely used: Cantu, the Colorado Medical Society, and the American Academy of Neurology. If the concussion is a grade 1, the athlete can usually return to play after 15 to 20 minutes without symptoms. If the athlete has a grade 2 concussion, he or she must stay out of play for 1 week even if he or she remains asymptomatic. Grade 3 concussions require immediate emergency room evaluation and 1 or 2 weeks without play depending on the injury. All guidelines agree that second concussion, even if minimal, requires at least 1 week out of play. A third concussion, even if mild, requires the player to terminate the season.

36. B

Although all of the choices have been advocated as a possible screening test, studies actually show no improved mortality. Lung cancer is the leading cause of cancer death in both men and women, surpassing breast cancer and prostate cancer. High-risk patients include those who currently smoke or have smoked within the past 15 to 20 years, patients older than 45 years, and patients with abnormal pulmonary function tests. There is a single study from Japan that advocates spiral CT screening, but more research is needed before this approach is adopted in the United States.

37. D

Melasma or chloasma is a characteristic darkening of the skin in response to estrogen. It often occurs in pregnancy and is called "mask of pregnancy." Many malignancies have associated skin disorders. Pruritis can accompany lymphoreticular cancers. A sudden onset of multiple seborrheic keratoses is called the sign of Leser–Trelat and can signify a cancer, especially adenocarcinoma of the GI tract. *Acanthosis nigricans* is most often associated with obesity and diabetes, but it is also associated with GI adenocarcinomas. Palmar–plantar keratoderma results in very thick, scaly skin and is usually familial but may indicate malignancy.

38. D

Urinary irritative symptoms such as urgency and frequency can occur in patients undergoing radiotherapy, along with colonic symptoms such as tenesmus and diarrhea. There are three common approaches to treating prostate cancer. Radical prostatectomy is usually offered to younger men and patients with tumor confined to the prostate. Complications are related to surgery, such as thrombosis and bleeding. In addition, there is a high risk of impotence and incontinence, both more common in older patients. Radiotherapy is a common alternative offered to older men who nonetheless have a life expectancy of at least 10 years. The radiation can be delivered either externally or through implanted radioactive "seeds." The main complications are a higher recurrence rate and bladder and bowel symptoms described previously. Watchful waiting or observation is reserved for elderly patients with comorbid conditions, whose life expectancy is less than 10 years, or those men with very small low-grade tumors. Obviously, there are no immediate risks, but metastasis will preclude any cure.

39. A

This is a classic epidermoid cyst, which is a thin-walled cyst derived from the hair follicle and contains keratin and lipids. Common terms include sebaceous cyst, epidermal inclusion cyst, and wen. It is usually present for many years and remains asymptomatic unless the thin walls rupture. The cyst contents are highly irritating and produce a strong inflammatory reaction. This reaction is often mistaken for infection. Treatment is removal of the cyst intact, including the connective pore, via a minor surgical procedure that can be performed in the office.

40. B

Keratosis pilaris is a common skin condition consisting of small perifollicular papules strongly associated with atopy. It occurs most often on the upper arms and thighs. In childhood, the face may be affected as well. Treatment is symptomatic with exfoliation and keratolytic agents, such as urea and lactic acid. Other than being a marker for allergic disorders, it is mainly of cosmetic concern.

41. B

A seborrheic keratosis is a raised lesion with multiple plugged follicles that give it a "warty" appearance. It is described as a "stuck on" plaque and can range from pale to dark. The most common benign skin tumor in adults, it occurs mainly on the trunk and face. Skin tags, or acrochordons, are polyps that come in all colors. These lesions occur more often in the elderly, in women, and especially in the obese in the intertrigal regions and the neck. Nevus sebaceous lesions occur almost exclusively on the scalp and are a raised plaque with orange color. In 10% of patients, these lesions can develop into basal cell carcinomas. Urticaria is a raised lesion also called a wheal, which by definition is temporary and occurs due to histamine release. Psoriasis is plaque with silver scale occurring most often at sites of daily trauma, such as over the knees, elbows, feet, and scalp. It is due to multiple defects that lead to a marked shortening of cell cycle resulting in overproduction of epidermal cells.

42. C

Actinic keratoses are irregular, scaly lesions that vary in size and color. They are related to cumulative sun exposure and are often called solar keratoses. These lesions have the potential to become squamous cell carcinomas. The treatment of choice is cryotherapy, although excisional biopsy is recommended if there is any question of the diagnosis or the lesion is larger than 5 mm. Other treatment options include curettage and 5-fluorouracil applied topically.

43. A

There are multiple risk factors for the development of SCC, the most significant of which are light complexion, Irish–Scottish ancestry, and cumulative sun exposure. In addition, areas of skin that have had chronic or prolonged inflammation, such as areas of burns, sinus tracts, or ulcers also lead to increased rates of SCC. This cancer is more common in men, people with previous SCC, and those who have used certain psoriasis treatments such as coal tar products and PUVA therapy. Family history is significant in melanoma but not SCC.

44. B

Basal cell carcinomas are usually treated by excision with narrow margins (2 to 5 mm), but some lesions are amenable to cryotherapy, which has the benefit of a more cosmetically pleasing result. The family physician can treat BCCs with cryotherapy if the lesion is less than 1.5 cm; does not occur near the eyes, nasolabial folds, scalp, or ear; and is of the nodular type. Recurrent BCCs are high risk and should be treated with Moh's micrographic surgery. Radiation therapy can be used in older patients if the lesion is in a difficult to treat area such as the eyelid margins. Sclerosing BCC is a particularly dangerous form of BCC because the tumor projects finger-like projections into the surrounding tissue; this lesion is best treated with Moh's surgery.

45. A

Halo nevi are depigmented areas around existing nevi. This is an immune reaction and the natural history of this lesion is resolution with disappearance of the original nevus over months to years. However, it may be a signal for a more serious problem, such as malignant melanoma or vitiligo. All halo nevi should be evaluated for any irregularity and biopsy should be performed for any concerning lesions. Even more important, a total body skin exam should be performed because the immune response might be derived from a melanoma in a different location. A halo nevus might also portend the development of vitiligo.

46. E

Although the rate of malignant melanoma in people of color is low, the rate of acral lentiginous melanoma is the same as that for all other ethnic groups. Almost 70% of melanomas in African Americans are acral melanomas, whereas the rate is only about 5% of all melanomas in whites. Most melanomas in whites are of the superficially spreading type or the nodular type, with lentigo maligna melanoma a distant third. Acral melanomas occur on the palm or sole and under the nail. They are usually slow growing and are often mistaken for plantar warts or subungual hematomas. Diagnosis is usually made when vertical growth (i.e., invasive growth) begins and the lesion becomes nodular or destroys the nail bed.

47. E

Tumor thickness is the most important prognostic indicator in malignant melanoma. All physicians should know about the ABCDEs of melanoma, referring to *a*symmetry, irregular *b*orders, *c*olor changes, *d*iameter greater than 0.6 cm, and *e*nlargement and *e*levation. However, this is only a tool to help identify lesions that need attention and biopsy. These characteristics have little relation to prognosis. For instance, superficially spreading melanoma may be 8 mm wide before the vertical or invasive growth begins. Nodular melanomas may be uniformly elevated with dark, even color, but these melanomas have a very early vertical growth and carry a poor prognosis. Although lesions on the extremities have a better prognosis, this is not a major determinant in survival. Both of the major grading tools for melanoma, Breslow's microstaging and Clark's level, use depth to predict survival. Breslow's microstaging describes the lesion in terms of millimeters and Clark's system describes the lesion by its histologic depth. See Figure 6-3.

48. B

Although the differential diagnosis for a scaling breast rash includes dermatitis, psoriasis, squamous cell carcinoma, impetigo, and seborrheic dermatitis, Paget's disease of the breast should always be at the top of the differential. Paget's disease can mimic all of the above lesions, but a unilateral rash involving the nipple and areola that does not respond to topical corticosteroids is highly suspicious. Although only one-half of patients with Paget's disease have a palpable breast mass, intraductal carcinoma is present in most patients. Mammography and skin biopsy can establish the diagnosis.

49. E

Dry skin or xerosis is one of the hallmarks of atopic dermatitis and a 12% ammonium lactate lotion is very effective in its treatment. Because pruritis is ubiquitous and often starts the vicious cycle that leads to the lichenified rash of eczema, its treatment is crucial. Topical corticosteroids are the mainstay of treatment but oral antihistamines, liberal application of emollients, and stress management are also effective. Since allergy evaluations rarely lead to any one allergen, RAS testing is not indicated. Topical antihistamines and

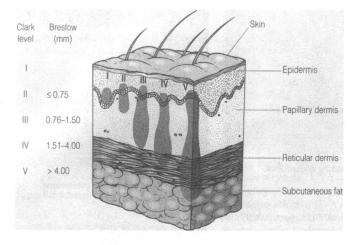

Figure 6-3. The Clark and Breslow classifications for melanoma. Reproduced by permission from Lawrence PF. Essentials of General Surgery. Baltimore: Williams & Wilkins; 1988:355.

HEPA filters are of limited to no use. Antibiotics are indicated only if there is impetigenous superinfection.

50. B

Psoriasis is relatively common, occurring in 2% of all Americans. Guttate psoriasis is a rare variant that occurs most often after a streptococcal pharyngitis but may also be a chronic variant. Guttate psoriasis consists of discrete papules that become confluent with typical silver scale. The lesions are concentrated on the trunk and spare the palms and soles. Antistreptolysin titer will often be high and the treatment is penicillin for the underlying strep infection. Guttate psoriasis will often clear spontaneously. If the lesions are a variant of chronic psoriasis, treatment is similar to that for the typical plaque psoriasis.

51. E

The Koebner phenomenon is a very important concept in many skin diseases, notably psoriasis and vitiligo. Lesions tend to occur at sites of trauma; hence, extensor surfaces of knees and elbows are most commonly affected. Lichen simplex chronicus is the skin lichenification or thickening associated with chronic scratching. Dermatographia occurs when histamine is released at the site where skin is stroked, resulting in urticarial lesions. Rhinophyma, or enlargement of the nose, occurs in rosacea and is the result of edema and hyperplasia of the skin of the nose.

52. A

Patients will often ask family physicians for advice on moles. The most common acquired lesions in Caucasians are nevocellular nevi, which can be classified into three categories: junctional, compound, and dermal. These lesions represent a continuum of development. Junctional nevi rest at the basement membrane and are epidermal. They are dark macules with uniform color. If the cells grow down into the papillary dermis, they are called compound nevi and have characteristics of both junctional and dermal nevi. Dermal nevi are intradermal dome-shaped papules that have less pigment, often becoming flesh colored. There may be a hair growing from the lesion. The decision to remove a lesion is based on the same warning signs as for malignant melanoma; itching, bleeding, or pain; and location such as mucus membranes, scalp, or genital region.

53. E

The lesion described is a giant congenital nevomelanocytic nevus (CNN), and in this distribution it is known as a bathing trunk nevus. During the exam of any newborn, particular attention should be paid to congenital nevi, a large majority of which are less than 3 cm. Up to 1% of newborns are born with CNN, but only 1 in 500,000 infants have a giant nevus. Lesions can become apparent in the first few weeks of life and are known as tardive lesions. Giant congenital nevi are actually associated with the development of small tardive lesions surrounding the giant nevus. The tragedy of this lesion is that it has a high risk of degeneration into malignant melanoma and the melanoma occurs half the time in children younger than 5 years of age. If malignant transformation occurs, the prognosis is poor. If the giant nevus occurs on the neck or upper back, there is a risk of meningeal involvement that can manifest as seizure or hydrocephalus.

54. C

Scheuermann's disease is associated with repetitive flexion, experienced in sports such as water skiing, especially when competition is started at a young age. It is characterized by kyphosis, anterior wedging greater than 5% in three consecutive vertebral bodies, vertebral endplate changes, Schmorl's nodes, and apophyseal ring fractures. This should be differentiated from juvenile postural round back, which may appear similar on initial physical exam but does not have the associated radiologic findings and requires different treatment.

55. D

TLSO bracing should be instituted in patients with Scheuermann's disease whose kyphotic curve exceeds 60 degrees. Overhead arm extensions can be used to treat juvenile postural round back. Upper trunk and postural exercises can be used in mild Scheuermann's disease. The surgical correction described is not appropriate treatment for Scheuermann's disease.

56. B

Seborrheic keratoses (SKs) are very common benign skin tumors most often seen on the trunk, face, and upper extremities. The tendency to develop these lesions is inherited in an autosomally dominant fashion. The differential diagnosis of SKs would include nevi, basal cell carcinoma (pigmented type), and malignant melanoma. However, SKs usually have a very characteristic appearance that allows diagnosis without biopsy. Most SKs require no treatment, but if the lesions are cosmetically unacceptable or are symptomatic, then liquid nitrogen, shave biopsy, or curettage are appropriate therapies.

57. B

Basal cell carcinoma (BCC) is the most common malignant skin cancer. When considering the management of BCC, one must consider the size of the tumor, cell type, and location of the tumor. For smaller and nodular BCC, electrodessication and curettage may work best, especially in areas such as the cheeks and the forehead. For large tumors with well-defined borders, excisional surgery may afford a good cosmetic result. Cryosurgery can be used. A BCC that is nodular or superficial has well-defined borders. Moh's procedure can be used for any type of BCC but is especially helpful in areas where recurrence is high or where the margins are ill-defined. This includes areas near the nose and around the eyes. Radiation therapy may be used in areas where skin preservation and good cosmetic results are of concern and also in the elderly. Because the dermis of the back and shoulders is thick, curettage is difficult and should not be used.

58. A

Seborrheic dermatitis is a very common condition affecting all age groups. However, a severe recurrent case of seborrheic dermatitis may be an early sign of HIV infection. Infants and adults have different areas of involvement. In infants, the scalp and eyebrows are often affected and it is often called "cradle cap." In adults, the scalp, eyebrows, nasolabial folds, external auditory canals, central chest, and groin are often involved. The lesions are described as greasy scales. The cause of "seb derm" is not fully understood but appears to be an abnormal reaction to a normal skin yeast called *Pityrosporum ovale*. The worldwide incidence is 3% to 5%, and it is treated either by reducing levels of the yeast through antifungals or by reducing inflammation with topical steroids. In AIDS, an overgrowth of the yeast and the abnormal response leads to especially severe and difficult to treat cases.

59. D

Hidradenitis suppurativa is the most likely diagnosis in this case. It involves the areas of the body with apocrine glands, namely the axilla; the area under the breasts in women; anal and genital regions; and the inner thighs. Patients will often describe frequent "blackheads" and large pores in the surrounding areas. The physician or patient may feel cordlike swelling that is quite tender, representing communicating inflamed glands. There is speculation that hydradenitis evolves from keratinous follicular plugs or apocrine duct blockage. These then progress to gland enlargement and rupture with subsequent inflammation and infection. Contrary to popular belief, deodorants, shaving devices, and depilatories are not involved in the development of this disorder. The mainstay of treatment is oral antibiotics. Isotretinoin may be used in some cases that are early without sinus tracts. Surgery is recommended if recurrent inflammation and infection occur.

60. A

Dysplastic nevi are important to identify because patients with this syndrome have a significantly higher chance of developing melanoma. These lesions can be large, even greater than 10 cm in size. They are most often located on the back and extremities. However, they can also be seen in sun-protected areas such as the breast, scalp, groin, and buttocks. The color of a dysplastic nevus can vary even within the same nevus from brown to red, black, or pink. The border of a dysplastic nevus is irregular and can appear to fade into the surrounding skin. These nevi are not present at birth and usually develop in late childhood. In dysplastic nevus syndrome, new nevi can appear anytime, in contrast to common nondysplastic nevi that do not develop after middle age. The management of dysplastic nevi includes a thorough history, physical exam, and an excisional biopsy to establish the diagnosis. The nevi can be followed by taking photographs of the entire body. Family members should be screened because it is inherited via an autosomal dominant pattern. Patients should be educated about performing self-examination and about the dangers of sun exposure. Recall the ABCDE acronym: asymmetry, boarder irregularity, color variation, diameter, and elevation.

61. C

This patient has a keloid scar that can be distinguished from a hypertrophic scar because it has expanded beyond the region of the original surgical scar. Keloids are more common in African Americans but have a similar incidence in men and women. Although this patient developed the keloid after surgery, almost any type of injury, even a very minor one, can cause keloid formation. Keloids can form anywhere on the body but are most common on the earlobes, shoulders, chest, and back. Patients may complain of pain or hyperesthesias in the surrounding area. The treatment of keloids is very difficult. Intralesional steroid injection can help reduce pruritis and pain but needs to be done at the time of the incision or soon after. If the scar is allowed to heal, it may become too thick to inject adequately. Other therapies include cryotherapy, compression, and even radiation. Surgery often causes the keloid to return even larger than before.

62. E

Family physicians who do procedures in the office should be familiar with the use of local anesthetics. Lidocaine (Xylocaine) is the most commonly used injectable anesthetic in the office. Allergies and reactions are rare. The maximal dose for lidocaine is 4 mg per kilogram and it provides $\frac{1}{2}$ to 2 hours of pain relief. On nonappendage areas of the body, especially in areas where hemostasis is needed, the practitioner may opt to use lidocaine with epinephrine. This formulation provides 2 to 6 hours of pain relief and up to 7 mg per kilogram may be injected. Other long-acting agents include bupivacaine (Marcaine) and etidocaine (Duranest). All of these techniques may be used to reduce the pain of the injection. Topical analgesics such as TAC (tetracaine, epinephrine, and cocaine), LET (lidocaine, epinephrine, and tetracaine), and EMLA (lidocaine and prilocaine) may also be used.

63. C

Impingement syndrome refers to tendonitis of the rotator cuff, which is made up of the supraspinatus, the infraspinatus, the subscapularis, and the teres minor. Although some rotator cuff tears are due to acute injury, they are most often the result of age-related changes and chronic tendonitis. If the tendonitis is acute, there may be difficulty differentiating between impingement and a full tear by exam alone. The Neer and Hawkins signs are positive in both disorders. Plain radiographs are not usually helpful in differentiating between the two. However, a simple office injection of the subacromial bursa will relieve the inflammation and allow the patient to have full range of motion. An MRI can also be performed to separate the two disorders, but this is much more costly and not instantly available.

64. A

Thoracic outlet syndrome occurs when the brachial plexus and subclavian vessels are compressed as they pass between the clavicle and first rib. There may be congenital anomalies involved, such as cervical ribs. There may also be abnormal fibrosis of the anterior scalene muscles. Symptoms vary depending on whether the brachial plexus is compressed or the vascular structures. The syndrome can often mimic ulnar nerve compression. When the arm is raised, the compression is increased and symptoms also increase. Carpal tunnel syndrome will affect the median nerve, resulting in numbness of the thumb, pointer, and middle finger. Impingement syndrome will also result in difficulty raising the arm, but it does not cause ulnar nerve symptoms. Shoulder subluxation will result in a "thunk" as the shoulder is lifted.

65. B

A very common scenario that family physicians face is the evaluation and "clearance" of patients for surgery. Age per se is not a risk factor, but it is considered a minor clinical predictor of risk simply because the elderly are more likely to have concomitant organ disease. Several studies show that elderly adults without comorbidities have complication rates similar to those of younger patients. Obesity is a risk factor for the development of pulmonary complications. This patient's weight loss is entirely appropriate. This patient's functional capacity is good, with both stair climbing and lawn mowing requiring more than four METs or metabolic equivalents of oxygen consumption. In addition, his cardiac status is known because he has had a stress test in the past 2 years with no clinical symptoms. His surgery is one of intermediate risk. High-risk surgeries include any emergency procedures and vascular procedures involving both peripheral vessels and the aorta.

66. E

Rabies cases in the United States are declining with improved domestic animal vaccinations, and most cases of rabies are due to either wild animal exposure or exposure in foreign countries. Approximately 16,000 to 39,000 people receive rabies prophylaxis yearly in the United States, which indicates a nonjudicious use of this resource. Rabies is a virus spread in the saliva of affected animals that invades the central nervous system. Significant exposure is one in which saliva is introduced into the mucus membranes or open areas on the skin through a bite or a cut. Nonbite exposure is extremely rare and occurs only if there is the possibility of large aerosolization of particles, such as in large bat caves. Other contact with animals, including petting, blood exposure, or feces exposure, is not a risk for rabies. Postexposure prophylaxis consists of rabies immune globulin (RIG), which provides a short period of passive immunity, and the injection of one of three rabies vaccines produced in the United States on days 0, 3, 7, 14, and 28, which will provide immunity in 7 to 10 days. The RIG has a half-life of 21 days and the rabies vaccine provides immunity for 2 years. Domestic animals may be observed for 10 days prior to the initiation of rabies prophylaxis. Hares and other small rodents carry an insignificant risk of rabies. Skunks, raccoons, foxes, and bats carry the highest risk of rabies and prophylaxis should begin immediately.

67. C

Floaters are a common and usually benign compliant. They occur because of normal aging as solid particles accumulate in the vitreous jelly. Myopia increases the risk of floaters because of premature vitreous aging. However, whenever a patient complains of floaters, a more serious cause should be ruled out. A rapid increase in the number of floaters, retinal flashes, eye surgery, and head trauma all suggest retinal detachment. The other pathologic condition associated with floaters is vitreous hemorrhage or inflammation, which occurs most often in patients with diabetes, hypertension, and sickle cell disease. Migraines are associated with scintillations or scotoma. Keratitis presents with pain, photophobia, and blurry vision. Strabismus presents with double vision. Corneal abrasion is associated with a foreign body sensation.

68. E

Most common in children, periorbital cellulitis usually originates from infected paranasal sinuses. Periorbital cellulitis can be divided into preseptal and postseptal, but differentiating them may be tricky. The division between pre and post is the orbital septum, a membrane that separates off of the orbital periosteum and inserts onto the tarsal plates of the eyelids. This septum exists to provide protection to the deeper eye structures. If the entire infection is anterior to this membrane, then it is classified as preseptal. Conversely, if the infection has breached the septum, it is called postseptal or orbital cellulitis. On presentation for both types of cellulitis, there is fever, pain, and eyelid swelling. On exam, the conjunctiva can be erythematous and palpation of the lids and globe may elicit tenderness. If there is decreased movement of the eye, proptosis, and/or visual loss, the cellulitis is likely to be postseptal. Treatment usually requires hospital admission with IV antibiotics to cover Strep species. In children, the typical organisms involved include *Streptococcus pneumoniae* and *Moraxella catarrhalis*. With the advent of immunizations, *Haemophilus influenzae* has become rare as an etiology. If trauma or surgery is involved, then *Staphylococcus aureus* is likely. As patients mature, the organisms become polymicrobial, and anaerobic organisms are frequently cultured along with the previously mentioned ones. A CT scan of the orbit and sinuses is helpful in diagnosing accompanying sinusitis, orbital abscess, and tumor and in differentiating between pre- and postseptal infection. *Mucormycosis* and *Aspergillosis* do occur in diabetic and immunocompromised patients, albeit rarely. Typically, the patient with fungal orbital cellulitis is a younger patient with poorly controlled diabetes.

69. E

Keratitis and uveitis, along with acute angle closure glaucoma, scleritis, and endophthalmitis, are among the causes of red eye that require emergent or urgent referral to an ophthalmologist. Without a slit lamp, diagnosis is difficult because many of the patient complaints and physical findings are similar. Uveitis, which is inflammation of the iris and ciliary muscles, is most often due to autoimmune reactions in ankylosing spondylitis, psoriasis, Reiter's syndrome, Behcet's disease, and herpes infections. Keratitis is inflammation of the cornea, most often due to infection, trauma, dry eyes, or contact lens use. Both can present with blurry vision, circumcorneal hyperemia (ciliary flush), photophobia, and pain. Uveitis has the additional finding of an irregular or constricted pupil due to adhesions between the iris and the anterior lens or posterior corneal surface.

70. A

This patient has medial epicondylitis or golfer's elbow, similar to but much less common than lateral epicondylitis or tennis elbow. The pain is distal to the medial epicondyle at the insertion of the flexor and pronator muscles of the forearm and wrist. With the repetitive motions seen in golfing, baseball pitching, and swimming, there is degeneration of the tendon with fibroblast and microvascular reparation. Treatment is first and foremost a modification or elimination of the repetitive motions. Nonsteroidal anti-inflammatory medications, elbow straps, and ice may also be used acutely. For persistent pain, a corticosteroid injection at the site of maximum tenderness may be helpful. If all else fails, surgery may need to be considered. Radial tunnel syndrome presents as lateral elbow pain more distal than tennis elbow. Radial head fracture will present with pain over the radial head and painful pronation and supination. Triceps tendonitis will present with pain above the olecranon process.

71. E

Radial head subluxation, also called nursemaid's elbow, occurs in children younger than 5 years old and is due to ligamentous laxity of the annular ligament that wraps around the head of the radius. It is the most common elbow injury in small children. Treatment consists of rapid reduction of the radial head by supinating the arm while putting mild pressure on the radial head. The child will then have full pronation and supination and begin to use the arm. This technique is easy to learn and should be taught to parents because the subluxation may recur. Splinting and casting are unnecessary. Referrals and x-rays are unnecessary unless the diagnosis is in question or reduction cannot be achieved. The only activity precaution is avoiding lifting children by outstretched arms.

72. D

Dislocation of the elbow is very common and usually occurs after a fall onto an outstretched hand. The dislocation is posterior in 80% of cases and has a number of associated injuries, including radial head fracture, olecranon fracture, brachial artery disruption, and median or ulnar nerve injury. Long-term complications include persistent decrease in range of motion, especially in extension. The elbow is extremely susceptible to decreased range of motion with any immobilization. Fractures and sprains need to be treated either with splints or with internal fixation in order to allow range of motion exercises. Other complications include development of arthritis and recurrent instability. Falls onto an outstretched hand can cause any number of injuries, including colles fracture of the wrist, radial head fracture, olecranon fracture, and scaphoid fracture.

73. C

This is a classic presentation for a felon, which is an infection in the pulp of the finger. The most common causative organism is

Staphylococcus aureus, which also causes paronychia, soft tissue infection around the nail. When no pus is seen, the preferred incision is a dorsal midaxial or hockey stick incision, performed after a digital block is given and a tourniquet is in place. Epinephrine containing anesthetic should not be used near the fingertip. If pus is seen, it is acceptable to incise the pulp of the finger. Nail removal is indicated for paronychia that are resistant to local measures and oral antibiotics. Herpetic whitlows can look like felons but there will be small vesicles at the site of infection. Felons should always be opened because undrained infections can lead to osteomyelitis and distal phalangeal reabsorption. The incision should always close by secondary intention.

74. D

Lateral femoral cutaneous nerve syndrome, also called meralgia paresthetica, occurs when this nerve is compressed, usually medial to the anterior superior iliac spine (ASIS). Patients who develop the syndrome are usually obese or wear tight waistbands or belts. The complaint is of pain, numbness, or dysesthesia along the anterior–lateral thigh. There is never any motor involvement because the nerve carries only sensory fibers. Treatment involves weight loss and/or removing the external compression. If needed, a corticosteroid injection can be performed near the ASIS. The family physician should note that in rare instances, a pelvic or abdominal mass can cause this syndrome. Any patient who does not respond to conservative measures should have further investigation by a CT scan.

75. B

Avascular necrosis occurs in association with a number of diseases, especially those that require long-term corticosteroid use such as systemic lupus erythematosus and rheumatoid arthritis. Also associated are traumas such as posterior dislocations and femoral neck fractures, alcohol use, chronic pancreatitis, sickle cell disease, Crohn's disease, and radiation therapy. It is not surprising that more than 10,000 new patients are diagnosed each year. Patients usually present with dull aching in the hip. Early x-rays may not reveal anything significant, although sclerosis of the femoral head is the first abnormality to be seen. If avascular necrosis is suspected, an MRI is the most useful imaging study. Total hip arthroplasty is used to treat a collapsed femoral head, but this surgery is avoided early in the disease process because the patients tend to be young (between 30 and 50 years old).

76. B

The most likely diagnosis in this age group is rotator cuff tear, and this patient's history is typical. Age-related degeneration and chronic impingement are the most common causes of rotator cuff tears in patients older than 60 years, but patients can often recall an injury after which they felt the pain. This patient would warrant initial conservative treatment of physical therapy and nonsteroidal anti-inflammatory medications. Patients should avoid overhead reaching. If these measures are not effective, the patient may receive a corticosteroid injection into the subacromial bursa. However, because of the steroids weakening effect on the tendon, this should be limited to three separate injections. If the patient continued to have pain and muscle weakness, an MRI would be warranted as well as referral for possible surgical repair. In a younger athletic patient, surgical repair would be indicated within 3 to 6 weeks of trauma for full recovery of muscle strength and agility.

77. C

Adhesive capsulitis, also known as frozen shoulder, results from thickening and contraction of the capsule around the gleno-humeral joint that causes loss of motion and pain. The hallmark of diagnosis is a marked reduction in both active and passive range of motion, with pain especially at the deltoid insertion. The cause is idiopathic, although there are a few medical conditions associated with this, such as type 1 diabetes mellitus, hypothyroidism, Dupuytren disease, Parkinson's disease, and cerebral hemorrhage. Pain is usually slow in onset and located near the deltoid inser-tion. During this early phase, there is a progressive loss of motion. Initial treatment consists of physical therapy and NSAIDs. The course of recovery is slow, with full motion restored only 1 or 2 years after symptoms start. If conservative measures fail, the patient may be taken to the operating room for manipulation of the shoulder under sedation. The other disorders can be differen-tiated from adhesive capsulitis by physical exam and x-ray. Osteoarthritis may be seen on radiograph. Impingement syndrome results in full range of motion but with pain on elevation of the arm. If a shoulder is dislocated anteriorly, the patient will support the arm in a neutral position and confirmatory x-rays can be taken. Rotator cuff tears cause loss of active range of motion but preserve passive range of motion.

78. C

The glenohumeral joint is the most commonly dislocated joint in the body secondary to lack of bony support. The glenoid is very shallow in order to allow great range of motion. The humeral head can dislocate anteriorly (95% of the time), posteriorly (4% of the time), inferiorly, and superiorly. In a true AP view, the x-ray beam is perpendicular to the plane of the scapula. Alone, this view can often appear normal and would miss posterior displace-ment at the level of the glenoid, and it may miss an anterior dis-location. However, an AP view of the shoulder in internal and external rotation may demonstrate dislocation. The standard views to diagnose dislocation radiologically are the Y view, Stryker notch, axillary, and West Point, which is a modified axil-lary view. Posterior dislocations are often missed or interpreted as rotator cuff tears. Radiographs are key in the diagnosis of poste-rior dislocation.

79. C

Low back pain is the second leading cause of presentation to the primary care provider. This patient presents with acute lumbar intervertebral disc prolapse that, based on his symptoms, can be identified as the L5 nerve root. The L5 nerve root (originating at the L4–L5 level) and the S1 nerve root (originating at the L5–S1 level) are most commonly affected. An L5 radiculopathy leads to weakness of dorsiflexion of the foot and toes accompanied by numbness and paresthesia of the accompanying nerve root distrib-ution. There is no associated reflex with L5. A diminished patellar reflex and medial foot numbness can diagnose a herniation at L4. If the herniation occurs at S1, the reflex affected is the one at the ankle and the numbness occurs in the lateral foot. See Table 6.3.

80. D

The majority of patients with disc prolapse will experience a sig-nificant improvement in pain within the first 2 weeks of recovery, although pain can remain for several months. With this history of acute injury and classic symptoms, plain films are unlikely to be helpful in diagnosis or treatment. Appropriate treatment may include 1 to 3 days of rest on a firm mattress, followed by return to activity as tolerated. Because sitting puts an increased strain on nerve roots, it should be avoided. Lying down and standing are more comfortable in this setting. Muscle relaxants, NSAIDs, and cold packs may help to decrease inflammation and pain initially, making it possible for patients to better tolerate activity and phys-ical therapy interventions. Time will often allow the herniated disc to retreat, resulting in improvement of symptoms.

81. B

Cervical spondylosis results from cervical disc degeneration with resultant herniation and calcification of disc material. The C5 and C6 nerve roots are most commonly affected, resulting in weakness of the deltoids, supraspinatus, infraspinatus, biceps, and brachio-radialis. Lateral flexion and rotation are often limited due to large osteophytes. Plain films are an appropriate test and may show osteophytes with encroachment on the intervertebral foramina, and joint space narrowing. They may also show subluxation of one vertebra onto another. These radiologic findings are sugges-tive, but not diagnostic, and must be interpreted in the setting of

Table 6.3 Impingement of nerve roots and symptoms

Level	Nerve Root	Deficits	Sciatica
L3–4	L4	Patellar jerk (reflex) Dorsiflexion of foot (motor) Medial aspects of tibia (sensory)	Uncommon
L4–5	L5	Extensor of great toe (motor) Dorsum of foot/base of first toe (sensory)	Common
L5–S1	S1	Ankle jerk (reflex) Plantar flexion (motor) Buttock, past thigh, cali, lateral Ankle and foot (sensory)	Common

other physical and historical findings because they may also be present in nonaffected individuals in this age group.

82. E

Cervical collar may help to restrict neck movements and relieve mild to moderate pain. Severe pain due to nerve root compression or persistent neurologic deficit may require operative treatment. Although pain medications may provide relief initially, NSAIDs, physical therapy, and muscle relaxants will not provide significant relief for patients with advanced cervical spondylosis because the pain is not primarily muscular in nature. The pain is neurogenic secondary to the narrowed neural foramen and spinal stenosis that occurs secondary to spurring, buckled ligament flavum, disc herniation, and subluxation of vertebral bodies. Surgery consists of decompressing the nerve roots and fusing the vertebrae.

83. E

Although this patient has a positive diagnosis for hemorrhoids, a polyp or cancer in the large bowel cannot be ruled out. A flexible sigmoidoscopy in addition to a double contrast enema or a colonoscopy alone should be performed. Of course, the hemorrhoids should be treated appropriately with Anusol, stool softener for constipation, and avoidance of irritating foods such as seeds, nuts, and corn. Referring the patient to a surgeon is appropriate after medical management fails. Despite the lack of personal or family history, or symptoms of a colon cancer, his age alone and history of rectal bleeding are indications for a workup to rule out a neoplasm.

84. E

Any family physician who performs suturing in the office needs to be familiar with various closure techniques and suture material. Because lipomas do not affect the skin above it, a simple incision is all that is needed. These incisions usually have no tension in them; therefore, they should be closed with simple interrupted sutures or possibly a subcutaneous suture. A mattress suture is used for wounds that have tension, that occur on areas with thick skin, or that require more eversion. Subcutaneous sutures are placed to closed dead space in deep wounds and provide more strength to a closure. Suture material falls into two broad categories: absorbable and nonabsorbable. Silk, nylon, polypropylene, polyester, and cotton are nonabsorbable sutures. A family physician is likely to use nylon, polypropylene, and polyester for skin closure. Subcutaneous sutures need to be absorbable, such as gut, polyglycolic acid (Dexon), polydioxanone (PDS), polyglactic acid (Vicryl), and polyglyconate (Maxon).

85. A

Painful subungual hematomas can involve both the fingers and the toes. Evacuation is a simple procedure that provides instant relief. A 1- to 2-mm perforation needs to be made over the hematoma with either a heated paper clip or a cautery unit. No anesthetic is needed because the procedure is painless and the nail does not have to be removed. A hematoma of greater than 50% suggests a laceration of the nail bed, which may require nail removal and suturing of the tear; evacuation works best with small hematomas. If the nail is cleaned adequately prior to making the perforation, no antibiotics are needed. Postprocedural care includes ice, elevation, and a simple bandage.

86. C

Because abscesses are acidic, local anesthetics work poorly. Injecting into the abscess will not provide anesthesia for the inci-

sion. There are multiple methods to anesthetize an abscess, including topical cryotherapy with liquid nitrogen, ethyl chloride, or a nitrous oxide unit. If that is unavailable, injection of diphenhydramine or lidocaine along the perimeter will allow painless incision. A cruciate incision is made with a number 11 scalpel and exploration of the cavity is necessary to break down any possible loculations. Postprocedural care involves packing the wound or using a drain to allow healing to occur from inside out. Daily soaking also helps keep the wound from closing prior to complete drainage and healing. Antibiotics are not needed because "incision cures the infection." However, if the area appears cellulitic or the patient is immunocompromised, a culture from inside the abscess should be obtained and appropriate antibiotic coverage may be begun.

87. C

Postoperative fever is extremely common. Knowing the common causes and the time frame when they appear will assist in making the correct diagnosis. In the first 24 to 48 hours post-op, fevers are usually attributable to inflammation from cytokine release. Recent research has shown that interleukin-1 and -6, as well as tumor necrosis factor, is responsible for almost all postoperative fever. Atelectasis was thought to be a cause of fever, but recent studies have failed to prove any association. Wound infections usually present after 3 to 7 days and appear erythematous with serous drainage or frank pus, but the incidence has decreased with current prophylactic therapy. Thrombophlebitis is also rarer now that DVT prophylaxis is universal, but if it does occur, usually it takes place 7 to 10 days postoperatively. It is important to check IV sites for phlebitis because this is commonly overlooked. Pneumonias occur after general surgery because both the intubation and the anesthetic interrupt the normal defense mechanisms of the lung. Abdominal abscesses also occur 7 to 10 days after surgery and require imaging to diagnose. Urinary tract infections are one of the most common infections, usually due to prolonged catheterization. Sinusitis can occur, especially in patients who are intubated or have prolonged nasogastric tube placement. Other causes of fever include drug fever, URIs, perirectal abscesses, prostatitis, myocardial infarction, alcohol withdrawal, and other concomitant diseases.

88. B

Diabetes mellitus is associated with a significant increase in postoperative complications. Hyperglycemia by itself is associated with poor wound healing, postoperative infection, and nutrient loss through polyuria. Hyperglycemia frequently occurs due to endogenous stress hormones, exogenous hormones such as steroids, exogenous pressors such as epinephrine, postoperative infection, and IV glucose infusion. Insulin is the best way to control glucose in the postoperative period, especially when the patient is NPO. A good rule of thumb is to provide half of the preoperative insulin to a patient, even if NPO. Diabetes itself predisposes patients to risks, such as myocardial infarction, pressure ulcers from neuropathy and atherosclerosis, hypotension, renal failure, and heart failure.

89. C

The "rule of nines" can quickly help the family physician estimate the extent of the burn. The body can be divided into 11 regions representing 9% of the total body surface area (TBSA), such as the arm, chest, abdomen, thigh, and lower leg, to provide a rough estimate of the size of the burn. A patient's entire palm area can also

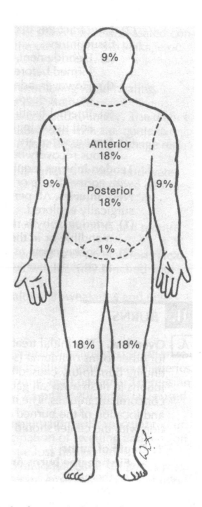

9%

Anterior
18%

9%   9%

Posterior
18%

1%

18%   18%

Figure 6-4. *Rule of nines. The body surface area (BSA) is divided into anatomic areas, each of which is 9% (or a multiple thereof) of the total BSA. This is a simple method of estimating the total burn surface.*

be used to estimate burns because it represents about 1% of the TBSA. Most superficial partial thickness burns present with blisters, weeping, and blanchable skin. There is pain, but scaring is unusual, although pigment changes can occur. The American Burn Association recommends hospital admission for patients who have burns that cover greater than 10% of the TBSA, that occur in children or the elderly, that involve high-voltage or inhalation injury, that are circumferential or involve the face or joints, and that occur in patients with other medical problems. See Figure 6-4.

90. A

All of the above are complications of a vasectomy, as all patients should be counseled. Sperm granuloma is the most common complication, with rates between 15% and 40%, although some believe that eventually all men will develop a sperm granuloma given enough time. This complication is increased with an open-end technique whereby the distal vas is separated from the proximal vas but not ligated or cauterized. The formation of a sperm granuloma actually decreases pressure in the epididymis, seminiferous tubules, and the testicle, but it also increases the risk of reanastamosis. Patients who develop sperm granulomas have the highest rate of success with reversal. Reanastomosis usually occurs within

6 months of the procedure. Anti-sperm antibodies form because the vas blood barrier is breached. There are no sequelae from the formation of antibodies, although there is speculation that it may reduce the chance of pregnancy if the vasectomy is reversed. Infection and hematoma formation are early complications. Hematoma formation is inversely proportional to the number of vasectomies the physician performs a year.

91. D

Burners are transient brachial plexus injuries involving the C5 and C6 nerve roots. They are caused by traction force when the shoulder is pushed down and away, and the head and neck are pushed in the opposite direction. This causes sharp burning pain radiating from the shoulder down the arm. The patient may also experience sensory loss, paresthesias, weakness, or paralysis. A detailed neurologic exam must be performed to assess if the injury is spinal, radicular, pre- or postganglionic plexus, or peripheral. Recurrent episodes may occur in patients with cervical stenosis. These people are at increased risk for spinal cord injury. With complete resolution of all signs and symptoms, the athlete may return to play. Those with prolonged or bilateral symptoms or recurrent episodes may not play until further evaluation is complete.

92. D

The Lachman maneuver is performed with the knee flexed to 30 degrees. With the femur stabilized, the tibia is gently pulled forward, grabbing the tibia from the medial side. The maneuver is considered positive for ACL tear when there is increased tibial motion with no solid end point. The anterior drawer test is negative in 50% of patients with ACL tears. Identifying hemarthrosis through knee aspiration is also quite helpful in affirming the diagnosis, but it is not specific for ACL tear. The other maneuvers do not test for ACL tears. The McMurray sign helps in diagnosing meniscal tears and the apprehension test is useful in diagnosing unstable patellae.

93. A

Younger patients tend to present more frequently with peripheral traumatic meniscal tears that disrupt the blood supply. These injuries secondarily cause effusions or hemarthroses. Elderly patients most often have degenerative tears involving the avascular central portion of the meniscus and may have minimal trauma history or effusion. Most tears occur in this avascular central area and thus are difficult to heal. The provocative McMurray test is positive when pain occurs upon forced flexion and circumduction of the knee. Treatment delays may cause osteoarthritis and progressive damage to the meniscus.

94. B

Causal associations for cataract formation and smoking, UV-B exposure, diabetes, and chronic steroid use have been found. The strongest predictors of cataract formation continue to be age and heredity. Cataract formation can be prevented if patients wear a hat and sunglasses when outdoors and stop smoking. Consuming a low-fat diet also helps because hyperlipidemia has also been implicated in cataract formation. Hypertension has not been associated with increased risk of cataract formation.

95. C

Normal saline or artificial tears may dilute the tear film allergen, and this alone may provide almost complete symptomatic relief. The air conditioners filter out allergen while glasses can block exposure. Histamine antagonists, especially topical forms including levocabastine (Livostin), emedastine (Emadine), and azelastine (Optivar), provide significant relief. Compared with systemic antihistamines, topical treatment avoids systemic side effects and also provides superior performance. Mast cell stabilizers, including nedocromil sodium (Alocril) and lodoxamide (Alomide), are also safe and effective. Topical corticosteroids may cause glaucoma and cataracts, and they are not recommended for the treatment of allergic conjunctivitis.

96. A

Hypothermia is classified in three grades: mild (core temperature, 90°F to 95°F or 32°C to 35°C), moderate (core temperature, 82°F to 90°F or 28°C to 32°C), and severe (core temperature, less than 82°F or 28°C). Passive rewarming should be attempted in all patients and may be sufficient for some mildly hypothermic patients. Active external rewarming techniques are indicated in patients with moderate hypothermia or in cases of mild hypothermia that do not respond to passive methods. External rewarming is a very effective noninvasive technique when invasive methods are not available, but care should be taken to prevent "after drop" in core temperature, when blood circulates through the previously vasoconstricted cold extremities and causes cold blood to return to the core. Peripheral vasodilation, venous pooling, and hypotension may then occur. Active core rewarming methods avoids these complications. Fluids should be warmed to 104°F (40°C) and humidified air should be less than 113°F (45°C). These methods are ideal. Hemodialysis is especially useful in patients who have drug intoxication. Gastric or colonic irrigation is not recommended because it may induce dysrhythmias or electrolyte disturbances. An extremely efficient method, extracorporeal blood rewarming, is used in cases of severe hypothermia.

97. B

Fractures of the distal phalanx may occur frequently; therefore, radiographs are routinely recommended. Subungual decompression, or trephination, is appropriate for subungual hematomas of any size as long as the nail may remain attached, and no fracture is suspected. If no complications are present, the finger should be splinted for 2 or 3 days. If greater than 50% of the nail surface is involved, a nail bed laceration is likely, and nail removal with bed repair is recommended. Antibiotics are not indicated unless the nail is removed.

98. E

Human bites contain multiple species of aerobic and anaerobic organisms. The most common culprits are *Streptococcus viridians*, *Staphylococcus aureus*, *Eikenella corrodens*, and *Haemophilus influenzae*, and these can result in cellulitis, osteomyelitis, or septic arthritis. The most common infecting organism in cats and dogs is *Pasteurella multocida*. If wounds presenting greater than 24 hours show no signs of infection, they may be observed without starting antibiotics. Controversy exists regarding wound closure if the patient presents within 8 hours. With extensive irrigation, debridement, and possibly prophylactic antibiotics, wounds may be closed in the head, neck, arms, and legs, but hand bites should be left open or loosely approximated to allow drainage. Rabies is only transmitted when it is introduced into a bite, open wound, or mucous membrane, not simply by touching urine, blood, or feces. Animals unavailable for confinement must be considered rabid and the bite victim should receive rabies prophylaxis.

99. C

Catgut and chromic are made from animal material. They are monofilament absorbable sutures that incite an inflammatory reaction in the tissue. Polyglactic acid (Vicryl) and polyglycolic acid (Dexon) are absorbable multifilament sutures that past 4 to 8 weeks and are most commonly used to approximate subcutaneous tissue. Nylon is a monofilament nonabsorbable suture that is biologically inert and induces little inflammatory reaction, resulting in a more acceptable scar. Thus, it is useful for skin closure.

100. C

Genu varum is a normal physiologic variation in children younger than 2 years of age. Some children overcorrect this normal variation so that by age 3 to 5 years, they actually have genu valgum. Both of these variations are part of normal development, which spontaneously correct. If either condition is extreme, rickets (vitamin D deficiency) or skeletal dysplasia must be ruled out. Blount disease, also called tibia vara, is a pathologic condition involving the proximal medial tibial growth plate. This causes increased varus angulation of the tibia and will lead to permanent varus (bowleg) angulation, knee growth disturbance, and arthritis if uncorrected. The cause of Blount disease is unknown, but increased compressive force on the medial knee is suspected. This explains why early walkers and obese children are at increased risk. Treatment if diagnosed before age 3 is bracing, and osteotomy is the treatment after 3 years of age.

101. B

Fluid replacement is vital in the prevention and treatment of burn shock. According to the American Burn Association guidelines, burns greater than 15% total body surface area should receive fluid replacement via an intravenous line. Controversy regarding the type of fluid replacement exists. A meta-analysis of 16 trials shows no advantage of hypertonic saline over isotonic saline. The solutions of Ringer's lactate and hypertonic saline and dextran have also been used, with the latter solution possibly reducing tissue edema and providing improved cardioprotection in some cases.

102. A

Furuncles are tender, erythematous, firm, fluctuant lesions arising from one hair follicle, and carbuncles arise from multiple follicles and drain from several tracts. When the lesion comes to a "head," incision and drainage is indicated. In fact, the only treatment necessary in patients with normal immune function is incision and drainage. If the patient has other risk factors or has a surrounding cellulitis, oral or IV antibiotics may be needed. Methods to prevent the reaccumulation of purulent material include wound packing with gauze, breaking up loculations that may hide walled-off lesions, daily soaking, and making the initial incision elliptical or cruciate instead of linear.

103. D

Osgood–Schlatter disease is the most common repetitive injury found in young athletes. It is caused by stress injury to the patellar tendon at its insertion into the tibial tubercle, which will be swollen in most cases. It is technically a traction apophysitis of the tibial tubercle. The syndrome in which patients describe pain just below the patella at the tendon origin is known as Sinding–Larsen–Johansson disease. Osgood–Schlatter disease is a self-limited condition occurring during adolescence, mostly in males. Treatment may also include icing after exercise and NSAIDs.

Although patients do not develop arthritis, they may develop a bone ossicle in the tendon, rarely requiring excision.

104. E

This patient most likely has De Quervain's tenosynovitis, given her difficulties with grasping and wrist pain. Finkelstein's test demonstrates pain from passive stretching of the thumb in flexion. In De Quervain's tenosynovitis, there is inflammation of the extensor and flexor tendons of the thumb secondary to overuse. This leads to rubbing and irritation of the snuffbox tendons as they course through the distal radial styloid. If left untreated, she can lose flexibility of the thumb in flexion, leading to stenosing tenosynovitis. Regional anesthetic block directly over the radial styloid confirms the diagnosis if relief of signs and symptoms occurs, which excludes the diagnoses of carpometacarpal and radiocarpal arthritis. Ice, rest, and buddy taping or a thumb spica splint may be used as initial treatment. If the condition persists beyond 3 or 4 weeks, a local steroid injection may be helpful. Physical therapy may also be helpful for chronic cases.

105. A

This patient has Gamekeeper's thumb, an injury named after royal court gamekeepers. They injured the ulnar collateral ligament of the metacarpal (MP) joint from twisting the necks of fowl hunted for the king. The contemporary version of this injury occurs in skiers who injure the ligament from ski pole accidents and repetitive use. The MP joint becomes unstable from this injury, resulting in poor pinching and thumb to finger opposition. The treatment of choice for acute injuries is to immobilize the thumb in a splint. It is important that the thumb is protected and completely rested for several weeks to allow the ligaments to reattach properly. Ice and NSAIDs will also be helpful but provide temporary relief for the acute injury. Orthopedic consultation and/or local corticosteroid injection are reserved until initial immobilization, physical therapy, and pain medications fail, resulting in an unstable thumb with compromised gripping and grasping function.

106. B

The patient most likely has trigger finger, which is inflammation of the flexor tendons of the finger as they cross the metacarpophalangeal (MCP) head in the palm. Overuse from gripping, grasping, or pressure over the palm causes tenosynovitis of these tendons. Over time, the flexor tendons lose their smooth motion under the specialized ligament (the A-1 pulley), which attaches the tendons to the bone. When the tendons swell, the finger can catch or lock, causing trigger finger. Tendon cysts appear after direct, nonpenetrating trauma damages the tendon or tendon sheath, leading to overproduction of fluid and formation of a cyst, which feels like a small marble or lump in the palm. There may be pain over the cyst to direct pressure, but locking or triggering is absent. Dupuytren contracture results from progressive fibrosis of the palmar fascia. The process is gradual, with pain, tenderness, and locking uncommon. Mallet finger results from stretching or partially tearing the extensor tendon of the finger from a hyperflexion injury.

107. C

This patient is in the early stages of Dupuytren contracture, with no interference of daily activities and mild flexion of the fingers. She will benefit from heated massage and stretching exercises in physical therapy. The scarring process is inevitable, and surgery is used in advanced cases to help restore function. Surgery is palliative only, and in some cases, repeat surgery is necessary for worsening progression. Corticosteroid injection is indicated if the patient has tenosynovitis, which may occur in Dupuytren contracture in about 5% of cases. Observation may be fine in this instance, but it is much more desirable to delay the process by keeping the flexor tendons flexible with physical therapy. Oral corticosteroid use has no role in this disease, although high-dose topical steroid cream has shown improvement in one case report.

108. A

There are many factors associated with epistaxis, one of which is cold dry air. Humidity decreases the risk of nosebleeds. Patients with septal deviation experience a greater incidence of nosebleeds, presumably due to the increased turbulence within the nasal passages, with resultant drying. Pregnancy, sinusitis, and renal failure are additional etiologies of epistaxis. The causes of epistaxis can be divided into environmental factors, including humidity, temperature, and irritants: trauma, especially nose picking; disease processes such as hypertension, coagulation defects, malignancy, and renal failure; and medications including NSAIDS, warfarin, and dipyridamole.

109. E

Initial management in a patient as described in question 108 is directed toward stopping the bleeding. The patient should be directed to sit up, leaning forward, to both decrease venous return and prevent swallowing of blood. Pressure should be held over Kisselbach's plexus, the main site for anterior nosebleeds, for 10 to 20 minutes in patients with persistent bleeding. Bleeding that fails to respond to pressure may be managed with epinephrine, neosynephrine, or silver nitrate. Severe bleeding that is brisk or does not respond to the previous measures may require packing or emergency referral. Only 5% of bleeding is posterior, but this is an emergency that requires packing with gauze or balloon such as a Foley catheter.

110. E

Musculoskeletal injuries account for 6% of family physician office visits and overuse syndromes can account for 60%. Sports-related injury is the most common injury that brings young patients to the family physician's office. Overuse syndrome is a blanket term for conditions caused by repetitive stress injuries as above and also include tennis elbow, Achilles and posterior tibial tendinitis, shin splints, exertional compartment syndromes, epicondylitis, flexor tendonitis, and generalized myofascial pain. When counseling athletes, particularly teen athletes, it is important to discuss the signs and symptoms of overuse.

111. A

Exposure to physical stresses such as repetition, force, temperature, vibration, or poor ergonomics puts people at risk for overuse syndromes. But psychosocial stresses such as monotony, fast work pace, depression, boredom, and relations with coworkers should not be underrated. Even compensation laws come into play. Treatment therefore not only involves medical management but also should include workplace modification of tasks and schedules and assessment for psychologic impairment.

112. D

Popliteal cysts, commonly called Baker's cysts, are synovial cysts that develop in the popliteal bursa of the knee. These cysts develop when trauma or synovitis causes tracking of excessive joint fluid into the popliteal bursa. They are commonly mistaken for soft tissue tumors or gastrocnemius strain. If the cyst ruptures, it is often mistaken for a deep vein thrombosis because of the significant calf swelling and tenderness that ensues. A patient with popliteal cysts should be evaluated for signs of intra-articular knee pathology such as inflammatory arthritis, meniscal, or ligamentous tears. Diagnosis is usually made by history and exam, but ultrasound and MRI may be necessary. The treatment is aimed at the underlying cause of the excessive synovial fluid. Aspiration is only a temporary solution because the fluid often reaccumulates. If the cause of the cyst is arthritis, cyst excision may be necessary. If an intra-articular derangement is present and is repaired, reoccurrence is rare.

113. C

Patellofemoral pain syndrome, otherwise known as chondromalacia patellae, describes diffuse anterior pain worse after climbing stairs, jumping, squatting, or prolonged sitting. While standing, signs of femoral anteversion (patellae pointing to each other) or genu valgum (knock-knees) may be present. The Q angle is the angle drawn from the anterior superior iliac spine to the patellar center, to the center of the tibial tubercle. In women, it should be less than 22 degrees in extension and 9 degrees in flexion. In men, it should be less than 18 degrees in extension and 8 degrees in flexion. When tracking the patella as the knee moves from flexion to extension, the knee moves laterally and sometimes subluxates. Tenderness at the inferior pole of the patella is indicative of patellar tendinitis.

114. D

Patellofemoral instability is primarily diagnosed by eliciting a positive apprehension sign in which the patient becomes anxious when the patella is manipulated, especially laterally. Knee x-rays, specifically axial (sunrise) views, show lateral articulation of the patella in relation to the femoral trochlea. Initial treatment is meant to approximate the torn supporting structures of the patella. The joint should be immobilized from 2 to 6 weeks. Patients with chronic recurrent symptoms may have to have surgery to realign the knee extensor mechanism.

115. A

Osteochondritis dissecans is the development of osteonecrosis of subchondral bone. The lesion is caused by overuse or repetitive stress to the bone. The blood supply is disrupted, and the bone necroses, weakens, and ultimately fractures. The bone fragments become loose bodies in the joint. Patients with osteonecrosis dissecans complain of knee swelling, pain, locking, giving out, and catching. They may walk with the affected foot rotated outward. The condition is diagnosed radiologically, but it may be suspected if there is a positive Wilson's test. This occurs when a supine patient has the hip and knee flexed 90°, the tibia is internally rotated, and pain is elicited when the knee is flexed from 20 to 30 degrees and is relieved when the knee is externally rotated.

116. B

The goal of drinking fluids during exercise is to maintain plasma volume and electrolytes, prevent abnormal heart rate elevation and core body temperature, and provide fuel to the working muscles. The ideal replacement fluid contains about

4% to 8% carbohydrate, which delays fatigue without impairing water delivery. Additionally, fluid intake should start early and be frequent, ideally every 15 to 20 minutes. Adequate amounts of fluid intake are essential to replace water lost in sweat. Drinking when thirsty will replace about two-thirds of the water lost in sweat, resulting in dehydration levels of 2 to 5. The correct answer is B, as recommended by the American College of Sports Medicine.

117. C

Graves' disease is an autoimmune disorder caused by thyroid-stimulating immunoglobulins. These immunoglobulins bind to the TSH receptor and hyperstimulate the thyroid gland. The clinical picture is that of goiter, exophthalmos, pretibial myxedema, coupled with signs and symptoms of hyperthyroidism. To confirm the diagnosis, a pattern of elevated T3 and T4 with suppressed TSH levels should be documented. Ultrasound of the thyroid and fine needle aspiration are utilized in the workup of thyroid nodules and suspected thyroid cancer. An electrocardiogram is useful because many patients with thyrotoxicosis can develop arrhythmias, particularly atrial fibrillation. Treatment options include antithyroid medications, radioactive iodine therapy, and subtotal thyroidectomy.

118. E

Well-controlled exercise-induced asthma does not warrant any further investigation. Asymptomatic MVP also does not require any further testing. HIV alone is not an indication for additional testing and does not preclude an athlete from participating in sports. Stress fractures are common in distance runners and do not mandate further testing on the preparticipation physical. A family history of sudden collapse and death is concerning for sudden cardiac death and certainly warrants additional evaluation. A very careful history that includes symptoms of exercise intolerance, exertional chest discomfort, syncope, near syncope, and palpitations is essential. Special attention should be given to the cardiac exam, especially listening for the classic murmur of hypertrophic cardiomyopathy (the number one cause of sudden cardiac death). This murmur will actually increase with the Valsalva maneuver and decrease with squatting. Additionally, one should look for the body habitus suggestive of Marfan's syndrome (arm span > height, pectus excavatum, and arachnodactyly). Additional testing may include ECG, echocardiogram, and exercise stress test as indicated clinically.

119. E

This is the classic presentation of cholecystitis. Cholelelithiasis is the presence of stones in the gallbladder, most of which are asymptomatic. Risk factors include female gender, obesity, multiparity, diabetes, and age older than 40 years. In the United States, most gallstones are composed of cholesterol. If a stone obstructs the neck of the gallbladder, inflammation and infection can arise. If a stone becomes lodged in the bile duct, the diagnosis is choledocholithiasis. Cholangitis is marked by Charcot's triad (fever, jaundice, and right upper quadrant pain) and progression to Raynaud's pentad (fever, jaundice, right upper quadrant pain, hypotension, and mental status changes). Pancreatitis can be a complication of cholelithiasis.

120. A

Sever disease typically occurs in prepubertal children, especially those engaging in sports in which hard cleats are worn. It is caused by overuse and repetitive trauma secondary to the pull of the Achilles tendon upon the calcaneal apophysis. Once the apophysis fuses to the main calcaneus around age 12 years, problems usually subside. Treatment includes short-term restriction or modification of activities, Achilles tendon stretching, and a heel lift or cushion worn in shoes. Achilles tendonitis would result in pain with any plantar flexion and would involve the length of the tendon. Plantar fasciitis presents with heal pain, but on exam the point of maximum pain would be at the insertion of the plantar fascia on the medial tubercle of the calcaneus. A Morton's neuroma presents with pain in the forefoot, and exam usually reveals tenderness between the third and fourth metatarsal heads.

Chapter 7

Geriatrics Questions

1. An anxious 80-year-old woman presents with multiple complaints. You perform a thorough evaluation of this patient, including laboratory work, stress testing with echocardiography, and pulmonary function testing. When evaluating this woman and her test results, which of the following is considered a normal finding for her age?
A. Decrease in creatinine clearance
B. Blood pressure of 160/80
C. Elevated FEV1 value on pulmonary function tests
D. Low-frequency hearing loss
E. Maximum stress test heart rate of 90

2. A 60-year-old male presents to your office for his physical examination. He is doing very well but has a history of hypertension, chronic obstructive pulmonary disease (COPD), and coronary artery disease. He has been considering long-term care insurance and wants to know how many elderly patients spend time in nursing homes at some time in their life. The percentage of patients 65 or older who require nursing home care during their lifetime is:
A. 1%
B. 5%
C. 20%
D. 40%
E. 80%

3. The majority of nursing home costs in the United States are covered by:
A. Out-of-pocket payments by patients
B. Medicare
C. Private insurance
D. Medicaid
E. Charity care provided by the nursing home

4. Which of the following is true regarding normal aging?
A. All individuals age and lose function at the same rate.
B. Reaction times are unaffected by aging.
C. Reasoning and learning are adversely affected by normal aging.
D. Personalities remain stable over time with normal aging.
E. Environmental influences have little effect on the aging process.

5. The daughter of an 81-year-old widowed male presents with concerns about her father. Recently when visiting him she noticed a lot of spoiled food in the refrigerator, various objects misplaced around the house, and that he had stopped balancing the checkbook. She states that he has become forgetful over the years. He has had no personality changes or difficulties with motor activity or ambulation. He has not seen a doctor for years and reports no significant past medical history. On examination, he has no focal findings and a mini-mental status score of 20. You order laboratory tests and a computed tomography scan of the brain. All tests are normal. You tell her that your findings support a diagnosis of dementia. The most likely cause for this patient's dementia is:
A. Multi-infarct dementia
B. Alzheimer's disease
C. Lewy body disease
D. Normal pressure hydrocephalus
E. Pick's disease

6. Which of the following activities would be categorized as an instrumental activity of daily living?
A. Using the toilet
B. Feeding oneself
C. Using the telephone
D. Bathing
E. Getting dressed

7. Routine vaccination of a 65-year-old would include which of the following?
A. Pneumococcal vaccine
B. Meningococcal vaccine
C. *Haemophilus influenzae* B vaccine
D. Hepatitis B vaccine
E. Varicella vaccine

8. An 80-year-old male presents with a laceration, while cutting vegetables, that requires suturing. Appropriate recommendations for tetanus vaccination include which of the following?
A. Administer the vaccine if not given within the past 10 years.
B. Elderly patients do not require tetanus vaccination.
C. If he had the primary series, he does not require reimmunization.
D. Administer the vaccine regardless of prior vaccination history.
E. Only tetanus immunoglobulin should be administered.

9. Which of the following is recommended for routine screening in patients older than age 65?
A. Carotid ultrasound
B. Stress testing
C. Abdominal aortic ultrasound
D. Serum CA-125
E. Cholesterol screening

10. A 72-year-old woman presents with questions about a newspaper article she read about advanced directives. She is unclear as to what advanced directives are. Which of the following most accurately describes advanced directives?

A. The hospital a patient would choose for his or her care

B. Funeral directives for the patient

C. Determines which family member decides the patient's care if the patient is unable

D. Living will and durable health care power of attorney

E. Decides in advance how the patient's possessions should be dealt with upon his or her death

11. You are called by a nurse regarding a 75-year-old male who has been hospitalized and recovering unremarkably from pneumonia. The nurse states that he has had a sudden change in his mental status and now seems quite confused and agitated. He had his Foley catheter discontinued today, and plans were in progress for discharge. He has had no other underlying medical conditions and was healthy prior to this bout of pneumonia. After reviewing his medications, you order a pulse oximetry and blood tests. While awaiting these results, another appropriate measure includes which of the following?

A. Sedation with 10 mg of intravenous diazepam

B. Straight catheterization of the bladder to assess for urinary retention

C. Donepezil 10 mg orally now and daily

D. Wrist and Posey restraints to prevent injury

E. Haloperidol 2 mg IM now

12. The wife of a 73-year-old male expresses concerns about her husband regarding forgetfulness, decreased appetite, and decrease in activity level during the past 6 weeks. He has a history of COPD, which has been well controlled over the past 5 years. His only medication is an albuterol metered-dose inhaler, which he uses as needed. Examination, including neurologic exam, is unremarkable. Upon performance of the mini-mental status examination, he scores 25 but fails to attempt several questions ("I don't know") and must be prodded to answer others. This patient's presentation is consistent with which of the following diagnoses?

A. Multi-infarct dementia

B. Pseudodementia

C. Parkinson's disease

D. Medication reaction

E. Seizure activity

13. A 75-year-old female presents with concerns about a change in her sleep pattern. She notes that she awakens a few times each night and awakens early every morning. She has no current medical problems and is taking hormone replacement therapy and calcium for osteoporosis prevention. She is active during the day and reports no problems with daytime alertness. She lives with her husband, who has noted no snoring or abnormal nocturnal movements. She denies any depressive symptoms. Which of the following is the most appropriate step in managing this patient?

A. Prescription of a benzodiazepine

B. Prescription of an antidepressant

C. Ordering a sleep study

D. Advise the patient to use over-the-counter diphenhydramine

E. Reassurance

14. Based on current demographics and future projected trends, the percentage of individuals older than age 60 in the United States in 2025 will be:

A. 10%

B. 15%

C. 25%

D. 35%

E. 50%

15. Laboratory changes that occur with aging include which of the following?

A. Increase in serum creatinine

B. Decrease in plasma glucocorticoids

C. Decrease in Westergren sedimentation rate

D. Decrease in serum cholesterol

E. Increase in blood glucose

16. Which of the following services are provided under Medicare Part A insurance coverage?

A. Physician services

B. Inpatient hospital care

C. Prescription medications

D. Durable medical equipment

E. 24-hour home caregiver

17. The daughter of an 85-year-old female presents with the patient for evaluation. She expresses concerns regarding the patient's forgetfulness and the fact that she is still living at home alone. The patient has poor short-term memory, poor insight, and has been noted to misplace objects and wander away from home and get lost. The daughter lives out of state and would like for the patient to be able to stay in this area but is concerned about her safety. You determine that she has a moderate dementia. An appropriate living environment for this patient would include which of the following?

A. Independent senior housing

B. Adult day care

C. Skilled nursing facility

D. Assisted living in dementia unit

E. Hire a caregiver for 8 hours per day

18. Which of the following statements is true regarding hospice?

A. Hospice care may be provided only in a hospice unit.

B. Hospice care may not be provided as part of hospital care.

C. Hospice is a portable service that follows the patient regardless of location.

D. In order to receive hospice care, a physician must certify that the patient will die within 30 days.

E. Hospice services are not covered by Medicare.

19. You suspect Parkinson's disease after examining a patient. Which of the following findings supports this diagnosis?

A. Hemiplegia

B. Stocking glove anesthesia

C. Memory loss

D. Bradykinesia

E. Action tremor

20. A 70-year-old male consults you for another opinion about a test result. He is currently asymptomatic and has been healthy with well-controlled hypertension. He has never had any neurologic complaints. He is a nonsmoker and exercises regularly. He recently had normal laboratory evaluation including lipid profile. On physical examination, he has a carotid bruit on the left. The physical examination is otherwise unremarkable. He wanted your opinion regarding what should be done for a carotid duplex that had a 60% lesion on the left side. You advise him to:

A. Take aspirin daily

B. Undergo angiography

C. Have a carotid endarterectomy performed

D. Begin vitamin E supplements

E. Recheck the carotid duplex in 1 month

21. Which of the following statements is true regarding recovery and prognosis following a stroke?

A. Diabetes does not affect prognosis.

B. Motor function recovery is usually complete within 6 months.

C. Speech and swallowing function usually recover within 2 months.

D. Advanced age correlates with worsened mortality rates and neurologic function.

E. Family support has no bearing on prognosis.

22. The percentage of patients requiring long-term institutional care following stroke is?

A. 10%

B. 30%

C. 50%

D. 70%

E. 90%

23. Age-related physiologic changes may affect pharmacologic activity, distribution, and clearance of medications. Which of the following is a normal physiologic change that occurs with age that may impact drug therapy?

A. Increased renal blood flow

B. Increased liver enzyme activity

C. Decrease in percentage body fat

D. Decrease in total body water

E. Increase in FEV1

24. A 72-year-old man with benign prostatic hypertrophy, diabetes, and chronic obstructive lung disease has recently been started on medications to treat his diseases. He notes that since the medication changes he has increased difficulty urinating. Which of the following medications may have these effects?

A. Oral glyburide

B. Oral metformin

C. Inhaled ipratroprium

D. Inhaled fluticasone

E. Oral prazosin

25. An 80-year-old male presents for follow-up on treatment of his hypertension. He has also noted claudication affecting his right leg. He has a blood pressure of 160/88. While evaluating his claudication, you wish to modify his blood pressure medications for better control. Which antihypertensive medication may adversely affect his symptoms of claudication?

A. Lisinopril

B. Amlodipine

C. Extended-release verapamil

D. Metoprolol

E. Doxasozin

26. Which of the following medications may cause drug-induced Parkinsonism?

A. Metoclopropamide

B. Ranitidine

C. Fluoxetine

D. Atovastatin

E. Citalopram

27. The most common cause for community-acquired bacterial pneumonia in the elderly is?

A. *Staphylococcus aureus*

B. *Streptococcus pneumoniae*

C. *Escherichia coli*

D. *Klebsiella pneumoniae*

E. *Legionella*

28. A decompensating nursing home patient with advanced Parkinson's disease and dementia is admitted to the hospital with altered mental status, tachypnea, and tachycardia. His initial examination reveals rhonchi in the right upper lobe, a pulse oximetry value of 88%, and a chest x-ray with an infiltrate in the right upper lobe. The cause for this patient's condition is most likely attributable to which of the following?

A. Pulmonary embolism

B. Community-acquired pneumonia

C. Acute myocardial infarction

D. Aspiration pneumonia

E. Congestive heart failure

29. Which of the following are indications for oxygen therapy in a patient with chronic obstructive lung disease?

A. pO_2 of 88 mmHg

B. pO_2 of 57 mmHg and P pulmonale on ECG

C. Clubbing of the nails

D. pCO_2 of 50 mmHg

E. Dyspnea on exertion

30. A 65-year-old male presents for follow-up and is noted to have a grade 3/6 systolic murmur along the left sternal border that does not vary with respiration and does not appear to radiate. He is asymptomatic. Which of the following is the most common type of valvular disease requiring surgical intervention in the elderly?

A. Mitral regurgitation

B. Mitral stenosis

C. Aortic stenosis

D. Aortic regurgitation

E. Pulmonic stenosis

31. You assume the care for a 72-year-old male with chronic atrial fibrillation. His rate is currently controlled with diltiazem and he has no symptoms or signs of congestive heart failure. He has never had a TIA or CVA. Which of the following is the most appropriate long-term treatment to lessen the risk of stroke in this patient?

A. Aspirin

B. Low–molecular-weight heparin

C. Observation and no medication

D. Coumadin

E. Clopidogrel

32. A 76-year-old presents with a syncopal episode and is found to be in atrial flutter. During the first 24 hours, she spontaneously converts to sinus rhythm at a rate of 42 beats per minute. Her heart rate remains in the 40s throughout her hospitalization and she continues to have paroxysms of atrial flutter. Which of the following is the most appropriate therapy for this patient?

A. Beta-blocker
B. Fludrocortisone
C. Pacemaker
D. Calcium channel blocker
E. Beta-blocker and pacemaker

33. An 80-year-old active male presents with pain in his right calf associated with walking that is relieved with rest. Examination reveals diminished pulses in the right dorsalis pedis and posterior tibial arteries. Which of the following would be the most appropriate recommendation for treatment of this patient?

A. Calcium channel blockers
B. Lower extremity exercise
C. Propranolol
D. Avoidance of lower extremity exercise
E. Oral nitrate therapy

34. An 85-year-old male presents with an exacerbation of COPD and is found to have a multifocal atrial tachycardia. He is hemodynamically stable and asymptomatic other than the shortness of breath and wheezing due to his COPD. Which of the following is recommended treatment of his arrhythmia?

A. Cardioversion
B. Treating his COPD
C. Beta-blocker for rate control
D. Pacemaker
E. Amiodarone

35. A 68-year-old male with a history of hypertension presents for physical examination. In the course of the examination, he is found to have a pulsatile abdominal mass, which on subsequent ultrasound is found to be 6 cm in size. Which of the following is true regarding this abdominal aortic aneurysm?

A. There is a 40% risk of rupture in the next 5 years.
B. He has a normal cardiac risk for surgery.
C. He should be monitored with yearly ultrasound.
D. Family members are at no increased risk for also having aneurysms.
E. Patients presenting with aneurysm rupture have survival rates of 60%.

36. Which of the following are supportive of a diagnosis of normal pressure hydrocephalus in a patient with dementia?

A. Bradykinesia
B. Perseveration
C. Cogwheel rigidity
D. Tremor
E. Ataxia

37. A 67-year-old woman with a history of chronic back pain presents with bilateral lower extremity pains and weakness associated with the upright position and walking. She notes that this pain is relieved by sitting or lying down. She has an intact neurologic exam of the lower extremities and 2+ and symmetric pulses of both lower extremities, including the femoral, popliteal, dorsalis pedis, and posterior tibial pulses. What is a likely cause for this patient's symptoms?

A. Peripheral neuropathy
B. Spinal stenosis
C. Peripheral vascular disease
D. Polymyalgia rheumatica
E. Guillain-Barre

38. A 75-year-old woman presents with a vesicular dermatomal rash on her trunk for the past 24 hours. The rash is uncomfortable and slightly pruritic. She has never had this rash before. She denies any other complaints and is currently only on atenolol for blood pressure control. Which of the following would be the most appropriate treatment for this patient?

A. Topical acyclovir
B. No treatment
C. Topical corticosteroids
D. Oral valcyclovir
E. Discontinue the atenolol

39. A 68-year-old female presents with complaints of headaches. Her physical examination is normal. You consider the diagnosis of temporal arteritis in the differential diagnosis. Which of the following is true regarding temporal arteritis?

A. It occurs most commonly in those younger than age 50 years.
B. Temporal arteriography is the test of choice for diagnosis.
C. Corticosteroids are contraindicated in this condition.
D. Hearing loss is a frequently associated symptom.
E. Erythrocyte sedimentation rate is a useful screening test.

40. Which of the following is the most common cause for tremor in the elderly?

A. Parkinson's disease
B. Cerebellar infarction
C. Wilson's disease
D. Essential tremor
E. Huntington disease

41. A 67-year-old with clinically suspected rheumatoid arthritis is sent for x-ray evaluation. Which of the following findings on x-ray examination is supportive of the diagnosis of rheumatoid arthritis?

A. Osteophytes
B. Loose body
C. Chondrocalcinosis
D. Bone erosions
E. Joint space narrowing

42. Which of the following is indicated for initial use as long-term disease modifying therapy of active rheumatoid arthritis in geriatric patients?

A. Cyclosporine
B. Methotrexate
C. Corticosteroids
D. Nonsteroidal anti-inflammatory medications
E. Acetaminophen

43. A 64-year-old obese female presents with medial right knee pain and stiffness. Clinically you suspect osteoarthritis and x-ray examination supports this diagnosis. What is the recommended first line of medication therapy for this patient's condition?

A. Acetaminophen

B. Methotrexate

C. Nonsteroidal anti-inflammatory medication

D. Corticosteroids

E. Cyclosporine

44. A 66-year-old female presents with a history of low-grade fever, malaise, and joint pains and stiffness. You suspect polymyalgia rheumatica. Along with an elevated erythrocyte sedimentation rate, which of the following provides additional support for this diagnosis?

A. Bony erosion on x-ray

B. Osteophytes

C. Calcified cartilage visible on x-ray

D. Proximal muscle tenderness

E. Proximal muscle weakness

45. A 70-year-old male presents with a past history of mildly elevated uric acid level. He has read about uric acid and its association with gout and renal disease. When counseling this patient regarding therapy, you recommend treatment to lower the uric acid in which of the following situations?

A. Repeat elevated uric acid

B. Recurrent episodes of gout

C. To prevent renal stones

D. To prevent kidney disease

E. After one episode of gout

46. Which of the following is the most common cause of chronic urinary incontinence in elderly patients?

A. Stress incontinence

B. Urge incontinence

C. Neurogenic overflow incontinence

D. Immobility

E. Vesicovaginal fistula

47. A 65-year-old male presents with complaints of difficulty with urination. He reports that he has difficulty initiating urination and that his urinary stream has less force than it used to have. He has some dribbling and awakens three times each night to urinate. His exam reveals an enlarged prostate with no masses. Urinalysis is normal. Which of the following therapies would be indicated to help provide relief of this man's symptoms?

A. Oxybutynin

B. Urecholine

C. Empiric therapy with ciprofloxacin

D. Tamulosin

E. Amitriptyline

48. You are evaluating a 75-year-old male in the emergency room for acute right lower quadrant abdominal pain. The abdominal pain is associated with loss of appetite. He notes nausea but no emesis, fever, or diarrhea. He reports no urinary or respiratory complaints. He has a history of mild COPD and hypertension. He has had no surgeries and is currently on verapamil SR 180 mg

daily. Physical examination reveals significant tenderness in the right lower quadrant. His white blood cell count is 7.5 and urinalysis is normal. Which of the following is true regarding the diagnosis of appendicitis in the elderly?

A. The elderly are at lower risk for appendiceal rupture than younger patients.

B. Absence of fever makes the diagnosis of appendicitis unlikely.

C. The elderly often have a normal white blood cell count with appendicitis.

D. Abdominal CT scan is not useful for evaluating for appendicitis in the elderly.

E. Anemia is a common finding associated with appendicitis in the elderly.

49. A 70-year-old male with chronic hypertension presents with shortness of breath and is diagnosed with congestive heart failure. He has no significant past medical history and is currently only on hydrochlorothiazide for treatment of his hypertension. His examination reveals no murmurs and an S4 is present. He has rales at the lung bases but no peripheral edema. His chest x-ray reveals mild pulmonary congestion. Electrocardiogram reveals sinus rhythm with no ischemic changes. His cardiac enzymes are normal and echocardiogram reveals mild LVH with normal wall motion and an estimated ejection fraction of 65%. Which of the following is the most likely etiology for this patient's congestive heart failure?

A. Valvular heart disease

B. Arteriovenous malformation

C. Systolic dysfunction

D. Diastolic dysfunction

E. Episode of unrecognized supraventricular tachycardia

50. Which of the following medications are recommended for routine long-term management of congestive heart failure?

A. Amlodipine

B. Amiodarone

C. Verapamil

D. Captopril

E. Clonidine

51. Which of the following interventions has been shown to prevent hospital admissions and lower health care costs for congestive heart failure?

A. Monthly chest x-rays

B. Coumadin therapy for target INR 2.0

C. Multidisciplinary care including daily weights

D. Care in a long-term residential facility

E. Echocardiography every 3 to 6 months

52. A 67-year-old female presents with vaginal itching and burning. She is currently on no medication other than calcium supplementation. Physical examination reveals thinning and pallor of the vaginal mucosa but no discharge. Wet prep from the scant material present is negative for any organisms. Which of the following will help in alleviating this patient's symptoms?

A. Estrogen vaginal cream

B. Topical corticosteroid cream

C. Metronidazole vaginal gel

D. Vinegar and water douche

E. Clotrimazole vaginal cream

53. An obese 75-year-old woman presents after sustaining a Colles' fracture to her left wrist. She is concerned about lessening her risk for future fractures. Her past medical history is significant for COPD for which she has required intermittent oral corticosteroid therapy in addition to inhalers. She quit smoking 10 years ago and drinks moderately. She has never been on hormone replacement therapy and has not taken calcium. She is 25 years postmenopausal. She engages in exercise by taking regular walks but is sometimes limited by her respiratory disease. Which of the following is a risk factor for osteoporosis in this patient?
A. Obesity
B. Chronic obstructive pulmonary disease
C. Walking as a form of exercise
D. Corticosteroid therapy
E. Beta agonist inhaler therapy

54. Which of the following is indicated for treatment of osteoporosis in the elderly?
A. Medroxyprogesterone 10 mg daily for 14 days per month
B. Calcium carbonate 500 mg daily
C. Risedronate (actonel) 5 mg daily
D. Alendronate (fosamax) 35 mg weekly
E. Tamoxifen 10 mg twice daily

55. Laboratory evaluation obtained from a 70-year-old woman during a routine physical examination reveals an elevated serum calcium. Repeat values are also elevated. She has no ongoing medical problems and her only medications are hormone replacement therapy. Which of the following is the likely cause for elevation of serum calcium in an asymptomatic elderly patient?
A. Excess dietary calcium
B. Hyperparathyroidism
C. Hypothyroidism
D. Malignancy
E. Excess vitamin D intake

56. A 60-year-old diabetic male presents for follow-up. He is currently on metformin with glucose values consistently in the 100s and a hemoglobin A1c value of 5.8%. He has a blood pressure of 138/86 and a normal physical examination, including lower extremity neurologic examination. He has had regular eye exams, showing no signs of retinopathy. In planning future treatment of this patient, which of the following would you recommend?
A. Adding an ACE inhibitor
B. No change in therapy
C. Adding beta-blocker therapy
D. Ambulatory blood pressure monitoring
E. Adding sulfonylurea oral therapy

57. A 75-year-old diabetic patient presents for follow-up with no current complaints. On physical examination, he is noted to have a blood pressure of 105/60 and a normal heart, lung, and neurologic exam. Review of his laboratory reveals a glucose of 134 (fasting), hemoglobin A1c 6.1%, triglyceride 140, cholesterol 203, HDL cholesterol 47, LDL cholesterol 128, creatinine 1.3, and urine negative for protein and microalbumin. His current medications include metformin and ramipril. What recommendation would you now make in caring for this patient?
A. Discontinue ramipril

B. Discontinue metformin
C. Begin atorvastatin
D. No change in therapy
E. Begin gemfibrozil

58. Which of the following is true regarding infection or colonization with methicillin-resistant *Staphylococcus aureus* (MRSA)?
A. Prior hospitalization increases risk.
B. Advanced age increases risk.
C. MRSA is more virulent than antibiotic-sensitive *Staphylococcus aureus*.
D. Colonization or infection with MRSA is unrelated to prior antibiotic use.
E. Nursing home patients colonized with MRSA require isolation.

59. An 80-year-old male presents with aches, fever, and congestion for the past 24 hours. He is in no acute distress and his lungs are clear. You suspect he has influenza. Appropriate measures at this time include which of the following?
A. Hospitalization for monitoring
B. Influenza vaccine
C. Levofloxacin 250 mg orally daily for 10 days
D. Olseltamivir 75 mg orally twice daily for 5 days
E. Chest x-ray to determine further therapy

60. An 83-year-old female with coronary artery disease and hypertension diagnosed 2 years ago presents for routine follow-up. She is currently being treated with metoprolol with good blood pressure control. Laboratory evaluation at the time of the visit reveals a creatinine of 1.7, which is increased from a value of 1.1 6 months ago. Which of the following is the most likely cause for the elevated creatinine?
A. Renal artery stenosis
B. Hypertension
C. Metoprolol
D. Advancing age
E. Simvastatin

61. Which of the following is true regarding heart failure in the elderly?
A. Valvular heart disease is the most common causative factor.
B. Hypertension is the most common cause in elderly women.
C. Systolic dysfunction is more common than diastolic dysfunction.
D. The incidence of heart failure is declining in the elderly.
E. New onset of heart failure is uncommon after age 65.

62. Which of the following is true regarding dental care in the elderly?
A. A common cause for tooth loss is periodontal disease.
B. Dentures restore 70% of chewing function.
C. Medicare coverage includes routine dental care.
D. Approximately 10% of Americans older than age 85 are edentulous.
E. Dentures are covered under Medicare Part B.

63. The leading cause for unintentional weight loss in the elderly nursing home population is:
A. Pulmonary disease
B. Gastrointestinal disease

C. Cancer

D. Medication effect

E. Psychiatric disease

64. Which of the following is true regarding alcohol abuse in the elderly?

A. The elderly must consume more alcohol than young adults to reach the same blood alcohol level.

B. Women abuse alcohol at a greater rate than men.

C. Elderly individuals who abuse alcohol are at low risk for suicide.

D. The elderly are more likely to require inpatient alcohol detoxification.

E. Lifetime prevalence of alcohol abuse is less than 1% in the geriatric population.

65. You are seeing a 75-year-old female with a past history of depression treated on five different occasions during her life. She now presents with a recurrence. In deciding treatment options, which of the following is true?

A. She should receive 6 months of antidepressant therapy.

B. Response to prior medications is not predictive of future response.

C. ECT is contraindicated in the elderly.

D. Methylphenidate may be used as short-term therapy.

E. Lithium is the preferred therapy in treating geriatric depression.

66. Which of the following is true regarding treatment of Alzheimer's disease?

A. Cholinesterase inhibitors restore patients to a normal level of cognitive function.

B. Cessation of cholinesterase inhibitors results in reversion to a level of function commensurate with never having been treated.

C. Anti-inflammatory medications improve cognitive function.

D. Ginko biloba use can prevent Alzheimer's disease.

E. Selegilene effectively prevents progression of disease.

67. Which of the following is the most common cause for severe vision loss in elder Americans?

A. Macular degeneration

B. Cataracts

C. Glaucoma

D. Diabetes mellitus

E. Amblyopia

68. A mildly demented 69-year-old male presents after falling. He sustained no apparent injuries and his mental status is unchanged. Which of the following is a routine test that should be ordered in patients who fall?

A. Head CT scan

B. Hemoglobin

C. Hip x-rays

D. Electroencephalogram

E. No routine testing

69. Which of these sleep disorders is most common in the geriatric population?

A. Narcolepsy

B. Obstructive sleep apnea

C. Idiopathic hypersomnia

D. Sleepwalking

E. Night terrors

70. Which of the following is true regarding myocardial infarction affecting patients older than age 70 years?

A. Men are affected three times more commonly than women.

B. PTCA and CABG are contraindicated in this age group.

C. Confusion may be the only presenting symptom.

D. Beta-blockers are of no benefit.

E. The risks of aspirin outweigh the benefits of aspirin in patients older than age 75 years.

71. A 68-year-old male with a history of diabetes mellitus presents with impotence. He is asking about using sildenafil. Which of the following is true regarding this treatment?

A. It is contraindicated in patients requiring nitrates.

B. It is contraindicated in patients requiring beta-blockers.

C. It should not be used following prostate surgery.

D. It should not be used in patients with peripheral neuropathy.

E. It is contraindicated in patients with vascular disease.

72. Which of the following is the leading cause of cancer death in the geriatric population?

A. Colon

B. Breast

C. Lung

D. Prostate

E. Pancreatic

73. A 65-year-old male presents with concerns regarding lung cancer and wants to know his risks. He is a former smoker of one pack per day for 20 years and he quit 10 years ago. Which of the following is true?

A. He is at no increased risk for lung cancer compared to a person who never smoked.

B. His risk will always remain greater than that of a person who never smoked.

C. His risk will always be equal to that of a person who currently smokes.

D. Quitting smoking lowers associated lung cancer risk but not cardiovascular risks.

E. Quitting smoking lowers cardiovascular risks but not lung cancer risks.

74. Which of the following is a significant risk factor for developing colon cancer?

A. Low fiber diet

B. Family history of colon cancer

C. Personal history of hyperplastic polyps

D. Personal history of irritable bowel syndrome

E. Personal history of chronic folate intake

75. An 85-year old male with severe COPD, history of congestive heart failure, and coronary artery disease presents for follow-up. He notes no urinary complaints but is concerned about being screened for prostate cancer. He has a slightly enlarged prostate but no nodules or masses. Which of the following should you now recommend?

A. No testing in the absence of symptoms

B. Annual PSA testing

C. Prostate ultrasound

D. Prostate biopsy

E. Alpha-blocker therapy with tamulosin

76. A healthy 80-year-old female with no significant past medical history presents for annual physical examination. She has had annual physical examinations for the past 10 years, including Pap smears, and all exams and tests have been normal. Which of the following is recommended for routine health screening in this patient?

A. Annual mammography

B. Pap smear every 2 or 3 years

C. Annual chest x-ray

D. Colonoscopy every 3 years

E. Annual DEXA scan

77. Presbycusis refers to which of the following?

A. Low-pitched hearing loss associated with vertigo

B. Aminoglycoside-induced hearing loss

C. Decreased taste sensation

D. Age-related high-pitched hearing loss

E. Hereditary hearing loss

78. Which of the following is a normal change in gait that is associated with aging?

A. Loss of arm swing

B. Widening of the base

C. Decreased stride length

D. Variable step lengths and height

E. Short, shuffling gait

79. A 75-year-old female presents with her daughter who expresses concerns about a decline in her mother's activity level. Her mother has become more dependent on others for performing activities that she recently performed. The patient has noted increased pain and stiffness in her right hip. She has had chronic osteoarthritis of her right hip but has not been on any therapy for this since prior to this it had not been very painful. Which of the following would you now recommend for treatment of this patient?

A. Prednisone 20 mg daily

B. Acetaminophen 1 g three times daily

C. Ibuprofen 800 mg three times daily

D. Referral for joint replacement

E. Hydrocodone 5 mg four times daily

80. Benign positional vertigo (BPV) is the most common cause for positional vertigo in the elderly. Which of the following is true regarding BPV?

A. Episodes typically last 60 to 90 minutes

B. Vertical nystagmus is a frequent finding

C. Tinnitus and hearing loss are common associated findings

D. Medication treatment is of little benefit

E. Positions that trigger symptoms should be avoided

81. Which of the following medications is associated with the highest risk for falls in the elderly?

A. Pseudoephedrine

B. Fludrocortisone

C. Buproprion

D. Acetaminophen

E. Lorazepam

82. Which of the following is the most common cause of death by injury in patients 65 to 74 years of age?

A. Motor vehicle accidents

B. Homicide

C. Burns

D. Falls

E. Drowning

83. An 83-year-old male is found to have been the cause of a motor vehicle accident. His family comes to you with concerns about whether he should be driving or not. He is currently on no medications. He denies significant alcohol use. His physical examination including vision exam and cognitive functioning appear normal. Which of the following should now be recommended?

A. The patient should no longer drive.

B. The patient should be referred to a program for formal driving assessment.

C. The patient should only drive during the day.

D. The patient should only drive during non-rush hour times.

E. The patient should only make short trips (less than 5 miles).

84. What percentage of 70-year-old men have erectile dysfunction?

A. 10%

B. 33%

C. 50%

D. 67%

E. 90%

85. Of the following, what is the most common sexual complaint in elderly women?

A. Vaginismus

B. Anorgasmia

C. Vaginal dyspareunia

D. Lack of a sexual partner

E. Low sexual desire

86. Which of the following is an indication for initiating therapy in Paget's disease?

A. Disease involving the pelvis

B. Disease involving the skull

C. Elevation in alkaline phosphatase

D. Elevation in serum calcium

E. History of congestive heart failure

87. The most common skin cancer occurring in the elderly is:

A. Squamous cell carcinoma

B. Malignant melanoma

C. Basal cell carcinoma

D. Seborrheic keratosis

E. Keratoacanthoma

88. An 80-year-old male with a history of mild COPD, dementia, and osteoarthritis suffers a hip fracture requiring surgical repair. Which of the following forms of prophylaxis is most effective in preventing deep venous thrombosis in this patient?

A. Aspirin

B. Compression stockings

C. Early ambulation

D. Subcutaneous unfractionated heparin

E. Subcutaneous low–molecular-weight heparin

89. An 84-year-old woman is nearing time for hospital discharge. She has a mini-mental status score of 23/30. Her daughter is her power of attorney for health care. In deciding this patient's future care, which of the following is true?

A. The daughter must make all decisions for her.

B. The patient may be able to make her own decisions.

C. The court must appoint someone to make decisions for her.

D. She requires neuropsychological testing to determine competency.

E. Her physician must make all medical decisions for her.

90. An 80-year-old male who suffers from dementia falls and fractures his hip. You are counseling the family about the impact of his injury on his future health. Which of the following most closely matches the 1-year mortality rate following a hip fracture in geriatric patients?

A. No effect on mortality

B. Less than 10% 1-year mortality

C. 15% to 30% 1-year mortality

D. 40% to 60% 1-year mortality

E. 90% 1-year mortality

91. Which of the following patients would be a poor candidate for participating in inpatient physical rehabilitation therapy?

A. A stable patient recovering from a CVA

B. A stable patient with moderate–severe dementia

C. A stable patient with diabetes mellitus

D. A stable patient with Medicare insurance

E. A stable patient with depression

92. An 80-year-old male presents with new-onset supraventricular tachycardia associated with palpitations, but no chest pain or shortness of breath. His examination reveals a regular tachycardia at a rate of 150 and a pulse oximetry reading of 98% on room air. He has a normal lung exam, no leg tenderness, and no peripheral edema. Initial evaluation of this patient's tachycardia should include which of the following?

A. Pulmonary arteriography

B. Stress testing

C. Thyroid-stimulating hormone

D. Chest CT scan

E. Arterial blood gases

93. A 60-year-old male presents with a history of repeated episodes of palpitations and near syncope that occur approximately every 2 weeks and last for 3 minutes. He has no significant past medical history and is currently on no medications. His physical examination, including orthostatic pulse and blood pressure check, is normal. His heart rate is 80 and regular with no murmurs detected. Which of the following tests would be most useful in determining the etiology of this patient's symptoms?

A. Electrocardiogram

B. Holter monitor

C. Tilt-table testing

D. CT scan of the brain

E. Event monitor

94. In order for Medicare to cover rehabilitation services in a nursing home, which of the following is true regarding length of hospital stay?

A. There are no time specifications regarding Medicare coverage of rehabilitation.

B. The patient must be hospitalized for at least 1 night.

C. The patient must be hospitalized for at least 3 nights.

D. The patient must be hospitalized for at least 1 week.

E. The patient must be hospitalized for less than 48 hours.

95. A 65-year-old female presents for review of her DEXA results. She has a T-score of −2.5. When interpreting this for her, you explain that:

A. Her bone density is 2.5 standard deviations below the mean for young women.

B. Her bone density is 2.5 standard deviations above the mean for young women.

C. Her bone density is 2.5 standard deviations below the mean for normal women her age.

D. Her bone density is 2.5 standard deviations above the mean for normal women her age.

E. Her bone density is 2.5% below the mean for all women.

96. In the course of evaluating a 75-year-old male for decreased libido and erectile dysfunction, he is found to have an elevated serum LH and FSH and a decreased serum testosterone and free testosterone. When planning treatment for this patient, which of the following is true?

A. Testosterone therapy is not indicated in geriatric patients.

B. His complaints and laboratory findings are part of normal aging.

C. Testosterone may improve his libido but may not resolve his erectile dysfunction.

D. Testosterone is unlikely to improve his libido but will resolve his erectile dysfunction.

E. Leuprolide therapy will resolve both his libido and erectile dysfunction.

97. A depressed-appearing 84-year-old female is found to have a TSH less than 0.003 and an elevated T3 and T4 during the course of her evaluation. Which of the following diagnoses is consistent with this patient's presentation and labs?

A. Iodine deficiency

B. Hyperthyroidism

C. Primary hypothyroidism

D. Secondary hypothyroidism

E. Clinical depression

98. Which of the following is the most common cause for hypothyroidism in geriatric patients?

A. Hashimoto's thyroiditis

B. Iodine deficiency

C. Thyroid carcinoma

D. Grave's disease

E. Secondary hypothyroidism

99. A 65-year-old female who is on hormone replacement therapy present with concerns about wanting to stop the therapy. However, in the past when she stopped the treatment, she experienced hot

flashes. Alternative treatment that may be beneficial in treating these symptoms includes which of the following?
A. Nifedipine
B. Propranolol
C. Medroxyprogesterone acetate
D. Raloxifene
E. Prazosin

100. A 79-year-old female is found to have an elevated MCV and MCH on a complete blood count. Follow-up labs included a vitamin B12 and folate level. The vitamin B12 was low but the folate was normal. Which of the following is the most common cause for vitamin B12 deficiency in geriatric patients?
A. Inadequate dietary intake
B. Crohn's disease
C. Parasite infestation
D. Ulcerative colitis
E. Pernicious anemia

101. Which of the following is a common risk factor for vitamin D deficiency in geriatric patients?
A. Increased sun exposure
B. Vigorous exercise
C. Urinary vitamin loss due to diuretic use
D. Decreased hepatic function
E. Limited dietary intake of vitamin D

102. A nursing home patient develops a 2-cm stage 2 decubitus ulcer on the sacrum without surrounding erythema, discharge, or odor. The wound looks clean. Which of the following therapies is most important in promoting healing of this lesion?
A. Oral antibiotics
B. Topical antibiotics
C. Protecting the area from pressure
D. Betadine irrigation
E. Daily application of hydrogen peroxide

103. Which of the following is the most common cause for chronic constipation in the elderly?
A. Hyperparathyroidism
B. Hypothyroidism
C. Reduced intestinal transit times
D. Colon carcinoma
E. Irritable bowel syndrome

104. Which of the following is true regarding fecal incontinence in geriatric patients?
A. It is a normal part of aging.
B. Incontinence is a leading cause for institutionalization.
C. There are no treatments available.
D. Dementia plays a limited role in causing incontinence.
E. Antimotility agents (e.g., loperamide) are the cornerstone of treatment.

105. Which of the following medications is associated with tardive dyskinesia as a side effect?
A. Levodopa/carbidopa
B. Pseudoephedrine
C. Metoclopropamide
D. Loratadine
E. Zolpidem

106. Elderly patients are more susceptible to developing hypothermia for which of the following reasons?
A. Increased shivering response
B. Increases in peripheral blood flow
C. Decreases in perception of temperature changes
D. Increases in baseline metabolic rates
E. More rapid metabolism of medications leading to altered mental status

107. Increases in which of the following laboratory results are most consistent with a diagnosis of iron deficiency anemia?
A. Ferritin
B. Serum iron
C. Reticulocyte count
D. Total iron binding capacity
E. Mean corpuscular volume

108. A 65-year-old male presents with bloody diarrhea and abdominal pain for the past 2 days. He has no identifiable risk factors, has not traveled, has not eaten raw or undercooked food, and has not recently had antibiotics. He has a significant past medical history of osteoarthritis, hypertension, and hyperlipidemia. He is currently taking over-the-counter anti-inflammatory medications, hydrochlorothiazide, and is a nonsmoker. He is nontoxic appearing. In considering the diagnostic possibilities, which of the following is true?
A. Ulcerative colitis is rare in geriatric patients.
B. Smoking is a risk factor for developing ulcerative colitis.
C. Nonsteroidal anti-inflammatory medications may cause colitis.
D. Ischemic colitis is not associated with bleeding.
E. Diverticular bleeding generally presents with diarrhea.

109. A 67-year-old with chronic respiratory complaints is found to have bronchiectasis on CT scanning. When further evaluating this patient, which of the following is commonly associated with bronchiectasis?
A. Pulmonary hypertension
B. Allergic bronchopulmonary aspergillosis
C. Pulmonary embolus
D. Asthma
E. Pulmonic stenosis

110. A 76-year-old male is found to have a gastric ulcer on esophagoduodenoscopy. When further evaluating this patient, which of the following is recommended?
A. *Helicobacter pylori* antibody testing
B. Anti-inflammatory medication to promote ulcer healing
C. Oral amoxicillin for 7 days
D. Follow-up endoscopy 6 to 8 weeks after therapy
E. Surgical resection of the ulcer

111. During cross-coverage for your partner, you are called with results from a urine culture obtained as part of routine nursing home admitting orders for an 84-year-old asymptomatic female. The culture showed greater than 100,000 of a gram-negative organism. Which of the following is the appropriate step in managing this finding?

A. Repeat the culture by obtaining a catheterized specimen.
B. Treat the patient and repeat the culture after treatment.
C. Treat the patient with no repeat culture.
D. No treatment is necessary.
E. Treat the patient and place in contact isolation.

112. An 80-year-old diabetic male has been well controlled on metformin and presents to establish himself as your patient. He has had mildly elevated blood pressure in addition to his diabetes and takes captopril 50 mg three times daily. His examination is unremarkable and his blood pressure is 120/74. Labs obtained at the visit reveal a glucose of 200, HgbA1c 6.4, serum creatinine 1.7, serum potassium 4.7, and a 1+ albumin on urine dipstick. Review of medical records reveals these all to be stable. Which of the following changes in medications should be recommended?
A. Increase metformin dose
B. Increase captopril dose
C. Decrease captopril dose
D. Discontinue metformin and substitute alternative therapy
E. Add rosiglitazone to current therapy

113. Which of the following classes of medications is associated with the least adverse effects on memory in geriatric patients?
A. Phenothiazines
B. Selective serotonin reuptake inhibitors
C. Benzodiazepines
D. Tricyclic antidepressants
E. Antihistamines

114. Which of the following patients has a relative contraindication for use of enoxaparin therapy and may require dosage adjustment if the medication is used?
A. An 85-year-old male who weighs 70 kg and has a serum creatinine of 1.5
B. An 80-year-old female who weighs 42 kg and has a serum creatinine of 1.0
C. A 70-year-old male with a normal protime and an SGOT and SGPT 1.5 times normal
D. A 65-year-old male who weighs 80 kg and has a serum creatinine of 2.0
E. A 75-year-old male s/p nephrectomy with a weight of 70 kg and creatinine of 1.2

115. A 65-year-old female presents with bunion deformity and pain of her left foot resulting from excessive pressure over the area of deformity. Examination reveals the presence of a bunion on the left foot with some mild thickening and redness of the overlying skin. There is an associated hallux valgus deformity. Which of the following is the most appropriate initial treatment?
A. Steroid injection into the left first MTP joint
B. Modification of the footwear
C. Surgery
D. Physical therapy
E. Narcotic pain medication

116. An 80-year-old male with a history of hypertension that has been well controlled presents for follow-up to discuss the finding of an elevated PSA of 5.8. His prostate exam is normal and he is asymptomatic. He is very anxious and fearful of cancer but also does not want to undergo any procedures or surgery. Which of the following is the next appropriate step in evaluating this patient?
A. Recommend ultrasound-guided biopsy
B. Recommend radiation treatment
C. Obtain a serum-free PSA
D. Advise him that he does not have cancer
E. Start him on finasteride

117. Which of the following is true when comparing community-acquired and nursing home-acquired pneumonias?
A. Gram-negative organisms are more common in nursing home patients with pneumonia.
B. Atypical organisms (e.g., mycoplasma, Chlamydia) cause most nursing home-acquired pneumonias.
C. Community-acquired pneumonias are more likely to have gram-negative organisms.
D. *Streptococcus pneumoniae* is uncommon in nursing home patients.
E. *Legionella* is the most common nursing home pathogen causing pneumonia.

118. A 75-year-old female is referred to you by her dentist for recommendations regarding antibiotic prophylaxis with dental work. The patient is being treated for type 2 diabetes mellitus and hypertension and had a total hip replacement 8 months ago, a myocardial infarction 3 years ago, and myocarditis as a child. She completed a course of antibiotics 4 weeks ago for a community-acquired pneumonia and is fully recovered. Which of the following is an indication for prophylactic antibiotic use in this patient?
A. Her age (75 years)
B. Her hip replacement less than 2 years ago
C. Her history of myocarditis
D. Type 2 diabetes mellitus
E. Recent antibiotic use

119. A 65-year-old female presents for follow-up evaluation of hair loss on the crown of her head. She has had no associated medical illnesses and currently is on no medications other than calcium and alendronate. Physical examination is within normal limits other than mild thinning of the hair on the scalp in the crown region. She has normal genitalia and no signs of virilization or hirsutism. Which of the following is indicated in evaluating this patient?
A. Abdominal CT scan
B. Serum DHEAS
C. Serum testosterone
D. Serum thyroid-stimulating hormone
E. Scalp biopsy

120. An 80-year-old male who lives with his daughter and her children and family presents for evaluation after a fall. He has mild dementia and a history of hypertension. He is taking lorazepam prn and hydrochlorothiazide. Other than a nontender contusion on his arm, his physical examination is normal. Regarding evaluation of falls, which of the following is true?
A. Exercise is beneficial in preventing falls.
B. Restraints decrease the number of falls.
C. Psychotropic medications are helpful in preventing falls.
D. Environmental factors rarely play a role in the etiology of falls.
E. Occupational therapy referral would likely not be useful in light of the patient's dementia.

Chapter 7

Answer Key

1.	A	43.	A	85.	E
2.	D	44.	D	86.	B
3.	D	45.	B	87.	C
4.	D	46.	B	88.	E
5.	B	47.	D	89.	B
6.	C	48.	C	90.	C
7.	A	49.	D	91.	B
8.	A	50.	D	92.	C
9.	E	51.	C	93.	E
10.	D	52.	A	94.	C
11.	B	53.	D	95.	A
12.	B	54.	C	96.	C
13.	E	55.	B	97.	B
14.	C	56.	A	98.	A
15.	E	57.	C	99.	C
16.	B	58.	A	100.	E
17.	D	59.	D	101.	E
18.	C	60.	A	102.	C
19.	D	61.	B	103.	C
20.	A	62.	A	104.	B
21.	B	63.	E	105.	C
22.	A	64.	D	106.	C
23.	D	65.	D	107.	D
24.	C	66.	B	108.	C
25.	D	67.	A	109.	B
26.	A	68.	E	110.	D
27.	B	69.	B	111.	D
28.	D	70.	C	112.	D
29.	B	71.	A	113.	B
30.	C	72.	C	114.	B
31.	D	73.	B	115.	B
32.	E	74.	B	116.	C
33.	B	75.	A	117.	A
34.	B	76.	A	118.	B
35.	A	77.	D	119.	D
36.	E	78.	C	120.	A
37.	B	79.	B		
38.	D	80.	D		
39.	E	81.	E		
40.	D	82.	A		
41.	D	83.	B		
42.	B	84.	D		

Chapter 7

Geriatrics Answers

1. A

There are many changes that occur normally as a result of aging. There is a decline in renal perfusion and functional glomerular units that results in a decline in creatinine clearance. This may clinically manifest as an increased susceptibility to medication side effects or toxicity. Definitions of hypertension do not change with age, and an elderly person with a blood pressure of 160/80 would be considered hypertensive. There is a decrease in FEV1 that occurs naturally as part of aging that is similar in effect but to a much lesser degree than occurs with smoking. High-frequency hearing loss is considered a normal finding in the elderly and may represent age-related cumulative high-frequency injuries to the hearing apparatus. The minimal acceptable heart rate response to stress testing is adjusted for age by the following formula: maximum heart rate = $(220 - \text{age}) \times 0.85$. Thus, in this patient, a heart rate response increasing to 119 beats per minute would be considered adequate for interpreting the stress test results. See Table 7.1.

2. D

Approximately 40% of individuals older than age 65 will require nursing home care at some point in their life. Of individuals who reside in nursing homes, one-half reside there permanently, one-fourth are there for rehabilitative services, and one-fourth have come there for end-of-life care. Approximately 5% of the geriatric population resides in nursing homes at any given time. Three-fourths enter nursing homes following hospitalization. The average age for a nursing home resident is 82 years. Predictors of needing nursing home care are dementia, requiring assistance with ADLs, lack of social supports, and being in a low-income group.

3. D

Medicaid is the major provider of nursing home costs. Medicaid covers approximately 47% of nursing home costs. Most of the remainder of costs are covered by out-of-pocket payments by patients and their families. Medicare covers only a small fraction of costs (4%) and private insurance accounts for less than 2% of nursing home funding. A more recent addition to the options for covering these services has been the purchasing, by individuals, of long-term care insurance. This allows individuals to protect their assets from the costs of long-term care.

4. D

Although there are general rates of decline in function that occur with aging, great variability in individuals' function occurs as a result of interplay of genetic and environmental influences. For example, although age-related decline in pulmonary function may occur, there is great variability between smokers and nonsmokers due to acceleration of the process in those who smoke. Reaction times do slow as a result of normal aging, but reasoning and learning are unaffected in

Table 7.1 Normal changes with aging

CNS/sensory
Presbyopia
Presbycusis
Slowed reaction times
Alteration in sleep efficiency

Gastrointestinal
Decreased number of taste buds
Slowed intestinal motility

Metabolism
Decreased hepatic blood flow
Decreased renal blood flow
Decreased creatinine clearance

Body composition
Increase in percentage body fat
Decrease in percentage body water
Decrease in muscle mass

Cardiovascular
Blood pressure tends to increase
Heart rate responses blunted
Left ventricular stiffness
Relative decrease in cardiac output with exercise

Pulmonary
Decrease in FEV1 and pO_2
Diminished cough reflex

Electrolytes/water balance
Decrease basal and stress-induced increase renin and aldosterone
Increased basal vasopressin
Decrease in ability to concentrate urine
Decrease thirst response to hyperosmolarity
Decrease in total body potassium

normal aging. Sensory input, including vision (through changes in the lenses) and hearing (presbycusis), and diminished peripheral sensory feedback are contributing factors affecting reaction time. Higher cortical functions, including one's personality, remain intact, and any changes in personality should be investigated for underlying disease, including depression.

5. B

A common presentation for patients with Alzheimer's disease is insidious decline in mental function with resultant gradual loss of the instrumental activities of daily living (e.g., preparing meals, buying groceries, and paying bills) followed by activities of daily living (e.g., continence, feeding, and bathing). Family members visiting from out of state may be surprised by the deficits that become apparent upon inspecting the living environment because in many cases, patients are able to interact socially and "cover up" their deficits. The score of 20 on the mini-mental status exam supports the diagnosis, and the presence of an otherwise normal neurologic examination as well as computed tomography make the other choices unlikely. The absence of movement difficulty would argue against Lewy body disease as a cause. Normal pressure hydrocephalus is characterized by the triad of incontinence, ataxia, and dementia. Multi-infarct dementia presents with a more abrupt and step-wise decline in function associated with focal neurologic deficits. Pick's disease is a type of frontotemporal dementia. Personality change, loss of inhibition, and decreased verbalization are some of the characteristic features. See Table 7.2.

6. C

Functional status of an elderly patient is usually described in terms of activities of daily living and instrumental activities of daily living. The instrumental activities of daily living (IADL) are those activities that are required for an individual to live independently without assistance. Examples include using the telephone, paying bills, shopping, cleaning, performing home repairs, doing laundry, and preparing meals. Individuals who are unable to perform or arrange for performance of these activities would require assistance and may be candidates for caregiver assistance, assisted living, or nursing home care. Using the toilet, feeding oneself, bathing, and getting dressed are all activities of daily living (ADL) and are more basic functions. When a patient is unable to perform ADLs, this generally signifies that greater assistance and care is needed. See Table 7.3.

Table 7.2 Types of dementia

Alzheimer's disease	Gradual onset; visual/spatial impairment and short-term memory affected early
Lewy body disease	Fluctuations in mental status; hallucination; parkinsonism
Frontotemporal	Disinhibition; loss of social skills; apathy; visual/spatial less affected early
Multi-infarct	More sudden onset in association with cerebrovascular event; focal deficits; risk factors for vascular disease
Depression	History of depression; other symptoms of depression; lack of attempt on testing; orientation intact

Table 7.3 Common tasks included in ADL and IADL scales

Katz Index of Activities of Daily Living
 Bathing
 Dressing
 Grooming
 Toileting
 Transfer
 Continence
 Feeding
 Communication

Lawton Instrumental Activities of Daily Living
 Shopping
 Cooking and meal preparation
 Laundry
 Using telephone
 Managing medication
 Transportation
 Household cleaning
 Managing finances

7. A

Routine vaccination of a 65-year-old patient includes diphtheria–tetanus every 10 years, pneumococcal vaccine, and annual influenza vaccination. Tetanus vaccination is frequently overlooked in this population of patients. Meningococcal, hemophilus, varicella, and hepatitis vaccinations are not routinely recommended for the geriatric population. See Table 7.4.

8. A

Tetanus vaccination should be provided routinely every 10 years after completion of the primary series regardless of age. The elderly are equally or more susceptible to tetanus following laceration injuries. With contaminated wounds, many authorities recommend vaccination following laceration if the interval since last vaccination is ≥5 years. Tetanus immunoglobulin is provided for contaminated wounds in unvaccinated individuals, along with the tetanus vaccine. The vaccine would not be required in either circumstance if the patient had been recently vaccinated.

9. E

Current recommendations call for routine screening of cholesterol, blood pressure, colon cancer, and breast cancer. Cardiovascular disease and cancer are the two leading causes of death in the geriatric population. Colon cancer and breast cancer increase incidence with age. The age at which colon and breast cancer screening may stop is controversial and in many instances determined by the presence of other underlying diseases and the overall health of the individual. However, many authorities recommend stopping after age 75. Ovarian cancer screening with serum CA-125 is not routinely recommended for any age group. Blood pressure screening and control has been shown to lower risk of cardiovascular disease in the geriatric population. Additional measures that may be helpful include counseling about smoking cessation and exercise. Cholesterol screening is recommended although

Table 7.4 Adult vaccination from CDC

Recommended Adult Immunization Schedule United States, October 2006–September 2007

Recommended adult immunization schedule, by vaccine and age group

Vaccine ▼ / Age group (yrs) ▶	19–49 years	50–64 years	≥65 years
Tetanus, diphtheria, pertussis (Td/Tdap)[1]*	1-dose Td booster every 10 yrs Substitute 1 dose of Tdap for Td		
Human papillomavirus (HPV)[2]*	3 doses (females)		
Measles, mumps, rubella (MMR)[3]*	1 or 2 doses	1 dose	
Varicella[4]*	2 doses (0, 4–8 wks)	2 doses (0, 4–8 wks)	
Influenza[5]*	1 dose annually	1 dose annually	
Pneumococcal (polysaccharide)[6,7]	1–2 doses		1 dose
Hepatitis A[8]*	2 doses (0, 6–12 mos, or 0, 6–18 mos)		
Hepatitis B[9]*	3 doses (0, 1–2, 4–6 mos)		
Meningococcal[10]	1 or more doses		

Recommended adult immunization schedule, by vaccine and medical and other indications

Vaccine ▼ / Indication ▶	Pregnancy	Congenital immunodeficiency; leukemia; lymphoma; generalized malignancy; cerebrospinal fluid leaks; therapy with alkylating agents, antimetabolites, radiation, or high-dose, long-term corticosteroids	Diabetes, heart disease, chronic pulmonary disease, chronic alcoholism	Asplenia (including elective splenectomy and terminal complement component deficiencies)[11]	Chronic liver disease, recipients of clotting factor concentrates	Kidney failure, end-stage renal disease, recipients of hemodialysis	Human immunodeficiency virus (HIV) infection[3,11]	Health-care workers
Tetanus, diphtheria, pertussis (Td/Tdap)[1]*	1-dose Td booster every 10 yrs — Substitute 1 dose of Tdap for Td							
Human papillomavirus (HPV)[2]*		3 doses for women through age 26 years (0, 2, 6 mos)						
Measles, mumps, rubella (MMR)[3]*			1 or 2 doses					
Varicella[4]*			2 doses (0, 4–8 wks)					2 doses
Influenza[5]*	1 dose annually			1 dose annually		1 dose annually		
Pneumococcal (polysaccharide)[6,7]	1–2 doses			1–2 doses			1–2 doses	
Hepatitis A[8]*		2 doses (0, 6–12 mos, or 0, 6–18 mos)			2 doses (0, 6–12 mos, or 0, 6–18 mos)			
Hepatitis B[9]*		3 doses (0, 1–2, 4–6 mos)				3 doses (0, 1–2, 4–6 mos)		
Meningococcal[10]		1 dose		1 dose				1 dose

* Covered by the Vaccine Injury Compensation Program

These recommendations must be read along with the footnotes, which can be found on the next 2 pages of this schedule.

Legend:
- For all persons in this category who meet the age requirements and who lack evidence of immunity (e.g., lack documentation of vaccination or have no evidence of prior infection)
- Recommended if some other risk factor is present (e.g., on the basis of medical, occupational, lifestyle, or other indications)
- Contraindicated

(continued)

Table 7.4 (continued)

Footnotes

1. Tetanus, diphtheria, and acellular pertussis (Td/Tdap) vaccination. Adults with uncertain histories of a complete primary vaccination series with diphtheria and tetanus toxoid–containing vaccines should begin or complete a primary vaccination series. A primary series for adults is 3 doses; administer the first 2 doses at least 4 weeks apart and the third dose 6–12 months after the second. Administer a booster dose to adults who have completed a primary series and if the last vaccination was received ≥10 years previously. Tdap or tetanus and diphtheria (Td) vaccine may be used; Tdap should replace a single dose of Td for adults aged <65 years who have not previously received a dose of Tdap (either in the primary series, as a booster, or for wound management). Only one of two Tdap products (Adacel® [sanofi pasteur, Swiftwater, Pennsylvania]) is licensed for use in adults. If the person is pregnant and received the last Td vaccination ≥10 years previously, administer Td during the second or third trimester; if the person received the last Td vaccination in <10 years, administer Tdap during the immediate postpartum period. A one-time administration of 1-dose of Tdap with an interval as short as 2 years from a previous Td vaccination is recommended for postpartum women, close contacts of infants aged <12 months, and all health-care workers with direct patient contact. In certain situations, Td can be deferred during pregnancy and Tdap substituted in the immediate postpartum period, or Tdap can be given instead of Td to a pregnant woman after an informed discussion with the woman (see http://www.cdc.gov/nip/publications/acip-list.htm). Consult the ACIP statement for recommendations for administering Td as prophylaxis in wound management (http://www.cdc.gov/mmwr/preview/mmwrhtml/00041645.htm).

2. Human Papillomavirus (HPV) vaccination. HPV vaccination is recommended for all women aged ≤26 years who have not completed the vaccine series. Ideally, vaccine should be administered before potential exposure to HPV through sexual activity; however, women who are sexually active should still be vaccinated. Sexually active women who have not been infected with any of the HPV vaccine types receive the full benefit of the vaccination. Vaccination is less beneficial for women who have already been infected with one or more of the four HPV vaccine types. A complete series consists of 3 doses. The second dose should be administered 2 months after the first dose; the third dose should be administered 6 months after the first dose. Vaccination is not recommended during pregnancy. If a woman is found to be pregnant after initiating the vaccination series, the remainder of the 3-dose regimen should be delayed until after completion of the pregnancy.

3. Measles, Mumps, Rubella (MMR) vaccination. *Measles component:* adults born before 1957 can be considered immune to measles. Adults born during or after 1957 should receive ≥1 dose of MMR unless they have a medical contraindication, documentation of ≥1 dose, history of measles based on health-care provider diagnosis, or laboratory evidence of immunity. A second dose of MMR is recommended for adults who 1) have been recently exposed to measles or in an outbreak setting; 2) were previously vaccinated with killed measles vaccine; 3) have been vaccinated with an unknown type of measles vaccine during 1963–1967; 4) are students in postsecondary educational institutions; 5) work in a health-care facility, or 6) plan to travel internationally. Withhold MMR or other measles-containing vaccines from HIV-infected persons with severe immunosuppression. *Mumps component:* adults born before 1957 can generally be considered immune to mumps. Adults born during or after 1957 should receive 1 dose of MMR unless they have a medical contraindication, history of mumps based on health-care provider diagnosis, or laboratory evidence of immunity. A second dose of MMR is recommended for adults who 1) are in an age group that is affected during a mumps outbreak; 2) are students in postsecondary educational institutions; 3) work in a health-care facility; or 4) plan to travel internationally. For unvaccinated health-care workers born before 1957 who do not have other evidence of mumps immunity, consider giving 1 dose on a routine basis and strongly consider giving a second dose during an outbreak. *Rubella component:* administer 1 dose of MMR vaccine to women whose rubella vaccination history is unreliable or who lack laboratory evidence of immunity. For women of childbearing age, regardless of birth year, routinely determine rubella immunity and counsel women regarding congenital rubella syndrome. Do not vaccinate women who are pregnant or who might become pregnant within 4 weeks of receiving vaccine. Women who do not have evidence of immunity should receive MMR vaccine upon completion or termination of pregnancy and before discharge from the health-care facility.

4. Varicella vaccination. All adults without evidence of immunity to varicella should receive 2 doses of varicella vaccine. Special consideration should be given to those who 1) have close contact with persons at high risk for severe disease (e.g., health-care workers and family contacts of immunocompromised persons) or 2) are at high risk for exposure or transmission (e.g., teachers of young children; child care employees; residents and staff members of institutional settings, including correctional institutions; college students; military personnel; adolescents and adults living in households with children; non-pregnant women of childbearing age; and international travelers). Evidence of immunity to varicella in adults includes any of the following: 1) documentation of 2 doses of varicella vaccine at least 4 weeks apart; 2) U.S.–born before 1980 (although for health-care workers and pregnant women, birth before 1980 should not be considered evidence of immunity); 3) history of varicella based on diagnosis or verification of varicella by a health-care provider (for a patient reporting a history of or presenting with an atypical case, a mild case, or both, health-care providers should seek either an epidemiologic link with a typical varicella case or evidence of laboratory confirmation, if it was performed at the time of acute disease); 4) history of herpes zoster based on health-care provider diagnosis; or 5) laboratory evidence of immunity or laboratory confirmation of disease. Do not vaccinate women who are pregnant or might become pregnant within 4 weeks of receiving the vaccine. Assess pregnant women for evidence of varicella immunity. Women who do not have evidence of immunity should receive dose 1 of varicella vaccine upon completion or termination of pregnancy and before discharge from the health-care facility. Dose 2 should be administered 4–8 weeks after dose 1.

5. Influenza vaccination: *Medical indications:* chronic disorders of the cardiovascular or pulmonary systems, including asthma; chronic metabolic diseases, including diabetes mellitus, renal dysfunction, hemoglobinopathies, or immunosuppression (including immunosuppression caused by medications or HIV); any condition that compromises respiratory function or the handling of respiratory secretions or that can increase the risk of aspiration (e.g., cognitive dysfunction, spinal cord injury, or seizure disorder or other neuromuscular disorder); and pregnancy during the influenza season. No data exist on the risk for severe or complicated influenza disease among persons with asplenia; however, influenza is a risk factor for secondary bacterial infections that can cause severe disease among persons with asplenia. *Occupational indications:* health-care workers and employees of long-term–care and assisted living facilities. *Other indications:* residents of nursing homes and other long-term–care and assisted living facilities; persons likely to transmit influenza to persons at high risk (i.e., in-home household contacts and caregivers of children aged 0–59 months, or persons of all ages with high-risk conditions); and anyone who would like to be vaccinated. Healthy, nonpregnant persons aged 5–49 years without high-risk medical conditions who are not contacts of severely immunocompromised persons in special care units can receive either intranasally administered influenza vaccine (FluMist®) or inactivated vaccine. Other persons should receive the inactivated vaccine.

Footnotes

6. Pneumococcal polysaccharide vaccination. *Medical indications:* chronic disorders of the pulmonary system (excluding asthma); cardiovascular diseases; diabetes mellitus; chronic liver diseases, including liver disease as a result of alcohol abuse (e.g.,cirrhosis); chronic renal failure or nephrotic syndrome; functional or anatomic asplenia (e.g., sickle cell disease or splenectomy [if elective splenectomy is planned, vaccinate at least 2 weeks before surgery]); immunosuppressive conditions (e.g., congenital immunodeficiency, HIV infection [vaccinate as close to diagnosis as possible when CD4 cell counts are highest], leukemia, lymphoma, multiple myeloma, Hodgkin disease, generalized malignancy, organ or bone marrow transplantation); chemotherapy with alkylating agents, antimetabolites, or high-dose, long-term corticosteroids; and cochlear implants. *Other indications:* Alaska Natives and certain American Indian populations and residents of nursing homes or other long-term–care facilities.

7. Revaccination with pneumococcal polysaccharide vaccine. One-time revaccination after 5 years for persons with chronic renal failure or nephrotic syndrome; functional or anatomic asplenia (e.g., sickle cell disease or splenectomy); immunosuppressive conditions (e.g., congenital immuno-deficiency, HIV infection, leukemia, lymphoma, multiple myeloma, Hodgkin disease, generalized malignancy, or organ or bone marrow transplantation); or chemotherapy with alkylating agents, antimetabolites, or high-dose, long-term corticosteroids. For persons aged ≥65 years, one-time revaccination if they were vaccinated ≥5 years previously and were aged <65 years at the time of primary vaccination.

8. Hepatitis A vaccination. *Medical indications:* persons with chronic liver disease and persons who receive clotting factor concentrates. *Behavioral indications:* men who have sex with men and persons who use illegal drugs. *Occupational indications:* persons working with hepatitis A virus (HAV)–infected primates or with HAV in a research laboratory setting. *Other indications:* persons traveling to or working in countries that have high or intermediate endemicity of hepatitis A (a list of countries is available at http://www.cdc.gov/travel/diseases.htm) and any person who would like to obtain immunity. Current vaccines should be administered in a 2-dose schedule at either 0 and 6–12 months, or 0 and 6–18 months. If the combined hepatitis A and hepatitis B vaccine is used, administer 3 doses at 0, 1, and 6 months .

9. Hepatitis B vaccination. *Medical indications:* Persons with end-stage renal disease, including patients receiving hemodialysis; persons seeking evaluation or treatment for a sexually transmitted disease (STD); persons with HIV infection; persons with chronic liver disease; and persons who receive clotting factor concentrates. *Occupational indications:* health-care workers and public-safety workers who are exposed to blood or other potentially infectious body fluids. *Behavioral indications:* sexually active persons who are not in a long-term, mutually monogamous relationship (i.e., persons with >1 sex partner during the previous 6 months); current or recent injection-drug users; and men who have sex with men. *Other indications:* household contacts and sex partners of persons with chronic hepatitis B virus (HBV) infection; clients and staff members of institutions for persons with developmental disabilities; all clients of STD clinics; international travelers to countries with high or intermediate prevalence of chronic HBV infection (a list of countries is available at http://www.cdc.gov/travel/diseases.htm); and any adult seeking protection from HBV infection. Settings where hepatitis B vaccination is recommended for all adults: STD treatment facilities; HIV testing and treatment facilities; facilities providing drug-abuse treatment and prevention services; health-care settings providing services for injection-drug users or men who have sex with men; correctional facilities; end-stage renal disease programs and facilities for chronic hemodialysis patients; and institutions and nonresidential daycare facilities for persons with developmental disabilities. *Special formulation indications:* for adult patients receiving hemodialysis and other immunocompromised adults, 1 dose of 40 μg/mL (Recombivax HB®) or 2 doses of 20 μg/mL (Engerix-B®).

10. Meningococcal vaccination. *Medical indications:* adults with anatomic or functional asplenia, or terminal complement component deficiencies. *Other indications:* first-year college students living in dormitories; microbiologists who are routinely exposed to isolates of *Neisseria meningitidis*; military recruits; and persons who travel to or live in countries in which meningococcal disease is hyperendemic or epidemic (e.g., the "meningitis belt" of Sub-Saharan Africa during the dry season [December–June]), particularly if contact with local populations will be prolonged. Vaccination is required by the government of Saudi Arabia for all travelers to Mecca during the annual Hajj. Meningococcal conjugate vaccine is preferred for adults with any of the preceeding indications who are aged ≤55 years, although meningococcal polysaccharide vaccine (MPSV4) is an acceptable alternative. Revaccination after 5 years might be indicated for adults previously vaccinated with MPSV4 who remain at high risk for infection (e.g., persons residing in areas in which disease is epidemic).

11. Selected conditions for which *Haemophilus influenzae* type b (Hib) vaccination may be used. Hib conjugate vaccines are licensed for children aged 6 weeks–71 months. No efficacy data are available on which to base a recommendation concerning use of Hib vaccine for older children and adults with the chronic conditions associated with an increased risk for Hib disease. However, studies suggest good immunogenicity in patients who have sickle cell disease, leukemia, or HIV infection or have had splenectomies; administering vaccine to these patients is not contraindicated.

This schedule indicates the recommended age groups and medical indications for routine administration of currently licensed vaccines for persons aged ≥19 years, as of October 1, 2006. Licensed combination vaccines may be used whenever any components of the combination are indicated and when the vaccine's other components are not contraindicated. For detailed recommendations on all vaccines, including those used primarily for travelers or that are issued during the year, consult the manufacturers' package inserts and the complete statements from the Advisory Committee on Immunization Practices (http://www.cdc.gov/nip/publications/acip-list.htm).

Report all clinically significant postvaccination reactions to the Vaccine Adverse Event Reporting System (VAERS). Reporting forms and instructions on filing a VAERS report are available at http://www.vaers.hhs.gov or by telephone, 800-822-7967.

Information on how to file a Vaccine Injury Compensation Program claim is available at http://www.hrsa.gov/vaccinecompensation or by telephone, 800-338-2382. To file a claim for vaccine injury, contact the U.S. Court of Federal Claims, 717 Madison Place, N.W., Washington, D.C. 20005; telephone, 202-357-6400.

Additional information about the vaccines in this schedule and contraindications for vaccination is also available at http://www.cdc.gov/nip or from the CDC-INFO Contact Center at 800-CDC-INFO (800-232-4636) in English and Spanish, 24 hours a day, 7 days a week.

Approved by the Advisory Committee on Immunization Practices, the American College of Obstetricians and Gynecologists, the American Academy of Family Physicians, and the American College of Physicians

somewhat controversial for patients without known cardiovascular disease. Carotid or aortic ultrasound and stress testing are not recommended as routine screening tests. See Table 7.5.

10. D

Advanced directives are a means of helping making decisions regarding health care should the condition of the individual preclude this decision-making capacity. Ideally, the document should be as detailed as possible and include instructions regarding resuscitation and artificial support (including ventilator use and tube feeding). Certainly, the document will not be able to cover all possible situations, and designation of a durable health care power of attorney can then determine who can make those decisions for patients when they are unable to make decisions for themselves. The durable health care power of attorney does not have to be a family member and should be someone who is familiar with the wishes of the patient.

Table 7.5 Table of recommended preventive services

Preventive Services Recommended by the USPSTF

The U.S. Preventive Services Task Force (USPSTF) recommends that clinicians discuss these preventive services with eligible patients and offer them as a priority. All these services have received an "A" (strongly recommended) or a "B" (recommended) grade from the Task Force.

Recommendation	Adults		Special Populations	
	Men	**Women**	**Pregnant Women**	**Children**
Abdominal Aortic Aneurysm, Screening[1]	✓			
Alcohol Misuse Screening and Behavioral Counseling Interventions	✓	✓	✓	
Aspirin for the Primary Prevention of Cardiovascular Events[2]	✓	✓		
Bacteriuria, Screening for Asymptomatic			✓	
Breast Cancer, Chemoprevention[3]		✓		
Breast Cancer, Screening[4]		✓		
Breast and Ovarian Cancer Susceptibility, Genetic Risk Assessment and BRCA Mutation Testing[5]		✓		
Breastfeeding, Behavioral Interventions to Promote[6]		✓	✓	
Cervical Cancer, Screening[7]		✓		
Chlamydial Infection, Screening[8]		✓	✓	
Colorectal Cancer, Screening[9]	✓	✓		
Dental Caries in Preschool Children, Prevention[10]				✓
Depression, Screening[11]	✓	✓		
Diabetes Mellitus in Adults, Screening for Type 2[12]	✓	✓		
Diet, Behavioral Counseling in Primary Care to Promote a Healthy[13]	✓	✓		
Gonorrhea, Screening[14]		✓	✓	
Gonorrhea, Prophylactic Medication[15]				✓
Hepatitis B Virus Infection, Screening[16]			✓	
High Blood Pressure, Screening	✓	✓		
HIV, Screening[17]	✓	✓	✓	✓
Lipid Disorders, Screening[18]	✓	✓		
Obesity in Adults, Screening[19]	✓	✓		

(continued)

Table 7.5 (continued)

Recommendation	Adults		Special Populations	
	Men	Women	Pregnant Women	Children
Osteoporosis in Postmenopausal Women, Screening[20]		✓		
Rh (D) Incompatibility, Screening[21]			✓	
Syphilis Infection, Screening[22]	✓	✓	✓	
Tobacco Use and Tobacco-Caused Disease, Counseling[23]	✓	✓	✓	
Visual Impairment in Children Younger than Age 5 Years, Screening[24]				✓

[1]One-time screening by ultrasonography in men aged 65–75 who have ever smoked.

[2]Adults at increased risk for coronary heart disease.

[3]Discuss with women at high risk for breast cancer and at low risk for adverse effects of chemoprevention.

[4]Mammography every 1–2 years for women 40 and older.

[5]Refer women whose family history is associated with an increased risk for deleterious mutations in BRCA1 or BRCA2 genes for genetic counseling and evaluation for BRCA testing.

[6]Structured education and behavioral counseling programs.

[7]Women who have been sexually active and have a cervix.

[8]Sexually active women 25 and younger and other asymptomatic women at increased risk for infection. Asymptomatic pregnant women 25 and younger and others at increased risk.

[9]Men and women 50 and older.

[10]Prescribe oral fluoride supplementation at currently recommended doses to preschool children older than 6 months whose primary water source is deficient in fluoride.

[11]In clinical practices with systems to assure accurate diagnoses, effective treatment, and follow-up.

[12]Adults with hypertension or hyperlipidemia.

[13]Adults with hyperlipidemia and other known risk factors for cardiovascular and diet-related chronic disease.

[14]All sexually active women, including those who are pregnant, at increased risk for infection (that is, if they are young or have other individual or population risk factors).

[15]Prophylactic ocular topical medication for all newborns against gonococcal ophthalmia neonatorum.

[16]Pregnant women at first prenatal visit.

[17]All adolescents and adults at increased risk for HIV infection and all pregnant women.

[18]Men 35 and older and women 45 and older. Younger adults with other risk factors for coronary disease. Screening for lipid disorders to include measurement of total cholesterol and high-density lipoprotein cholesterol.

[19]Intensive counseling and behavioral interventions to promote sustained weight loss for obese adults.

[20]Women 65 and older and women 60 and older at increased risk for osteoporotic fractures.

[21]Blood typing and antibody testing at first pregnancy-related visit. Repeated antibody testing for unsensitized Rh (D)-negative women at 24–28 weeks gestation unless biological father is known to be Rh (D) negative.

[22]Persons at increased risk and all pregnant women.

[23]Tobacco cessation interventions for those who use tobacco. Augmented pregnancy-tailored counseling to pregnant women who smoke.

[24]To detect amblyopia, strabismus, and defects in visual acuity.

11. B

This patient has an acute episode of confusion, often termed delirium, for which the underlying cause should be determined. Sedation may interfere with assessment of the patient and may put the patient at risk for falls or other injuries as well. Donepezil is a long-term therapy for Alzheimer's disease and would have no role in this situation. Wrist and Posey restraints should be used as a last resort. Supervision and reassurance of the patient along with assessing for underlying causes for the change in status are warranted. Urinary retention could be a potential cause for this patient's change and can be assessed by straight catheterization while awaiting other test results. See Tables 7.6 and 7.7.

12. B

Patients presenting with features of dementia that have developed over a relatively short period of time should be investigated for other potential causes. In this particular patient, a decrease in appetite and activity should heighten one's suspicion for depression as the underlying cause. In addition, failing to attempt to answer questions is typical of depression, whereas patients with

Table 7.6 Differentiating delirium from dementia

Delirium	Dementia
Abrupt, precise onset	Gradual, ill-defined onset
Altered level of consciousness	Normal alertness until end stage
Short attention span	Normal attention span until late stages
Hallucinations common	Hallucinations uncommon until late stages (except Lewy body dementia)
Loss of orientation early	Orientation preserved in early stages
Psychomotor changes common (agitation or lethargy)	Psychomotor changes uncommon until late stages
Usually reversible if cause found and treated	Usually irreversible

Table 7.7 Causes for delirium

Systemic hypoperfusion: anemia, cardiac disease, pulmonary disease
Fluid/electrolyte imbalance
Endocrine disease: vitamin deficiency, thyroid disease, diabetes
Infection
Renal or liver disease
Medications
Neurologic disease: CVA, seizure, tumor, trauma
Acute pain
Psychiatric disease: mood disorder, alcohol withdrawal

dementia attempt to answer questions but are more commonly incorrect. In the elderly, depression can masquerade as dementia and thus in this instance is termed " pseudodementia." The absence of neurologic findings on physical examination would lead one to consider diagnoses other than Parkinson's disease or multi-infarct dementia. Albuterol may cause anxiety and palpitations as a side effect, but it is not associated with depression. Although seizure activity can affect mental status, the absence of documented "spells" or seizure-like motor activity would make depression a much more likely diagnosis.

13. E

Although the patient reports a change in her sleep pattern, she is having no functional difficulties related to this change. She denies difficulties with alertness, activities, or depression. Her husband has noted no abnormalities during her sleep. The changes this patient is describing are consistent with normal changes that may occur with aging. Increased nocturnal awakening, earlier bedtimes and awakening, less efficient sleep, and spending more time in bed with less actual sleep time are all consistent with normal age-related changes in sleep patterns. In addition, decreased rapid eye movement sleep and deep sleep and increased sleep latency occur with aging. Diphenhydramine, although sedating, can lead to excess sedation and other anticholinergic side effects.

14. C

The geriatric population is the fastest growing segment of the U.S. population. The number of patients older than the age of 60 is expected to grow from its current proportion of 17% to 25% by 2025. In addition, an even larger percentage increase is projected for the numbers of minority individuals older than the age of 60, creating more ethnic diversity among the elderly. This surge in geriatric population may create some stress to our health care system both financially and in terms of meeting their health care needs.

15. E

Although renal perfusion and renal function show a decline with aging, there is a concomitant decrease in muscle mass that results in a slight decline or no change in serum creatinine. Plasma glucocorticoids do not change with normal aging. The Westergren sedimentation rate increases significantly with aging, and these values must be interpreted with adjustment for age. Cholesterol tends to show a slight increase with aging, as does plasma glucose. For a variety of reasons, activity levels tend to decrease with aging, which along with a gradual weight gain into the 50s and 60s may explain, in part, the age-related increase in serum glucose and the increased incidence of type 2 diabetes in the elderly. See Table 7.8.

16. B

Medicare Part A provides for inpatient hospital care. Coverage for physician services and durable medical equipment is through

Table 7.8 Laboratory values with aging

CBC	No change
Sedimentation rate	Increased
Serum creatinine	No change
Creatinine clearance	Decreased
Glucose	Increased
Albumin	Decreased
Cholesterol	Increased
Plasma glucocorticoids	Unchanged
TSH	Unchanged
T3	Decreased

Medicare Part B. Prescription medication coverage is available through Medicare Part D. Medicare Part A is funded by the Social Security tax and is automatically provided to all older persons who are eligible for Social Security. Medicare Parts B and D are not automatically provided to all individuals, and individuals must enroll and pay a premium in order to be covered under Medicare Parts B and D.

17. D

This scenario is not at all uncommon. Families often live in separate cities or states and during the course of a visit begin to notice that their elderly mother or father is beginning to struggle to care for herself or himself independently. Safety concerns frequently prompt decisions regarding hiring caregivers or seeking out assisted living or nursing home placement. In patients with Alzheimer's disease, special assisted living units have been developed that prevent wandering and provide environmental clues and activities geared toward maximizing independence and function. This particular individual has no acute skilled care needs. Assuming her activities of daily living are intact, she would be a candidate for a 24-hour caregiver or an assisted living environment if the family is unable to care for her. If the patient or family do not have the financial resources for these options, then nursing home placement may be the best option. In a nursing home, supervision and care can be provided, and once personal funds are exhausted, patients may apply for Medicaid to provide payment for continuing care.

18. C

There are many misconceptions regarding hospice care. Hospice is not a place but is a philosophy that focuses on comfort for the patient. Hospice may be provided in the home, in a hospice unit, in the hospital, or in a nursing home environment, thus following the patient wherever he or she may be. Hospice services are generally provided by special nurses trained in this philosophy of care. The hospice medical director or the patient's personal physician or both may supervise this nursing care and provide medical care. Hospice services are covered by Medicare Part A. Appropriate candidates for hospice are those patients who the physician certifies as terminal, having a life expectancy of 6 months or less to live.

19. D

The cardinal features of Parkinson's disease are resting tremor, rigidity, bradykinesia, and postural instability. Frequently, early in the course of the disease, the patient may not have all of these findings and a period of observation may be warranted before labeling the patient with this disease. The disease is very often asymmetric in its presentation. For example, a patient may present initially with a unilateral pill rolling resting tremor but not have rigidity or bradykinesia. Tremor may cause concern but may not significantly impair function, whereas bradykinesia, rigidity, and postural instability will eventually lead to functional limitations and initiation of drug therapy. Hemiplegia and stocking glove anesthesia are not found with Parkinson's disease. The tremor with Parkinson's disease is typically resting and pill rolling in nature. Action tremor most commonly represents essential tremor. Memory loss is not a feature that is diagnostic of Parkinson's disease. However, 30% or more of patients with Parkinson's disease will also develop a dementia.

20. A

There is some controversy and debate over optimal management of patients with asymptomatic carotid bruits. The presence of a carotid bruit generally suggests that there is at least a 50% narrowing of the involved artery. Thus, the presence of a carotid bruit does signify the presence of atherosclerotic vascular disease and increased risk for stroke and heart disease. However, the increased risk for stroke does not correlate with the occurrence of stroke on the side ipsilateral to the bruit. Current management recommendations for asymptomatic carotid bruits generally include management of risk factors (smoking, lipids, blood pressure, and diabetes), use of aspirin, and advising the patient to promptly report any neurologic symptoms. Stroke is preceded by transient ischemic attacks (TIAs) in 50% to 70% of patients. When TIAs are present in concert with carotid artery stenosis, then surgical management is recommended in patients with high-grade lesions (70% to 99%). Surgery may also benefit those with lesions of a moderate degree (50% to 69%). For those with lower grade lesions, surgery has not been of proven benefit. Factors to consider in recommending surgical therapy for a symptomatic patient include underlying medical condition, expected longevity (more than 5 years), the presence of concomitant cardiac disease, and the complication rate of the surgical team (ideal, less than 2.5%).

21. B

Most people with stroke survive, and stroke is the most common problem that leads to a patient needing rehabilitation therapy. Predictors of recovery have been identified, and age has not been a predictor of recovery from stroke. Predictors of poor recovery include absence of any motor return by 1 month, neglect, impaired cognition, bowel incontinence, coma at stroke onset, persistent urinary incontinence, fever, and diabetes mellitus. Motor recovery will be complete by 6 months post-stroke; however, it may take up to 2 years for maximal recovery of speech and swallowing functions.

22. A

Following a stroke and rehabilitation, 10% of survivors will have a full recovery, 40% will be left with mild deficits, 40% will have significant deficits, and 10% will require long-term institutional care. Other factors that are important in determining the need for long-term care include whether or not there is an underlying dementia as well as the social and financial supports available to the patient. Other predictors of poor recovery include the absence of any motor return by 1 month, neglect, impaired cognition, bowel incontinence, coma at stroke onset, persistent urinary incontinence, fever, and diabetes mellitus. Age alone has not been found to be a predictor of stroke recovery.

23. D

There are many changes that occur in body composition and organ function with advancing age. Many of these may also affect drug metabolism and distribution. With advancing age, there is a decrease in renal and hepatic blood flow along with a significant decline in renal function and a slight decrease in hepatic enzyme activity. This may result in a decrease in drug metabolism and clearance in the elderly for those medications metabolized through the liver and kidney. In addition, there is a decrease in muscle mass and increase in body fat that may result in accumulation of fat-soluble medications in the adipose tissue. This may result in prolonged medication effects. Finally, there is a decrease in percentage body water, which may result in higher levels, or overdosage, of water-soluble medications when "usual" doses are prescribed in the elderly. FEV1 declines slightly as individuals age and would be expected to have no impact on medication therapy. See Table 7.9.

Table 7.9 Potential age-related physiologic changes influencing pharmacotherapy in the elderly

Increases	Decreases
Gastric pH	Splanchnic blood flow
α_1-Acid glycoprotein concentrations	Surface area of the small intestine
Adipose tissue	Hepatic blood flow
	Total body water
	Hepatic metabolism (phase I)
	Renal tubular secretion
	Lean muscle mass
	Glomerular filtration rate

24. C

As patients age and are placed on an increasing number of medications, the risk of side effects and drug interactions increases. A patient's therapy for one condition may adversely impact another condition. Review of medications is an important element in assessing a change in the status of a patient's condition. Of the medications listed, inhaled ipratropium may impact urinary flow in patients with benign prostatic hypertrophy. Ipratropium has anticholinergic activity that may cause urinary retention. Glyburide, metformin, and fluticasone have no effects on the urinary system. Prazosin is an alpha-adrenergic blocker and is useful in relaxing the bladder sphincter and for treatment of benign prostatic hypertrophy.

25. D

When selecting therapy for an existing or newly diagnosed condition, review of the patient's medications and other underlying conditions is important in order to avoid drug interactions and/or undesirable side effects. In following current hypertension treatment guidelines, beta-blockers are recommended as one of the first-line choices for patients with hypertension. However, therapy should not be prescribed without examining the patient's other underlying medical conditions. In this case, beta-blocker therapy may aggravate his peripheral vascular disease by blocking the B-receptors and peripherally allowing alpha-adrenergic vasoconstriction to dominate. Lisinopril, amlodipine, doxazosin, and verapamil would be better alternatives in this patient since they would either have no effect or have a vasodilatory action on the peripheral vasculature.

26. A

Parkinsonism may be present with Parkinson's disease, related neurologic disorders, or medication-induced symptoms. When medication induced, withdrawal of the medication may result in resolution of the patient's symptoms. Medications may cause parkinsonism by blocking dopamine receptosrs or by depleting stores of dopamine in the central nervous system. Commonly used medications that block dopamine receptors include the antipsychotic drugs (e.g., haloperidol) as well as metoclopropamide. Ranitidine, fluoxetine, atorvastatin, and citalopram do not affect dopamine stores or receptors.

27. B

The most common organism causing community-acquired bacterial pneumonia is *Streptococcus pneumoniae*. This is true for both younger adults and the elderly. *Streptococcus pneumoniae* accounts for approximately 60% of community-acquired pneumonias. *Staphylococcus aureus* is a less common cause and may occur as a complication of a viral pneumonia or as a nosocomial infection. *Escherichia coli* is a rare cause for pneumonia but may occur with nosocomial infections. *Klebsiella* is associated with pneumonias developing in alcoholic patients, nursing homes, and with nosocomial infections. *Legionella* is one of the atypical pneumonias. The bacillus is found in contaminated soil and water and may be spread by the aerosol route. This infection occurs less frequently than infection with *S. pneumoniae*; however, the elderly may be more susceptible than younger adults to infection with *Legionella*.

28. D

The most likely cause for this patient's symptoms and x-ray findings is aspiration pneumonia. Patients with Parkinson's disease as well as dementia may exhibit difficulties in swallowing that place them at great risk for aspiration. The localized lung findings and right upper lobe lung infiltrate provide further support for this diagnosis. Because of his immobility, the patient would be at risk for deep vein thrombosis and pulmonary embolism. Pulmonary embolism may cause tachycardia, tachypnea, and oxygen desaturation but would not be expected to present with localized findings on lung exam and usually the chest x-ray is normal in appearance. Community-acquired pneumonia may present with similar findings, although the infiltrate in the right upper lobe, along with the patient's underlying medical condition and lung findings, is very suggestive of aspiration as the cause. Congestive heart failure may cause oxygen desaturation but would not account for the localized x-ray and lung exam findings. Acute myocardial infarction would not be expected to cause oxygen desaturation in the absence of pulmonary edema and congestive heart failure, and it would not account for the localized x-ray and lung exam findings.

29. B

Indications for oxygen therapy with chronic obstructive pulmonary disease include pO_2 less than 55 mmHg or pO_2 less than 59 mmHg and evidence of cor pulmonale. The pO_2 of 88 mmHg is not low and thus does not warrant oxygen therapy. Clubbing of the nails may occur independently due to causes other than COPD (e.g., biliary cirrhosis, inflammatory bowel disease, and lung cancer) and with COPD is not used in determining the need for oxygen therapy. The pCO_2 of 50 suggests that the patient is a CO_2 retainer and that the patient's respiratory drive is provided by the presence of hypoxemia. Although oxygen therapy may be indicated in such a patient, the pCO_2 is not the determining factor. Great care must be exercised in utilizing oxygen therapy in such patients since without some degree of hypoxemia, patients' respiration may be suppressed and they may develop CO_2 narcosis and respiratory failure. Dyspnea on exertion may have causes other than hypoxemia and should be assessed prior to considering oxygen therapy.

30. C

Calcified aortic valvular disease is the most common valvular lesion in the elderly. Thickening and calcification of the aortic valve, termed aortic sclerosis, is present in 25% of individuals older than age 65 and up to one-half of those older than age 75. By definition, aortic sclerosis is not associated with significant obstruction. However, it is believed to be an active disease process and not an inevitable consequence of aging. Aortic stenosis, on the other hand, is associated with left ventricular outflow obstruction and represents the more severe extreme of this same disease process. Hemodynamically significant aortic stenosis is present in up to 9% of the geriatric population and calcific aortic stenosis is the underlying cause for up to 90% of all aortic valve replacements. Mitral annular calcification is similar in nature to aortic sclerosis and occurs in 20% to 30% of individuals by age 80. One-half of those with calcification have associated mitral regurgitation, which is managed medically and rarely requires surgery. Rheumatic heart disease is the most common cause for mitral stenosis and generally presents by middle age, rarely in the elderly. Aortic regurgitation occurs in up to 25% of the elderly in association with aortic sclerosis or from aortic root dilation resulting from hypertension or atherosclerosis. Aortic regurgitation is managed medically, rarely requiring surgery in the elderly population.

31. D

The risk of stroke for patients with chronic atrial fibrillation is five times higher than that in patients of similar age who are in sinus rhythm. The incidence of stroke with chronic atrial fibrillation has been reported to be as high as 10% per year. Studies in these patients using coumadin to lessen the risk have shown a decrease in risk for stroke of up to 68%. In patients who have experienced symptoms of TIA or stroke, the risk for recurrent stroke is 19% per year. Coumadin lessens this risk for recurrent stroke to 4%. Because of the potential risk for bleeding complications, some clinicians have advocated for use of aspirin or clopidogrel as a safer alternative for stroke prevention, particularly in patients older than age 75. Although treatment with coumadin is associated with a slight increased risk for bleeding complications, this risk is more than offset by the benefits of stroke risk reduction, and thus coumadin is generally recommended, especially for symptomatic patients.

32. E

Sick sinus syndrome, also known as bradycardia–tachycardia syndrome, is especially common among the geriatric population. This syndrome is thought to be caused by diffuse degenerative or inflammatory changes in the conduction system of the heart involving the SA node, AV node, as well as the bundle of His. The resulting manifestations may be bradyarrhythmias, sinus arrest, conduction disturbances, or alternating paroxysms of bradycardia and atrial tachycardia. Symptoms that may occur include palpitations, angina, congestive heart failure, dizziness, or, as occurred in this patient, syncope. Patients with bradycardia only who are not symptomatic may not warrant therapy unless the heart rate falls below 40. In symptomatic bradycardic patients, pacemaker therapy is warranted. For those with both bradycardia and tachycardia, a pacemaker along with medication to control the tachycardia is recommended. Fludrocortisone is a useful medication in treating syncope related to orthostatic hypotension, but it would have no role in treating the patient presented, whose syncope is arrhythmia related. See Table 7.10.

33. B

This patient exhibits symptoms consistent with claudication of the right lower extremity, supported by the physical sign of diminished pulses. Peripheral vascular disease is a common clinical entity encountered by family physicians. Risk factors for developing peripheral vascular disease are similar to those for developing coronary artery disease, namely hypertension, smoking, diabetes mellitus, and hyperlipidemia. Therapy for peripheral vascular disease involves risk factor modification, such as smoking cessation; treatment of hyperlipidemia, diabetes, and hypertension; and exercise. Exercise is a cornerstone of therapy and leads to symptom

Table 7.10 Indications for pacemaker therapy

Third-degree heart block
Symptomatic second-degree heart block

Bifascicular or trifascicular block and
    Intermittent third-degree heart block or
    Type II second-degree heart block or
    Alternating bundle branch block

Patients after myocardial infarction with:
    Persistent second-degree heart block and bilateral bundle branch block
    Third-degree heart block
    Persistent symptomatic second or third-degree heart block

Symptomatic sinus node dysfunction
Pause-dependent ventricular tachycardia with or without QT prolongation
Recurrent syncope associated with carotid sensitivity
Carotid sensitivity resulting in ≥3-second pauses

From the American College of Cardiology (www.acc.org).

resolution and improved exercise tolerance. Exercise is thought to improve muscle metabolism, red blood cell movement, and alter pain thresholds. Prognosis for patients with peripheral vascular disease presenting with claudication is very good with regard to the limb. Only 3% of patients with peripheral vascular disease presenting with claudication lose their limb in the subsequent 5 years, and none of those who quit smoking lost their limbs. Increased mortality with peripheral vascular disease is associated with concurrent cardiac, cerebrovascular, and aortic disease. Vasodilators, calcium channel blockers, and beta-blockers do not lead to symptom improvement and may actually worsen symptoms because vasoconstriction plays little or no role. Vasoconstrictors, on the other hand, may worsen or aggravate symptoms. See Table 7.11.

34. B

Multifocal atrial tachycardia is an atrial tachycardia that is irregular, has a rate between 100 and 200 beats per minute, and arises from different foci within the atria. P waves are identifiable before each QRS and have differing morphology and PR intervals. This arrhythmia arises due to underlying medical disease, commonly COPD, or medication toxicity (e.g., theophylline or digitalis). Therapy for multifocal atrial tachycardia is directed toward the underlying disease. In those who are hemodynamically unstable and require rate control, calcium channel blockers, such as diltiazem or verapamil, may be used. Beta-blockers can potentially aggravate this patient's COPD, which is the underlying cause for his multifocal atrial tachycardia. There is no role for pacemaker or amiodarone therapy in patients with pure multifocal tachycardia (i.e., no bradycardia or bradycardia–tachycardia syndrome). See Table 7.12.

35. A

Abdominal aortic aneurysms are reported to cause approximately 9,000 deaths per year in the United States. Ninety-five percent of

Table 7.11 Therapy for peripheral vascular disease

Exercise
Smoking cessation
Control blood pressure
Optimize lipid status
Optimize diabetes therapy
Avoid trauma to feet including well-fitting shoes

Medications
  Platelet inhibitor: aspirin, clopidogrel, ticlopidine
  Viscosity lowering agents: pentoxyphylline or cilastazol

Surgery
  Large vessel occlusive disease: bypass grafting or angioplasty
  Small vessel disease: amputation for limb or life-threatening disease

Table 7.12 Common causes for multifocal atrial tachycardia

Chronic obstructive pulmonary disease
Congestive heart failure
Renal failure
Medications (e.g., digoxin)
Electrolyte disturbances (including hypomagnesemia)
Hypoxia

these deaths occur in the elderly population. Early detection can lead to closer monitoring and elective repair of the aneurysm. Of those with undiagnosed aneurysms that rupture, only 18% reached a hospital and survived surgery. There are no recommendations for routine screening in asymptomatic adults without risk factors. However, abdominal ultrasound has a nearly 100% sensitivity in diagnosing aneurysms in those with pulsatile masses on abdominal examination. Prognosis and management of abdominal aortic aneurysms depend on the size of the aneurysm. As aneurysms enlarge, the risk of rupture increases, such that for those with aneurysms greater than 5 cm the risk of rupture is 40% over the subsequent 5 years. Most vascular surgeons advise surgical repair of aneurysms 5 cm or greater since the risks of surgery are considerably less than that of rupture. These patients have a high incidence of coronary artery disease and thus are at high cardiac risk for surgery. Risk factors for abdominal aortic aneurysm include increasing age, male gender, family history of aneurysms, tobacco use, hypertension, and peripheral vascular disease. See Table 7.13.

Table 7.13 Recommendations for surveillance and screening for abdominal aortic aneurysm

Screening
  Males 60 years or older with sibling or parents with AAA
  Males 65–75 years of age who have ever smoked

Surveillance
  2.5–3.0 cm diameter ecstatic aorta: recheck every 5 years
  3.0–4.0 cm diameter: recheck annually
  4.0–4.9 cm diameter: recheck every 6 months

36. E

Initial workup of a patient with dementia is performed with the goal of finding a reversible cause. In general, only about 5% of patients will have a reversible cause. Normal pressure hydrocephalus is a rare but potentially reversible form of dementia with the triad of symptoms of dementia, incontinence, and ataxic gait. Findings on computed tomography scanning of the brain that are consistent with a diagnosis of normal pressure hydrocephalus are ventricular enlargement disproportionate to atrophy and enlargement of the sulci in other areas of the brain. Reversibility of the symptoms of this disease depends on the duration of symptoms and may be predicted by symptom improvement upon removal of cerebrospinal fluid through lumbar puncture. Definitive treatment would involve placement of a ventricular shunt. Cogwheel rigidity, tremor, and bradykinesia are findings consistent with Parkinson's or related diseases. Perseveration is a feature of dementia but is not specific to the type of dementia. See Table 7.14.

Table 7.14 Causes for dementia

Potentially Reversible	Irreversible
Alcohol	Alzheimer's
Depression	Lewy body disease
Medications	Frontotemporal
Autoimmune disease	Vascular (multi-infarct)
Vitamin B12 deficiency	Huntington's disease
Hypothyroidism	Parkinson's-related dementia
Tertiary (CNS) syphilis	Postanoxic
Trauma	Trauma
Encephalopathy	Encephalopathy (including AIDS-related)
CNS tumor	Progressive supranuclear palsy
Normal pressure hydrocephalus	Creutzfeldt–Jakob disease

37. B

This patient's presentation is very characteristic of lumbar spinal stenosis. This disease is common in the elderly population and occurs as a result of foraminal and lateral recess stenosis in the lumbar spine. The underlying cause in the elderly is usually degenerative osteoarthritis and less commonly spondylolisthesis. The disease occurs less commonly in younger patients and in these instances may be due to congenitally acquired disorders such as achondroplasia or spondylolisthesis. The classic presentation is that of a patient with a chronic history of back pain who notes pain in the back, buttocks, and upper thighs, usually bilaterally, in association with the upright position. The pain is relieved by sitting or lying down. If the patient maintains the upright position or continues to walk, he or she may note sensory and then motor symptoms in the lower extremities. The pain and symptoms may be relieved if the patient leans forward, termed a positive "stoop test." The pain may also be relieved in the sitting position by leaning forward. The physical examination, including neurologic exam and straight leg raise, is often normal. The symptoms of lumbar spinal stenosis may be confused with vascular insufficiency and hence have been labeled "pseudoclaudication." Important distinguishing features are the absence of diminished pulses, symptoms occurring independently of walking or exercising but in association with the upright position, and relief of symptoms by stooping over. Vascular claudication is usually precipitated by walking some distance and relieved by stopping and standing. Peripheral neuropathy symptoms occur independent of activity and frequently are worse at night. In addition, patients will often have an abnormal lower extremity sensory examination as well as an underlying disease, such as diabetes, that may lead to developing a neuropathy. Polymyalgia rheumatica causes a proximal muscle pain and stiffness, most commonly of the shoulders. Symptoms may also occur in the thighs. The symptoms may be worse in the morning and occur independent of position. An elevated sedimentation rate and prompt response to a trial of steroids help confirm the diagnosis. Guillain-Barre syndrome is an acute demyelinating polyneuropathy resulting in muscle weakness, classically in an ascending fashion.

38. D

The rash and symptoms this patient is experiencing are consistent with herpes zoster, also known as shingles. Shingles is a reactivation of the chickenpox virus from its dormant site in a nerve root ganglion. Reactivation may occur at any time and may be triggered by illness or immunosuppression and is more common with advancing age. Patients commonly experience a prodrome of tingling, itching, or pain prior to eruption of a papular rash that subsequently forms vesicles. The vesicles become pustular and then scab and resolve. The rash is unilateral along a single dermatome, occasionally with slight overlap with neighboring dermatomes. The virus may be spread to others by direct contact, in contrast to primary chickenpox infection, which has airborne transmission. Therapy for shingles is slightly controversial. People older than age 50 with severe pain or with trigeminal nerve or ophthalmic involvement should be provided with oral antiviral therapy. Patients with suspected or potential ophthalmic involvement should be referred to an ophthalmologist. Antiviral therapy will hasten resolution of the rash and may lessen the likelihood of developing postherpetic neuralgia if patents present within 48 to 72 hours of onset. Oral steroids may also be of benefit in prevention of postherpetic neuralgia, although this is also controversial. There is no role for use of topical acyclovir or topical steroids in patients with shingles.

39. E

Temporal arteritis occurs most commonly in the geriatric population, with an average age of onset of 70 years. Patients commonly present with headache and vague systemic symptoms, such as fatigue, myalgias, anorexia, and possibly even weight loss. The disease typically has a gradual onset and the time from development of symptoms to diagnosis is, on average, 7 months. Scalp tenderness, jaw claudication, and visual complaints are classic symptoms of temporal arteritis. Hearing loss is not one of the frequently reported symptoms. The erythrocyte sedimentation rate is a useful screening test and is usually significantly elevated, with values often more than 100 mm/hour. C-reactive protein is also often elevated and may be useful as a screening test with this disease. Definitive diagnosis requires biopsy of any artery with suspected involvement. Common sites for biopsy are the temporal, occipital, or facial arteries. Arteriography frequently does not delineate arterial changes well and can not be relied on for the diagnosis. In patients with suspected temporal arteritis, corticosteroids are the treatment of choice and should be started promptly without awaiting biopsy results in order to prevent potential visual complications. Biopsy can be obtained after starting corticosteroids and may be positive for up to 2 weeks or more after commencing therapy with corticosteroids. After initiation of steroid therapy, therapy with steroids is titrated and monitored through use of the erythrocyte sedimentation rate and C-reactive protein. Therapy is tapered as these measures normalize. Therapy may be required for 2 years or more.

40. D

The most common form of tremor is the essential tremor, which is a postural tremor occurring in 2% to 5% of the population. It is a tremor that involves alternating flexion and extension and may affect the extremities, head, neck, and voice. There is a bimodal peak of occurrence, with individuals affected during adolescence as well as approximately age 50 years. There is a form of this tremor with autosomal dominant inheritance leading to use of the term familial tremor interchangeably with essential tremor. The other diseases listed occur less commonly but may also cause different forms of tremors or movements. Parkinson's disease involves supination and pronation and is a resting tremor. Cerebellar tremors, also referred to as intention tremors, are brought out by a goal-directed limb movement in which the shaking occurs most notably as the patient reaches the end point of his or her goal. Patients with Wilson's disease may exhibit coarse postural tremors that have been described as "wing beating" in nature. Huntington's disease is associated with nearly constant chroreiform or writhing movements.

41. D

Rheumatoid arthritis is an inflammatory form of arthritis that leads to soft tissue edema, synovitis, and destruction of bone and cartilage. X-ray findings may show soft tissue edema along with the joint space narrowing and bone erosions indicating cartilage and bone destruction from the inflammatory process. Juxta-articular osteopenia is also characteristic of the inflammatory arthropathies. Other findings consistent with rheumatoid arthritis include subluxation of the MCP and interphalangeal joints and rheumatoid nodules. Osteophytes are found on x-rays in patients with osteoarthritis and represent bone overgrowth from the mechanical stresses on the bone associated with osteoarthritis. Joint space narrowing and sclerosis of the juxta-articular bone also occur with osteoarthritis. Loose bodies represent displaced bone or cartilage that are within the joint space. They may become symptomatic and are not specific to any of the arthritides. Chondrocalcinosis represents calcification of the cartilage and most patients with this finding are asymptomatic or may have mild arthritic symptoms.

42. B

Methotrexate is the preferred and first-line disease-modifying therapy for patients with active rheumatoid arthritis. Methotrexate therapy should be started early in the disease process since much of the joint damage occurs within the first 2 years of the disease. Methotrexate has been safe, effective, and relatively inexpensive. Contraindications for its use include pregnancy, liver disease, underlying immunodeficiency, and blood dyscrasias. The other therapies listed would be considered adjunctive therapies. Acetaminophen, nonsteroidal anti-inflammatories, and corticosteroids can be used early on for pain control. Corticosteroids should not be used as long-term therapy due to their potential toxicity. The goal for the disease-modifying therapy is to eliminate the need for significant use of these therapies. Cyclosporine is one of the second-line therapies used as a disease-modifying agent, but it would not typically be used as a first-line medication.

43. A

Acetaminophen has been recommended as a first-line choice for treatment of osteoarthritis. In regularly scheduled doses, it is efficacious, safe, and inexpensive. Doses up to 4 g daily may be used. The primary toxicity to monitor is liver toxicity, which is associated with concomitant alcohol use as well as excessive dosing. Methotrexate is used primarily for psoriatic arthritis and rheumatoid arthritis, but not for osteoarthritis. Nonsteroidal anti-inflammatory medications are commonly used for osteoarthritis but are not recommended as first-line agents due to the associated gastrointestinal side effects and their generally greater cost. Corticosteroids should not be used as long-term therapy for osteoarthritis due to their potential toxicity, and cyclosporine currently has no role in treatment of osteoarthritis.

44. D

Polymyalgia rheumatica is a common nonarticular rheumatologic disease that more commonly affects individuals older than age 50 and females at a 2:1 ratio. The disease presents with bilateral pain and stiffness, especially in the morning, of the neck, shoulders, and, in some cases, the hips and thighs. Patients may also have nonspecific systemic symptoms, such as low-grade fever, weight loss, and fatigue. The affected areas are often tender, but muscle weakness does not occur. X-rays will not be helpful in diagnosing polymyalgia rheumatica since this is a nonarticular disease. Helpful in the diagnosis is the characteristic finding of an elevated erythrocyte sedimentation rate, which is often found to be more than 40 mm/hour.

45. B

With automated blood testing, the finding of asymptomatic hyperuricemia has become more common. This has sparked some debate over management of results. However, many experts do agree that the therapies do have potential toxicity (up to 10% of patients taking probenecid and 25% taking allopurinol will have adverse drug reactions). In addition, the elevated uric acid alone may have no potential consequences. Thus, recommendations are to treat those individuals with recurrent episodes of gout or with evidence of uric acid renal stones. There are no data to suggest that therapy is warranted to prevent renal disease, kidney stones, or correct asymptomatic hyperuricemia.

46. B

Detrusor overactivity is the most common cause of urinary incontinence in the elderly and causes what is termed urge incontinence. This occurs because bladder contractions are not inhibited and the patient will experience a sudden strong urge to void accompanied by urine loss, usually of large volume. Underlying causes should be investigated since urinary tract infections, carcinoma, and stones may all contribute to this detrusor overactivity. Stress incontinence is also common in older women and is due to incompetence of the bladder outlet leading to leakage of small amounts of urine with increases in intra-abdominal pressure. Neurogenic overflow incontinence occurs when bladder contraction does not occur and the bladder fills until it eventually overflows with continuous leakage of small amounts of urine. Immobility alone is not thought to be a cause of incontinence but may compromise the individual's ability to compensate for a pre-existing condition. For example, someone may have urge incontinence but can no longer get to the bathroom

Table 7.15 Incontinence characteristics and treatment

Type	Characteristics	Treatment	Other Considerations
Urge	Large volume, urgent frequent voiding	Oxybutynin, Tolterodine, imipramine	UTI, BPH, fecal impaction
Stress	Small volumes, induced by increased abdominal pressure	Alpha-agonists, Kegal exercises, surgery	Inflammation (e.g., UTI), use of alpha-blockers
Overflow	Small volume, continuous dribbling, frequent, urgent urination	Alpha-blockers, treat underlying causes, catheter	Anticholinergics, alpha-agonists, opioids, urethral stricture, uterine prolapse, prostate cancer or BPH, neuropathy or spinal lesion
Functional	Large volumes, inability to respond to normal urge to void	Treat underlying cause	Anticholinergics, sedative medications, diuretics, osteoarthritis

in time due to worsening osteoarthritis. Vesicovaginal fistulae can cause continual leakage of urine from the vaginal opening. These fistulae can occur in younger women as a complication from childbirth and in older women as a result of cancer, surgery, or radiation therapy. See Table 7.15.

47. D

The patient presented with symptoms consistent with benign prostatic hypertrophy and incomplete bladder emptying. In treating this patient, medication should be provided to attempt to lessen the bladder outlet obstruction that is present. Oxybutynin is a smooth muscle relaxant that is commonly used to treat urge incontinence and may worsen this patient's condition. Likewise, the anticholinergic activity of amitriptyline would cause bladder relaxation and may worsen his urinary retention. Urecholine is used for individuals with detrusor underactivity in an attempt to enhance bladder contractions and emptying. Urecholine would not be useful in this scenario, in which the patient has an outlet obstruction. A normal urinalysis and nontender prostate examination suggest that empiric therapy with ciprofloxacin would not be beneficial. Tamulosin is an alpha-adrenergic blocker that may help in relaxing the bladder outlet to allow more complete bladder emptying. Tamulosin was developed as a selective agent to minimize the effects on blood pressure associated with other agents that also have been used to treat benign prostatic hypertrophy, such as prazosin, terazosin, and doxazosin.

48. C

Although appendicitis is most common in children and young adults, it is still common in the geriatric population, occurring in up to 14% of cases of acute abdomen. Classic signs and symptoms of appendicitis include right lower quadrant abdominal pain, rigidity, and periumbilical abdominal pain that migrates to the right lower quadrant. Patients frequently present either with no fever or with low-grade elevation of temperature. If perforation has occurred, then fever is more common, occurring in up to 40% of patients. Evaluation of patients with abdominal pain and suspected appendicitis frequently includes white blood cell count and urinalysis. Abdominal CT scan is a valuable tool for assessing abdominal pain in patients of all ages. The geriatric population has a higher incidence of appendiceal rupture and higher mortality from appendicitis than patients in other age groups. Anatomically, there is less blood flow to the appendix in elderly patients, and the lumen and walls of the appendix are thinner, making them more prone to rupture. In addition, geriatric patients tend to present later in the disease process and may have atypical findings at presentation. For example, geriatric patients are more likely to present with a diffuse abdominal pain and often have a normal white blood cell count. Thus, several factors make the diagnosis and management of appendicitis in geriatric patients more challenging.

49. D

Congestive heart failure is prevalent among the geriatric population. Congestive heart failure may be due to either systolic or diastolic dysfunction. Systolic dysfunction is present in 50% to 60% of cases and is associated with an ejection fraction of 40% or less. Diastolic dysfunction as a cause for congestive heart failure occurs in 40% to 50% of cases and is suggested when the ejection fraction is normal or high-normal. Underlying etiologies for congestive heart failure also need to be considered in the evaluation of the patient and include hypertension, ischemic heart disease, and valvular heart disease. In the patient described, the findings of LVH and an ejection fraction of 65% along with congestive heart failure are consistent with diastolic dysfunction. In this patient, hypertensive heart disease is the likely underlying etiology, although consideration and evaluation for coronary artery disease may also be warranted.

50. D

Therapy for congestive heart failure is tailored initially toward reestablishing fluid balance through use of diuretics. Subsequently, therapy is aimed at maintaining fluid balance and interrupting the underlying mechanisms contributing to the heart failure. ACE inhibitor therapy is a mainstay of therapy and interrupts the renin–angiotensin–aldosterone response to limited systemic perfusion that promotes fluid retention. In addition, ACE inhibitors may reduce preload and afterload, thus promoting more optimal cardiac contractility. Beta-blockers are also of benefit and improve survival, particularly in those with underlying ischemia. Spironolactone also has been shown to provide benefit, possibly by limiting the effects of aldosterone on fluid and sodium retention. Digoxin is a second line of therapy that may be used to augment cardiac contractility and has been shown to help lower hospitalization rates. Antiarrhythmic medications, such as amiodarone, are not part of routine therapy but are useful for patients with underlying arrhythmias. Amlodipene, verapamil, and clonidine are antihypertensive agents that have not been shown to provide direct benefit to treatment of congestive heart failure.

51. C

Interventions targeted toward improving management of a patient's heart failure have focused on attempting to identify worsening of the patient's condition before the onset of symptoms and the need for hospitalization. Success in achieving these goals has been through use of multidisciplinary teams that involve physicians, nurses, and the patient. Monitoring of daily weight is one of the cornerstones of this approach and allows adjusting the patient's medications at the first signs of worsening CHF, before clinical symptoms may develop. Monthly chest x-rays and routine echocardiography are not part of this approach and there are no data to support their routine use. Coumadin has a role in preventing stroke complications in those with prosthetic heart valves or atrial fibrillation, but it is not a routine part of CHF management. Care in a long-term residential facility could in theory provide some of the benefits of a multidisciplinary team approach; however, this would not be suitable for many patients and would incur costs associated with long-term care.

52. A

Atrophic vaginitis may present with vaginal itching, burning, pain, dryness, or dysparunia. In the absence of estrogen, the vaginal mucosa thins, has diminished blood supply and vaginal secretions, and there can be loss of connective tissues that provide pelvic support. Treatment of the postmenopausal woman for atrophic vaginitis includes replacing estrogen, either orally or topically with vaginal creams. Vaginal creams may help in alleviating local symptoms but do not provide enough systemic absorption to be relied on for the beneficial effects of estrogens on osteoporosis. Oral estrogens must be used in concert with progesterone in order to avoid the risks of endometrial hyperplasia and cancer in women with an intact uterus. Before providing oral estrogen therapy, careful consideration of the risks and benefits should be discussed with the patient. Potential risks include cardiovascular and venous thromboembolic disease as well as slight increased risk for both endometrial and breast cancer. Topical corticosteroids, metronidazole gel, clotrimazole cream, and douching provide no benefit in treating atrophic vaginitis.

53. D

In the United States, up to one-half of all geriatric patients have either osteopenia or osteoporosis. By the age of 80, a woman's risk for sustaining an osteoporotic fracture approaches 40%. There is substantial morbidity and mortality that occur in conjunction with osteoporotic fractures, particularly hip fractures. Identifying and treating these individuals can lower these risks. Risk factors for osteoporosis have been identified. Family history of osteoporosis, thin body build, history of fractures, cigarette smoking, alcohol abuse, white or Asian race, physical inactivity, chronic corticosteroid therapy, and early menopause are the major risk factors. Obesity and performance of weight-bearing exercise are protective factors. Chronic obstructive pulmonary disease and beta agonist inhaler therapy have no effect on risk unless they cause the patient to be inactive or to require other medications that increase risk.

54. C

Therapies that are available for treatment of osteoporosis include estrogen replacement, selective estrogen receptor modulators (SERMs), bisphosphonates, and calcitonin. Calcium supplementation is an important part of therapy. Calcium should be used in doses of 1 to 1.5 g along with vitamin D supplementation. Estrogen replacement, SERMs, and the bisphosphonates can result in increased bone density in both the spine and the hips, and all have been shown to reduce the incidence of fractures. Calcitonin has effects on bone density in the spine but has not been shown to lower risk for hip fracture. Risedronate and alendronate are bisphosphonates that may be used for therapy in patients with osteopenia or osteoporosis. Risendronate at 5 mg per day or 35 mg once weekly is appropriate treatment for either osteoporosis or osteopenia. Alendronate is also available in a once weekly formulation, 35 mg weekly for osteopenia and 70 mg weekly for osteoporosis. A newer agent, ibandronate, may be administered at a dose of 150 mg once per month for either prevention or treatment of osteoporosis. Medroxyprogesterone will have no beneficial effects in treating women with osteoporosis but is used in conjunction with estrogen therapy to lessen the risk of endometrial cancer associated with unopposed estrogen therapy. Tamoxifen does appear to have beneficial effects on bone but at this time is not indicated for treatment or prevention of osteoporosis.

55. B

With the advent of chemistry panels for laboratory testing in adults, the finding of elevated serum calcium has increased nearly fourfold. Many of these patients may be asymptomatic or have nonspecific complaints, such as fatigue or musculoskeletal aches and pains.

Hyperparathyroidism is the most common cause for the finding of hypercalcemia in these patients. Malignancy is the second most frequent cause for hypercalcemia, with breast, lung, and renal cancers being most common. Other potential causes include familial hypocalciuric hypercalcemia, sarcoidosis, hyperthyroidism, immobilization, Addison's disease, and medication use (lithium, theophylline, and thiazide diuretics). Diabetes and hypothyroidism are not associated with hypercalcemia. Excess dietary calcium intake would be extraordinarily rare; however, excess calcium supplementation (3 or more grams) in conjunction with excess vitamin D intake (50,000 IU) can result in elevated calcium levels and has been reported to occur with the increasing health consciousness of the public and the desire to prevent osteoporosis.

56. A

Adding an ACE inhibitor would be the recommended treatment for this patient. Although his diabetes is well controlled, he is still at risk for developing diabetic nephropathy. His urine should be screened for microalbuminuria at least annually. ACE inhibitors are recommended to limit the progression of renal disease in those with evidence of compromised renal function or microalbuminuria, even if the patient is normotensive. Data suggest that ACE inhibitors may be useful in preventing the development of microalbuminuria. In addition, his blood pressure is in the high-normal range and the target blood pressure for diabetic patients is to achieve a normal blood pressure of 120/80 or less. Because of the renal protective effects, ACE inhibitors are the first line of therapy recommended for diabetic patients.

57. C

This patient's diabetes is well controlled, as is his blood pressure. Since he is having no problems tolerating his medications, they should be maintained to continue this success. Evaluation of his lipids does reveal an LDL of 128 and current lipid guidelines consider diabetes to be a heart disease equivalent. Thus, in this patient, the target LDL value would be less than 70. His HDL value is acceptable, as are his triglycerides. The most reasonable first choice would be to add a statin. After initiation of statin therapy, repeat lipid evaluation and monitoring of liver enzymes should occur in 6 weeks. Once the target LDL value is achieved, then re-evaluation every 3 to 6 months should occur. See Table 7.16.

58. A

Methicillin-resistant *Staphylococcus aureus* (MRSA) has been recognized since the late 1960s. Its significance is not in the virulence of the organism but in the fact that intravenous antibiotics are

Table 7.16 Recommendations for lipid therapy

Risk Level	Target LDL level	Lifestyle Modifications	Medication
High (CHD or equivalent)	<70 mg/dL	>70 mg/dL	>100 mg/dL and consider for >70 mg/dL
Moderate high risk (multiple risk factors)	<100 mg/dL	>100 mg/dL	>130 mg/dL
Moderate risk	<130 mg/dL	>130 mg/dL	>160 mg/dL
Low risk	<160 mg/dL	>160 mg/dL	>190 mg/dL

often required for therapy. MRSA exhibits the same level of virulence as methicillin-sensitive *Staphylococcus aureus*. The antibiotic resistance and the need for more complicated and expensive antibiotic therapy have led to efforts to limit the spread of MRSA from one patient to another. Risk factors for infection or colonization with MRSA have been identified and include prior hospitalization, impaired functional status, recent broad-spectrum antibiotic use, exposure to an active MRSA infection, chronic diseases leading to wounds or skin breakdown, and need for medical devices such as urinary catheters, IVs, or feeding tubes. Advanced age alone is not a risk factor. Patients with active infections should be isolated, but those who are colonized need not be isolated. Routine patient care measures, such as good hand washing, good housekeeping measures, and use of gloves with exposure to open wounds or body fluids, can limit the spread of this organism.

59. D

Influenza outbreaks occur every winter and the overall impact of these outbreaks will vary from year to year. Patients who are at risk for increased morbidity and mortality associated with influenza infections include those with heart disease, lung disease, diabetes, immunocompromising diseases, and the elderly. Annual influenza vaccines for these high-risk groups provide one effective means of limiting the impact of influenza infections. The vaccine must be given at least 2 weeks before exposure in order to be effective. In those who have contracted the disease, vaccination will not be of benefit. In the case of active infection, therapy may be provided with amantidine, rimantidine, oseltamivir, or zanamivir. Chest x-rays are not a routine test in patients with suspected influenza but should be ordered as indicated by the signs and symptoms exhibited by the patient. Antibiotics are not indicated except to treat bacterial complications such as pneumonia. Patients with significant respiratory symptoms, dehydration, or other complications may require hospitalization. Routine hospitalization to monitor patients with influenza is not warranted.

60. A

Renal artery stenosis is a common cause for progressive renal insufficiency in elderly hypertensive patients. It is often bilateral and may be present even with good blood pressure control. In the geriatric population, the underlying etiology for renal artery stenosis is usually atherosclerosis and thus concomitant disease such as peripheral vascular and coronary artery disease are often also present. Well-controlled hypertension of short duration, as in this patient, would not be expected to result in progressive renal insufficiency. Poorly controlled hypertension of long duration can result in impaired renal function. Metoprolol and simvastatin do not have adverse renal effects. Advancing age results in gradual decline in creatinine clearance, but due to an associated decline in muscle mass, the serum creatinine either remains unchanged or decreases.

61. B

Heart failure is a common disease of the elderly. Over 75% of patients are older than age 65 years. The incidence and prevalence of heart failure are increasing due to improved survival rates with cardiovascular disease. Hypertension is the leading cause of heart failure in women, whereas coronary artery disease is the most common cause for men. Many of the elderly have heart failure associated with normal or near normal systolic function. This type of heart failure is termed diastolic dysfunction. Diastolic dysfunction occurs more commonly in the elderly and accounts for over 50% of cases of heart failure in those older than age 75 years, compared to

Table 7.17 Causes of congestive heart failure

Diastolic dysfunction
  Cardiac ischemia
  Hypertension
  Infiltrative disease (e.g., amyloidosis, sarcoidosis)
  Valvular heart disease
  Constrictive pericarditis

Systolic dysfunction
  Myocardial infarction
  Cardiac ischemia
  Dilated cardiomyopathy
  Toxins
  Valvular heart disease
  Infection

Extracardiac
  Anemia
  AV fistula
  Renal failure
  Hyperthyroidism

less than 10% of those younger than age 65 years. Other factors that may contribute to onset of heart failure in the elderly include age-related changes in the cardiovascular system that limit cardiac reserve, lead to heart disease, and alter neurohormonal responses to various cardiac stressors. See Table 7.17.

62. A

Dental disease is common among elderly patients. Lack of dental coverage and resources for preventive care is a major contributing factor. Medicare coverage does not include dental care. Rather than undergo costly restorative care, many elderly patients opt for tooth removal. The most common causes for tooth loss include lack of resources to pay for repairs, periodontal disease, and previous loss of other teeth that hinders prosthetic restoration. Thus, approximately 50% of Americans older than age 85 years are edentulous. Dentures are not covered by Medicare. Patients without resources may forego denture use and those who have dentures may not get new dentures when they are needed. Dentures restore only about 15% of chewing function and thus the diet must be modified. This may ultimately result in nutritional compromise.

63. E

Unintentional weight loss occurs commonly in the geriatric population. In the nursing home population, it is associated with increased morbidity and mortality. Causes for unintentional weight loss are similar among patients in the community and those in long-term care facilities; however, the frequencies of the various causes differ. In the general elderly population, depression, cancer, and gastrointestinal disease are the most common causes. Psychiatric disease is present in approximately 17% of these patients. Twenty-five percent have no identified cause. In nursing home patients, psychiatric disease is the underlying cause 58% of the time. Neurologic disease (15%), medication effects (14%), cancer (7%), and gastrointestinal (3%) are other common causes. Only 3% of nursing home residents are considered to have no identifiable cause. See Table 7.18.

Table 7.18 Causes of weight loss in geriatric patients

Psychiatric disease
Neurologic disorders
Medications
Malignancy
Gastrointestinal disease
Infection
Hyperthyroidism
Diabetes mellitus

64. D

Alcohol abuse is common in the geriatric population, with a lifetime prevalence of 14% in men and 1.5% in women. Alcohol abuse is a significant risk factor for excess medical morbidity and hospitalization. In addition, individuals who abuse alcohol are at significant risk for depression and suicide. Potential problem alcohol use in the elderly is defined as more than one drink per day. The reason for this is that the elderly achieve higher alcohol levels than younger individuals who consume the same amount of alcohol. Thus, elderly patients may suffer from complications at lower levels of consumption. Treatment of elderly alcoholic patients must consider their overall medical condition. Due to concomitant medical and psychiatric diseases, elderly patients are more likely to require inpatient alcohol detoxification.

65. D

Antidepressant therapy is warranted in elderly patients with moderate to severe depression, persistent symptoms, or in those in whom depression interferes with day-to-day life. When choosing therapy, antidepressants should be selected with several factors in mind. Medication selection should be individualized with consideration of comorbid condition, side effect profile of the medication, and prior response to medication. A prior positive response to a particular medication is predictive of future responses. Medication should be started at low dosages and titrated upward every 6 to 8 weeks depending on the response. For first episodes of depression, therapy may be continued for 6 to 12 months. For those with three or more episodes, severe or life-threatening disease, or persistent symptoms of depression between episodes of worsening, lifetime therapy may be warranted. For patients refractory to typical medication therapy, cautious use of lithium is an option. Additionally, methylphenidate is commonly used for short-term therapy in medically ill anergic patients. For those who do not respond to medical therapy, electroconvulsive therapy may be beneficial.

66. B

Alzheimer's disease is the most common form of dementia affecting the geriatric population. The prevalence of dementia increases with age, doubling every 5 years after the age of 60 years. It is estimated that up to 30% of individuals older than age 85 years have Alzheimer's disease. In addition to supportive care, medication therapy has been developed to slow the progression of Alzheimer's disease. A cholinergic deficit is thought to be part of the pathology of Alzheimer's disease, and cholinesterase inhibitors, such as donepezil, rivastigmine, and galantamine, may be used as therapy. Another

agent that may slow the progression of Alzheimer's disease is memantine, an N-methyl-D-aspartase (NMDA) receptor antagonist. Its mechanism of action is thought to result from limiting calcium influx into cells and thus slowing neuronal injury. These agents will not normalize cognition but can slow progression of the disease and may result in slight improvement in cognition after 6 to 12 months of therapy. Data suggest that using cholinesterase therapy along with NMDA antagonist therapy provides additive benefits. Cessation of therapy, however, will result in regression to a curve that follows the normal disease progression without therapy. Vitamin E may be useful in slowing disease progression but is associated with potentially adverse effects, including cardiovascular events, and thus vitamin E is no longer recommended for Alzheimer's disease. Anti-inflammatory medications may lessen the risk for developing Alzheimer's disease. There are mixed data for and against the use of estrogens for lowering Alzheimer's risk, and the risks of estrogen use outweigh any potential benefit. There are conflicting data on the effects of ginkgo biloba on patients with Alzheimer's disease, and there are currently no data suggesting that it can prevent the disease. Selegilene is indicated for early Parkinson's disease, and a transdermal form has been developed for use in depression.

67. A

One-third of individuals older than the age of 65 years will suffer from vision loss. Cataracts may eventually develop in up to 50% of the geriatric population, and though it is the leading cause for vision loss worldwide, the ready availability of surgical correction limits its impact in the United States. Age-related macular degeneration affects approximately 10% of individuals older than age 65 and is the leading cause for vision loss for geriatric patients in the United States. Macular degeneration causes a central loss of vision and can be debilitating and contribute to a lower quality of life. There are two forms of macular degeneration, exudative and nonexudative. Nonexudative accounts for 90% of cases but only 10% of severe vision loss. The exudative variety is associated with neovascularization and is more aggressive, and though it accounts for only 10% of cases of macular degeneration, it accounts for most of the associated vision loss. Glaucoma is a significant cause for vision loss and is the leading cause for blindness in African Americans. Diabetic retinopathy is the leading cause for new blindness in middle-aged Americans, and ambylopia affects predominantly children.

68. E

There are no recommended routine tests to perform after a patient falls other than a history and physical examination. The circumstances surrounding the fall and determining whether the event represents a syncopal or near-syncopal episode are most important. Geriatric patients may exhibit an unsteady gait and fall as a result of systemic illness or infection. In patients with suspected infection or anemia, a complete blood count may be useful. In those with suspected arrhythmias or syncope or near-syncope, an ECG is warranted. If orthostatic blood pressure changes are present, assessment for anemia and volume status by ordering a hemoglobin and basic metabolic panel may be helpful. Medication should be reviewed and determination of need for or adjustment of dosages of narcotics, sedatives, diuretics, and vasodilators should be considered. In patients with suspected head injury, altered mental status, neurologic findings, or painful extremities, x-rays, CT scan, or EEG may be ordered to assess for seizures or further injuries.

69. B

Obstructive sleep apnea and nocturnal myoclonus are the two most common sleep disorders affecting the geriatric population. Obstructive sleep apnea affects 2% to 4% of adults and a greater percentage of geriatric patients. Nocturnal myoclonus may be present in up to 35% of individuals older than age 65 years. Obstructive sleep apnea occurs as a result of narrowing of the upper airway and is manifest as snoring, apneic episodes, and daytime somnolence. Treatment of this disorder is important because of the oxygen desaturation that occurs resulting in secondary complications such as hypertension, cardiovascular disease, and motor vehicle accidents. Nocturnal myoclonus is the occurrence of limb movements with (restless legs syndrome) or without (periodic limb movement disorder) leg discomfort. In either case, nocturnal myoclonus may disrupt sleep and lead to daytime somnolence. Narcolepsy and idiopathic hypersomnolence are related disorders that affect younger adults, with onset in the teens and twenties. Night terrors affect children and are associated with abrupt awakening from sleep in a fearful state, with no subsequent recall of the event.

70. C

Coronary artery disease is more prevalent in the elderly population than in younger patients. More than 85% of patients who die from coronary artery disease are older than 65 years of age. The elderly are more likely to present with atypical symptoms, such as confusion, stroke, and painless infarction. Men are affected more often than women, but it is only about 1.5 times more common in men. PTCA and CABG are treatment options in the elderly as well as younger patients. Although the elderly as a group have more complications with procedural intervention as well as fibrinolytic therapy, concomitant disease plays a role in these complications. Beta-blockers and aspirin are of benefit in all age groups, and the benefits of aspirin therapy outweigh the risks in the general geriatric population with cardiovascular disease.

71. A

Sildenafil has added greatly to treatment of erectile dysfunction by offering effective oral therapy. Sildenafil acts by inhibiting GMP phosphodiesterase enzyme, thus increasing cGMP in the smooth muscle of the corpus cavernosum, resulting in vasodilation, increased blood flow, and erection of the penis. Sildenafil is effective in men with diabetes, hypertension, vascular disease, spinal cord injury, and those who have had prostate surgery. Sildenafil's side effects include headache, flushing, nasal congestion, dyspepsia, and temporary visual changes of increased light sensitivity and a blue tinge to the vision. There have been reports of permanent visual loss associated with sildenafil use, although cause and effect are yet to be determined. An absolute contraindication is use of nitrates since sildenafil will potentiate the hypotensive effects of nitrates. Relative contraindications include recent myocardial infarction, stroke, or arrhythmias as well as uncontrolled hyper- or hypotension, unstable cardiac disease, and any predisposition to priapism. Sildenafil may be used in patients on beta-blockers or with peripheral neuropathy who have no other contraindications.

72. C

Cancer is the second leading cause of death in the United States. Fifty-eight percent of all cancers and two-thirds of all cancer deaths occur in patients older than 65 years of age. In order, the leading causes of cancer death in women are lung, breast, colon, and pancreas. In men, this order is lung, prostate, colorectal, and pancreas. The number of deaths from lung cancer outnumbers deaths from breast, prostate, and colorectal cancer combined. Despite advances in diagnosis and treatment of many types of cancer, there has been very little improvement in survival associated with lung cancer. See Table 7.19.

Table 7.19 Cancer diagnosis and mortality

Most commonly diagnosed cancers	
Males	Females
Prostate	Breast
Lung	Lung
Colorectal	Colorectal
Bladder	Uterine
Non-Hodgkins lymphoma	Ovarian
Most common causes for cancer death	
Males	Females
Lung	Lung
Prostate	Breast
Colorectal	Colorectal
Pancreas	Pancreas
Leukemia	Ovarian

73. B

Tobacco use is the major risk factor for developing lung cancer. Ninety-five percent of lung cancers are associated with smoking. Other risk factors include radon, asbestos, and exposure to materials such as coal and uranium dust. Although the risk for lung cancer lessens with time since quitting smoking, the risk never returns to that of a nonsmoker. After 20 years of not smoking, the risk is substantially reduced. Smoking cessation, in addition to lowering the cancer risk somewhat, has other benefits. Lung function will improve somewhat after smoking cessation and, importantly, further lung damage will be limited. In addition, risks for future cardiovascular disease are reduced after smoking cessation. Efforts to limit the effects of smoking on health must be directed not only at smoking cessation but also toward preventing teens and young adults from starting a smoking habit.

74. B

Colorectal cancer is one of the leading causes of cancer-related morbidity and mortality in the United States. Although most colon cancers occur in patients with no identifiable risk factors, the presence of risk factors increases an individual's chances of developing colon cancer. In recent years, research has provided much insight into some of the important factors associated with a patient's risk for developing colon cancer. Genetic factors have been shown to be a major factor in risk for colon cancer. Several oncogenes have been characterized, and mutation in the APC gene is thought to play an important role in predisposing patients to formation of adenomatous polyps and colon cancer. Thus, positive family history places a patient in a high-risk group. Dietary risk factors include excess alcohol and fat intake, inadequate folate and calcium intake, and possibly low-fiber diet. However, recent research has shown that dietary fiber intake has no effect on the incidence of colon cancer. Ulcerative colitis also increases the risk for developing colon cancer; however, irritable bowel syndrome is not considered to place a patient at increased risk. Hyperplastic polyps do not place patients at increased risk and are not considered neoplastic.

75. A

Currently, the U.S. Preventive Services Task Force does not recommend routine screening for prostate cancer and suggests that if screening is performed, it should be targeted toward those with a life expectancy of more than 10 years. The American Cancer Society and the American Urologic Society recommend annual prostate exams beginning at age 40 and PSA testing beginning at age 50 in low-risk groups and at age 40 in high-risk groups (e.g., positive family history or African American men). The decision to test the elderly should consider their comorbidities and the risks that would be associated with any subsequent procedures. Many men develop prostate cancer and develop few, if any, symptoms and die of another cause. In the patient presented, his age, cardiovascular disease, pulmonary disease, absence of symptoms, and normal exam would make any further testing unnecessary and potentially harmful.

76. A

Routine health care recommendations for geriatric patients include recommendations for mammography, colonoscopy, osteoporosis screening, and Pap smear testing but do not include recommendations for annual chest x-rays. Mammography is recommended for all women between ages 40 and 70 annually. There is no conclusive age at which to stop screening, and this may be determined by the patient's comorbid conditions. Since breast cancer and breast cancer deaths do increase with age, continuing screening in this otherwise healthy woman is appropriate. Pap smear testing can be discontinued in this patient, who has had regular screening and normal test results. Experts agree that after age 65, screening may be discontinued provided the patient has had regular screening in the past with normal results. Colonoscopy is recommended every 10 years in patients with no risk factors. The optimum interval for DEXA screening for osteoporosis is ill-defined; however, screening intervals less than every 2 years are unlikely to detect appreciable changes in bone density.

77. D

Hearing loss affects up to one-fourth of patients older than the age of 65 years. Presbycusis is a sensorineural hearing loss that is associated with aging. It is typically a high-pitched hearing loss that is symmetric and gradual in onset. It is not generally associated with vertigo. Other causes of sensorineural hearing loss include noise-induced, drug-induced, Meniere's disease, trauma, acoustic neuroma, and hereditary syndromes. Impairment in taste sensation is referred to as dysguesia and may occur with facial nerve or olfactory disturbances. See Table 7.20.

Table 7.20 Causes of hearing loss

Conductive	Sensorineural
Cerumen impaction	Presbycusis
Otitis media/externa	Noise-induced
Middle ear effusion	Autoimmune
Otosclerosis	Perilymphatic fistula
Cholesteatoma	Meniere's disease
	Acoustic neuroma

78. C

Changes in gait may occur as part of the normal aging process or may signify underlying disease. With normal aging, there may be slight stooping of the posture, decrease in stride length, diminished dorsiflexion and plantar flexion of the foot, and less shoulder flexion and elbow extension noted with arm swing. Loss of arm swing, along with a bent forward posture, and short shuffling gait are characteristic of Parkinson's disease. Widening of the base occurs with vestibular and cerebellar disturbances. Variability in step length and height is a feature of the foot slapping or stomping gait that occurs with sensory ataxia and loss of proprioceptive feedback.

79. B

Therapy for osteoarthritis is directed toward pain relief and physical therapy. Although there may be some inflammation associated with osteoarthritis, it is not an inflammatory arthropathy and the presence of inflammation does not correlate with pain. Thus, the first-line agent recommended for analgesia is acetaminophen because of its effectiveness and safety profile. Some people may not respond to acetaminophen, and other medications such as NSAIDs, opioids, or intra-articular steroid or hyaluronic acid injections may be tried. Systemic steroids are not indicated for treatment of osteoarthritis. Referral for possible joint replacement is an option when all other therapies have failed. Thus, in this patient, medication and physical therapy should be tried initially.

80. D

Benign positional vertigo (BPV) is a common cause of vertigo in the elderly thought to be caused by the presence of otoliths in the semicircular canals. These otoliths move about the vestibular apparatus with head movement and cause hyperstimulation of the sensory hair cells. Episodes of vertigo last seconds to a minute and may be associated with nystagmus that is horizontal or rotatory. Tinnitus and hearing loss are not features of BPV. Treatment of BPV involves exercises that utilize one of the diagnostic features of BPV—namely, extinguishability. Repetitive exercises that duplicate the maneuver that brings on symptoms can also help relieve the patient's symptoms. In addition, therapy for benign positional vertigo may be undertaken in the office by performance of the Epley maneuver. This maneuver is performed by rotating the patients through a series of positions attempting to relocate the debris in the semicircular canal into the vestibule of the labyrinth. The Epley maneuver is reported to have a success rate approaching 80%. Medication therapy tends to provide little benefit to patients with BPV.

81. E

Medication use can place elderly patients at increased risk for falls. Medications that alter sensorium, such as benzodiazepines, antipsychotics, and some antidepressant medications (e.g., amitriptyline), have been shown to be associated with increased risk for falling. Other medications that cause sedation as a side effect or that may produce hypotension as a side effect may also increase risk. Examples of medications in this category include the alpha-adrenergic blockers (e.g., terazosin), nitrates, antihypertensives, and medications used for seizures or peripheral neuropathy (e.g., gabapentin and phenytoin). Pseudoephedrine is an alpha-adrenergic agonist that should not affect sensorium and may have a tendency to elevate blood pressure. Fludrocortisone is a corticosteroid that promotes sodium retention and is used to treat orthostatic hypotension. Buproprion is an antidepressant and neither it nor acetaminophen have sedative or blood pressure-lowering effects.

82. A

Motor vehicle accidents are the leading cause for injury-related death in older adults aged 65 to 74 years. In adults older than age 75 years, motor vehicle accidents are second only to falls. Despite a decline in overall accident rates in the United States, there has been a significant increase in accidents involving geriatric drivers. Although geriatric drivers do not drive as many miles per year as younger drivers, they have higher accident rates. Assessment of an older patient's capacity for driving is thus an important role for the patient's primary care physician. See Table 7.21.

83. B

Healthy older adults have the potential to be as good or better drivers than younger drivers. As individuals age, they may develop medical diseases, sensory impairments, or cognitive decline that may interfere with their driving abilities. In addition, medication use may affect their overall alertness. However, medical disease alone has not been a reliable predictor for driving difficulties, and a better measure seems to be functional status and cognitive abilities. Thus, a patient with very mild dementia but no other limitations may safely drive, whereas a patient with intact cognitive abilities but limited vision or mobility may be unsafe. These factors along with a review of medications can allow the physician to provide a judgment on driving ability. In cases in which there is any doubt, formal assessment in a driving program can help further determine whether a particular patient may safely drive. In the patient presented, the fact that he has been involved in an accident and that his family has serious concerns should prompt a more formal evaluation. Advising patients only to drive during certain times of the day or to make short trips does not fully address whether the patient can safely drive, and forbidding the patient from driving based on one accident may be excessively punitive and inappropriate.

Table 7.21 Most common causes of death

Ages 65–74	Ages 75–84
Malignancy	Cardiovascular disease
Cardiovascular disease	Malignancy
Respiratory disease (chronic)	Respiratory disease (chronic)
Cerebrovascular disease	Cerebrovascular disease
Diabetes mellitus	Diabetes mellitus
Accidents	Alzheimer's disease
Renal disease	Influenza and pneumonia
Chronic liver disease	Renal disease
Influenza and pneumonia	Accidents
Septicemia	Septicemia

84. D

Erectile dysfunction is one of the most common sexual complaints or problems in geriatric men. Some degree of erectile dysfunction is present in 52% of men between the ages of 40 and 70 years. The prevalence increases with age. Complete impotence is present in 15% of 70-year-old men and some degree of erectile dysfunction is present in 67%. The most common secondary cause for erectile dysfunction is vascular disease. Other risk factors for erectile dysfunction include diabetes mellitus, hypertension, smoking, elevated lipids, medication use, depression, and pelvic surgery (particularly prostate). Medications that may cause erectile dysfunction include sedatives, antipsychotics, antidepressants, antihypertensives, spironolactone, H2 blockers, seizure medications, and long-term alcohol use. Prior to initiating testing and therapy for erectile dysfunction, medication use should be reviewed.

85. E

With aging, sexual desire lessens in both men and women. Low sexual desire is the most common sexual complaint in postmenopausal women. Maintenance of sexual activity is influenced by many factors, including general medical health and marital status. In men, poor health and medication use are the most commonly cited reasons for decline in sexual activity. For women, lack of a partner is the most common reason cited for decline in sexual activity. Only 5% of unmarried women report being sexually active, in comparison to 56% of married women. Approximately one-half of patients age 60 or older remain sexually active and two-thirds to three-fourths consider this an important part of their partner relationship. Vaginal dysparunia is the second most commonly reported sexual complaint in geriatric women. This occurs as a result of urogenital atrophy secondary to the hypoestrogenic state. Oral or vaginal estrogen may help in alleviating these symptoms.

86. B

Paget's disease is a disease of bone remodeling that results in high bone turnover and haphazard formation of new bone that has diminished strength. The new bone is weaker and more susceptible to deformity and fracture. This disease is of unknown cause and affects approximately 3% of patients older than age 55 years. Patients with Paget's disease may present with pain in the affected area or may be found to have the disease incidentally through x-ray findings or elevation of the serum alkaline phosphatase. Not all patients with Paget's disease require therapy. Indications for therapy include pain, involvement of the hip, long bones, skull or vertebral bodies, and significant elevation of the serum alkaline phosphatase (greater than two to three times). Due to the increased blood flow to affected areas, extensive disease has been associated with high-output congestive heart failure. Involvement of the skull or vertebral bodies can lead to neurologic insult. The hip and long bones affected by Paget's disease are susceptible to fracture or deformity. Asymptomatic disease in the pelvis may not require therapy.

87. C

Basal cell carcinomas (BCCs) are the most common skin cancers found in the elderly. Squamous cell cancers are also common, but BCC is approximately four times more common. BCCs may be nodular or ulcerative and are characterized as papules or nodules with a central depression and a waxy or pearly border with telangectasia within the lesion. They most commonly occur on sun-exposed areas. Squamous cell carcinomas are erythematous, keratotic, scaling nodules that also generally occur on sun-exposed areas. The incidence of malignant melanoma has been increasing in patients of all ages. Malignant melanoma is a pigmented lesion and must be distinguished from other benign pigmented lesions. Asymmetry, irregular borders, irregular coloration, and size greater than 6 mm should raise concern that a lesion may be melanoma. Although usually present on sun-exposed areas, malignant melanoma may occur in other areas as well. Seborrheic keratosis is a benign lesion that is very common in the elderly. It is a keratotic brown or brown-black lesion with the classic "stuck-on" appearance. They are not sun related and occur most commonly on the trunk and face. Keratoacanthoma is a benign skin nodule that is firm and erythematous with a central depression that appears as a scab. They generally occur on the extremities.

88. E

Deep venous thrombosis (DVT) develops in 60% to 70% of patients who suffer a hip fracture or those who undergo hip surgery. In order to lessen the risks for pulmonary embolism, prophylactic therapy to prevent or limit DVT is recommended for all patients requiring hip surgery. Aspirin is only minimally effective in lowering the incidence of DVT and is clearly less effective than the heparins or coumadin. Compression stockings lessen the risk but are best used along with other more effective measures. Unfractionated heparin provides some benefit but is not as effective as either low-molecular-weight heparin or coumadin, which are the most effective methods available. Low–molecular-weight heparins are generally begun postoperatively and are indicated for use for up to 3 weeks. There is a 1% to 3% risk of bleeding associated with its use and the risk for thrombocytopenia is approximately 1%. Blood counts should be monitored during therapy. In patients who are obese, weigh less than 45 kg, or who have renal insufficiency, the effects of low–molecular-weight heparins are less predictable and dosage may need to be adjusted. See Table 7.22.

89. B

The issue of competency is not always straightforward and requires judgment on the part of the physician or individual assessing the patient's decision-making ability. Although by mini-mental status testing the patient has mild dementia, she may be able to make some, or all, decisions by herself. The understanding and thought process that revolve around an issue are the key items that should be assessed. A mini-mental status test may fluctuate and should be reassessed when the patient is well and in her usual living environment. If deemed unable to rationally make decisions, then her daughter should exercise her power of attorney. If the daughter should want guardianship, then the courts may become involved. Neuropsychiatric testing may provide insight into underlying disease processes, such as dementia or depression, and may support any determination but does not substitute for the physician's judgment.

90. C

Hip fractures account for a significant percentage of all hospital admissions in the United States and account for over $8 billion in health care expenditures. The two most common fractures that affect the geriatric population are intertrochanteric and femoral neck fractures of the proximal femur or hip. After medical stabilization, prompt surgical treatment and mobilization can lessen the morbidity and mortality associated with hip fractures. Intertrochanteric fractures are generally repaired with internal fixation, whereas femoral neck fractures often are repaired with hemiarthroplasty. The tenuous blood supply to the femoral head can be interrupted with femoral neck fractures, thus resulting in non-union or avascular necrosis of the femoral head when repaired by means other than hemiarthroplasty. Due to the complications that can arise from decreased mobility, along with other concomitant medical problems, the 1-year mortality rate associated with either type of hip fracture is approximately 15% to 30%.

91. B

Physical rehabilitation therapy does not usually begin until a patient is medically stable. Stable patients recovering from a CVA, diabetes, or other medical conditions would be suitable candidates provided their mental status is appropriate. During therapy, the patient must be able to follow directions and learn new tasks. This often will prevent patients with moderate or severe dementia from being suitable rehabilitation candidates. Patients with depression may be suitable candidates with appropriate medication, support, and counseling. Good social support can help in caring for the patient and in maintaining patient motivation for continuing therapy. Finally, the resources to pay for therapy services must be in place. For patients with Medicare, therapy is a covered benefit in the rehabilitation unit, nursing home, or home settings. For those not covered by Medicare, private insurance may provide coverage.

92. C

In a patient presenting with a new-onset supraventricular tachycardia, a search for underlying causes should be part of the evaluation

Table 7.22 Prophylactic therapy for DVT prevention

Low risk (medical patient without risk factors)[a]	Gradient compression stocking and ambulation
Moderate risk (minor surgery or medical patient with risk factors)	Low-dose heparin subcutaneously or low–molecular-weight heparin; can use with gradient stockings and/or pneumatic compression stockings
High risk (multiple risk factors or high-risk surgery)	Low–molecular-weight heparin or fondaprinux or coumadin; can be used with gradient stocking and/or pneumatic compression stockings

[a]Risk factors include age older than 40, obesity, cancer, prior DVT, major trauma, orthopedic lower extremity surgery, recent travel, congestive heart failure, family history of hypercoaguable condition, estrogen therapy, or contraception.

and treatment. Cardiac causes for supraventricular tachycardia include cardiac ischemia, cardiomyopathy, valvular heart disease, and pericarditis. Noncardiac causes that may trigger supraventricular tachycardia include hyperthyroidism, pulmonary disease, venous thromboembolism, and toxins such as stimulant medications and alcohol. Basic initial assessment for these underlying causes should be undertaken. Common initial laboratory evaluation includes complete blood count, electrolytes, serum creatinine, cardiac enzymes, and thyroid-stimulating hormone. A D-dimer test is also commonly ordered to screen for possible venous thromboembolic disease. This test is very sensitive but not specific. Thus, a negative test virtually excludes this condition and a positive test requires further evaluation. In addition to an electrocardiogram, a chest x-ray and echocardiogram are often also ordered as initial tests to evaluate supraventricular tachycardias. Chest CT or pulmonary arteriography may be indicated to evaluate for pulmonary embolism if warranted by the initial testing. Arterial blood gases would not be warranted in this patient with no pulmonary symptoms and a normal pulse oximetry. Stress testing also would not be indicated initially in this patient but may be warranted on follow-up after therapy depending on the results of his cardiac enzymes and echocardiogram.

93. E

Syncope and near syncope occur when there is a global change in cerebral perfusion or metabolism. The priority in evaluation of syncope and near syncope is a search for cardiac etiologies. The prognosis for patients with these symptoms and an underlying cardiac etiology is much worse than for those with noncardiac etiologies. One-year mortality rates for those with a cardiac etiology are reported to be as high as 33% compared to approximately 10% for those with noncardiac or unexplained syncope. Mortality rates in the elderly are thought to be higher than for younger patients. Cardiac causes have been reported in 9% of patients undergoing syncope evaluation in the general population, compared to 33% of geriatric patients. Thus, in addition to evaluating hemoglobin and electrolytes, cardiac testing including an electrocardiogram, echocardiogram, and cardiac monitoring are of prime importance. Cardiac monitoring may be in the form of an event monitor or a 24-hour Holter monitor. Important factors in deciding which of these modalities to choose are the frequency of occurrence of symptoms and the ability of the patient to capture an event. For example, if patients have daily symptoms, then a Holter monitor should provide useful information. If patients have infrequent symptoms, then carrying an event monitor for 30 days or more may be more informative. With an event monitor, the patient must wear or place the monitor over the chest and activate and then transmit the information to the providers. Since the patient is currently asymptomatic and has infrequent symptoms, an electrocardiogram or Holter monitor are unlikely to be beneficial. A CT scan would not likely be of any benefit in this patient with recurrent palpitations who likely has a cardiac source for his symptoms. Tilt-table testing would be beneficial if there were orthostatic symptoms.

94. C

The majority of nursing home costs are paid for by Medicaid (58%) or private funds (38%). The next largest payer for nursing home care is Medicare. In order for a patient to be covered by Medicare in a nursing home, he or she must require skilled nursing care and rehabilitation following a hospital stay of at least three nights for a condition related to the need for rehabilitation.

Medicare will then provide coverage for the lesser of 100 days per year or until the patient's condition has stabilized.

95. A

Dual energy x-ray absorptiometry (DEXA) is considered the gold standard for assessing bone density due to its precision and low radiation exposure. The World Health Organization has developed definitions of osteoporosis based on bone density. Osteopenia is defined as a bone density of 1.0 to 2.5 standard deviations below the mean for young adults. Osteoporosis is defined as a bone density of 2.5 or more standard deviations below the mean for young adults. These values are reported as T scores, with a negative value reflecting a diminished bone density and a positive indicating a higher bone density. Another score that is commonly reported is the Z score. The Z score is a comparison of the individual to the age-matched mean. The T score is most clinically useful and is what the definitions are based on. For each standard deviation below the mean T score, an individual's risk for fracture increases two to three times.

96. C

Testosterone levels diminish with increasing age after attaining a peak in the teens or early adulthood. For many men, the low or low-normal testosterone levels may have no clinical manifestations. Conversely, low testosterone levels may cause decrease in muscle mass, bone mass, energy, libido, as well as erectile dysfunction. Testosterone therapy may reverse many of these effects but commonly does not resolve erectile dysfunction. Attaining penile erections is dependent on many factors, and compromised vasodilatory function of the penile vessels most commonly underlies erectile dysfunction; thus, testosterone replacement may not restore erectile function. Primary hypogonadism is not considered a part of normal aging and can be detected by the findings of elevated LH and FSH along with decreased testosterone levels. Replacement therapy is indicated when these findings are present along with symptoms. Patients should be evaluated for hyperprolactinemia, prostate cancer, breast cancer, polycythemia, and sleep disorders before starting therapy.

97. B

Hyperthyroidism is present in up to 1% of the geriatric population and will commonly present with classic findings of heat intolerance, nervousness, weight loss, and palpitations that also occur in younger patients. Older patients may also present more commonly with atypical symptoms such as anorexia, constipation, and apathy. Apathetic hyperthyroidism may be mistakenly diagnosed as depression if other physical signs or symptoms are not present and the thyroid is not assessed. Atrial fibrillation, congestive heart failure, or increasing angina are other ways that a hyperthyroid patient may present. If the diagnosis is considered, then a thyroid-stimulating hormone should be obtained. Newer generation tests are very sensitive and if suppressed should be investigated by assessing both T4 and T3 levels. Up to 10% of elderly patients may have hyperthyroidism due to T3 toxicosis, and in some of the patients, only the free T3 is found to be elevated. Iodine deficiency would cause hypofunction of the thyroid and is rare in the United States since foods are supplemented with iodine. Primary hypothyroidism refers to hypofunction of the thyroid gland and laboratory assessment would find an elevated TSH and decreased T4 and T3. Secondary hypothyroidism would occur due to disease in the pituitary–hypothalamic system and would manifest with decreased TSH as well as T4 and T3 values.

98. A

Hypothyroidism is present in up to 6% of the geriatric population. Patients may present with classic symptoms of diminished energy, cold intolerance, and constipation. Elderly patients may also present nonspecifically with decline in physical or mental function, gait disturbances, or weakness. In many cases, these symptoms are attributed to normal aging. Hypertension can also be a manifestation of hypothyroidism, present in up to one-third of patients. Treatment may result in normalization of blood pressure. Ninety-five percent of cases of hypothyroidism are either due to radioablation of the thyroid to treat hyperthyroidism or are caused by an autoimmune destruction of the gland, termed Hashimoto's thyroiditis. Detection of primary hypothyroidism is through finding an elevated serum TSH in association with low total or free T4 levels. In such instances, replacement therapy should be initiated and testing for antibodies directed at the thyroid is not indicated. Further investigation should be pursued in those cases with both decreased TSH and T4 levels, indicating a secondary hypothyroidism of pituitary or hypothalamic origin.

99. C

Both medical practitioners and the public have voiced increasing concern about continuing hormone replacement therapy since increased risk for cardiovascular and cancer complications have been found in recent studies. Indications for use of hormone replacement are for preservation of bone mass and treatment of vasomotor symptoms, referred to as hot flashes. In women who are reluctant to continue with HRT, alternative treatments for hot flashes can be tried, although estrogens are the most effective therapy, resulting in improvement in 95% of cases. Other treatments and their effectiveness include medroxyprogesterone acetate (60% to 85%), clonidine (30% to 40%), and Bellergal (50%). Soy flour may also provide some symptom relief but requires further study. Raloxifene, a selective estrogen receptor modulator, may worsen or cause symptoms of hot flashes and also is associated with increased risk for developing deep vein thrombosis. Propranolol may help with cardiovascular symptoms of menopause, such as palpitations, but would not be likely to help with hot flashes. Nifedipine and prazosin would not be expected to affect the occurrence of hot flashes.

100. E

Vitamin B12 deficiency can lead to development of a megaloblastic anemia as well as neuropsychiatric disease. Vitamin B12 deficiency may be present in up to 10% of individuals older than age 70 years. Vitamin B12 (cobalamin) is present in foods of animal origin but is not present in plants. Vitamin B12 is released from the animal proteins in the stomach by the acidity and action of pepsin. It then attaches to the cobalamin binding protein and passes to the duodenum. In the duodenum, pancreatic proteases degrade the binding factor, thus allowing intrinsic factor, produced by the stomach, to bind and transport the vitamin B12 to the terminal ileum, where it is absorbed. Pernicious anemia is the most common cause for vitamin B12 deficiency. Up to 50% of individuals older than age 70 have evidence of decreased gastric acidity, pepsin secretion, and intrinsic factor, all of which may contribute to decreased vitamin absorption. Inadequate dietary intake may occur in strict vegetarians. Because of liver stores and reabsorption of vitamin B12 secreted in bile, it may take over 10 years of a vegetarian diet to result in vitamin B12 deficiency. Ingestion of multivitamins may increase this time further. Crohn's disease may affect the terminal ileum and thus impair vitamin B12

absorption, but it occurs less commonly than pernicious anemia in geriatric patients. Fish tapeworms may cause impairment of vitamin B12 absorption. Ulcerative colitis generally does not affect vitamin B12 absorption.

101. E

Older patients are at risk for osteoporosis not only due to hormonal changes affecting bone metabolism but also because of inadequate calcium intake and deficiency of vitamin D. Sources of vitamin D include oral intake and generation of vitamin D in the skin from sun exposure. Both of these sources tend to be inadequate in many geriatric patients, and thus supplementation should be provided. Individuals at highest risk for vitamin D deficiency are those residing in nursing homes, living in the Northern Hemisphere, requiring chronic anticonvulsant therapy, and those who are housebound. Vitamin D precursors are metabolized in the liver and the kidney into the final product, 1,25-dihydroxyvitamin D. Renal insufficiency and decreased renal conversion of 25-hydroxyvitamin D to 1,25-dihydroxyvitamin D is another common cause for vitamin D deficiency. Hepatic function generally is not a limiting factor in vitamin D metabolism. Exercise would have no effect on vitamin D levels and diuretic use would not be expected to affect vitamin D metabolism.

102. C

Decubitus ulcers are common in patients with limited mobility. Prevention by frequent turning to minimize the pressures that may lead to decubitus formation is a major focus of hospital and nursing home personnel caring for immobile patients. When an ulcer has formed, debridement of the lesion and limiting the pressure on the site are the most important aspects of care to promote healing. The wound base should be kept moist, with care to prevent maceration of surrounding skin. Limiting contact with feces and urine is also important. Antibiotics should be reserved for those wounds with suspected infection since overuse of antibiotics will promote colonization and infection with resistant organisms. Signs of infection include erythema and warmth of surrounding skin as well as purulent, malodorous wound discharge. When wound irrigation is necessary, normal saline is the preferred irrigant since chemicals such as povidine iodine (betadine) and hydrogen peroxide can impair new tissue growth. For diabetic ulcers that are refractory to healing, becaplermin (regranex), a growth factor, can be used topically to promote new tissue growth. Routine use of this material is limited by the high cost.

103. C

Although all these conditions may cause constipation, the most common causes are functional and are related to decreased intestinal transit times. This results in slowing of the movement of material through the intestines and less frequent bowel movements. If bowel movements do not occur on a daily basis, many older adults are concerned and equate that with constipation. If the bowel movements are soft and easily passed, the patient can be reassured that this is a normal variant. However, with slower transit times more water may be absorbed from the stool resulting in harder bowel movements, and evaluation and treatment should then be recommended. Evaluation for underlying medical diseases, such as hypothyroidism and hyperparathyroidism, should be performed. Colorectal cancer screening is recommended for all patients older than age 50. In the absence of an underlying cause, initial treatment measures generally call for increasing the dietary fiber by diet changes or supplementation. See Table 7.23.

Table 7.23 Causes for constipation

Dietary factors (e.g., low fiber, water)
  Decreased mobility
  Dementia
  Depression
  Other medical/neurologic condition

Medications
  Laxative abuse
  Anticholinergics, narcotics, calcium channel blockers

Mechanical
  Colonic lesions such as stricture or carcinoma
  Rectal lesions such as hemorrhoids, fissures, stricture

Metabolic/endocrine
  Diabetes with neuropathy
  Hypothyroidism
  Hyperparathyroidism
  Hypercalcemia, hypokalemia

104. B

Fecal incontinence is not a normal part of aging and is a leading cause for institutionalization of the elderly. There are treatments available; however, treatment will depend on the underlying cause as well as the underlying condition of the patient. Dementia plays a major role in fecal incontinence, and in many instances the presence of dementia will limit the ability to institute behavioral forms of treatment. In these cases, either stimulated defecation or use of diapers may be the only options. Dietary modification by increasing fiber content and use of opioid medications, such as loperamide or diphenoxylate, may also be tried. Medications may be more useful when frequent, liquid stools are present. Constipation may result from misuse of these agents.

105. C

Antipsychotic medications, such as trifluoperazine and haloperidol, are associated with development of tardive dyskinesia, involuntary repetitive movements of the mouth, tongue, and lips associated with facial grimacing and other head movements. Other medications that have been implicated in this disorder include the phenothiazine antiemetics and metoclopramide. Cessation of therapy will not lead to immediate reversal of symptoms, which may be present for many years. Levodopa or carbidopa is not associated with tardive dyskinesia, but chorea is a common effect and may be part of the on–off phenomenon alternating with akinesia. Loratidine, zolpidem, and pseudoephedrine are not associated with movement disorders.

106. C

Geriatric patients, particularly those older than age 75 years, are more vulnerable to developing hypothermia. Hypothermia may develop during any season of the year and does not necessarily require extreme cold exposure. Often, hypothermia will develop gradually and present with nonspecific symptoms or a change in mental status. The elderly have a decreased perception of temperature changes along with decreased shivering response, metabolic rates, and peripheral blood flow. Socioeconomic factors and medications may also play significant roles in many cases. Recognition is of paramount importance so that patients undergo thorough assessment and receive the appropriate rewarming for their clinical status and degree of hypothermia.

107. D

With iron deficiency anemia, there is a hypochromic microcytic anemia along with decrease in iron stores as indicated by a low serum ferritin value. Other findings consistent with iron deficiency anemia include a low or low-normal serum iron, a low reticulocyte count, and an elevated total iron binding capacity. Serum ferritin values are the most reliable blood tests in assessing iron status but may be falsely elevated with liver disease or inflammatory conditions. Serum iron and total iron binding capacity cannot be relied on for the diagnosis because these values tend to fluctuate greatly in association with a variety of diseases and serum iron levels decrease somewhat with age. In those cases in which serum laboratory findings are inconclusive, bone marrow stores can be assessed by aspiration. See Figure 7-1.

108. C

The differential diagnosis for bloody diarrhea includes inflammatory bowel disease, infectious diarrhea, and other forms of colitis such as medication-induced or ischemia. Colon cancer, diverticular bleeding, and colonic angiomas do not typically present with diarrhea. Most clinicians think of inflammatory bowel disease as a disease of younger patients; however, there is a bimodal incidence of ulcerative colitis with a second peak in the 60s. Smoking is associated with a decreased risk for developing ulcerative colitis. Nonsteroidal anti-inflammatory medications are a potential cause for colitis. Patients with bloody diarrhea require evaluation for the different causes and any possible medications that may be contributing to symptoms should be discontinued. Typically, a complete blood count and evaluation of the stool for leukocytes, *Clostridium difficile*, and bacterial pathogens is ordered. In the absence of an identified cause, colonoscopy and biopsy are often also performed. If no definite cause is found, treatment for the colitis is commonly provided with agents such as corticosteroid or 5-aminosalicyclic acid administered orally or by enema.

109. B

Bronchiectasis is an abnormal dilation of the bronchi resulting from destruction of the muscular and connective tissue components of the bronchial walls. The causes for bronchiectasis are untreated infection and bronchial obstruction. Common diseases associated with development of bronchiectasis include tuberculosis, foreign body, cystic fibrosis, primary ciliary dyskinesia, alpha-1-antitrypsin deficiency, and bronchopulmonary aspergillosis. Viral infections, such as influenza, measles, and adenovirus, may also play a role by altering ciliary motility. Other conditions that are associated with development of bronchiectasis include immunodeficiencies, such as HIV, and rheumatoid arthritis. Pulmonary hypertension may occur as a secondary effect in patients who have associated hypoxemia, but it would not itself cause bronchiectasis.

110. D

Peptic ulcer disease affects up to 10% of the population at some point in their lives. Common causes for peptic ulcer disease include *Helicobacter pylori* infection, use of nonsteroidal anti-inflammatory medication, stress-induced ulcers, and, rarely, hypersecretory states such as Zollinger–Ellison disease. *Helicobacter pylori* infections more commonly cause duodenal ulcers, but they can also cause

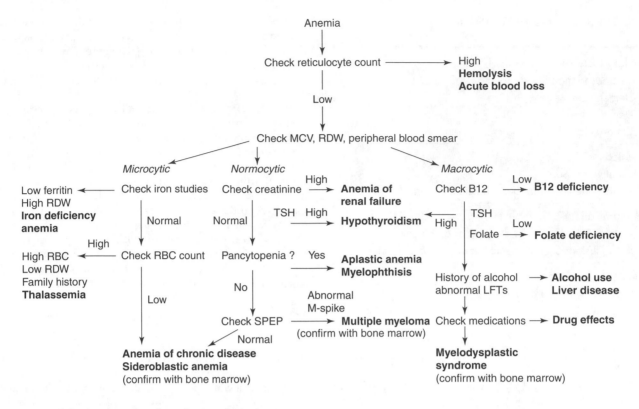

Figure 7-1. *An approach to the evaluation of anemia.*

gastric ulcers. During endoscopy, tissue obtained can be tested for urease or sent for pathologic identification of the organism. *Helicobacter pylori* testing is very sensitive, but many older patients are positive for the antibody, which cannot distinguish new from old infection. Thus, *H. pylori* antibody testing would not be indicated in this patient. Nonsteroidal anti-inflammatory medications should be stopped since they may be the cause or aggravate existing ulcers. Proton pump inhibitors may facilitate healing. Follow-up endoscopy should be performed for gastric ulcers to document healing since some gastric cancers can present as ulcers and may not be identified on biopsy specimens. See Table 7.24.

Table 7.24 Peptic ulcer disease

H. pylori-positive disease
- 7 to 14 days of antibiotics: clarithromycin and ampicillin or metronidazole; bismuth subsalicylate, metronidazole, and tetracycline
- 4 to 8 weeks of H2 blocker or proton pump inhibitor therapy for duodenal ulcers and 6 to 12 weeks for gastric ulcers
- Follow-up EGD to document eradication of gastric ulcers

H. pylori-negative disease
- H2 blockers or proton pump inhibitor therapy as for *H. pylori*-positive disease
- Follow-up EGD as for *H. pylori*-positive disease
- Removal of causative agents (e.g., NSAIDs)
- Misoprostal can help prevent NSAID-induced ulcers

111. D

Urinary infections are the most common type of bacterial infection in geriatric patients. Symptoms that may suggest infection include fever, dysuria, urinary frequency, urinary urgency, and, in some patients, nonspecific symptoms such as weakness, fatigue, or change in mental status. In the absence of symptoms, the presence of bacteria in the urine at a concentration greater than 100,000 colonies is termed asymptomatic bacteriuria. This may occur transiently and often there is lack of the presence of white blood cells in the urine. In these asymptomatic cases, treatment is not indicated. Likewise, repeating the urine culture in the absence of symptoms would not be warranted. Asymptomatic bacteriuria occurs in up to 10% of community males and 30% of women. This incidence increases approximately 1.5- to 2-fold in nursing home residents. Patients with indwelling catheters will have colonization of the bladder and urine by multiple organisms such that by the time the catheter has been in for 3 or 4 weeks, 100% of patients are bacteruric. In the absence of symptoms, these patients should not be treated.

112. D

Captopril or another ACE inhibitor are excellent choices for antihypertensive therapy in a diabetic patient and are also used in normotensive patients to limit the effects of diabetes on the kidney. In geriatric patients who are started on ACE inhibitor therapy, the serum creatinine and potassium must be monitored. The addition of captopril does not appear to be causing any renal compromise in this patient with renal insufficiency since the creatinine has remained stable. His blood pressure is controlled and thus the captopril dose should be maintained at its current level. Metformin is an excellent insulin sensitizer that acts through the liver to decrease hepatic gluconeogenesis and glycogenolysis. Adverse effects of metformin are primarily gastrointestinal and include a metallic taste, abdominal discomfort, and diarrhea. A less common but potentially very serious side effect is that of lactic acidosis. Metformin must be excreted through the kidney. In individuals with renal compromise (elevated serum creatinine), metformin excretion is impaired and they are at risk for developing lactic acidosis. In the patient presented, metformin is contraindicated. An alternative diabetes medication should be prescribed.

113. B
Cognitive side effects are common in those medications in which the primary action is on the central nervous system. The diseases that these agents are aimed to treat may also be an underlying cause for memory impairment; thus, a high index of suspicion and an awareness of the data available in terms of cognitive side effects are important in targeting treatment to the elderly patient. Studies have indicated that the selective serotonin reuptake inhibitors (SSRIs) have the least adverse cognitive effects among the antidepressant medications, thus accounting for their popularity in this group of patients. Rarely, elderly demented patients may suffer mental status changes due to an SSRI. Drugs in the phenothiazine, benzodiazepine, tricyclic antidepressant, and antihistamine classes all have been shown to adversely effect memory and performance of different measured tasks and to cause sedation.

114. B
In geriatric patients the primary reason for adjusting the dose of a low-molecular-weight heparin or for using alternative therapy is impaired renal function. Low-molecular-weight heparins are cleared primarily through the kidneys and thus with renal insufficiency will accumulate and place the patient at increased risk for bleeding complications. Studies indicate that enoxaparin may be safely used when the creatinine clearance is more than 30 mL/min. For patients with lower creatinine clearances, those who are obese or less than 45 kg, or who require prolonged therapy (months), it is recommended that anti-Xa activity be monitored (4 hours after dose). Mild elevation in liver enzymes would not be a contraindication for use of a low–molecular-weight heparin. Creatinine clearance is less than 30 mL/min in patient B, and her weight falls below the lower limit for recommended unmonitored use. Creatinine clearance is calculated as weight $\times$ (140 − age)/72 $\times$ serum creatinine.

115. B
Bunions are a common foot disorder among both younger and older patients. The cause for bunion deformities has not been precisely defined but they are thought to be related to genetic predisposition, flat-feet, as well as footwear selection (e.g., narrow toe boxes and high heels). Commonly, there is an associated hallux valgus deformity that creates a widening of the width of the foot and pain resulting from pressure of the shoes. Steroid injections play no role in therapy. Physical therapy will not correct any anatomic deformity. Narcotic medication may help relieve some of the pain, but it must be used judiciously, if at all, and will not correct the underlying problem. Initial therapy should be provided by modification of the footwear to shoes with widened toe box. Orthotics may benefit some patients with flat-feet or metatarsalgia. For patients refractory to these initial measures, surgery may be necessary.

116. C
There is controversy over PSA screening regarding at what age testing should no longer be performed. Some have defined specific ages (e.g., 75 years) and others life expectancy (more than 10 years) as cutoffs for further PSA testing. PSA values increase with age, and using age-adjusted PSA values as a guide, this

patient would fall into the 4.5 to 6.5 ng/mL that is considered normal for the 70- to 80-year age range. Thus, initial efforts may be to educate the patient regarding the effects of age, to review his past testing, and to reassure him that in the absence of symptoms and a normal exam he does not have any significant disease. The PSA value reported and a normal physical examination, although reassuring, do not prove that he does not have prostate cancer. Of the choices listed, the best choice in a patient who cannot be reassured by lesser efforts may to be offer free PSA testing. If the free PSA to total PSA is high (greater than 0.25), then his chances of the elevation of PSA being due to prostate cancer are less than 10% and this may reassure him. If the values are lower, then he may choose to undergo further testing, such as ultrasound or ultrasound-guided biopsy. There would be no basis for radiation therapy or use of finasteride in this patient at this time.

117. A
Pneumonia and influenza are leading causes of mortality from infectious disease in the elderly. Geriatric patients have a fivefold increased chance for developing pneumonia compared to young adults. Underlying medical diseases, such as COPD and cardiovascular disease, are partly responsible. Etiologies of pneumonia in community and nursing home residents are similar, with the exception of a much greater percentage of mixed and gram-negative infections in nursing home patients. *Streptococcus pneumoniae*, *Haemophilus influenzae*, and *Moraxella catarrhalis* are common community and nursing home organisms, but *Klebsiella* and *Escherichia coli* are also found commonly in nursing home residents. Atypical organisms may cause pneumonia in the geriatric population but occur less frequently than other bacterial pathogens.

118. B
With the increasing size of the geriatric population, more patients are undergoing surgery that results in prosthetic implants. These implants may, in some instances, become infected due to bacterial seeding from bacteremia from dental work or another source. Most prosthetic joint infections occur due to organisms from nonoral sources, commonly staphylococcus. Indications for coverage with antibiotics prophylactically include prosthesis implanted

Table 7.25 Conditions requiring prophylactic antibiotic coverage for endocarditis and prosthetic joint infections

Endocarditis
 Prior history of endocarditis
 Prosthetic heart valve
 Valvular heart disease
 Hypertrophic cardiomyopathy
 Mitral valve prolapse with regurgitation

Prosthetic joint infections
 Device implanted within past 2 years
 Rheumatoid arthritis
 Systemic lupus erythematosis
 Immunosuppression
 Type 1 diabetes
 Prior prosthetic joint infection
 Malnutrition

less than 2 years ago, immunosuppression, type 1 diabetes, prior joint infection, malnutrition, lupus, and rheumatoid arthritis. See Table 7.25.

119. D

Up to 50% or more of men and 37% of women will experience hair loss consistent with male pattern baldness. The history and physical examination are the primary means of evaluation and determine the need for further testing. Family history and the presence

Table 7.26 Differential diagnosis for baldness

Telogen effluvium
Postpartum
Medications
Stress
Medical illness/malnutrition
Scarring (cicatrical) alopecia
Skin infection
Inflammatory skin disease (e.g., discoid lupus)
Skin cancer
Chemical agents
Androgenic alopecia
Hereditary
Senescent
Androgenic endocrine abnormality (e.g., adrenal, ovarian, pituitary)
Androgenic medications
Alopecia areata
Traction alopecia
Tinea capitus

of virilizing features and hirsutism are important pieces of information. In this patient, the differential diagnosis for her hair loss primarily includes androgenic alopecia, senescent alopecia, or telogen effluvium. The absence of virulization or hirsutism obviates the need for testosterone or DHEAS levels at this time. An abdominal CT scan would be ordered to assess for an androgen-secreting tumor and thus is also not necessary. In the absence of scarring or skin abnormalities in the scalp, a biopsy would not be warranted. Senescent alopecia and androgenic alopecia may present with a similar male pattern of hair loss, but with androgenic alopecia there is usually a family history of baldness and earlier age of onset (before age 50). No laboratory will confirm these diagnoses and topical minoxidil may be helpful in both cases. Finasteride has also been used for androgenic alopecia. Telogen effluvium is a diffuse hair loss generally associated with an underlying traumatic event, medical illness, or medications. The primary approach is to search for underlying medical diseases, such as anemia or hypothyroidism, and treat any identified disease. In persistent cases without an identified cause, topical minoxidil has been used to shift the follicles into an anagen phase. See Table 7.26.

120. A

Physicians should obtain a fall history on geriatric patients on at least an annual basis. Office assessment of balance and gait should occur following a fall. For a patient with recurrent falls or gait difficulties, the best approach to evaluating and trying to prevent falls is a multidisciplinary one. The medical evaluation should include review of medications, orthostatic blood pressure and pulse, cardiac exam, and neurologic exam including cognitive assessment. Several medications, notably psychotropic medications, have been implicated in increasing the risks for falling in geriatric patients. Referral for physical therapy for exercise and gait training has been shown to be of benefit. Evaluation for use of assistive devices may also be of benefit. Occupational therapy assessment of the home environment can identify factors that might increase the risks for falling as well as lead to provision of preventive devices, such as raised toilet seats or handbars. Use of restraints has consistently been shown to increase the risk for injury and thus should be avoided.

Chapter 8

Community Medicine Questions

1. A true statement concerning disability is which of the following?
A. Disability is determined solely by physical impairment.
B. There is a single system for determining disability.
C. Disability is an administrative concept.
D. The definition of disability is fixed and unchanging.
E. Impairment is a subjective determination that can be medically documented.

2. The U.S. Preventive Services Task Force recommends that all sexually active women be screened for disease based on risk assessment. In high-risk women, which of the following is not recommended screening?
A. Syphilis
B. Chlamydia infection
C. Hepatitis C infection
D. Genital herpes simplex virus

3. A true statement concerning the material safety data sheet (MSDS) is:
A. Required by the FDA for all pharmaceutical products
B. Includes all possible health effects
C. Lists all active ingredients
D. Includes a phone number to contact the manufacturer for further information
E. Does not include information about the physical characteristics and reactivity properties

4. Which of the following is true?
A. After acute infection with parvovirus B19, no further evaluation of the fetus is required.
B. Parvovirus B19 has a long incubation period, with patients becoming symptomatic 21 to 28 days following exposure.
C. Maternal parvovirus IgM and IgG should be checked 2 weeks after exposure to determine if acute infection has occurred.
D. More than 90% of women have immunity to parvovirus B19 during the childbearing years secondary to childhood exposure to the virus.
E. The most common presentation of acute infection parvovirus B19 in adults is fever with a facial rash that gives a "slapped cheek" appearance.

5. An absolute criterion for the commercial drivers license (CDL) includes which of the following?
A. Vision must be 20/40 or better without corrective lens.

B. Hearing loss must be no greater than the average of 40 dB at 500; 1,000; and 2,000 Hz in the better ear without aids.
C. Disqualified by a clinical diagnosis of type 2 diabetes mellitus controlled with an oral agent.
D. Disqualified by a history of heart disease.
E. Each hand must possess five normal fingers.

6. You are a medical director of a nursing home from which a number of patients were recently transferred to the hospital with complications of influenza. In deciding whether to order prophylactic treatment for all other residents in the nursing home, you rely primarily on predicting the likely benefit of prophylaxis in all patients, balanced with the potential adverse effects that your treatment may cause. This approach to decision making best illustrates which of the following ethical theories?
A. Kantian theory
B. Utilitarian theory
C. Deontological theory
D. Theory of prima facia duties

7. The recommendation of the U.S. Preventive Services Task Force regarding the routine use of aspirin for primary prevention of myocardial infarction in asymptomatic adults is best categorized by which of the following?
A. Insufficient evidence to recommend for or against aspirin use
B. Recommended for men, but against its use in women
C. Recommended for women, but against its use in men
D. Recommend for patients at increased risk for coronary heart disease
E. Treatment should be limited to only 5 years.

8. All of the following are true of patients exposed to an index case of meningococcal meningitis *except*:
A. Household contacts of the index case should receive prophylaxis.
B. Cipro 500 mg PO in a single dose is adequate prophylaxis for adults.
C. Day care contacts exposed to the index case 2 weeks prior to the onset of symptoms should receive prophylaxis.
D. Hospital personnel having casual contact with the patient should not receive antibiotic prophylaxis.
E. Rifampin PO bid × 4 doses can be used for prophylaxis of children.

9. Which of the following is a true statement concerning respirator use in the workplace?

A. The Occupational Safety and Health Administration (OSHA) requires that anyone who uses respiratory protection at work to be screened annually to ensure they can wear it safely.

B. No OSHA standards exist for respiratory exposure to specific substances.

C. Respiratory protection standards apply to masks used to prevent tuberculosis transmission.

D. The use of a self-contained breathing apparatus reduces workload.

E. Masks are made so one size fits all.

10. Which of the following chest x-ray patterns would you expect to see in a patient with inhalational anthrax?

A. No chest x-ray evidence of infection

B. Prominent mediastinum with pleural effusions in the absence of parenchymal involvement

C. Parenchymal consolidation

D. Alveolar interstitial pattern

E. Pulmonary edema

11. Which of the following is false?

A. Casual sexual relationships are more common among travelers.

B. Using alcohol is a risk factor for an STD.

C. Use condoms for sexual intercourse with new partners.

D. Begin ciprofloxacin prior to travel to reduce the risk of acquiring gonorrhea.

E. Commercial sex workers are at higher risk of HIV infection.

12. Factors associated with thromboembolism and air travel include all of the following *except*:

A. Coach seating

B. Recent surgery

C. A history of prior deep venous thrombosis

D. High fluid intake

E. Alcohol ingestion

13. An advantage of case–control studies over prospective cohort studies includes which of the following?

A. Less expensive to complete

B. Provide more accurate estimates of risk

C. More useful for studying common conditions

D. Have fewer problems with recall bias

E. Multiple disease outcomes can be studied

14. A true statement concerning routine health care of a 45-year-old lesbian includes which of the following?

A. A Pap smear is not needed if her current partner is a woman.

B. The risk of human papillomavirus is negligible.

C. Fewer than 10% of lesbians have had intercourse with men.

D. Mammography is not recommended.

E. The risk of alcohol and substance abuse may be greater.

15. The Hippocratic Oath includes statements that apply directly to all of the following *except*:

A. Abortion

B. Physician-assisted suicide

C. Sexual relations with patients

D. Confidentiality

E. Refusing to care for certain patients

16. A true statement concerning the Americans with Disabilities Act (ADA) is:

A. The ADA is designed to screen for disabilities and limit such individuals from working.

B. By definition, a person is disabled if he or she has a physical or mental impairment that substantially limits work ability.

C. The ADA prohibits inquiries about a disability before a job offer is made.

D. The ADA prohibits assessment about disability after a job offer is made.

E. The ADA allows testing of skills unrelated to job performance.

17. A true statement concerning workers' compensation and Social Security is which of the following?

A. Workers' compensation requires that an individual establish employer negligence.

B. Lost work expenses usually comprise approximately two-thirds of the cost of a workers' compensation claim.

C. Social Security disability is for conditions severe enough to prevent a person from working for at least 1 month.

D. The Social Security Administration and Supplemental Security Income Program cover families of workers injured on the job.

E. Coverage by workers' compensation is voluntary.

18. A 72-year-old male is taking ibuprofen for pain from metastatic prostate cancer. He asks you for a stronger medication to relieve his pain and wonders whether meperidine (Demerol) is a good choice. He remembers having good relief of postoperative pain from Demerol injections in the past. Which of the following is true regarding the use of oral meperidine for this patient?

A. Parenteral and oral doses are equianalgesic.

B. It offers a longer therapeutic half-life that most other oral opioids.

C. Toxic levels of its metabolite can accumulate.

D. It is less addictive than morphine.

E. It provides better relief of "bone pain" than other opioids.

19. A true statement concerning OSHA is which of the following?

A. OSHA requires only businesses that employ more than 1,000 workers to keep a written log of work-related illnesses and injuries.

B. A log of injuries must include all events, even those involving only first aid.

C. Hepatitis B vaccination after blood-borne pathogen exposure is an exception to the record-keeping requirement.

D. OSHA monitors workplace logs and inspects sites that have increased work-related illness and injury.

E. The definition of workplace injury is the same as for workers' compensation.

20. Mr. G is a 68-year-old male who presents to your office for an initial history and physical examination. He smokes one pack of cigarettes each day and used to take a medication for hypertension until he "ran out" 6 months ago. He rides a bicycle once a week for exercise. His physical exam reveals a blood pressure of 170/102, a dark, flat 1-cm pigmented skin lesion on his back, and no other significant abnormalities. Which of the following would be considered a *secondary* prevention task or intervention for Mr. G?

A. Advising him about smoking cessation to prevent lung cancer

B. Treating his hypertension to prevent a stroke

C. Advising him to wear a bicycle helmet to prevent injury

D. Screening for prostate cancer with a prostate-specific antigen (PSA) test

E. Advising him about a healthy diet

21. Which of the following is true regarding the use of child restraints in motor vehicles in the United States?

A. All but a few states have laws regarding the use of child restraints.

B. Safety standards for car seat manufacturers are regulated by federal law.

C. Mandatory use of car seats for infants is regulated by federal law.

D. In most states with child restraint laws, 3-year-old children may use adult seat belts.

E. Newborn transportation seats are equally effective in both forward- and rearward-facing configurations.

22. Outrage over the lack of informed consent in a single observational research study in the United States prompted the establishment of institutional review boards and federally regulated ethical standard for medical research. The research study that prompted these policy changes was designed to document (choose one):

A. The effects of radiation exposure

B. The natural history of syphilis

C. The outcomes of illegal abortions

D. The effects of poverty on infant health

E. The course of untreated tuberculosis

23. A true statement concerning occupational hearing screening includes which of the following?

A. Occupational hearing loss is usually conductive in nature.

B. Audiometric testing is unable to quantitatively assess the success of a hearing conservation program.

C. Speech hearing is reflected primarily in the range of 4,000 Hz and above.

D. Ninety percent of workers who are exposed to excessive noise levels of 90 dB or greater (equivalent to a subway) will eventually suffer hearing loss.

E. Noise-induced hearing loss is most severe around 4,000 Hz and may mimic presbycusis.

24. Current U.S. Preventive Services Task Force recommendations for breast cancer screening found which of the following to have the strongest evidence for patient benefit?

A. Breast self-examination

B. Clinical breast examination

C. Mammograms every 1 or 2 years starting at age 40

D. Baseline mammogram at age 35

E. Genetic screening for breast cancer risk

25. Which of the following is *true* regarding pinworm infection?

A. It is unnecessary to repeat testing after definitive treatment because reinfection is uncommon.

B. Abdominal pain, anemia, and diarrhea are common symptoms.

C. The pinworm larva burrows through the host skin to infect the host, occasionally causing a local, pruritic inflammatory reaction.

D. Eggs are only infective for several hours after they are shed by the host.

E. The diagnostic test of choice is a "Scotch tape" test of the perianal region because O&P is often falsely negative.

26. The following patients are candidates for postexposure empiric therapy with isoniazid *except*:

A. Children younger than 5 years old with known tuberculosis exposure, even if the PPD is negative

B. HIV-positive patients with positive PPD and negative CXR

C. Patient with positive PPD and an upper lobe infiltrate

D. Health care worker with recent PPD conversion

27. Family physicians frequently counsel patients to increase physical activity and exercise to improve their health. The strength of scientific evidence for counseling in primary care to promote physical activity shows:

A. Strong evidence to counsel adults

B. Strong evidence to counsel both adults and adolescents

C. Strong evidence, but only to counsel adults with obesity

D. Insufficient evidence to recommend for or against counseling

E. Benefits of obesity counseling in children have been well studied

28. Which of the following research designs will provide the most accurate estimate of disease incidence in the study sample?

A. A nationwide telephone poll survey

B. A large case–control study

C. A series of case reports

D. A comprehensive meta-analysis

E. A prospective cohort study

29. You have uncovered a probable lung cancer on chest film of one of your favorite patients. An appropriate approach to delivering this "bad news" might include:

A. Discussing the finding in professional jargon

B. Arranging a referral and suggesting the patient does not need to see you again

C. Keeping your feelings to yourself

D. Minimizing the problem and suggesting it is unlikely to be serious

E. Assessing and responding to the patient's emotional state

30. Which of the following is *false* regarding oral creatine dietary supplementation?

A. Creatine is most beneficial for aerobic endurance exercise.

B. Creatine recommended maintenance dose is 2 or 3 g per day.

C. Creatine's most common side effects are muscle cramping, GI disturbance, and renal dysfunction.

D. Creatine's effects are dose related without a ceiling effect.

E. Creatine users may gain weight due to water retention.

31. In the event of a biologic terrorist attack, botulinum toxin may be used as a potential weapon. The following is *true* concerning botulinum toxin:

A. The toxin is heat stable and can withstand temperatures up to 100°C for 30 to 60 minutes.

B. The toxin affects primarily sympathetic nerve terminals, leading to profound hypotension, salivation, and incontinence.

C. Inspiratory pressure and vital capacity should be closely monitored because respiratory failure requiring mechanical ventilation occurs in 30% of victims.
D. If wound botulism has occurred, it is not necessary to debride the wound if it appears to be well healing.
E. Antibiotics are the mainstay of treatment in infant botulism.

32. A true statement concerning shift work includes which of the following?
A. Shift rotation should proceed from night to evening to day.
B. Shift workers are just as well rested as non-shift workers.
C. Workers older than age 40 adjust better to shift work.
D. Shift workers have higher rates of heavy drinking and job loss.
E. Complete adaptation to shift work occurs in most individuals given enough time.

33. Mr. T is a 72-year-old male with hypertension but otherwise in good health who is admitted to the hospital with sudden onset of left-sided weakness, slurred speech, and difficulty swallowing. Four days later, after being transferred to a rehabilitation unit with a nasogastric feeding tube in place, he develops aspiration pneumonia and fever. That night, his dyspnea worsens, he experiences acute respiratory arrest, and he dies despite resuscitation attempts. Causes of death on Mr. T's death certificate would most accurately be listed as (choose one):
A. Immediate cause: cerebrovascular accident (CVA); secondary to hypertension
B. Immediate cause: respiratory arrest; secondary to CVA
C. Immediate cause: respiratory failure; secondary to aspiration pneumonia
D. Immediate cause: aspiration pneumonia; secondary to CVA
E. Immediate cause: CVA; secondary to cerebrovascular atherosclerosis

34. A true statement concerning Medicare and Medicaid is which of the following?
A. Medicare is a federal program for children of impoverished families.
B. Medicaid coverage varies by state and has only partial federal funding.
C. Medicare covers outpatient prescription drugs provided they are on a select Part C formulary.
D. Medicaid benefits are set federally and do not vary by state.
E. Medicare benefits vary by state.

35. All of the following are true regarding ciguatera food poisoning *except*:
A. Grouper, red snapper, amberjack, and barracuda are the most common species of fish implicated in ciguatera food poisoning.
B. Ciguatoxic fish look, smell, and taste normal.
C. Ciguatoxin is unaffected by normal cooking procedures.
D. Breast-feeding infants are unaffected by maternal ciguatoxin ingestion.
E. Clinical manifestations include gastrointestinal manifestations, paresthesias, bradycardia, hypotension, and rash.

36. Which of the following is true regarding obesity?
A. Orlistat is an oral medication whose mechanism of action is appetite suppression by inhibiting reuptake of norepinephrine.
B. Bariatric surgery is a recommended option for patients whose BMI is greater than 30.

C. Weight loss of 0.5 kg/week can be obtained by decreasing daily intake by 1,000 kcal below the intake required to maintain current weight.
D. An overweight patient is defined as a person with a BMI greater than 20.
E. Fenfluramine was withdrawn from the market primarily because of its lack of efficacy.

37. Which of the following is true?
A. Medicare was begun as a demonstration project for FDR's New Deal.
B. Medicare covers all medical expenses.
C. Medicare Part A covers hospital services and some hospice, nursing home, and skilled care.
D. Medicare payment to hospitals is based on a usual and customary basis.
E. Medicare pays over 90% of health care expenses of elders.

38. In order to enroll a patient in a clinical trial of a new medication, the patient must read, understand, and voluntarily sign an informed consent statement (ICS). Federal regulations mandate that certain elements be included in the ICS. These elements include all of the following *except*:
A. Description of the purpose of the research
B. Potential risks from participating in the study
C. Alternative treatments or intervention
D. Encouragement to complete study procedures
E. Description of payments or reimbursement to participants

39. "Tertiary prevention" is best represented by which of the following?
A. Preventive efforts in an acute hospital setting
B. Physical therapy for gait training following a stroke with hemiplegia
C. A vaccine program to prevent pneumococcal pneumonia in nursing home patients
D. Screening for coronary artery disease using new helical CT scanning technology
E. International efforts to eradicate polio

40. Disease X is most accurately diagnosed with an expensive, invasive endoscopy procedure. A simple screening blood test is available with a positive value considered any value over 140. Approximately 10% of people with disease X have a value between 120 and 140, and 10% fall below 120. An expert panel decides to recommend lowering the cutoff for a "positive" screening test to 120. The effect(s) of this recommendation will be?
A. Increased specificity of the screening test
B. Increased sensitivity of the screening test
C. Fewer false-positive screening test results
D. An increase in the positive predictive value of the screening test
E. A shift in the receiver-operating characteristic (ROC) curve for the screening test

41. Which of the following is true?
A. The Omnibus Budget Reconciliation Act (OBRA) of 1987 requires spouses to sell the family home to meet the Medicaid asset test prior to nursing home entry.
B. Medicaid is prohibited from developing prospective capitation-based programs and HMO alternatives for its enrollees.

C. Medicaid provides up to one-half of payments for long-term care.

D. Medicare recipients cannot receive Medicaid benefits.

E. Medicaid benefits are explicitly specified by the federal government and cannot vary by state or plan.

42. A patient is traveling to Southeast Asia and is concerned about the risk of dengue fever. You advise:

A. The risk of dengue in Southeast Asia is very small.

B. Avoid rats and other potential vectors of dengue.

C. Begin ciprofloxacin daily beginning 1 week prior to travel.

D. Most cases of dengue are self-limited.

E. Vaccination is recommended.

43. The "gate control theory" is probably the most widely known theory designed to understand mechanisms of pain. Which of the following is true about the gate control theory of pain?

A. Helps explain variations in individual responses to similar painful injuries

B. Centers on serotonin "pain gates" in the brain

C. Explains the mechanisms of pain control generated by opioid medications

D. Centers on the differences between sharp, light touch, and position sense

E. Emphasizes dopamine-based "pain control gates" in the hypothalamus

44. A true statement concerning hospice care is which of the following?

A. Medicare coverage for hospice care is on a fee-for-service basis.

B. To be eligible for hospice benefits, a physician must certify that the life expectancy is less than 1 month.

C. A 20% copayment is required for hospice care.

D. Most drugs are covered by Medicare for hospice care.

E. The median length of hospice care is 6 months for patients under Medicare hospice coverage.

45. The results of one portion of the Women's Health Initiative study were widely reported in medical journals and the popular press in 2002. The results of this study suggest that in counseling postmenopausal women regarding hormone replacement therapy (HRT), physicians should:

A. Advise all postmenopausal women to use HRT

B. Advise primarily women at high risk for cardiovascular disease to use HRT

C. Advise women at risk for colorectal cancer to stop taking HRT

D. Weigh the risks and benefits of HRT for each woman before advising treatment

E. Advise against HRT for most women because the study showed an increase in mortality in the HRT treatment group

46. A true statement concerning elders in the community includes which of the following?

A. The majority of elderly men live with their spouse.

B. Most elderly men are widowers.

C. Over 95% of elders older than age 85 report functional impairment.

D. The life expectancy of a woman age 65 is 5 years.

E. Over 50% of elders (older than age 65) live in nursing homes.

47. The primary duty of an institutional review board is to:

A. Review the results of research studies

B. Review the scientific validity of proposed research

C. Detect scientific misconduct of researchers

D. Facilitate the proper reporting of research results

E. Ensure adequate informed consent of research subjects

48. The following treatments are appropriate for calcium channel blocker overdose in an adult *except*:

A. Glucagon 5 to 15 mg IV bolus

B. Calcium chloride 2 mg IV, slowly

C. Amiodarone 150 mg IV

D. High-dose insulin infusion (1 U/kg/hour) with D10W

E. Activated charcoal 50 to 100 g PO

49. A 70-year-old male is receiving home-based hospice care for advanced pulmonary fibrosis. He does not want to be intubated or receive mechanical ventilation. He requires oxygen by nasal cannula and his medication regimen includes inhaled bronchodilators, prednisone, and lorazepam. Despite these medications, he complains of severe symptoms of dyspnea. At this point, the addition of oral morphine to his regimen would be:

A. Contraindicated due to sedative affects

B. Contraindicated due to respiratory depression affects

C. Contraindicated due to adverse interactions with his other medication(s)

D. Indicated as trial to control dyspnea

E. Contraindicated due to inadequate supporting literature

50. All the following are potential pulmonary risk factors for patients undergoing surgery *except*:

A. Preoperative FVC less than 20

B. Confusion on neurologic assessment

C. pH of 7.28 on arterial blood gas

D. Postoperative ambulation expected no sooner than 48 hours

E. History of controlled hypertension

51. Which of the following is *true* regarding the treatment of obesity?

A. The National Institutes of Health (NIH) recommends that herbal supplements be used as adjuncts for weight loss.

B. Xenical (Orlistat) has no effect on the absorption of fat-soluble vitamins.

C. NIH guidelines state that nonpharmacologic therapies should be used for 6 months before considering weight-loss drugs.

D. Bupropion (Wellbutrin), metformin (Glucophage), and topiramate (Topamax) are all currently approved by the FDA for the pharmacologic treatment of obesity.

E. Ephedrine has no serious side effects when used for the treatment of obesity.

52. A true statement concerning antipsychotic drug use in the nursing home is which of the following?

A. An antipsychotic may be used to control noise making.

B. An antipsychotic may be prescribed to control insomnia.

C. An antipsychotic cannot be used to control delusional disorders.

D. An antipsychotic must be used in cases of schizophrenia.

E. Antipsychotics must be monitored regularly for safety and efficacy, and dosage reduction efforts must occur regularly.

53. In formulating guidelines for preventive services, panels such as the U.S. Preventive Services Task Force consider the strength of evidence from published studies and other sources. Different types of research design carry more weight than others when determining the strength of evidence for a particular preventive intervention or screening test. In the hierarchy of evidence considered by the U.S. Preventive Services and other groups, which of the following would be considered "stronger" evidence than a case–control study?

A. A National Institutes of Health consensus panel

B. Multiple case reports

C. Expert opinion

D. Randomized controlled trial

E. Cohort study

54. Which of the following is appropriate advice for travelers?

A. Advise patients with diabetes to pack all syringes in their checked luggage; current FAA regulations preclude the carrying of such items.

B. A patient with a room air PaO_2 of 70 mmHg should be advised to use supplemental oxygen.

C. Pregnant travelers should restrict fluids and remain seated throughout the flight.

D. Patients with well-controlled seizure disorders should increase their antiseizure medication 3 days prior to travel.

E. Pregnant travelers should not travel by air after the first trimester because of the increased risk of premature labor.

55. Which of the following is *false*?

A. Hispanics are more likely to be uninsured and less likely to see a physician than the general population.

B. Two-thirds of migrant adults test positive for tuberculosis exposure.

C. Three-fourths of the people in the United States who have difficulty paying their medical bills have some form of insurance.

D. Women and minorities are less likely to be diagnosed with angina when presenting with the same symptoms as men.

E. Homeless children have a higher incidence of ear infections, diarrhea, and asthma than the general population of children.

56. The following test is recommended for a 35-year-old, previously well woman undergoing sinus surgery:

A. Chest x-ray

B. Liver function tests

C. Electrocardiogram

D. Creatinine

E. None of the above are routinely required.

57. Medicare covers all of the following preventive interventions *except*:

A. Routine tetanus vaccinations

B. Pap smears

C. Mammograms

D. Fecal occult blood screening

E. Screening colonoscopy

58. For a 75-year-old female with pain from metastatic breast cancer, you have prescribed 30 mg of sustained-release oral morphine every 12 hours, with 5 mg of immediate-release oral morphine every 3 hours as needed for "breakthrough pain." A home health nurse calls to report that the patient has started taking 10 mg of the "breakthrough" morphine every 2 hours. You should initially (choose one):

A. Ask the nurse to warn the patient about oversedation and to follow the prescription.

B. Ask the nurse to assess the patient's level and pattern of pain.

C. Change the breakthrough medication to oxycodone or another longer acting opioid every 3 hours.

D. Discontinue the breakthrough prescription and increase the sustained-release oral morphine dose.

E. Add a nonsteroidal anti-inflammatory drug.

59. All of the following are true *except*:

A. Campylobacter is the most common cause of bacterial food poisoning in the United States.

B. Ciguatera fish poisoning is the most commonly reported food-borne disease associated with eating fish in the United States.

C. *Staphylococcus aureus* is the most common cause of toxin-related food poisoning in the United States.

D. Norwalk virus is the most common viral cause of dysentery in infants in the United States.

E. Salmonella growth can be controlled by refrigeration below 40°F.

60. The fundamental elements of the patient–physician relationship described in the American Medical Association's Code of Medical Ethics state that a patient has the right to all of the following *except* (choose one):

A. Information from physicians regarding treatment

B. Confidentiality

C. Timely attention to his or her health care needs

D. Continuity of health care

E. Treat all patients presenting for treatment

61. According to the U.S. Preventive Services Task Force guidelines, chemoprophylaxis to prevent tuberculosis should be considered in patients with a positive Mantoux (PPD) skin test. The interpretation of the PPD depends, in part, on the risk profile of the patient for TB. A positive Mantoux test for patients at low risk, high risk, and very high risk, respectively, are induration of (choose one):

A. Low risk, 5 mm; high risk, 10 mm; very high risk, 10 mm

B. Low risk, 10 mm; high risk, 10 mm; very high risk, 15 mm

C. Low risk, 15 mm; high risk, 10 mm; very high risk, 10 mm

D. Low risk, 15 mm; high risk, 10 mm; very high risk, 5 mm

E. 10 mm is the criteria for all risk levels.

62. In order to prevent injuries from hot water in the household, patients should be advised to set their hot water temperature to (choose one):

A. Less than 100°F

B. Less than 118°F

C. Less than 120°F

D. 120°F to 130°F

E. Less than 140°F

63. Of the following, the leading preventable cause of death while traveling is:
A. Boating accidents
B. AIDS
C. Motor vehicle accidents
D. Hepatitis B
E. Ebola virus

64. Which of following preventive services can be recommended based on effectiveness demonstrated in large randomized, controlled trials?
A. Prostate cancer screening using PSA testing
B. Colorectal cancer screening using fecal occult blood testing (FOBT)
C. Advising the use of child restraints in motor vehicles
D. Counseling older adults how to prevent falls
E. Screening for diabetes mellitus in teenagers

65. Rifampin is the drug of choice for postexposure prophylaxis for household contacts of a patient with:
A. *Escherichia coli* sepsis
B. *Haemophilus influenzae* type B disease
C. West Nile virus
D. Streptococcal meningitis
E. Staphylococcal skin infections

66. Which of the following statements is true for patients who access the Medicare hospice benefit?
A. All medication costs are covered under hospice care.
B. Under Medicare rules, the patient may only receive hospice care for 6 months.
C. Two physicians must agree that a patient is eligible for the hospice benefit.
D. Patients with end-stage heart failure must meet specific congestive heart failure criteria.
E. Acute hospitalization is not covered by the Medicare hospice benefit.

67. Which of the following is *true* about treatment success for smoking cessation?
A. Physician advice to quit results in no greater success rates than a patient going cold turkey.
B. Buproprion is the most successful aid to cessation.
C. Nicotine replacement therapy coupled with counseling is the most successful intervention for cessation.
D. Using more than one form of nicotine replacement is no more effective than a single form.
E. A quit rate of 50% is the goal with any intervention.

68. The following is *true* concerning lead toxicity in children:
A. Dimercaprol therapy is instituted immediately for lead levels between 10 and 15 μg/dL.
B. After dimercaprol is administered, gut decontamination is not necessary if lead fragments are present in the stomach.
C. Dimercaprol should be administered orally at least 4 hours after gut decontamination.
D. Lead toxicity produces a typical pattern mimicking iron deficiency anemia, characterized by hypochromia and microcytosis.
E. Diarrhea is a common presenting symptom.

69. The mother of a 10-year-old child calls on Saturday night because of concern about rabies exposure. Her child was bitten by a squirrel earlier in the day while he was playing in the park. The squirrel was "acting strangely" according to the child's report. You should:
A. Send the child to the emergency department immediately for human rabies immune globulin (HRIG).
B. Advise that HRIG should be given, but that it can wait until your office is open on Monday.
C. Consider immediate HRIG but only based on the size of the wound.
D. Recommend a rabies vaccine series rather than HRIG.
E. Reassure the mother that rabies is not associated with squirrel bites.

70. A new published study reveals a statistically significant increase in the incidence of breast cancer among postmenopausal women who take hormone replacement therapy. In order to decide whether this new evidence should influence his or her approach to counseling female patients, a physician should especially consider all of the following factors *except*:
A. The study population
B. The "p values" from statistical analysis were very small (less than 0.01)
C. The outcomes of other similar previous studies
D. The study design (case–control, prospective cohort, etc.)

71. When considering how published studies impact the practice of medicine, the acronym POEM stands for:
A. Problem-oriented effective management
B. Patient-oriented evidence that matters
C. Published objective evidence for management
D. Peer-reviewed objective evidence in medicine
E. Primary care-oriented effective medicine

72. If a 45-year-old man comes into the office with his 5-year-old son, planning to take him to Honduras, what medication might you give his son for traveler's diarrhea prophylaxis?
A. Ciprofloxacin
B. Doxycycline
C. Azithromycin (Zithromax)
D. Cephalexin
E. Penicillin

73. Which of the following clinical findings do methanol and ethylene glycol ingestion have in common?
A. Hypocalcemia
B. Retinal edema
C. Fluorescent urine with Wood's lamp examination
D. Kussmaul respirations
E. Elevated formic acid level

74. Disease X is a newly discovered fatal infectious disease diagnosed by a researcher on an isolated Pacific island that is home to 10,000 residents. In Figure 8-1, "A" represents the onset of disease, and "B" represents death from the disease for the first 10 cases of disease X diagnosed on the island. Which of the following is true?
A. The 1-month incidence during February was 4 in 10,000.
B. The prevalence on April 1 was greater than the prevalence on May 1.

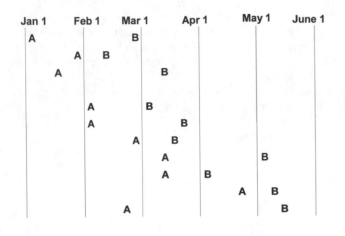

Figure 8-1. *The onset of disease (A) and death from the disease (B) for the first 10 cases of disease X, a newly discovered fatal infectious disease diagnosed by a researcher on an isolated Pacific island with 10,000 inhabitants.*

C. A new treatment that greatly lengthens the time from onset until death would tend to decrease prevalence of disease X.

D. Prevalence of disease X steadily increased from February 1 through May 1.

75. During the initial years of the AIDS epidemic, there were no specific antiviral treatments available for the HIV virus. In the U.S. population, more recent advances in antiretroviral treatments have resulted in (choose one):

A. A decreased incidence of HIV infection

B. An increased incidence of HIV infection

C. A decreased prevalence of HIV infection

D. An increased prevalence of HIV infection

E. No significant affect on HIV incidence or prevalence

76. For some patients with terminal illness in the past few hours or days before death, the "death rattle" is often:

A. A sign of infection

B. Associated with gastrointestinal symptoms

C. Disturbing to caregivers

D. Caused by brief, focal seizures

E. Accompanied by coughing

77. In providing palliative care for a patient with terminal illness near the end of life, the principle of "double effects" is best represented by which of the following procedures:

A. Using escalating doses of opioids to adequately control pain, even if it may hasten death

B. Providing spiritual counseling to both the patient and her family

C. Treating two different infections with a single antibiotic

D. Using oxygen for both dyspnea and angina

E. Prescribing two different types of pain medication

78. Which of the following statements is not true regarding malaria prevention?

A. Insect precautions, such as the use of protective clothing, mosquito nets, and 30% to 50% DEET, confer about 85% protection.

B. Ninety percent of patients that get malaria have no symptoms until returning home.

C. Medication prophylaxis is about 75% to 95% effective.

D. Mefloquine can have neuropsychiatric side effects such as hallucinations and paranoia.

E. Malarone (proguanil + atovaquone) is the cheapest antimalarial available.

79. Which of the following is *true* regarding phenylketonuria in pregnancy?

A. Phenylketonuria predisposes pregnant women to hyperemesis gravidarum.

B. An indiscriminate diet in a pregnant woman with phenylketonuria can lead to fetal anomalies.

C. Phenylketonuria is a risk factor for gestational diabetes.

D. A pregnant woman with phenylketonuria has a 50% chance of having an infant who is clinically affected.

80. The leading cause of mortality in U.S. travelers is:

A. Infection

B. Injury

C. Cancer

D. Cardiovascular

E. Suicide or homicide

81. Which of the following is false regarding babesiosis?

A. Babesiosis resembles malaria in that it causes fever, fatigue, and hemolytic anemia.

B. Babesiosis may be transmitted by blood transfusions.

C. Babesiosis may be transmitted to a fetus in utero.

D. Babesiosis is a zoonotic infection transmitted by a mosquito vector.

E. Babesiosis is diagnosed by the presence of ring-forms within erythrocytes.

82. One of the most important ethical principles in medical practice is the physician's duty to keep patient information confidential. In some cases, however, laws require physicians to break confidentiality in areas of public health or protection of vulnerable persons. All states have laws that require reporting of all of the following *except*:

A. Gonorrhea

B. Tuberculosis

C. Spousal abuse

D. Child abuse

E. Syphilis

83. Which of the following is the expected result of successful treatment of severe acute cyanide toxicity?

A. Hemolysis

B. Myoglobinuria

C. Methemoglobinemia

D. Hemoptysis

E. Hepatitis

84. Which of the following is false regarding the diet of vegetarians?

A. Vegetarians exhibit a lower rate of obesity, coronary artery disease, hypertension, and diverticular disease than omnivores.

B. Children following a strict vegetarian diet have lower growth velocity and lower total growth potential than age-matched omnivores.

C. Avoidance of all animal foods and milk places vegetarian children at risk for vitamin D and B12 deficiency.

D. There is an increased risk of anorexia nervosa and disordered eating among adolescent vegetarians compared to omnivore counterparts.

E. It may cause increased incidence of Wiscott–Aldrich syndrome.

85. Which of the following constitutes a positive PPD test?

A. Erythema greater than 5 mm in an HIV-positive patient

B. Induration 6 mm in diameter in an HIV-negative IV drug user

C. Erythema greater than 10 mm in a recent immigrant from Russia

D. Induration greater than 10 mm in a diabetic patient

E. 5 mm of erythema in a 3-year-old

86. All of the following concerning Dengue fever are true *except*:

A. The virus is transmitted to humans through a day-biting *Aedes aegypti* mosquito.

B. Symptoms include high fever, macular rash, and severe bone pain.

C. Laboratory findings include hemoconcentration and thrombocytosis.

D. Corticosteroids are not helpful.

E. Dengue fever patients may develop Dengue hemorrhagic fever.

87. Which of the following has good evidence to be included in routine screening for all asymptomatic adults older than the age of 50?

A. Routine screening for cutaneous melanoma

B. Routine screening for osteoporosis

C. Routine screening for lung cancer

D. Routine screening for depression

E. Routine screening for hepatitis B antibodies

88. Which of the following is the appropriate amount of folic acid for a patient contemplating pregnancy who has had a previous child with spina bifida?

A. Folate 0.1 mg daily

B. Folate 0.4 mg daily

C. Folate 1.0 mg daily

D. Folate 4.0 mg daily

E. Folate 10.0 mg daily

89. A 62-year-old male with progressive pain from metastatic prostate cancer is taking a sustained-release oral morphine preparation for pain control. During an office visit he asks about "a pain patch" he heard about and whether it offers any advantages over his current treatment. The advantages of a transdermal fentanyl patch for this patient might include which of the following?

A. Lower cost

B. Less constipation

C. Less chance of drug dependence

D. Once-daily dosing

E. Increased risk of hallucinations

90. Which of the following is not a covered service under the Medicare hospice benefit?

A. Home health aide services

B. Homemaker services

C. Physical therapy

D. Laboratory testing

E. Transportation for physician office visits

91. Mr. F. is a 54-year-old asymptomatic male with a 40 pack-year history of cigarette smoking who presents to your office for a routine physical examination. Ordering a chest x-ray to screen for lung cancer for Mr. F. would be best described as which of the following?

A. Primary prevention; supported by U.S. Preventive Services Task Force (USPSTF) guidelines

B. Primary prevention; not supported by USPSTF guidelines

C. Secondary prevention; supported by USPSTF guidelines

D. Secondary prevention; not supported by USPSTF guidelines

92. The ability of a test to detect disease when the disease is truly present is a description of which of the following?

A. Sensitivity

B. Specificity

C. Positive predictive value

D. Negative predictive value

E. Selection bias

93. In a study to determine the accuracy of fecal occult blood testing (FOBT) to detect polyps in the colon, 1,100 adults older than age 65 completed a six-card FOBT screening, followed by a full colonoscopy 1 week later to detect polyps. From the results listed in Table 8.1, which of the following is true?

A. Sensitivity of FOBT equals 60/60 (50%).

B. Specificity of FOBT equals 40/60 (67%).

C. Positive predictive value of FOBT equals 60/940 (6%).

D. Negative predictive value of FOBT equals 940/980 (96%).

E. The prevalence of polyps cannot be determined.

94. Which of the following procedures is an indication for subacute bacterial endocarditis prophylaxis in a susceptible patient?

A. Routine dental filling

B. Circumcision

C. Cardiac catheterization

D. Root canal

E. Tympanostomy tube insertion

95. The Goldman scale helps determine the cardiac risk of noncardiac procedures. All of the following are risk factors *except*:

A. Age older than 70 years

B. Signs of congestive heart failure

Table 8.1

	Poly No.		Total
	p(s) Present	Polyps Present	
FOBT			
Positive	60	60	120
Negative	40	94	980
Total	100	1000	

C. Aortic operation

D. Premature atrial contractions

E. Recent myocardial infarction (less than 6 months ago)

96. Appropriate perioperative medication management includes which of the following?

A. For patients with well-controlled diabetes, administer the full dose of insulin the morning of surgery.

B. Never augment the dose of a corticosteroid in a patient on long-term corticosteroid therapy.

C. Continue beta-blockers the morning of surgery with a sip of water.

D. Unless a patient quits smoking for 1 year, there is no advantage to perioperative smoking cessation.

E. Discontinue aspirin use the day before surgery to diminish the chance of bleeding.

97. The Public Health Service recommends five steps to effective smoking cessation counseling. Which of the following is not one of the recommended steps?

A. Asking a patient about tobacco use at every visit

B. Advising all tobacco users to quit

C. Assessing readiness to quit

D. Administering the Fagerstrom nicotine dependence assessment

E. Arranging follow-up

98. Which of the following is *true* regarding transmission of tuberculosis?

A. Patients with extrapulmonary tuberculosis are rarely infectious.

B. More than 1,000 bacilli are required to initiate a primary infection.

C. Infection is not possible without coming into direct contact with the patient.

D. A patient is only considered infectious if three consecutive sputums contain acid-fast bacilli.

E. PPD will turn positive within 48 hours of initial exposure.

99. A 29-year-old construction worker seeks a disability opinion from you regarding low back pain from a recent accident. Your examination is normal and you believe the patient is malingering. An appropriate response might include which of the following?

A. A prescription for long-acting opioid analgesic

B. Refusal to complete the disability form

C. Discussion with the patient and family to explore job satisfaction

D. A referral to a pain clinic

E. Prescription of an SSRI

100. When considering a living will or a durable power of attorney for health care, which of the following is true?

A. The contents of both documents are regulated by federal law.

B. A living will allows the patient to choose a health care proxy for decisions.

C. Either one can be easily revoked by the patient, either orally or in writing.

D. A living will takes precedence over the durable power of attorney in most cases.

E. Both a living will and a durable power of attorney must be executed by a judge to be legally accepted.

Chapter 8

Answer Key

1.	C	43.	A	85.	D
2.	C	44.	D	86.	C
3.	D	45.	D	87.	D
4.	C	46.	A	88.	D
5.	B	47.	E	89.	B
6.	B	48.	C	90.	E
7.	D	49.	D	91.	D
8.	C	50.	E	92.	A
9.	A	51.	C	93.	D
10.	B	52.	E	94.	D
11.	D	53.	D	95.	D
12.	D	54.	B	96.	C
13.	A	55.	B	97.	D
14.	E	56.	E	98.	A
15.	E	57.	A	99.	C
16.	C	58.	B	100.	C
17.	B	59.	D		
18.	C	60.	E		
19.	D	61.	D		
20.	D	62.	D		
21.	B	63.	C		
22.	B	64.	B		
23.	E	65.	B		
24.	C	66.	C		
25.	E	67.	C		
26.	C	68.	D		
27.	D	69.	E		
28.	E	70.	B		
29.	E	71.	B		
30.	A	72.	C		
31.	C	73.	D		
32.	D	74.	A		
33.	D	75.	D		
34.	B	76.	C		
35.	D	77.	A		
36.	C	78.	E		
37.	C	79.	B		
38.	D	80.	D		
39.	B	81.	D		
40.	B	82.	C		
41.	C	83.	C		
42.	D	84.	B		

Community Medicine Answers

1. C

Disability is an administrative concept defined by the agency or organization administering the program. The definition of disability may change and conditions may be added or deleted that are considered disabling. Impairment is an *objective* physical finding that can be documented. Physical impairment is only one factor in determining disability; others include age, training, and education.

2. C

The U.S. Preventive Services Task Force (USPSTF) strongly recommends that clinicians routinely screen all sexually active women at increased risk for infection. The USPSTF found no evidence that screening for HCV infection in adults at high risk leads to improved long-term health outcomes.

3. D

The MSDS is required by the Occupational Safety and Health Administration (OSHA) for hazardous chemicals. It includes the chemical components of the material, not necessarily "trade secret" ingredients. Also included are a manufacturer's phone number; the material's physical characteristics; reactivity properties; and spill, containment, and cleanup procedures. Although the MSDS may not list every potential health complication, it provides an informative resource for the health professional confronting an exposed or contaminated patient.

4. C

Parvovirus B19 viremia occurs about 7 days after exposure. If there is no prior immunity, IgM becomes positive 10 days after exposure. A positive IgM indicates acute infection, although false positives can occur. Parvovirus B19 is highly infectious and up to 35% of reproductive age women do not have protective immunity. With evidence of acute infection, ultrasound monitoring of the fetus for hydrops is performed for at least 10 to 15 weeks. Adults rarely develop the "slapped cheek" appearance that is common in children. Arthralgias, vasculitis, and malaise are more common presentations of parvovirus B19 in adults.

5. B

Absolute criteria for the CDL include the following: Vision must be 20/40 or better in each eye, with or without glasses, and peripheral vision must be at least 70 degrees; hearing loss must be no greater than 40 dB at 500; 1,000; and 2,000 Hz in the better ear without aids; there must be no history of diabetes mellitus requiring insulin; and there must be no history of epilepsy. There is no requirement

regarding the number of fingers. If these criteria are not met, the individual is disqualified regardless of the examiner's judgment.

6. B

Utilitarianism considers primarily the consequences of alternative actions in ethical decision making. The other theories listed are "duty-based" theories or deontologic approaches that maintain that the basis of duties and/or rights can be found in something other than evaluating the consequences of our actions.

7. D

The task force found good evidence that aspirin decreases the incidence of coronary heart disease in asymptomatic adults who are at increased risk for heart disease. There is also evidence that aspirin increases the incidence of gastrointestinal bleeding and the incidence of hemorrhagic strokes. No such 5-year limitation recommendation exists. The balance of benefits and harms is most favorable in patients at high risk of coronary heart disease but is also influenced by patient preferences.

8. C

Household contacts and day care contacts of the index case within the prior 7 days should receive antibiotic prophylaxis. Any person having contact with oral secretions of the patient should also receive prophylaxis. Hospital personnel who have had only casual or indirect contact with the patient do not require prophylaxis.

Rifampin can be used for all age groups for prophylaxis; ciprofloxacin is acceptable treatment for adults older than 18 years. Ceftriaxone can also be used for prophylaxis.

9. A

OSHA regulates respiratory protection in the workplace. Specific standards exist for such substances as arsenic, formaldehyde, and lead. The self-contained breathing apparatus is used in conditions of low or no oxygen. These devices substantially increase workload. Masks need to be fitted to the individual.

10. B

Inhalational anthrax will produce a chest x-ray with minimal to no parenchymal involvement. The primary radiographic finding is a prominent mediastinum with or without pleural effusions.

11. D

Advice for international travelers with regard to sexual relations is similar to that given to all patients. Up to 60% of individuals abroad will have a casual sexual relationship and in many areas of the world, especially Southeast Asia and Africa, HIV is extremely prevalent. Abstinence remains the best prevention; if sexual intercourse with a new partner occurs, the use of condoms is recommended. Individuals should not engage in sexual activity with commercial sex workers. Alcohol is known to lower inhibitions and is associated with STD. There is no chemoprophylaxis recommended for gonorrhea.

12. D
Many factors are associated with thromboembolism and air travel, including history of DVT, malignancy, recent surgery, cigarette use, immobility, coach seating, alcohol ingestion, and insufficient and poor fluid intake.

13. A
Case–control studies are less expensive since they involve data collection at only one point in time, compared with prospective cohort studies that follow participants over time, sometimes for multiple years. They are useful for studying rare conditions. "Case" definitions describe a single illness or injury that has already occurred, and participants are asked to recall previous risk exposures. Risk estimates are less accurate from case–control studies.

14. E
More than two-thirds of lesbians have had sexual intercourse with men. Routine Pap testing is still important. HPV DNA testing is positive in up to one-fifth of women reporting no prior sex with men. Mammography is now recommended for women age 40 to 50 years and lesbians are no exception. The risk of heavy alcohol use and substance abuse may be greater, and routine counseling is appropriate.

15. E
The Oath, dating from 4th-century Greece, includes statements that preclude physicians from performing abortions, giving a "deadly drug if asked for it," or from any sexual relations with patients or patients' family members. It includes a strong statement regarding patient confidentiality. It does not include any directive about refusing to care for certain patients or any promise to care for all patients who ask for assistance.

16. C
The ADA was enacted to ensure employment of people with disabilities. By definition, a person is disabled if he or she has a physical or mental impairment that substantially limits one or more major life activities (not just work-related). The ADA prohibits inquiries about a disability prior to job offer; however, a standard test of skills or aptitudes related to the essential functions of a job is permissible.

17. B
Workers' compensation is based on fair, no fault compensation, with mandatory coverage. Generally, workers and employees cannot be sued for work-related injuries. Lost work expenses comprise approximately two-thirds of the cost of a workers' compensation case. Social Security disability covers conditions severe enough to prevent an individual from working 1 year or longer. The SSI program covers the aged, blind, and disabled.

18. C
A number of qualities make meperidine a less desirable choice than other opioids for treatment of chronic pain. The oral form has poor bioavailability, a short therapeutic half-life, and toxic metabolites can accumulate with repeated dosing or in patients with renal insufficiency. The equianalgesic oral dose of meperidine is three times the parenteral dose.

19. D
OSHA requires businesses that employ 10 or more individuals to keep a written log of work-related illnesses and injuries. Those involving simple first aid are excluded, but these guidelines are somewhat arbitrary. Postexposure hepatitis B vaccination is considered a loggable medical intervention. The definition of injury may differ substantially from the state workers' compensation definition. OSHA does monitor logs to target workplace inspections.

20. D
Secondary preventive efforts are those that detect a condition that is present but has not yet caused symptoms, with the hope of improving treatment effectiveness (early detection of prostate or skin cancer by screening). Primary prevention is an action or intervention that decreases the risk of developing a condition—in this case preventing the onset of lung cancer, injury, or stroke.

21. B
All 50 states and the District of Columbia have laws governing the use of child restraints. Whereas safety standards for manufacturing child restraint devices are regulated by federal law, laws that regulate the use of child restraints are at the state level. Age requirements vary from state to state, but only six states have some provision for children younger than the age of 4 to use adult seat belts. Most states allow the use of adult seat belts starting somewhere between ages 4 and 6 years. Child seat manufacturer instructions need to be carefully followed. Many newborn child safety seats require a rearward-facing orientation for safe use.

22. B
The Tuskegee syphilis experiment was a longitudinal, observational study conducted by the U.S. Public Health Service from 1932 to 1972 to study the long-term effects of untreated tertiary syphilis among a group of African American men. Study patients, many of whom died from syphilis during the course of the study, were not informed of what disease they had, how serious the disease was, or about available treatments.

23. E
Noise-induced hearing loss (NIHL) is usually sensorineural and most severe around 4,000 Hz. It initially spares higher frequencies unlike presbycusis. Speech discrimination falls within the 500 to 2,000 Hz range and will eventually deteriorate with ongoing noise exposure. Individuals will often complain of difficulty comprehending speech against background noise. Approximately 25% of people will develop NIHL when exposed to noise above 90 dB habitually. OSHA regulates noise exposures above 85 dB over an 8-hour period. Serial audiometry provides a quantitative, reliable measure of a hearing conservation program's effectiveness.

24. C
The task force recommends mammograms every 1 or 2 years for women starting at age 40, but there is no good evidence to include a baseline mammogram at an earlier age. There is insufficient evidence to recommend for or against breast self-examinations or clinical breast examinations. The task force has not reviewed evidence regarding genetic screening.

25. E

Enterobius vermicularis (pinworm) infection is most common in young children and in their household contacts and parents. The transmission of this worm parasite is via the fecal–oral route with ingestion of the eggs leading to direct infection of the colon. The infection is often asymptomatic, with perianal itching the most common presenting complaint. Abdominal pain, anemia, and diarrhea are extremely rare and are usually only seen in patients with other bowel wall comorbidities such as ulcerative colitis. The female worm migrates to the anus to lay eggs, which can remain infective for weeks. O&P is notoriously poor at diagnosing pinworm infection due to false-negative studies. Because reinfection is common, retesting treated individuals is recommended 3 weeks after definitive therapy with mebendazole.

26. C

Candidates for postexposure empiric therapy with INH include:

- Patients younger than 35 years old with positive PPD
- HIV-positive patients with positive PPD
- Anergic patients with recent known contact to a patient with active TB
- Children with known TB exposure even if the PPD is negative
- Health care workers with recent PPD conversion or contact to an individual with active TB
- Health care workers with a medical condition that predisposes to risk of progression to active disease

A patient with a positive PPD and abnormal chest x-ray suggests active tuberculosis and warrants more aggressive management.

27. D

The USPSTF found that evidence is insufficient to recommend for or against counseling in primary care settings to promote physical activity and exercise. There is insufficient evidence to determine whether counseling leads to sustained increases in physical activity among adult patients. There are no completed trials with children or adolescents that compared primary care counseling to promote exercise with usual care practices.

28. E

A prospective cohort study is the only one listed that will allow determination of disease incidence by prospectively counting new diagnoses in the study group. A nationwide survey would be best to measure prevalence (a "snapshot" in time). Case–control, meta-analysis, and case report techniques do not follow subjects over time or determine incidence rates.

29. E

Delivering bad news can be challenging. Physicians can "hide" behind professional jargon and not clarify the gravity of the situation. Rather, physicians should be honest and forthright, clear, and remain available to their patients. While being honest about the probable gravity of the situation, physicians should offer hope. It is important to acknowledge the patient's emotional response and appropriate to share your own sadness.

30. A

Creatine is most beneficial for anaerobic short-duration exercise. In controlled laboratory studies, oral creatine supplementation has been shown to be effective in repeated stationary cycling sprints, weight lifting, and repetitive sets of muscle contractions such as knee extensions. Creatine's most common side effects are muscle cramping, GI problems, and renal dysfunction.

31. C

The botulinum toxin is a heat labile toxin that is quickly inactivated at a temperature of 80°C. The toxin affects primarily cholinergic nerve terminals causing a descending paralysis of the cranial and spinal nerves. The sympathetic nervous system and sensory nerves remain intact. In wound botulism, the wound should be debrided and anti-toxin injected directly into the wound. Antibiotics are not recommended in the treatment of infants with botulism because cell lysis may result in the release of more toxin.

32. D

Shift work stresses the body's normal circadian pattern. Roughly one-third of workers never adapt to shift work at all, and the majority never fully synchronize their circadian functions. Individuals older than age 40 adjust less well. Shift rotation should proceed around the clock: from day to evening to night. Higher rates of job stress, heavy drinking, and accidents have been reported.

33. D

For purposes of tracking vital statistics and the causes of death, a distinction is made between "causes" (specific diseases, pathologic conditions, and injuries) and "mechanisms" of death. A physiologic event such as cardiac or respiratory arrest is a mechanism of death rather than a cause and should not be listed on the death certificate. In this case, the cause that occurred closest to the time of death and contributed to death was aspiration pneumonia (immediate cause). This was due to changes from CVA, which occurred 4 days earlier (secondary cause).

34. B

Medicare is a federal program administered through CMS and covers the aged, certain blind and disabled individuals, and others such as renal dialysis patients. Medicaid covers individuals who are poor or fit into select aged, blind, or disabled categories. Medicare benefits are set by the federal government, whereas Medicaid benefits vary widely from state to state beyond a core set of services. Medicare does not cover outpatient prescription drugs, although this element is the subject of much debate and political proposals. Major gaps in Medicare include many routine evaluations; outpatient medications; hearing, vision, and dental tests; and prolonged custodial or hospital care. Recent legislation has enhanced the Medicare benefits to include some pharmaceuticals. The new section named "Part D" (not Part C) has provided prescription benefits to seniors under the Medicare program.

35. D

Ciguatoxin is most common in fish from Hawaii and southern Florida. The toxin is concentrated in the head and viscera of the fish; therefore, these parts should never be consumed. Children are most sensitive to the effects of the toxin. The toxin is a naturally occurring poison found in algae-associated microorganisms that live in coral reefs. These algae are consumed and concentrated by fish. Breast-feeding mothers with ciguatera toxin consumption have reported excessive nipple pain and diarrhea in their infants. Treatment of ciguatera toxin exposure is symptomatic and supportive. Neurologic symptoms may be treated with mannitol (1 g/kg), which is most effective if given within 48 hours of symptoms.

36. C

Orlistat is a lipase inhibitor that prevents the uptake of approximately one-third of fat intake in the intestine. Bariatric surgery should not be considered unless the patient has a BMI greater than 40 or greater than 35 with obesity-related medical complications. An overweight person is defined as a patient with a BMI between 25 and 29.9 and obesity is defined as a BMI greater than 30. Fenfluramine was withdrawn from the market due to dangerous side effects, including pulmonary fibrosis and valvular heart disease.

37. C

Medicare began in 1965 as part of Title XVIII of the Social Security Act. Medicare only finances a little more than 50% of all personal health care expenses of its enrollees, and older patients pay approximately 25% of their health care expenses. Medicare Part A pays for most hospital services on a prospective payment (DRG) system. Hospice care and some nursing home and skilled nursing care is also covered. Part B covers medical physician services, certain mental health services and immunizations, and many other additional health expenses.

38. D

An ICS should not include statements that would encourage or coerce participants to remain in a study. In fact, a required element in every ICS is to state the right of participants to withdraw from the study at any time.

39. B

Tertiary prevention describes interventions that help limit disability or prevent disease progression once a patient has experienced an illness or injury. The other listed options are primary (vaccines) or secondary (screening) prevention efforts. All types of prevention may occur in the hospital setting.

40. B

Lowering the cutoff for the screening test will increase its ability to detect disease X since a greater proportion of those with disease X will have a "positive" screening result (the 10% with values of 120 to 140 will now be "positive"). Increasing the sensitivity of a test by changing the cutoff value almost always decreases the specificity of the test, will increase the number of false-positive screening results, and thus will decrease the positive predictive value. A ROC curve reflects the trade-off between sensitivity and specificity for all possible values of the screening test and does not change or shift when a new cutoff is chosen.

41. C

Medicaid covers aged, blind, and disabled patients and the indigent. States have wide discretion over coverage and many have turned to capitated plans and HMOs to control costs and utilization. In general, the spouse of a patient entering a nursing home does not have to sell the family home to meet the Medicaid asset test. Medicaid does provide about 50% of the payments for long-term care. Dual eligible patients can receive both Medicare and Medicaid benefits. Benefits from Medicaid vary by state and can also vary within plans within a given state.

42. D

Dengue is a viral illness epidemic in Southeast Asia, South America, and the Caribbean. It is transmitted by the *Aedes aegypti* mosquito. Most cases of dengue are characterized by headache, fever, rash, and malaise. Although potentially life-threatening, the vast majority of cases are self-limited. There is no specific vaccination or chemoprophylaxis recommended.

43. A

The "gate control theory" of pain hypothesizes that "gates" through large- and small-diameter fibers in the dorsal horn of the spinal cord are influenced by a complex, dynamic interaction of the type of pain stimulus, affect, cognition, and other central factors. The gate control theory provides a framework for a biopsychosocial understanding of why different people respond differently to similar painful stimuli.

44. D

To receive hospice benefits, a physician must certify a life expectancy of less than 6 months. Provider reimbursement is capitated and patient care is 100% covered, with no copayment. Most drugs are covered under the hospice benefit. Despite the broad coverage, the average coverage under hospice was approximately 1 month.

45. D

The largest arm of the Women's Health Initiative study published in 2002 showed a statistically significant increase in rates of breast cancer, cardiac events, and stroke in the HRT treatment group when compared to placebo in a randomized, double-blind, placebo-controlled trial in postmenopausal women who had not had a hysterectomy. The trial showed a protective effect of HRT in preventing fractures and colon cancer. There was no increase in mortality in the treated group.

Although differences between the groups were statistically significant, the absolute differences were small, with approximately one additional adverse event occurring per year for every 500 women in the HRT treatment group. These risks and potential benefits, including treatment of postmenopausal symptoms, should be reviewed with patients before initiating HRT.

46. A

Over 95% of individuals age 65 or older continue to live at home. Seventy-five percent of men live with their spouse, but only slightly more than 40% of women live with a spouse. In 1990, the life expectancy of men at age 65 was 15 years, and that for women was 19 years. Approximately 50% of elders older than age 85 report functional impairment.

47. E

The primary duty of the IRB is to ensure that persons who consent to participate in a research study do so only after being clearly informed of critical facts about the research, particularly those that impact patient safety and risks to the study participant. The IRB may also complete some of the other tasks while promoting ethical research standards, but the central task of the IRB is related directly to adequate and proper informed consent and the safety of research subjects.

48. C

Calcium channel blocker (CCB) overdose can cause profound hypotension and bradycardia. Hypotension can lead to decreased cerebral and mesenteric perfusion causing seizures, mental status changes, and bowel ischemia. Appropriate treatments for CCB overdose include glucagon, calcium chloride, atropine, and dopamine to reverse hypotension. Gut decontamination can be carried out with activated charcoal and sorbitol once the patient's airway is secured. High-dose insulin infusion with D10W or D25W, keeping glucose levels within normal limits, can be effective at reducing the effects of CCB. Transcutaneous pacing may also be required in refractory cases.

49. D

Severe dyspnea near the end of life is best managed with opioid drugs. A trial of small oral doses of morphine can be initiated in this patient, titrating the dose until dyspnea is relieved. Careful clinical assessment and judgment are necessary to achieve relief of distressing symptoms while avoiding adverse effects of oversedation and respiratory depression. Hospice literature has documented the benefits of therapy to alleviate suffering.

50. E

Pulmonary risk factors include significant abnormalities on the expiratory spirogram such as post-bronchodilator FEV1/FVC less than 50%, preoperative FVC less than 20, and % FVC + % FEV1/FVC less than 150. Although controlled hypertension and distant history of myocardial infarction (more than 2 years ago) are not risk factors, dyspnea on exertion and symptoms of angina or congestive heart failure are perioperative pulmonary risk factors. Abnormalities of mental status and significant muscle weakness are also concerning. Metabolic abnormalities on the arterial blood gas or a PCO_2 greater than 50 or PO_2 less than 60 on room air and bed rest for more than 36 hours are other risk factors.

51. C

The NIH recommends against the use of herbal supplements in the treatment of weight loss due to the lack of reliability of their preparation and the lack of randomized controlled trials proving efficacy. Xenical (Orlistat) decreases the absorption of fat-soluble vitamins; vitamin supplements are recommended during treatment with xenical. Bupropion (Wellbutrin), metformin (Glucophage), and topiramate (Topamax) all have weight loss side effects and are currently undergoing clinical trials for the indication of weight loss but are not currently FDA approved. Ephedrine has notable side effects, including cardiovascular and central nervous system events, hypertension, cardiac arrhythmia, stroke, seizure, myocardial infarction, and death.

52. E

The Omnibus Budget Reconciliation Act regulates the way antipsychotics are used in long-term care facilities. Antipsychotic agents cannot be used to control noise making, insomnia, or wandering. They may be used for diagnoses such as schizophrenia, delusional disorders, and dementias complicated by significant psychotic symptoms. Regular monitoring must occur and dosage reduction efforts must occur every 6 months.

53. D

The U.S. Preventive Services Task Force and others use the following hierarchy of evidence, listed from strongest to weakest, when measuring the strength of evidence for preventive guidelines: randomized controlled trials, nonrandomized controlled trials, cohort studies, case–control studies, uncontrolled experiments, descriptive studies (including case reports), and expert opinion. NIH consensus panels are another form of expert opinion.

54. B

Most patients with medical illness can travel safely by air. Individuals with diabetes can travel with syringes and needed equipment (a doctor's note is recommended). Individuals with COPD generally do not need supplemental oxygen unless they are hypercapnic or have a PaO_2 of less than 70 mmHg. Pregnant individuals should drink plenty of fluids and get up regularly during the flight to reduce the risk of deep venous thrombosis. Guidelines suggest refraining from travel in pregnancy during the last 4 to 8 weeks. Patients with well-controlled seizure disorders are not at increased risk for seizures and should not increase their anti-seizure medication.

55. B

Hispanics and African Americans more often use the emergency room as their regular source of medical care than the general population. They are more likely to be uninsured and less likely to have a personal physician. Migrant farm workers, immigrants, and refugees are at particular risk for health disparities. Nonetheless, even the insured or partially insured often have difficulty paying their health-related bills. Three-fourths of people in the United States who have difficulty paying their medical bills have some form of insurance. Even when insured, women and minorities are less likely to be diagnosed with angina when presenting with the same symptoms as men. Homeless children are at risk for a wide range of problems and have a greater incidence of otitis media, diarrhea, and asthma. Among migrant adults, almost one-third test positive for tuberculosis exposure.

56. E

No routine testing is universally recommended for a young, healthy woman in these circumstances. Most authorities recommend a pregnancy test in women of childbearing years to avert medications that might affect a growing fetus. Some experts would recommend a hemoglobin, particularly if a procedure might have a high risk of blood loss. An electrocardiogram is recommended by some authorities after age 40 for men and age 50 for women. Routine chest x-ray, clotting studies, liver function testing, and creatinine are not recommended preoperatively in younger individuals unless suggested by a complete history and physical.

57. A

Medicare has included coverage of answers B, C, and D for many years. A more recent change in policy includes colonoscopy as a covered screening option for colorectal cancer. In most states, Medicare covers influenza, pneumoccal, and hepatitis B vaccinations. Tetanus prophylaxis and other routine vaccinations are generally not covered.

58. B

This patient is most likely taking more medicine than prescribed because her pain is not well controlled. The first step is to assess the level of pain and pattern of pain during the day in order to adjust her medication appropriately. If pain is not well controlled, and the patient is taking more than 25% of her daily morphine as "rescue" or "breakthrough" doses, the next step is to increase the dose of her sustained-release morphine and reassess her pain control within a few days. Rescue doses of morphine can be given as often as every 1 or 2 hours.

59. D

Norwalk virus is usually transmitted through poorly cooked or raw shellfish. Contamination often occurs when these shellfish filter untreated infectious sewage. Outbreaks of Norwalk virus occur year-round and affect older children and adults but not infants or young children. Symptoms begin 24 to 48 hours after ingestion and include rapid onset of nausea, vomiting, abdominal cramping, headache, malaise, and non-bloody diarrhea. Fever and leukocytosis may occur. Complications are rare and most patients make a full recovery. Bismuth subsalicylate has been shown to decrease the duration of symptoms.

60. E

The AMA code of ethics does state that patients have "a basic right to have available health care" but does not address compensation for disability. Answers A through D are all included as basic patients' rights in the code of ethics. The AMA code also states, "A physician shall, in the provision of appropriate patient care, except in emergencies, be free to choose whom to serve, with whom to associate, and the environment in which to provide medical care."

61. D

A positive Mantoux cut-off for number of millimeters of induration is based on the risk for TB or complications from TB: low risk, 15 mm; high risk, 10 mm (e.g., immigrants, medically underserved low-income populations, injection drug users, nursing home residents, infants, and children younger than 4 years of age); and very high risk, 5 mm (e.g., HIV infection, abnormal chest x-ray, and recent contact with infected persons).

62. D

According to the U.S. Preventive Services Task Force Guide to Clinical Preventive Services, patients should be advised to set water heaters to 120°F to 130°F to help prevent hot water injuries.

63. C

Despite the risk of infectious disease, motor vehicle accidents remain the most common cause of preventable deaths while traveling. Seat belt use and appropriate child restraints should be recommended.

64. B

The effectiveness of FOBT screening for colorectal cancer has been tested in some of the largest randomized trials of preventive interventions ever conducted. The results of large randomized studies to evaluate PSA screening are not yet available. The National Cancer Institute PLCO trial seeks to establish the effectiveness of PSA and several other screening tests in reducing mortality. A randomized trial of child restraints would be unethical given results of observational studies that have demonstrated effectiveness in reducing injuries and mortality from motor vehicle accidents. There is insufficient evidence to recommend for or against routine counseling to prevent falls or for diabetes screening in teens.

65. B

Rifampin is the drug of choice for postexposure prophylaxis for household contacts of any patient with serious *Haemophilus*

influenzae type B disease. Rifampin is also used in postexposure prophylaxis regimens for contacts of patients with tuberculosis and meningococcal infections.

66. C

The only criteria to be met for a Medicare patient to select the hospice benefit is that the patient's physician and a physician from the hospice organization certify that the patient has a terminal condition with a 6-month or less prognosis based on "the physicians' clinical judgment regarding the normal course of the individual's illness." There are no special requirements for heart failure or other specific diagnoses, and a patient may receive the benefit indefinitely if the primary definition of "terminally ill" continues to be met. Hospitalization for palliative care is covered. Only medications used to treat symptoms related to the terminal diagnosis and related conditions are covered.

67. C

There are many effective aids to smoking cessation, and the choice of one particular intervention will largely hinge on patient preference. The most successful is nicotine replacement therapy (NRT) coupled with counseling. Using more than one form of nicotine replacement is more effective than using a single form of NRT. Physician advice is about equivalent to NRT alone and better than going cold turkey. Buproprion is about equivalent to the use of more than one form of NRT. A goal of 15% to 20% quit rate is considered very good.

68. D

Lead toxicity produces a hemogram pattern that mimics iron deficiency anemia with hypochromia and microcytosis. An elevated whole blood lead level is the gold standard of diagnosis. Free erythrocyte protoporphyrin levels may be increased in lead toxicity due to lead's effect on blocking ferrochetalase. Irritability, lethargy, headaches, constipation, and abdominal pain are common presenting symptoms. Diarrhea is not usually associated with lead toxicity. Dimercaprol is an intramuscular medication. It is utilized for acute, symptomatic lead toxicity, and it usually is not necessary until lead levels are higher than 25 μg/dL. Gut decontamination is important for lead toxicity if lead fragments are present in the intestinal tract regardless of the decision to administer dimercaprol.

69. E

Rabies has not been associated in the United States with bites by squirrels, chipmunks, or other rodents. Greater concern for rabies exposure should be based on the type of animal (e.g., carnivorous wild animals and bats), the circumstances of the attack (e.g., an unprovoked attack), whether the animal was captured or can be observed or examined (e.g., a neighborhood pet), and the type of exposure (e.g., extent of the bite wound). Specific guidelines for HRIG and rabies vaccine use are available from local and state health departments.

70. B

To evaluate whether a particular published study is important enough to change practice patterns, one must consider, among other things, the strength of the study design, whether the study population is similar to patients in one's own practice, and whether consistent findings have been described from other studies. Although "p values" listed from statistical tests are important in showing that differences between study groups were not due to chance, very small p values may primarily reflect the size of the study rather than the absolute difference between study groups and the level of importance to patients.

71. B

The acronym POEM (patient-oriented evidence that matters) refers to published studies that provide scientifically sound evidence for clinical decisions.

72. C

Zithromax would be the most appropriate antibiotic to use in this case. Cephalexin and penicillin would not cover the most likely bacterial causes, and doxycycline and ciprofloxacin should not be used in children.

73. D

Ethylene glycol ingestion is characterized by hypocalcemia, renal failure due to calcium oxalate crystal deposition, and mental status changes. Methanol ingestion results in retinal edema and visual changes. Urine from these patients may smell like formaldehyde. Both methanol and ethylene glycol ingestions can cause an elevated osmolal gap, elevated anion gap, and metabolic acidosis that leads to Kussmaul respirations.

74. A

Incidence is the number of new cases during the period of interest divided by the population at risk. Four new cases of disease X were diagnosed during February. Prevalence is the proportion of the population at one point in time that has the condition. There were three cases on the island on April 1 and three cases on May 1. Any treatment that would cause people with disease X to live significantly longer would tend to increase prevalence since prevalence (number of current cases) is influenced by both the incidence of disease (rate of new cases) and the duration of the disease.

75. D

Prevalence (the proportion of a population with the condition at one point in time) is influenced by the incidence (rate of new cases diagnosed) and duration of the condition. Any new treatment that greatly increases the average duration of a condition, HIV infection in this case, will tend to increase the prevalence of the condition.

76. C

The "death rattle" is a noise generated with each breath caused by respiratory secretions and partially collapsed airways in a terminal patient in semi- or deep coma who has lost the cough reflex. It is a common occurrence in dying patients that rarely causes acute distress for the patient. If no one has helped caregivers to anticipate and understand the causes of the death rattle, it is often disturbing and commonly assumed to be an indication of choking or other distress for the patient.

77. A

The ethical principle of "double effects" allows for treatments or actions that run the risk of a significant deleterious effects (e.g., a treatment that may hasten death) if the intent of the treatment is to provide a beneficial effect (e.g., an adequate relief of severe suffering).

78. E

Actually, malarone is the most expensive antimalarial, with mefloquine being the second most expensive. The other statements are true.

79. B

A woman with phenylketonuria should remain on a phenylalanine-free diet from birth through the childbearing years. Although the effect of phenylalanine on neurologic function significantly decreases after childhood, neurologic dysfunction may still occur in adulthood. Phenylketonuria is transmitted in an autosomal recessive manner. Therefore, children will have a 50% chance of being a carrier. Since phenylketonuria only occurs in 1 in 10,000 births, the actual chance of having an affected infant is much lower and depends on the carrier status of the father of the infant. Even in noncarrier, unaffected infants, an indiscriminate maternal diet can lead to mental retardation and cardiac anomalies.

80. D

Cardiovascular causes are present in 40% to 50% of cases. Injury is the cause of approximately 20%, and cancer is the cause of 6% of cases.

81. D

Babesiosis is a zoonotic infection transmitted by Ixodes ticks. Babesia organisms invade erythrocytes and cause hemolytic anemia. Patients present similarly to those who are infected with malaria. Fever, chills, fatigue, hemolytic anemia, and hemoglobinuria are common manifestations. The infection is definitively diagnosed by the presence of ring-forms of babesia within red blood cells. Patients often exhibit elevated sedimentation rates, lymphopenia, and thrombocytopenia. The disease is rarely fatal in patients with intact splenic function. Treatment regimens include clindamycin and quinine.

82. C

All states have enacted laws that require reporting of infections important to public health and for cases of suspected child abuse. A minority of states require reporting of spousal abuse or domestic violence.

83. C

Intravenous sodium nitrate induces the formation of methemoglobin, which has a greater affinity for cyanide than the cytochrome system. After infusion of sodium nitrate, sodium thiosulfate is given to create sodium thiocyanate, which is excreted. Methemoglobin levels are maintained between 20% and 30% until the metabolic acidosis caused by cyanide has resolved. The level of methemoglobinemia can be controlled with 1% methylene blue.

84. B

Studies have shown that growth among children following a vegetarian diet is equal to that of children who eat meat. Vegan and broader vegetarian diets do not impair a child's growth as long as inadequacies in calories, protein, vitamins B12 and D, calcium, iron, and zinc are supported in the diet. Wiscott–Aldrich syndrome is not associated with a vegetarian diet.

85. D

Interpretation of a PPD depends on the risk of the patient being exposed to tuberculosis.

A PPD is positive when the following criteria are met:

5-mm induration

- HIV-positive patient
- Recent close contact with a patient with active TB
- Patient with chest x-ray consistent with healed TB

10-mm induration

- IV drug user
- Patient with chronic illness (silicosis, chronic renal disease, diabetes mellitus, chronic steroid use, and malignancy)
- Children younger than 4 years old
- Immigrants from endemic areas
- Residents of long-term care facilities (nursing homes and prisons)
- Medically underserved, low-income patients

15-mm induration

- Positive in all patients

Erythema alone without induration does not constitute a positive test.

86. C

Dengue fever is a viral illness transmitted to humans through the *Aedes aegypti* mosquito. Typical laboratory findings in Dengue fever include hemoconcentration, thrombocytopenia, leukopenia, electrolyte imbalances, acidemia, elevated BUN, and elevated transaminases. Disseminated intravascular coagulation is not seen unless the patient has developed Dengue hemorrhagic fever.

87. D

The U.S. Preventive Services Task Force found good evidence that screening improves the accurate identification of depressed patients in primary care settings and that treatment of depressed adults identified in primary care settings decreases clinical morbidity. Routine screening for osteoporosis is recommended for women ages 65 years and older. There is no good evidence to include routine screening for melanoma or lung cancer in periodic examinations of asymptomatic adults. Testing for hepatitis B antibodies is not recommended unless the patient is at high risk for disease based on factors unrelated to age.

88. D

For women who have previously had a neural tube defect (NTD)-affected pregnancy, the Centers for Disease Control and Prevention recommends increasing the intake of folic acid to 4,000 μg per day beginning at least 1 month before conception and continuing through the first trimester.

89. B

The transdermal fentanyl patch is less likely to cause significant constipation compared to sustained-release oral morphine but is more expensive. Drug tolerance, dependence, and addiction issues are similar for the two preparations. Transdermal fentanyl patches are changed every 3 days.

90. E

The hospice benefit covers all testing, treatment, medications, and home-based support services necessary for palliative care of the terminal illness. Transportation costs are not covered.

91. D

Numerous studies have shown routine chest x-rays to not be beneficial in screening for lung cancer. Screening for asymptomatic disease is considered secondary prevention.

92. A

The sensitivity of a test reflects its ability to detect disease when the disease is present. For example, if a "rapid strep test" is positive in 80 out of 100 patients with culture-proven streptococcal pharyngitis, the sensitivity of the rapid test is 80/100 or 80%.

93. D

Colonoscopy is considered a "gold standard" test for colonic polyps and determines the prevalence of polyps in the study group (100/1,100). Sensitivity, the ability of FOBT to detect polyps when they are present, is 60/100 or 60%. Specificity, the ability of FOBT to indicate nondisease when no polyps are present, is 940/1,000 or 94%. Positive predictive value indicates what proportion of patients with positive FOBT actually have polyps, 60/120 or 50%. The only correct answer is for negative predictive value, the proportion of patients with a negative FOBT who do not have polyps, 940/980 or 96%.

94. D

Subacute bacterial endocarditis (SBE) prophylaxis is recommended in patients at increased risk for bacterial endocarditis undergoing many common procedures. Patients at highest risk include those with complex cardiac abnormalities (e.g., tetralogy of Fallot), prosthetic valves, and surgically constructed shunts. Patients with problems such as hypertrophic cardiomyopathy, mitral valve regurgitation, and rheumatic heart disease are at moderate risk. Procedures likely to cause bacteremia include dental procedures (including routine cleaning and root canal) and surgery of the respiratory, gastrointestinal, and genitourinary tracts.

SBE prophylaxis is not required for routine dental filling, x-rays, or fluoride treatments; cardiac catheterization; circumcision; intubation; flexible bronchoscopy; or pressure equalization tube insertion.

95. D

The Goldman scale is a multifactorial index of cardiac risk in non-cardiac surgical procedures. Risk is increased most with recent myocardial infarction, signs of congestive heart failure, more than five premature ventricular contractions per minute, and rhythm other than sinus or premature atrial contractions. Risk is increased somewhat less dramatically with age older than 70 years, significant aortic stenosis, general debilitation, major surgery, or an emergency operation.

96. C

Patients with well-controlled diabetes should typically hold short-acting insulin and take one-half to two-thirds of their intermediate or long-acting insulin on the morning of surgery. Corticosteroids should be increased to reflect the stress of surgery, both perioperatively and postoperatively. Cardiac and antihypertensive medications can be given with a sip of water on the morning of surgery. Smoking cessation is valuable, even if it is only 6 weeks prior to surgery (and although less well proven, many authorities would recommend cessation if only for shorter periods). Aspirin and nonsteroidal anti-inflammatory drugs ideally should be stopped 1 week prior to surgery.

97. D

Although assessing nicotine dependence may play a role in smoking cessation, it is not part of the routine steps suggested by the Public Health Service. The other step is assisting the patient in quitting.

98. A

Transmission of tuberculosis occurs primarily through inhalation of aerosolized bacilli. These bacilli can exist in droplet nuclei that can remain suspended in a room even if the patient is no longer present. As few as 1 to 10 bacilli entering an alveolus can cause infection. A single sputum sample containing acid-fast bacilli is diagnostic of active or recurrent tuberculosis.

99. C

Developing rapport with a patient seeking disability or workers' compensation can be challenging. However, overzealous referral, inappropriate medicalization through overuse of tests and medications, and inadequate attention to job satisfaction and psychosocial issues can jeopardize longer term functional outcomes. Job satisfaction is highly associated with return to work and functional outcomes. Exploration of the psychosocial aspects of the patient's life, including family relationships, substance use, and psychiatric symptoms, is important. The physician should emphasize functional outcomes and address underlying problems.

100. C

The content of advance directives documents is regulated by state laws. The durable power of attorney for health care allows patients to choose someone they trust to make health care decisions for them if they are unable to do so. A patient can easily and immediately revoke either document with a simple oral statement. The two documents serve different purposes in health care decisions, and one does not take precedence over the other.

Chapter 9

Clinical Set Problems

The questions in the clinical set problems are designed to assess clinical problem-solving skills. Please answer each either T for true or F for false.

Problem 1. A 55-year-old man presents to your office with intermittent blurred vision accompanied by pain in the right eye and headache for the past 2 days. He is nauseated and vomited this morning. At this point, when considering how to evaluate and manage this patient, which of the following should you consider?

1. This patient may have a migraine.
2. A stat MRI and CT of the brain are indicated to rule out a mass lesion.
3. The patient should be referred to an ophthalmologist immediately for a dilated exam to rule out retinal or optic nerve pathology.
4. This patient should follow-up with an ophthalmologist in 1 week since the visual symptoms are most likely related to migraine.
5. This patient may need an immediate surgical procedure.

The patient describes seeing colored halos around lights during the past 2 days. On examination, you note a fixed mid-dilated pupil and a red eye on the right. He can only see your hand move in front of that eye. Which of the following regarding this patient are true?

6. An oral osmotic is indicated.
7. Oral acetazolamide (Diamox) is indicated.
8. Oral ergotamine is indicated.
9. The patient's right eye pressure is probably very high.
10. The patient is at risk of losing most of his vision in the right eye within hours.
11. The patient should recover with medical therapy.
12. The patient's other eye is probably at risk for a similar episode.
13. Surgical intervention in the left eye will probably be necessary in the future.

Problem 2. A 7-year-old female presents to the emergency room with a 2-day history of diarrhea and decreased appetite. She feels nauseated but denies vomiting. Over the past 24 hours she has had seven partially formed stools. No one else is sick in the family. Her only medicine is Tylenol, which she took for fever. Which of the following statements are true?

1. The most likely cause of this patient's symptoms is Norwalk virus.
2. Milk products will aggravate the patient's symptoms.
3. A Sudan fat stain is likely to be negative in this patient.

On physical exam, the child appears to be mildly dehydrated. Temperature is 38.1°C, blood pressure is 80/50 mmHg, and the pulse is 90. The abdomen is soft with increased bowel sounds and mild diffuse tenderness. No masses or rebound tenderness is appreciated. Appropriate steps could include which of the following?

4. Checking a stool smear for white blood cells
5. Obtaining a stool specimen for *Clostridium difficile*
6. Checking the stool for ova and parasites
7. Checking the stool for occult blood
8. Obtaining an abdominal flat plate
9. Prescribing a fluoroquinolone
10. Prescribing diphenoxylate (Lomotil)
11. Treating the child with clear liquids only for 24 to 48 hours

Problem 3. A 15-year-old female presents with her mother for her yearly physical exam. She has no previous medical problems. Her mother recently remarried, and they have moved to a new town. Her last immunizations were done at the pre-kindergarten age. Which of the following statements are true regarding consent and confidentiality?

1. Any discussion with the adolescent regarding mental health is strictly confidential.
2. The physician may test and treat an adolescent for sexually transmitted diseases without parental consent.
3. The physician is required to notify the parents if their adolescent child requests emergency contraception.

You perform the physical exam. You note that she is now menstruating and that her pubertal development is appropriate. Which statements are true regarding the physical exam?

4. A pelvic exam is a routine part of the physical once a patient starts menstruating.
5. A patient with dense curled but not abundant pubic hair and breasts with areola and papillae forming a round projection from the breast contour is in Tanner stage 3.
6. The typical sequence of female pubertal growth is as follows: (a) initial growth spurt, (b) breast development begins, (c) peak height velocity, and (d) menarche.

You now perform preventive screening and counseling. Which statements are true regarding counseling and screening?

7. The number one cause of death among 12- to 24-year-olds is unintentional injuries, with drowning the most common cause.
8. Of the approximately 1 million teenage pregnancies yearly, approximately 50% are unintended.
9. A cholesterol test should be performed at least once on every patient during his or her adolescent years.
10. A sexually active adolescent female should be screened for chlamydia and gonorrhea and have a Pap smear.
11. The patient requires vaccines against tetanus and hepatitis B if not already completed.

Problem 4. A 45-year-old male comes to the office requesting a checkup. He shares with you that his wife is concerned about his drinking. In evaluating this patient, which of the following are true?

1. More than 100,000 Americans die each year from alcohol-related problems.
2. One "yes" answer on the CAGE questionnaire has a sensitivity of 75%.
3. The patient does not have an increased risk of hypertension.
4. Males are more susceptible to alcohol-related liver disease than females.
5. The patient should be screened for depression.
6. An elevated aspartate amino transferase is the most sensitive liver abnormality in alcoholic patients.

The patient admits to drinking several shots of whisky a day to relax. Although he feels the need to cut down on his drinking, he does not want to do so at this time. He does not show up for his follow-up appointment. Six months later, you get a call because the patient shows up in the emergency room complaining of nausea and shakiness. His last drink was yesterday when he decided to give up drinking. His vital signs are: P, 102; RR, 26; BP, 170/110 mmHg; and T, 99.2°F. The patient appears anxious, moderately shaky, and sweaty. The patient complains of nausea and while oriented to person and place has trouble remembering the exact date. Physical examination is otherwise unremarkable except for some mild mid-epigastric tenderness. Appropriate actions include which of the following?

7. Admit the patient for alcohol intoxication.
8. Obtain serum glucose and electrolyte levels.
9. Obtain a serum magnesium level.
10. Give 15 mg of diazepam (Valium) orally.
11. Give 3 mg of lorazepam orally.
12. Give 100 mg of thiamine orally to prevent Korsakoff's psychosis.
13. Give 2 mg of haloperidol (Haldol) intramuscularly.

Problem 5. A 25-year-old female comes into your office in June with complaints of sneezing, itchy and watery eyes, and nasal congestion. Her past medical history is significant for childhood asthma. She has tried a variety of over-the-counter medications but continues to have daily symptoms. She has also taken a course of antibiotics that failed to provide any relief.

PE: Ht: 5'4''
     Wt: 50kg
     RR = 14
     T = 98.3°F orally

HEENT: Sclera slightly injected bilaterally. Oral pharynx reveals cobble-stoned appearance. Nasopharynx reveals swollen, pale, boggy turbinates. The tympanic membranes are unremarkable and the chest is clear. Which of the following statements are true?

1. The patient's symptoms most likely are secondary to allergic rhinitis.
2. Patients with allergic rhinitis more frequently have a history of asthma.
3. Patients with allergic rhinitis usually have nasal polyps.
4. Appropriate treatment of allergic rhinitis can improve asthma symptoms.

5. Perennial allergic rhinitis is caused predominately by outdoor allergens.
6. Benadryl (diphenhydramine) is less effective in relieving symptoms than newer medications.
7. The patient's symptoms are easily confused with an upper respiratory infection.

Which of the following steps might be appropriate in diagnosing this patient?

8. Examine a smear of nasal secretions for eosinophilia.
9. Test the patient with intradermal allergens to determine a pattern of allergy.
10. Send a blood sample for in vitro IgE testing to determine a pattern of allergy.
11. Order limited CT of sinuses.
12. Order full pulmonary function tests.

Allergy testing reveals that the patient is allergic to golden rod pollen.

13. Avoidance of allergens is a mainstay of therapy.
14. Second-generation antihistamines are generally longer acting than over-the-counter counterparts.
15. Decongestants should not be used in combination with an antihistamine.
16. Intranasal corticosteroids treat congestion but do not improve itchiness.
17. Intranasal corticosteroids should not be used in children because of the potential for growth retardation.

Problem 6. S.M. is a 16-year-old male complaining of shortness of breath for 5 days that started with a runny nose and cough. In the past 2 days his cough has worsened, especially at night. Today in gym class, his chest felt tight and he wheezed while running. He has a history of asthma since age 9, requiring emergency department visits approximately "once a year or so." He normally uses an albuterol inhaler approximately 3 or 4 times per week and used it twice today with only minimal relief. Review of systems is otherwise noncontributory. With regard to this patient's disease, the following are true:

1. It is less common in those with a history of eczema.
2. It is characterized by airway inflammation, which leads to an irreversible obstruction of airflow.
3. Common symptoms include chest tightness and cough.
4. It is associated with gastroesophageal reflux disease (GERD).
5. It is associated with exposure to cockroaches.
6. It often improves with exercise.
7. Death rates from it are highest in Caucasians.
8. It is more common in children whose parents smoke.

Physical examination reveals an adolescent male in mild respiratory distress. Vital signs are: P, 102; RR, 26; BP, 120/70 mmHg; and T, 36.9°C. His lung examination is significant for bilateral wheezing with a prolonged expiratory phase. Appropriate management currently includes the following:

9. Pulse oximetry
10. Determination of peak expiratory flow
11. Use of inhaled corticosteroids
12. Use of oral corticosteroids
13. Chest x-ray
14. Nebulized albuterol followed by repeat evaluation
15. Amoxicillin 250 mg PO tid ×10 days
16. Oral albuterol

17. Pulmonary function testing

The patient does well and follows up in your office 2 weeks later. Appropriate management at this point might include which of the following?

18. Education of patient and caregivers
19. Daily use of leukotriene inhibitor
20. Daily use of inhaled corticosteroids
21. Inhaled corticosteroids for 2 weeks as needed for asthma exacerbations
22. Annual flu shot
23. Daily use of inhaled salmeterol

Problem 7. T.J., a pleasant but extremely active 8-year-old, is brought in by his mother, who tells you his teacher believes he is "hyperactive." In the exam room, T.J. is unable to sit still, repeatedly jumping on the scale and attempting to pull the stethoscope from your neck. He has been having trouble at school with grades of C's and D's this year. He is easily distracted by outside stimuli and often loses things needed for tasks in school, such as assignments, pencils, or books. He is unable to sit still for stories or meals yet remains glued to the television when watching his favorite show. Which of the following is true?

1. Attention deficit hyperactivity disorder (ADHD) is the most common pediatric behavioral problem.
2. Girls are affected more commonly than boys.
3. There is rarely a family history for ADHD in affected children.
4. ADHD occurs at all intellectual levels.
5. Symptoms are less likely to be seen in group settings.
6. Children with ADHD generally grow out of it by early adulthood.
7. Neuroimaging studies support a central role of the prefrontal lobes and basal ganglia in ADHD.
8. Specific diagnostic tests are available.

Physical examination including neurologic testing is all normal. However, during the exam you notice T.J. found it difficult to listen to what was being said to him, had a difficult time following instructions. and made careless mistakes in answering questions. Which of the following are true?

9. An EEG and thyroid studies should be part of the evaluation of ADHD.
10. Blood lead levels and hematocrit screening should be ordered in preschool children.
11. Vigilance testing is often helpful.

After reading T.J.'s teacher's concerns and further discussion with his mother, you arrive at the conclusion that T.J. has ADHD. The mother had concerns regarding treatment. In advising her, which of the following are true?

12. Parents often feel that they have caused this disorder.
13. Mental health referral for management strategies and behavior modification is not beneficial.
14. Drug treatment is equally effective as behavior modification.
15. Fifty percent to 80% of children respond to stimulant drug therapy.
16. Stimulant medications act by increasing serotonin.
17. The response to medication can be used as a test for confirming the diagnosis of ADHD.
18. Stimulants have the potential for exacerbating motor tics in Tourette's syndrome.
19. Stimulants lower the seizure threshold.

20. Treatment is best started with short-acting medication.
21. Monitoring medication is essential and comments from teachers are very helpful.
22. Blood levels are useful in monitoring stimulant treatment.

Problem 8. P.J., a 40-year-old female, presents to the office with complaints of a nonpainful breast mass that has fluctuated in size over the past several weeks. There is no history of trauma and her periods are regular, lasting for approximately 5 days. Her last period ended approximately 2 weeks ago. She is in good health and denies a family history of breast cancer or ovarian cancer.

Physical examination reveals a minimally tender 2-cm mass in the upper outer quadrant. The mass is firm and easily movable. There is no erythema or increased warmth to the lesion. The rest of her physical exam is unremarkable. Which of the following statements are true?

1. The risk factors for breast cancer include age, family history, early menarche, late menopause, and nulliparity.
2. Approximately one-fourth of breast cancers occur in women aged 30 to 50 years.
3. The most likely diagnosis in this patient is fibrocystic changes.
4. Physical examination can usually distinguish a cyst from a solid mass.
5. The management of this patient includes an ultrasonography or aspiration.

After obtaining the patient's consent, you decide to aspirate the mass. The aspirate is nonbloody, and following aspiration the mass is no longer palpable. Appropriate management could include which of the following?

6. Consult surgery for evaluation and treatment of possible cancer.
7. Send the aspirate for cytology.
8. Recommend that the patient avoid caffeine.
9. Prescribe danazol.

The patient returns in 6 weeks and upon examination you find a mass in the same location as before. You aspirate the fluid again with resolution of the mass. At subsequent follow-up 4 weeks later, the mass is still there. Which of the following is true?

10. Surgery should be consulted to do a biopsy.
11. Cysts require surgical biopsy only if the aspirated fluid is bloody, the palpable abnormality does not resolve completely after the aspiration of fluid, or the same cyst recurs multiple times in a short period of time.

The biopsy reveals a benign mass. Two years later, the patient returns with another breast lump that is nontender. Attempted fluid aspiration is unsuccessful. You decide to do an ultrasound, and the radiologist reads it as a solid mass. Management of this patient includes:

12. Mammography more to rule out other lesions rather than to assess the palpable mass
13. Consultation with surgery for biopsy
14. Fine needle aspiration for cytology
15. Observation for 6 months if the mammogram indicates that the mass is benign

Problem 9. A social worker brings a 7-year-old who was recently placed in foster care in for an assessment because of possible physical abuse. In evaluating the patient, signs and symptoms that increase the likelihood for child abuse include:

1. Weight less than fifth percentile for age

2. Bruises found on the shin

3. Bruises of various coloration

4. History of a greenstick fracture following a fall when the child was 6 years old

5. History of a femoral fracture when the child was 9 months old

6. Torn frenulum

7. Bilateral black eyes following a fall

8. History of the parents recently divorcing

When taking the patient's history, which of the following should increase your suspicion of abuse?

9. An overly concerned parent

10. Injuries that do not match the child's history

11. Failure to obtain necessary immunizations

12. History of aggressive behavior at school

Examination reveals multiple bruises in various stages of healing. There also appears to be a lesion on the back of the hand consistent with a cigarette burn. Appropriate action at this time includes:

13. Recommending the child not be photographed to avoid further distress

14. Providing a detailed description of the injuries

15. Documenting a detailed description of the injuries

16. Arranging for a family conference to resolve the abuse

17. Requesting medical records from previous providers

18. Recommending evaluation of the child's siblings

Problem 10. A 53-year-old male was sent fecal occult blood test cards by his insurance company. He returned three stool samples and the insurance company notifies you that one of the three stool specimens is positive for occult blood. He makes an appointment for further evaluation. He reports feeling well and denies any rectal bleeding, melena, weight loss, or change in bowel habits. Physical examination reveals a small hemorrhoid that is not actively bleeding. Your physical examination is otherwise normal. The stool is brown and tests Hemoccult negative in the office. Appropriate tests at this time include which of the following?

1. Repeat Hemoccult testing after advising the patient to avoid red meat

2. A CBC

3. A carcinoembryonic antigen (CEA)

4. A CT scan of the abdomen

5. Referral for colonoscopy

The patient is very concerned that he may have colon cancer. Which of the following is true?

6. Having a first-degree relative with colon cancer doubles his risk.

7. Aspirin reduces the risk of colon cancer.

8. A high-fat, low-fiber diet increases the risk of colon cancer.

9. One in four patients with a Hemoccult positive stool will have colorectal cancer.

Evaluation reveals a 4-cm mass in the sigmoid colon. At surgery, the mass is removed, and the pathology report identifies it as an adenocarcinoma of the colon. One of 12 lymph nodes is positive. Which of the following are true?

10. The patient has a Duke's stage B tumor.

11. The patient has a 75% 5-year survival rate.

12. The patient will need chemotherapy.

13. The patient will need a follow-up colonoscopy in 6 months.

14. The patient is at greater risk than average for having a second colon cancer in the future.

Problem 11. D.L. is a 72-year-old male who presents to your office with complaints of gradually worsening shortness of breath. He states that over the previous 6 months he has been getting more short of breath when walking up stairs and now has to stop after 5 or 6 steps to catch his breath. He also notes mild swelling in both of his legs and that he is sleeping on three pillows at night. His past medical history is significant for long-standing hypertension. Medications include a "water pill" which he ran out of 2 months ago. The remaining history is unremarkable. With regard to the patient's condition, which of the following statements are correct?

1. Exacerbations of congestive heart failure are the most frequent cause of hospital admissions in the elderly.

2. Hypertension is the most common underlying cause of systolic dysfunction.

3. Poor compliance of the left ventricular wall is not a contributing factor.

4. The overall 5-year mortality of men who suffer from it is roughly 25%.

5. Alcoholism is not an established cause of this condition.

6. This condition may be seen in those with amyloidosis.

On physical examination the patient is moderately short of breath. Vital signs include: P, 100 and regular; BP, 155/110 mmHg; and RR of 24. Pulse oximetry is 95% on room air, and the patient is afebrile. There is jugular venous distention, bibasilar rales, and 2+ pitting edema of both lower extremities. Cardiac examination reveals an S3 and no murmurs.

You decide to admit the patient to the hospital. Appropriate testing and intervention include which of the following?

7. Rapid CT scan of the chest

8. Cardiac enzymes

9. CBC

10. CXR

11. Echocardiogram

12. Intravenous furosemide

13. Monitoring daily weight

The patient improves with treatment and after 2 days is ready for discharge. Review of the chart gives the following information: Echocardiogram reveals an ejection fraction of 53% and mild LVH. Serum cholesterol is 155 mg/dL with an LDL of 90 mg/dL. An ECG reveals a strain pattern and demonstrates LVH by voltage criteria. The remainder of the workup is normal. Appropriate therapy includes which of the following?

14. Lipitor 20 mg PO qid

15. Digoxin 0.125 mg PO daily

16. Metoprolol 25 mg PO four times a day

17. Lisinopril 5 mg PO daily, increase as tolerated to maximum dose

18. Bed rest and avoidance of exercise

Problem 12. A 64-year-old female developed severe constipation about 3 weeks ago. She complains of feeling bloated but denies the presence of blood in her stools, nausea, abdominal pain, or a previous history of constipation. She has a history of depression and hypertension for which she takes diltiazem (Cardizem) and sertraline (Zoloft). She is otherwise healthy and her only other complaint is mild fatigue. Which of the following statements are true about the patient's condition?

1. Constipation is a normal finding in elderly adults.

2. The patient's constipation is most likely functional.

3. Sertraline (Zoloft) is commonly associated with constipation.

4. Diltiazem (Cardizem) is commonly associated with constipation.

5. A careful neurologic examination is indicated.

Physical examination reveals a mildly overweight female with a blood pressure of 110/70. Her abdomen is soft with good bowel sounds without evidence of a mass or organomegaly. On rectal examination, there is a small amount of hard brown stool, which is heme negative. Appropriate steps at this time include:

6. Discontinuing the diltiazem

7. Ordering electrolytes

8. Ordering serum calcium

9. Ordering a TSH

10. Checking CBC

11. Requesting the patient check her stools for occult blood at home

The patient is instructed to stop her diltiazem and to increase her dietary fiber and fluid intake. All her lab work, including her CBC, is normal. Adjusting her diet and stopping the diltiazem improves her constipation but has caused her to complain of more gas. One of her three stool specimens for occult blood was positive. Which of the following steps are indicated?

12. Repeating three more stool specimens to determine if the stool remains heme positive

13. Scheduling a colonoscopy

14. Ordering an abdominal CT

15. Ordering a CEA level

16. Reducing the dietary fiber to improve the gas

17. Prescribing a daily stool softener

Problem 13. J.M., a 65-year-old male, presents to your office with a productive cough and worsening dyspnea over the past week. He denies having fever, chills, nausea, or chest pain. The past medical history is significant for a 10-year history of moderately severe chronic obstructive pulmonary disease (COPD). Medications include occasional Tylenol and "some inhaler." Social history includes a 60 pack-year history of smoking. Which of the following statements regarding this patient's condition are true?

1. Cigarette smoking is the cause of more than 80% of cases of COPD.

2. COPD exacerbations occur more often in the summer months.

3. Use of bronchodilators easily reverses the condition.

4. Exacerbations are defined by increased sputum production, more purulent sputum, or worsening dyspnea.

5. Chronic inflammation of the bronchiolar airways leads to difficulty clearing secretions.

6. Alpha-1-antitrypsin deficiency is a common cause.

Physical examination revealed the following:

Ht: 6′ 1″
Wt: 75 kg
RR = 20   T = 99.2°F
P = 95   BP = 125/80 mmHg

The patient appears mildly short of breath. Examination reveals a barrel-shaped chest accompanied by prolonged expiratory phase, expiratory wheezing, and scattered rhonchi. Heart sounds are distant with a regular rhythm and rate. Extremity exam reveals no cyanosis or edema. Appropriate tests at this time might include:

7. A chest x-ray

8. Pulmonary function tests

9. Arterial blood gas

10. CBC

11. CT scan of chest

12. Pulse oximetry

J.M.'s test results reveal the following:

Chest X-ray: flattened diaphragm and mild hyperinflation
WBC = 8.7   Hgb = 16.8
Pulse oximetry = 94% on room air
ABG: pCO_2 = 49 PO_2 = 78   %Sat = 94 HCO_3 = 29

Pulmonary function tests obtained 12 months prior show moderate reduction in FEV1 and ratio of FEV1/FVC.

Appropriate management at this point might include:

13. Salmeterol inhaler

14. Oral corticosteroids

15. Intravenous steroids

16. Oral antibiotics

17. Home oxygen

18. Influenza vaccine

19. Pneumococcal vaccine

Problem 14. D.N. is a 53-year-old obese female who presents to the emergency department with 30 minutes of left-sided chest "pressure and squeezing," accompanied by shortness of breath, diaphoresis, and nausea. She has a past medical history of hypertension and hypercholesterolemia. Family history is significant for a brother who had a myocardial infarction at age 48 and a father who died of a heart attack in his 50s. Medications include hydrochlorothiazide 25 mg PO qid and fluvastatin 20 mg PO qhs. Social history is significant for having a "stressful job" and smoking one pack of cigarettes per day. In this patient, the following are absolute risk factors for the development of coronary artery disease:

1. Family history

2. Obesity

3. Hypertension

4. Hypercholesterolemia

5. Stress

Physical examination reveals an obese female in mild distress secondary to chest discomfort. Her vital signs are as follows: P, 85; RR, 22; BP, 145/95 mmHg; and T, 97.1°F.

Test results include:

Chest x-ray—within normal limits
ECG—normal sinus rate with ST segment elevation in leads V2–V5, lead 1 aVL; depressions in II, III, and aVF
Troponin and myoglobin within the normal range

Appropriate intervention at this time includes the following:

6. Administering an intravenous calcium channel blocker

7. 5 mg of atenolol IV

8. Applying 1 in. of nitro paste

9. Having the patient chew one aspirin

10. Morphine intravenously

11. Atropine intravenously

The patient undergoes coronary angiography and angioplasty of the LAD. The patient is stabilized and has an uneventful hospital course. Labs obtained during hospital stay include an LDL of 135, HDL of 30, and HgbA1C of 5.5. The patient follows up in your office 1 week after discharge and is without complaints. Her BP 110/70 mmHg and her P is 60. Appropriate therapy for this patient includes the following:

12. Oral beta-blocker
13. Daily aspirin
14. Tobacco cessation
15. Continue fluvastatin at 20 mg PO daily
16. Coumadin with titration to INR between 2 and 3
17. An ACE inhibitor

Problem 15. A 42-year-old white female presents to your office as a new patient with complaints of fatigue, profuse muscle aches, insomnia, marital problems, and occasional flushing. She complains of dry skin despite liberal use of moisturizing creams and would like to start exercising but claims that she is too tired. Her periods are regular and she denies smoking or illicit drug use but admits to drinking three or four beers a day to help her relax. There is no family history of drug or alcohol abuse. On physical examination, the patient makes poor eye contact and appears to be on the verge of tears throughout the exam. She is 5'1'' and weighs 165 lbs. There is some muscular tenderness, including the trunk and distal and proximal limb muscles. The ear, nose, and throat exam is normal. Her thyroid is within normal limits. The pulmonary and cardiac examination is also normal. The neurologic exam demonstrates subjective weakness secondary to muscular discomfort but no objective findings of weakness.

Tests that might be helpful at this time include:

1. TSH
2. A fasting lipid profile
3. Chemistry panel
4. FSH
5. LH
6. CBC
7. CPK

All lab tests are normal except for her lipid profile of total cholesterol 232 mg/dL, LDL-C 150 mg/dL, and an HDL-C 50 mg/dL. Appropriate recommendations at this point include:

8. Discussing the patient's feelings and problems with possible usage of an antidepressant
9. Starting Synthroid 0.025 mg per day
10. Starting Lipitor 10 mg in the evening
11. Starting Prempro 0.625 mg daily
12. Advising the patient to begin an exercise program
13. Recommending discontinuing the use of alcohol

Problem 16. M.R. is a 68-year-old African American female with a 10-year history of type 2 diabetes mellitus. She has always been about 20% above her ideal weight. Although her blood sugars were well controlled in the past with a sulfonylurea, she is developing polyuria, nocturia, and fatigue despite maximum doses of her medication. She was also diagnosed with hypertension about 3 years ago and currently takes hydrochlorothiazide, 25 mg a day. Which of the following statements are true about the patient's condition?

1. African Americans are more at risk for developing type 2 diabetes.
2. The patient's difficulty with blood sugar control is most likely due to progressive insulin resistance.
3. An elevated HbA1c level would confirm the diagnosis of type 2 diabetes.

4. It is likely that without adjusting her treatment regime she will develop ketoacidosis.
5. Cardiovascular disease accounts for the majority of excess mortality in type 2 diabetes.
6. Insulin levels will most likely be elevated in this individual.

Physical examination revealed the following:

Ht: 5' 3'
Wt: 65 kg
BP: 135/88

Physical examination revealed a nonproliferative retinopathy, decreased pedal pulses, and a right femoral bruit. On neurologic examination, she has absent ankle reflexes and decreased vibration sense. Touch sensation was normal. Appropriate tests at this time might include:

7. An MRI of the lumbosacral spine
8. A fasting lipid profile
9. A fasting insulin level
10. A glucose tolerance test
11. A chest x-ray
12. An electrocardiogram

M.R.'s blood work included the following results:

Urinalysis: 1+ glucose; otherwise normal
Random plasma glucose: 220 mg/dL
HbA1c: 8.8%
Total cholesterol: 239 mg/dL
LDL-C: 160 mg/dL
HDL-C: 30 mg/dL
Triglycerides: 290 mg/dL

Appropriate treatment options include the following:

13. Discontinuing the sulfonylurea and starting metformin
14. Adding bedtime 70/30 insulin
15. Starting a statin
16. Starting an angiotensin converting enzyme inhibitor
17. Referring the patient to an ophthalmologist
18. Starting 325 mg of aspirin a day
19. Influenza vaccination
20. Further reduction in the patient's blood pressure

Problem 17. A 6-month-old Caucasian male infant is being seen for his 6-month well child visit. He is the product of a term normal spontaneous vaginal delivery with a birth weight of 4 lbs 8 oz. He has been exclusively breast-fed and is on vitamin D supplementation. You note that his height (24 in.) is at the fourth percentile and his weight (12 lbs 0 oz) is at the second percentile on the growth chart. On a visit at 4 months of age, his height was at the eighth percentile and his weight was at the fifth percentile. The mother expresses no concerns and denies any recent illness, vomiting, or diarrhea. Which of the following are true about the patient's condition?

1. Intrauterine growth retardation (IUGR) is not a cause for small stature in a 6-month-old infant.
2. Children with IUGR may not attain their full intellectual potential.
3. Assessment of growth should be adjusted for parental height.
4. In older children approaching puberty, any investigation or treatment should be deferred because they will soon experience a growth spurt that will usually bring them up to normal adult height.

5. Hypothyroidism is a relatively common cause of organic failure to thrive.

6. Gastroesophageal reflux is a relatively common cause of organic failure to thrive.

Examination reveals an alert child without dysmorphic features. Temperature is 99.5°F rectally, P is 125 and regular, BP is 75/50, and RR is 30. The anterior fontanelle is soft and the tympanic membranes are gray and intact. The oropharynx shows no erythema of exudate. S1 and S2 are audible with no murmurs or extra sounds. Femoral pulses are present. There are no chest wall deformities and the lungs are clear to auscultation. The abdomen is without hepatosplenomegaly or masses. The infant moves all extremities and is up to date on developmental milestones.

Appropriate tests or further investigations at this time would include which of the following?

7. CBC with differential
8. Basic metabolic profile
9. Karyotype
10. Urine assay for organic acids
11. Wrist x-rays
12. No laboratory testing pending dietary treatment if there appears to be inappropriate oral intake

All of the above studies and further investigations are normal. Which of the following would be appropriate next steps in management?

13. Have an evaluation done by a lactation nurse, dietitian, and social worker
14. Begin subcutaneous growth hormone injections each evening
15. Hospitalization of infant to ensure adequate intake

Problem 18. A 23-year-old female comes to the office requesting oral contraceptives. She will be married in 1 month and wants to delay having a child until she finishes graduate school. In discussing contraception with this patient, which of the following are true?

1. The theoretical effectiveness of oral contraceptives is over 99%.
2. Oral contraceptive pills increase the risk of hepatic adenomas.
3. Oral contraceptive pills increase the risk of thrombophlebitis.
4. Oral contraceptive pills increase the risk of breast cancer.
5. Oral contraceptive pills increase the risk of ovarian cancer.

The patient is started on a low-dose estrogen–progesterone combination pill. After 1 month she returns to the office complaining of some intermenstrual spotting. She denies missing any pills and otherwise is without complaints. Appropriate actions include:

6. Stopping the pill and using a barrier method or contraception for 1 month
7. Reassuring the patient and continuing the same pill
8. Changing the pill to a higher estrogen dose pill
9. Changing to a pill with stronger progesterone
10. Advising patient to use a backup method of birth control on days she spots

Problem 19. A mother brings in her 4-year-old daughter for a visit. She is worried because 6 months ago her daughter had a nonfocal febrile seizure that lasted about 10 minutes. The mother is concerned because her previous doctor did not do an EEG. In discussing this with the mother, which of the following are true?

1. Febrile seizures occur in about 2% to 5% of children.
2. The child has less than a 50% chance of having another febrile seizure.

3. An EEG is indicated to determine if the child will develop epilepsy.
4. CT scan is indicated to rule out a focal lesion.
5. The child's long-term risk for having a seizure disorder is about 1%.
6. The child should not receive an aDTP.
7. The child should receive influenza vaccine.
8. The mother should be given a prescription for phenobarbital elixir to start at the first sign of infection.

The child's neurologic examination is completely normal. However, you note a heart murmur. Which of the following suggests the need for further evaluation?

9. A crescendo decrescendo murmur
10. The presence of a thrill
11. A diastolic murmur
12. Radiation of the murmur to the right carotid artery
13. A family history of early atherosclerosis

Problem 20. A 6-month-old male is brought to the emergency room with a 1-day history of fever. He has been eating poorly and is irritable. There has been no congestion, cough, vomiting, diarrhea, or rashes. He has had no known exposures to sick individuals. His past medical history reveals a normal birth and development. The physical examination reveals an irritable, inconsolable crying male with no localized findings. His temperature is 103°F and his heart rate is 160 and regular. No rash is noted. In addition to a CBC, initial assessment should include:

1. Abdominal CT scan
2. Urinalysis and urine culture
3. Gallium nuclear medicine scan
4. Blood culture
5. Lumbar puncture for cerebrospinal fluid analysis

After receiving acetaminophen and ibuprofen, his temperature is 99.6°F, and the infant is no longer irritable and is now consolable. His CBC reveals normal hemoglobin and platelet count and a WBC of 17,000 with 80% polymorphonuclear leukocytes. The remaining studies ordered are pending. Appropriate management at this point may include:

6. Intravenous ceftriaxone
7. Oral amoxicillin
8. Hospitalization for monitoring and observation
9. Discharge with follow-up in 24 hours

Problem 21. A 40-year-old white female in good general health complains of progressively worsening midepigastric pain for the past 3 months. The pain usually develops suddenly and lasts about 2 hours. She has tried several over-the-counter medications for indigestion but so far nothing has helped. She denies any fever, chills, or night sweats.

On physical examination, she is a moderately obese female who is afebrile with a blood pressure of 136/80 mmHg. There are normal bowel sounds and there is no abdominal tenderness or mass. The rest of her physical exam is unremarkable. Which of the following are true?

1. Only about one-third of patients with gallstones experience symptoms.
2. Biliary colic usually lasts less than 3 hours.
3. Fatty foods increase the likelihood of biliary colic.
4. An ultrasound is 85% sensitive and specific for gallstones.

5. The pain of biliary colic is due to spasm of the cystic duct when obstructed by a gallstone.
6. Fasting improves the sensitivity of ultrasound testing for gallstones.

A diagnostic test reveals gallstones. Which of the following statements about biliary colic are true?

7. In patients with biliary colic, 40% to 50% will have recurrent episodes within the next year.
8. The best test for choledocholithiasis is an endoscopic retrograde cholangiopancreatography (ERCP).
9. The risk of developing complications from gallstones is 1% to 2% per year.
10. The patient should be scheduled for a cholecystectomy.
11. Bile duct injury is less common with an open cholecystectomy.
12. Nonsurgical therapies for gallstones include ursodiol and shock wave lithotripsy.
13. Ursodiol is useful for calcified cholesterol stones less than 5 mm in size.

Problem 22. A 65-year-old Caucasian woman complains of a sudden loss of vision in the right eye after noting intermittent episodes of diplopia during the previous week. She denies eye pain but complains of a right-sided headache and tenderness around her ear when brushing her hair. She has a history of high blood pressure for which she takes atenolol (Tenormin). Which of the following are true?

1. She should follow up with her ophthalmologist in 2 weeks for a cataract check.
2. Her left eye is at significant risk of a similar episode.
3. She is at risk for myocardial infarction.
4. She is at risk for a stroke.
5. With treatment, her vision should improve.
6. You should obtain a CT of the optic nerve to rule out a compressive tumor.
7. Treatment would provide no benefit.

During your examination, you discover that she can only see the number of fingers you are holding up in front of the right eye. The left eye appears normal with about 20/30 vision. Which of the following should you do?

8. Start steroid drops in the right eye immediately.
9. Obtain a stat Westergren erythrocyte sedimentation rate (ESR).
10. Start 80 mg of oral prednisone at once.
11. Make arrangements for a temporal artery biopsy.
12. Withhold treatment until test results are available.
13. Discontinue treatment if biopsy results are negative.

Problem 23. J.S., a 34-year-old male with a history of HIV diagnosed 5 years ago, presents with diarrhea and weight loss despite a good appetite. Although he takes antiviral medications, he frequently misses doses. He denies any other medical problems and has no known drug allergies. Vital signs reveal a blood pressure of 124/86 mmHg, respirations 18, pulse 72 and regular, and temperature of 98.4°F. Physical examination of the oral mucosa shows a white plaque-like material on the tongue that bleeds when removed. His lungs are clear to auscultation. Which of the following are true statements?

1. The patient should be treated with amphotericin.
2. Oropharyngeal candidiasis is predictive of CD4 counts less than 500/mm.

3. Prophylactic fluconazole for candidiasis is indicated in this patient.
4. Chronic use of fluconazole is associated with development of drug-resistant candida.
5. Prophylaxis for *Pneumocystis carinii* is indicated in this patient.

Several weeks later, the patient comes in with a history of a nonproductive cough and shortness of breath for the past 3 days. The patient denies chest pain but does complain of chills and night sweats. On physical examination, the patient's temperature is 102°F and he appears to be tachypneic. His lungs are clear to auscultation and the heart sounds are regular without a murmur or gallop. You suspect *P. carinii* pneumonia. Which of the following are true?

6. Trimethoprim-sulfamethoxazole (TMP-SMZ) for 3 weeks is effective therapy for Pneumocystis pneumonia.
7. Pentamidine is an alternative treatment for Pneumocystis for patients allergic to sulfa medications.
8. The prophylactic agent of choice for *P. carinii* is pentamidine.
9. Patients with life-threatening adverse reactions to TMP-SMZ may be switched to dapsone.
10. Prophylactic TMP-SMZ for Pneumocystis will also protect against toxoplasmosis encephalitis.
11. Patients responding to antiviral medications may stop TMP-SMZ if their CD4 count improves to more than 200 cells/mm^3 for 3 to 6 months.

Problem 24. While you are reviewing labs for your partner who is away on vacation, you come across the lab results for a 32-year-old female patient who has a serum calcium level of 11.7 mg/dL. After looking through her chart, what actions are important in managing the patient?

1. Discontinuing her oral contraceptives
2. Stopping the furosemide that the patient takes as needed for premenstrual edema
3. Telling her to avoid sun exposure
4. Asking her if she is constipated
5. Reviewing the results of a previous electrolyte panel
6. Reviewing the results of a previous CBC
7. Inquiring about her family history

After talking with the patient you find out that she feels well except for some occasional joint pains, headache, and mild fatigue. Her only medication is a multivitamin that she takes a few times per week. She makes an appointment for the following week. Examination reveals a thin African American female with a blood pressure of 140/100 and pulse of 96 but otherwise unremarkable. A repeated ionized calcium level confirms the elevated level. At this time, appropriate studies might include:

8. A serum iPTH level
9. A chemistry panel
10. A head CT scan
11. A mammogram
12. A chest x-ray
13. A serum TSH

Laboratory testing confirms the diagnosis of hyperparathyroidism. Factors that favor surgical intervention include which of the following?

14. Allergy to hydrochlorothiazide
15. Intolerance to bisphosphonates
16. Intolerance to calcitonin
17. A history of kidney stones

18. Age younger than 50
19. An abnormal DEXA scan

Problem 25. A 26-year-old previously normotensive female is found to have a blood pressure of 165/100 mmHg in both arms. She is asymptomatic and has no significant past medical history. She is on no medications and she does not smoke, drink alcohol, or use drugs. Her parents and siblings have no history of hypertension. She returns for two repeat blood pressure measurements and the readings are unchanged. Initial evaluation of this patient should include:

1. Complete blood count
2. Serum creatinine
3. Serum catecholamines
4. Serum calcium
5. Electrocardiogram

Initial laboratory studies are within normal limits and the patient is started on medication. She has appropriate follow-up but her blood pressure remains elevated despite being on maximal doses of three medications. Which of the following tests are useful in identifying secondary causes for hypertension?

6. Parathyroid scan
7. Plasma aldosterone:renin ratio
8. Renal magnetic resonance angiography
9. Thyroid ultrasound
10. Urine for VMA and metanephrines

All lab tests are normal and the patient wants to try changing her diet before taking medication. After 6 month of adhering to a low-salt diet and following an exercise regimen, her blood pressure is 145/92.

11. She should be continued on nonpharmacologic therapy alone.
12. An ACE inhibitor is a good choice for this patient.
13. A calcium channel blocker is a good choice for this patient.
14. Diuretics should be avoided because of the risk of hypokalemia.

Problem 26. A 42-year-old female notes a 10-lb weight gain over the past year. She is also concerned because of increasing fatigue, muscle aches, and heavy periods. She has not been sleeping well and feels a little blue. Laboratory tests that would be helpful in the initial evaluation of this patient include:

1. Anti-nuclear antibodies (ANA)
2. Serum TSH level
3. A CBC
4. Serum estrogen levels
5. A lipid profile
6. A dexamethasone suppression test to rule out depression
7. Lyme disease titers

In further discussion with the patient, she believes her sadness is because of her physical complaints and she is happy with her job and home life. Lab tests reveal a TSH of 34, a T4 of 4.2, and a CBC, which is within normal limits. A lipid profile reveals a cholesterol level of 232, HDL of 42, and a LDL of 150. Which of the following are true?

8. TSH is the most sensitive test for hypothyroidism.
9. Hypothyroidism is a common consequence of I_{131} treatment.
10. There are no laboratory markers for Hashimoto's thyroiditis.
11. Postpartum thyroiditis symptoms resolve spontaneously and do not occur with subsequent pregnancies.
12. Hashimoto's thyroiditis is the most common cause of primary hypothyroidism.

13. Hypothyroidism can cause carpal tunnel syndrome and obstructive sleep apnea.
14. Ibuprofen can cause hypothyroidism.
15. Patients with hypothyroidism may exhibit loss of the medial aspect of their eyebrows.
16. Primary treatment of hypothyroidism is levothyroxine.
17. Older patients should be started on higher doses of thyroid replacement in order to correct their hypothyroidism quickly.

Problem 27. A.B., a 49-year-old white male, presents to your office complaining of right knee pain that developed rapidly over the past 24 hours. The pain is moderately severe and awakened him from sleep. A.B. takes no medications and is otherwise in good health. He drinks between three and six beers per night and has never used intravenous drugs. Physical examination reveals a mildly obese male with a temperature of 100.5°F and a warm, swollen, erythematous, and diffusely tender right knee. There is no evidence of joint instability. Which of the following are appropriate diagnostic tests?

1. CBC
2. ESR
3. MRI of right knee
4. Arthrocentesis with gross and microscopic evaluation of joint fluid
5. Arthrocentesis with culture and Gram stain of joint fluid
6. Rapid strep test
7. Serum rheumatoid factor

Lab results include the following:

ESR 41 mm/hour; white blood cell count is 11 cell/mm^3 with a normal differential. Joint fluid: negatively birefringent crystals. Gram stain: no organisms.

The following are appropriate interventions:

8. Encourage ambulation
9. Indomethacin 25 to 50 mg every 8 hours
10. Hydrochlorothiazide 25 mg PO daily
11. Colchicine 0.6 mg PO every hour until pain is gone, independent of side effects
12. Allopurinol 100 mg PO tid

The patient responds to treatment and 3 weeks later is without complaints. Appropriate therapy now includes:

13. Indomethacin 25 mg PO very 6 to 8 hours
14. Counseling to stop drinking alcohol
15. High-purine diet
16. Counseling to lose weight

With regard to this patient's disease, the following statements are correct:

17. The disease does not occur in women.
18. It is more common in those older than the age of 30.
19. Most individuals who suffer from it also suffer from kidney stones.
20. It may occur in patients being treated for lymphoma or leukemia.
21. It is a metabolic disease characterized by either undersecretion or overproduction of uric acid.

Problem 28. M.L., a 42-year-old male, comes into the office complaining of back pain for 1 week. The pain began the evening after M.L. helped a friend move into a new apartment. Although he tried to rest the back over the weekend, the pain has gotten worse. The pain is a constant, dull ache that is worsened by bending or twisting. Lying down and flexing the knees improves the pain. Which of the following statements are true about the patient's condition?

1. Approximately 75% of adults experience back pain at some time in their lives.
2. Approximately 10% of individuals with lower back pain have a serious underlying cause, such as a fracture, neoplasm, or infection.
3. Mechanical low back pain worsens at nighttime.
4. Back pain from spinal stenosis worsens with standing.
5. The presence of sciatica usually indicates a disc herniation.

On physical examination, M.L.'s vital signs are within normal limits. Examination reveals a mildly overweight individual in moderate distress. There is diffuse tenderness along the right paravertebral muscles. Straight leg raising to more than 45 degrees produces pain that radiates down the right leg. Neurologic exam reveals a slight decrease in strength in right foot dorsiflexion. Reflexes are symmetrical and equal. Which of the following statements are true?

6. The patient most likely has a herniated disc at L4–L5.
7. Disc herniation most commonly occurs at the L4–L5 level.
8. Lumbosacral spine films are helpful in confirming the diagnosis.
9. Strict bed rest should be prescribed to this patient for a 2-week period.
10. This patient will benefit from early surgery.
11. Muscle relaxants in combination with NSAIDs are more effective than NSAIDs alone.
12. Spinal manipulation can be helpful in patients without radiculopathy.
13. An MRI should be scheduled immediately.
14. If the patient does not return to work within 6 months, there is less than a 50% chance that the patient will work again.

Problem 29. A 38-year-old female comes in the office complaining of no menses for the past 8 months. She had regular periods starting at age 18 but about 2 years ago noted that they were lighter. She is married and her husband uses condoms for birth control. She has had two previous uncomplicated pregnancies and is in good general health. She denies a history of vaginal discharge, pelvic pain, or any previous surgeries. Physical examination reveals a mildly overweight female (BMI 27) with normal vital signs. Her remaining examination including gynecologic examination is normal. What tests would be useful in an initial evaluation of this patient?

1. A serum TSH
2. A urine HCG
3. A serum prolactin level
4. A morning serum cortisol level
5. A pelvic ultrasound with a vaginal probe to assess the uterus
6. Serum estrogen levels

All laboratory tests are normal. Which of the following are appropriate next steps to assess for withdrawal bleeding?

7. Starting a low-dose combination oral contraceptive
8. Giving medroxyprogesterone acetate (Provera) 10 mg orally for 7 days
9. Administering medroxyprogesterone 100 mg IM

After initiating withdrawal therapy the patient does not have any bleeding. After receiving 3 weeks of estrogen followed by progesterone, the patient experiences bleeding. Which of the following statements are true?

10. The patient may have Asherman's syndrome.
11. The patient may have pituitary dysfunction.
12. The patient may have ovarian failure.
13. The patient may have polycystic ovarian disease.

Problem 30. C.F., a 30-year-old white female, presents at a follow-up visit for renewing her oral contraceptives complaining of throbbing headaches occurring in the left frontal area and accompanied by photophobia with nausea and vomiting. She denies drinking alcohol, drug use, or smoking but she admits that she frequently eats one or two chocolate candy bars with nuts a day.

1. This patient most likely has classic migraines.
2. Migraine headaches are twice as common in women than in men.
3. A positive family history is present in over 80% of patients with migraines.
4. Tension headaches are often band-like and usually bilateral.
5. Jaw clenching and bruxism associated with headaches are symptoms of temporomandibular joint dysfunction.
6. Oral contraceptives can trigger migraines.
7. The severity of the pain is of value in evaluating chronic headache.

C.F. denies any weakness, fever, or neck stiffness. She denies any visual changes and says that she has had these headaches for the past several years. Which of the following are true?

8. An MRI scan is likely to be normal.
9. Acute headaches in patients older than age 50 years associated with tenderness over the temples suggest a cerebellar hemorrhage.
10. Acute onset of a frontal headache with fever and upper respiratory congestion suggests sinusitis.
11. Headache worsened by cough or bending is characteristic of an intracranial mass.

Management of this patient might include which of the following?

12. A small daily dose of triptans may be used to reduce headache frequency.
13. Chest pain associated with triptans is usually from coronary artery spasm.
14. Ergotamines should not be used since the patient uses oral contraceptives.
15. Daily dosing of acetaminophen may benefit this patient and reduce the need for more potent pain relievers.

Problem 31. A 42-year-old female comes to the office requesting your help to lose weight. She has been overweight throughout her life but has recently gained about 20 pounds. Both her parents were also overweight. She is 63 inches in height and weighs 175 lbs. Her BMI is 31 kg/m². Her blood pressure is 130/90, pulse 82, temperature 37°C, and respirations 14. The remainder of her physical examination is within normal limits. She has a family history of a sister with type 2 diabetes.

When considering how to evaluate and manage her complaint, which of the following should you take into account?

1. Her BMI meets the definition for obesity.
2. Her obesity is due to a genetic condition.
3. If her waist-to-hip ratio is greater than 1, she is at increased risk for developing cardiovascular disease.
4. She is at increased risk for developing sleep apnea.
5. Weight loss might help lower her blood pressure.
6. Her obesity places her at greater risk for osteoporosis.

7. Rapid weight loss increases the risk of gallstones.

8. A calorie deficit of 500 to 1,000 calories per day should result in a 1 or 2 lb per week weight loss.

Appropriate options for initial management include:

9. Checking a fasting blood sugar

10. Checking a fasting lipid profile

11. Recommending a 10% reduction in body weight over the next 6 months

12. Recommending an increase in exercise

13. Scheduling a follow-up appointment in 3 months

14. Starting sibutramine at 5-mg daily dose

15. Referring for evaluation for possible bariatric surgery

Problem 32. A 78-year-old Asian American female presents to the emergency room complaining of right groin pain after falling. Her x-ray reveals a right intertrochanteric hip fracture requiring pinning. You are asked by her daughter about the likely outcome. Which indicators predict a patient's likelihood for a good recovery?

1. The bone density prior to fracture

2. The patient's mental status prior to fracture

3. The nutritional status of the patient

4. The surgical skill of the orthopedic physician

5. Ensuring that the patient gets physical therapy

6. Early ambulation

The patient does well postoperatively and is transferred on day 4 to a long-term care facility for rehabilitation and physical therapy. Two days later, the nurse notes some bilateral lower leg edema, which is slightly worse on the right side. The patient has no other complaints, the lungs are clear, and the cardiovascular examination is unremarkable. Appropriate orders include:

7. Obtaining venous duplex scans of the lower extremities

8. Ted hose to above the knee

9. Asking the nurses to check daily weights

10. Obtaining a chest x-ray

11. Starting furosemide 40 mg a day

The patient returns to your office for follow up after discharge from rehabilitation. Her DEXA shows a T score of -2.8 and her Z score is -1.0. She is very concerned about preventing another similar fracture. Which of the following would you order?

12. A consultation for secondary causes of osteoporosis

13. Calcium intake of 1,500 mg a day

14. Weight-bearing exercise as tolerated

15. Alendronate (Fosamax) 70 mg weekly

Problem 33. A.M. is a 5 year-old male who presents to the office with a 3-day history of an upper respiratory infection (URI) and low-grade fever. Today his temperature is 101°F and he complains that his right ear hurts. Physical examination reveals an alert male in no acute distress. He has a bulging, red tympanic membrane and the remainder of the exam is unremarkable. Which of the following are true about the patient's condition?

1. Most cases of acute otitis media (AOM) are preceded by a viral illness.

2. About 90% of AOM cases have a bacterial etiology.

3. *Haemophilus influenzae* is the most common bacterial cause.

4. A history of low birth weight increases the risk of ear infection.

5. Most cases occur between 6 and 36 months of age.

6. Living with parents who smoke increases the risk of infection. Preferred management options at this time include:

7. Tympanocentesis

8. An oral decongestant

9. Oral ibuprofen as needed for pain

10. Topical antipyrine and benzocaine (Auralgan otic) as needed for pain

11. Oral amoxicillin (40 mg/kg/day)

12. Erythromycin if the patient is allergic to penicillin

13. Ceftriaxone 125 mg intramuscularly

14. Oral cefazolin (10 mg/kg/day)

After 48 hours, A.M.'s parents call to let you know that he is much better. You schedule a follow-up appointment in 4 weeks. At this visit, A.M. no longer has symptoms but on examination you note decreased mobility and fluid behind the eardrum. At this time, appropriate options include:

15. High-dose amoxicillin (80 mg/kg/day) orally for 2 weeks

16. A 2-week course of an antihistamine or decongestant

17. Inhaled nasal steroids

18. Referral to an otolaryngologist

19. Re-examination in 8 weeks

Problem 34. A 62-year-old male comes to the office because of two falls during the past 2 weeks. His wife notes that he has a slight tremor and shuffles when he walks. You believe that the falls may be related to Parkinson's disease. Which of the following are true regarding Parkinson's disease?

1. Individuals with Parkinson's disease have an intention tremor.

2. A unilateral tremor virtually excludes Parkinson's disease.

3. Parkinson's disease can cause dementia.

4. Depression is associated with Parkinson's disease.

5. Signs of decreased sensation in the lower extremities are common.

6. The patient is outside the usual age range for Parkinson's disease.

7. The patient's children are at increased risk for Parkinson's disease.

8. Carbidopa-levodopa (Sinemet) delays the progress of Parkinson's disease.

You recommend treating with carbidopa–levodopa to the patient and his family. In advising the patient about treatment, which of the following are true?

9. Carbidopa–levodopa (Sinemet) is more effective for tremor than rigidity.

10. Carbidopa–levodopa should be started if symptoms interfere with the patient's employment.

11. Nausea is a common side effect of carbidopa–levodopa.

12. Carbidopa is important because it increases the absorption of levodopa.

13. Dyskinesias are a potential side effect of carbidopa–levodopa.

The patient improves markedly with carbidopa–levodopa. However, after 2 years he begins having a less predictable response to the medicine. Options at this time include:

14. A drug holiday for a week and then resuming carbidopa–levodopa

15. Adding a dopamine antagonist to the patient's regiment

16. Taking the carbidopa–levodopa with a high-protein meal

Problem 35. J.S., a 72-year-old female, comes in complaining of fatigue, weakness, and stiffness for the past 2 months in the shoulder and hip girdles. Although it usually takes her a little time to get going in the morning, on a recent camping trip she noticed that the stiffness had increased significantly. She denies feeling depressed or being under extra stress. Physical examination reveals normal vital signs and some degenerative changes in her distal interphalangeal joints. Her neurologic examination is normal. She has no muscle tenderness or joint effusion. Appropriate lab tests at this time include which of the following?

1. CBC
2. ESR
3. TSH
4. Uric acid level
5. *Borrelia burgdorferi* antibody titers

Medication therapy that may help this patient includes:

6. Naprosyn 370 mg PO bid
7. Prednisone 20 mg PO qid
8. Colchicine 0.6mg PO bid
9. Cyclobenzaprine at night and as needed for stiffness
10. Doxycycline 100 mg PO bid for 14 days

At a follow-up visit in 2 weeks, the patient reports that she feels much better. Then about a month later she complains of a throbbing right-sided headache and scalp tenderness. Appropriate steps to take at this time include:

11. Increasing prednisone to 60 mg PO daily
12. Scheduling a biopsy of the temporal artery
13. Scheduling a cerebral angiogram
14. Giving sublingual ergotamine to abort the headache

Problem 36. A 52-year-old male in good general health presents to the office with a 1-day history of fever, headaches, myalgia, and a cough productive of greenish sputum. He complains of mild shortness of breath and decreased appetite, but he is able to ambulate and keep fluids down. On physical exam, he is alert and oriented. Vital signs are: BP, 130/90 mmHg; T, 102.4°F; P, 88; and RR, 20. A pulse oximeter reading in the office is 94%. Lung exam reveals a few coarse rhonchi. Which of the following are true?

1. A chest x-ray is necessary to determine if this patient has pneumonia.
2. A chest x-ray can help distinguish an atypical pneumonia from a bacterial pneumonia.
3. A Gram stain can confirm if this patient has pneumonia.
4. An arterial blood gas is indicated in this patient.
5. A sexual history is important in evaluating this patient.
6. An IGM mycoplasma antibody is greater than 1:64 diagnostic for mycoplasma pneumonia.
7. A negative urinary antigen can rule out *Legionella*.

A chest x-ray reveals an upper lobe infiltrate. The white blood cell count is 12,800 with 72% neutrophils and 2% bands. The hemoglobin level and platelet counts are normal. A sputum Gram stain reveals many white blood cells, a few epithelial cells, and no organisms. A basic metabolic profile is within normal limits. At this time, appropriate management steps include:

8. Admitting the patient to the hospital
9. Starting high-dose amoxicillin
10. Prescribing a course of doxycycline
11. Prescribing a course of cefuroxime
12. Prescribing a course of amoxicillin and clavulanate
13. Prescribing a course of clarithromycin

Problem 37. A 12-year-old white female presents to your office with a chief compliant of "sore throat" for 2 days. She also has had a fever of 102.5°F. Which of the following statements are true regarding group A beta hemolytic strep pharyngitis?

1. It is most common between ages 5 and 15 years.
2. Symptoms include enlarged tonsils with erythema, exudates, and vesicular lesions on the posterior pharynx.
3. Cough is a prominent symptom.
4. Petechiae on the soft palate are often seen.
5. It accounts for about one-half of all sore throats seen by physicians.

The patient is in no acute distress and is well hydrated. You perform a rapid step test, which is positive. Which of the following statements are true?

6. Rapid strep tests have a significant false-negative rate, so true strep cultures must always be performed.
7. Antibiotic treatment will shorten the duration of symptoms by 50%.
8. Broad-spectrum antibiotics are recommended to cover highly resistant strains of group A strep.
9. Patients may stop antibiotic therapy 48 hours after the resolution of symptoms.
10. Family members with pharyngitis should be treated.
11. Erythromycin is a drug of choice for penicillin-allergic patients.

The patient's mother calls 24 hours later and reports that her child now has a red fine rash and that the other symptoms have not changed. Which of the following statements are true?

12. Antibiotic therapy must be extended to 21 days.
13. Scarlet fever indicates a more serious group A strep infection.
14. The symptoms of strep throat may last 5 to 7 days.
15. The likelihood of peritonsillar abscess is higher in this patient.
16. Antibiotic treatment reduces the incidence of glomerulonephritis.

Problem 38. An 84-year-old woman requests "medical clearance" for an elective cholecystectomy. Her past medical history is significant for hypertension and coronary artery disease, for which she takes atenolol 50 mg/day, lisinopril 10 mg/day, atorvastatin 10 mg/day, and aspirin. She does not smoke and is very active, walking 2 to 3 miles 3 or 4 days per week. She denies recent chest pain, dyspnea, and after complaining of some dizziness 18 months ago had a stress test that was normal. Which of the following are true regarding this patient based on her history?

1. Her age increases her risk for surgery.
2. She is at high risk for cardiac complications.
3. Abdominal surgery increases her risk for pulmonary complications.
4. Her functional capacity is associated with lower cardiac risk.

On physical examination, blood pressure is 160/94 mmHg, pulse 64 and regular, and respiratory rate 12. She is 5'4" tall and weighs 165 lbs. Her lungs are clear and her heart has a regular rate and rhythm without murmurs. She has no peripheral edema and 2+ peripheral pulses. Which of the following tests are recommended preoperatively in this patient?

5. Echocardiogram
6. Electrocardiogram
7. Stress test
8. Prothrombin time
9. Complete blood count
10. Basic metabolic profile

Her preoperative ECG shows normal sinus rhythm with Q waves in the inferior leads, unchanged from prior electrocardiograms. Her chest x-ray is normal. A complete blood count and basic metabolic profile are within normal limits. In addition to the previous recommendations, you would now also recommend which of the following?

11. Preoperative education about using incentive spirometry
12. Compression stockings and subcutaneous heparin postoperatively
13. Hold aspirin for a minimum of 3 days before surgery
14. Continue beta-blocker therapy

Problem 39. B.S., a 76-year-old male, was transferred to a rehabilitation center following a stroke, which left him with right-sided hemiparesis. He also has a history of atrial fibrillation with a well-controlled ventricular rate. Medications include coumadin 2 mg per day and atenolol 50 mg every morning for his atrial fibrillation and high blood pressure. In preventing bed sores in this patient, which of the following are true?

1. Urinary incontinence increases the risk of pressure ulcers.
2. Pressure ulcers can develop in as little as 1 hour.
3. Aging increases the risk of pressure ulcers.
4. Prescribing zinc sulfate will reduce the risk of pressure ulcers.
5. Coumadin increases the risk of pressure ulcers.

Despite precautions, the nurse at the rehabilitation center calls you because the patient has developed a 2-cm open area over the sacrum. Nurses report that there is fat tissue visible in the ulcer crater and that there is a small amount of yellowish discharge, but no erythema around the wound. Which of the following are true?

6. The patient has a stage 2 ulcer.
7. A wound culture is indicated.
8. Wet-to-dry dressings and wound irrigation are indicated.
9. The area should be cleansed daily with povidone iodine.
10. The patient's diet should contain 20 to 25 kcal/kg/day.
11. Antibiotics will improve wound healing in this patient.

Problem 40. A 43-year-old white male with no previous medical problems presents via ambulance to the emergency room with sudden onset of severe difficulty breathing and pleuritic chest pain. The patient appears pale and diaphoretic. His blood pressure is 85/50 mmHg, pulse is 112 and regular, and his respiratory rate is 32. A pulse oximetry reveals 83% saturation. On exam, the patient has elevated neck veins, a loud P2, and a right ventricular heave. Lung exam reveals bilateral rales. An arterial blood gas performed on room air shows a PO_2 of 55. Which of the following statements are true?

1. This patient has signs and symptoms of acute left-sided ventricular dysfunction and pulmonary hypertension.
2. The ECG pattern of S1Q3T3 is the most common abnormality for patients with a documented pulmonary embolus.
3. A normal PO_2 rules out a pulmonary embolus.

With the preceding clinical information, pulmonary embolism is suspected, but further testing must be performed to solidify the diagnosis.

4. If the patient is clinically unstable, ventilation perfusion lung scanning is the best diagnostic option.
5. A normal spiral (helical) CT scan result may be interpreted in the same way as a low probability V/Q scan.
6. Pulmonary angiography is the safest and most specific test available in diagnosing pulmonary embolism.

7. In patients with nondiagnostic V/Q scans or helical CT scans, compression ultrasonography of the deep proximal leg veins is sufficient to effectively rule out pulmonary embolism.
8. The negative predictive value of the D-dimer test is 99% in patients with nondiagnostic lung scans and low or moderate pretest probability.

A pulmonary embolism has been positively diagnosed in this patient. Which of the following are true?

9. Low–molecular-weight heparin does not require an aPTT laboratory monitoring.
10. Low–molecular-weight heparin is appropriate initial therapy for patients with pulmonary embolism.
11. An advantage of low–molecular-weight heparin is that it does not cause thrombocytopenia.
12. Thrombolytics are indicated when the patient develops shock, severe respiratory failure, or right ventricular dysfunction.
13. Thrombolytics are absolutely contraindicated in patients with a history of GI bleeding.
14. A patient with recurrent pulmonary embolism on anticoagulation should get an inferior vena caval filter.

Problem 41. A previously healthy 18-month-old presents to your office with a 1-day history of cough, congestion, rhinorrhea, and low-grade fever. He had difficulty sleeping due to the cough. On exam, the child appears well, with respirations of 20 to 25 per minute, pulse of 110, and normal ear, throat, and lung findings. You diagnose the patient with a viral upper respiratory infection and recommend symptomatic treatment.

The next morning, the patient returns with difficulty breathing. He now has respirations of 40 to 45, audible wheezes, tracheal tugging, and intercostal refractions. The lung exam reveals inspiratory and expiratory wheezes, decreased air entry, and pulse oximetry is 93% on room air. You now suspect respiratory syncytial virus (RSV) bronchiolitis. Which of the following are true?

1. Patients from low-income families are twice as likely to require hospitalization for RSV bronchiolitis.
2. The most important means of infection control is hand washing.
3. Typical chest radiograph findings in RSV bronchiolitis include hyperinflation, atelectasis, peribronchial thickening, and diffuse interstitial infiltrates.
4. The diagnosis can be confirmed by rapid RSV assays using sputum specimens.
5. An oxygen saturation less than 95% correlates with more severe disease.

You decide to hospitalize this patient. Which statements regarding management of RSV are true?

6. Bronchodilators should be used routinely in the management of RSV bronchiolitis.
7. Racemic epinephrine has been shown to improve oxygenation.
8. The use of corticosteroids is not supported in the literature.
9. Empiric use of antibiotics to prevent secondary bacterial infection is indicated in hospitalized patients.
10. Ribavirin is recommended for patients requiring hospitalization.
11. Palivizumab (Synagis) is recommended for patients born prior to 35 weeks gestation.
12. Infection with RSV early in life predisposes a child to develop asthma.
13. A previous infection with RSV confers immunity against future infections.

Problem 42. A 52-year-old female comes to the office requesting a checkup. Her last checkup was more than 10 years ago. The patient smokes one pack per day and drinks one glass of wine per week. She denies any illicit drug use and her past medical history is pertinent for an appendectomy at age 16. According to the current U.S. Preventive Task Force, what screening tests are indicated?

1. Fecal occult blood testing
2. Flexible sigmoidoscopy
3. Measuring blood pressure
4. An ECG
5. A chest x-ray
6. Pulse oximetry
7. A mammogram
8. A Pap smear

Problem 43. A 62-year-old male comes into the office complaining of constant left-sided chest pain that has been increasing over the past 2 days. On physical examination, you notice a vesicular rash that goes from his back to the midline of his chest that follows two dermatomes. Otherwise, his physical examination is normal. Which of the following is true about his condition?

1. The pain from this condition usually precedes the rash.
2. Thoracic dermatomes are the most common site of involvement.
3. A chronic neuralgia occurs in about one-half of patients.
4. A Tzank smear taken from a lesion is likely to be negative.
5. The patient should be evaluated for an underlying malignancy.

Appropriate treatment options at this time include which of the following?

6. Prescribing acetaminophen with codeine as needed for the pain
7. Applying calamine lotion to the rash
8. Starting acyclovir 200 mg five times a day
9. Starting prednisone at 60 mg per day and tapering over a 3-week period

The patient complies with his prescribed regimen and the rash resolves. However, although the pain in the chest is much better, it still remains after several months and interferes with the patient's sleep. Treatments that may help the patient at this time include:

10. Amitriptyline 25 mg PO at night
11. Gabapentin 300 mg three times a day and titrating the dose upward if needed
12. Topical capsaicin ointment
13. Supplemental vitamin B12

Problem 44. A 12-year-old male is brought to the office by his mother because of a 2-day history of nasal congestion and fever up to 101°F. His mother is concerned because the nasal discharge has turned yellowish-green. The child denies a headache or earache and is eating well. Which of the following are true about the child's condition?

1. The average child experiences more than twice as many colds than an adult does.
2. About 25% of children with a cold develop bacterial sinusitis.
3. Children are less likely to develop bacterial sinusitis following a URI than adults.
4. A bacterial sinus infection can be reliably differentiated from a viral infection by clinical means.
5. Sinusitis is unlikely if the sinuses transilluminate.
6. Radiographs can reliably diagnose bacterial sinusitis.

Management options at this time include:

7. Amoxicillin 40 mg/kg/day orally for 10 days
8. An oral antihistamine
9. A topical decongestant for up to 3 days
10. Saline nasal spray

Problem 45. A 55-year-old man is brought in by his wife because of heavy snoring and restlessness while sleeping. The patient complains of feeling tired during the day. Which of the following are true?

1. Alcohol will worsen the patient's condition.
2. As people age, they will tend to spend less time in stage 3 sleep.
3. The patient may experience hypoxemia at night.
4. The patient may retain carbon dioxide at night.
5. The patient is likely to experience hallucinations just after falling asleep.

On examination, the patient has a BMI of 32 and blood pressure of 180/100 mmHg. There is a soft systolic murmur and a loud S2, which is paradoxically split. Appropriate action is to include which of the following?

6. Arranging a sleep study
7. Periodic nighttime monitoring of O_2 saturation
8. Starting O_2 2 L per nasal cannula at night
9. Obtaining a serum TSH level
10. Recommending weight loss
11. Recommending tonsillectomy and uvula plasty to improve apnea
12. Prescribing theophyline to improve respiratory drive
13. Having the patient sleep on his side

Problem 46. A 66-year-old male with chronic stable angina smokes about one pack of cigarettes per day. His only medication is phenytoin (Dilantin), which he takes for seizures. In counseling this man about smoking cessation, which of the following statements are true?

1. Smoking is the leading cause of preventable death in the United States.
2. After 2 years of smoking cessation, the rate of decline in FEV1 will be reduced to that of a nonsmoker.
3. It is unlikely that he will gain weight trying to stop smoking.
4. After age 65 there is no significant overall improvement in survival associated with smoking cessation.
5. Nicotine replacement therapy doubles the quit rate.
6. Nicotine patches should not be used because of the patient's history of angina.
7. Typical quit rates are about 50% at 1 year.

The man decides he wants to quit smoking. Appropriate treatment options include:

8. Setting an exact quit date
9. Prescribing nicotine replacement therapy
10. Buproprion therapy for 2 to 4 weeks
11. Nortriptyline started 3 days before a quit date
12. Benzodiazepines to help with nicotine withdrawal symptoms

Problem 47. A 26-year-old man presents to the office with a history of discomfort urinating. This morning he noted a small amount of discharge from his penis and some staining of his underwear. Which of the following organisms could account for this patient's symptoms?

1. Gonorrhea
2. *Chlamydia trachomatis*
3. *Ureaplasma urealyticum*
4. Mycoplasma
5. Trichomonas
6. Candida
7. Syphilis
8. *Haemophilus ducreyi*

On examination, the patient has a mucoid discharge but has no visible lesion or lymphadenopathy. The patient's testes and scrotal exam are also within normal limits. A Gram stain of the discharge reveals numerous white blood cells with gram-negative intracellular diplococci. At this time, appropriate steps include:

9. Culturing for *Neisseria gonorrhoeae*
10. Direct immunoflourescent antibody testing for chlamydia
11. Obtaining a RPR
12. Obtaining a CBC
13. HIV testing
14. Checking to determine if the patient is HLA-B27 antigen positive
15. Prescribing 3 g of amoxicillin plus 1 g of probenecid
16. Prescribing ofloxacin 500 mg orally plus doxycycline 100 mg bid for 7 days
17. Recommending that the patient's partner be treated

Problem 48. A 21-year-old female college student complains of dysuria for the past 2 days. She denies nausea, vomiting, fever, flank pain, or hematuria. This is her fourth episode in the past 6 months. The last episode was 6 weeks ago. Prior to 6 months ago, she never experienced a UTI. She has been sexually active with a single male partner for the past 7 months. She uses a spermicide in addition to his condom use for contraception. Her last menstrual period was last week, which was normal and on time. Which of the following are true about this patient's condition?

1. This patient is likely to have a structural abnormality of the urinary tract.
2. *Staphylococcus saprophyticus* causes 20% to 30% of cystitis in this age group.
3. Recurrent cystitis is usually caused by highly resistant bacterial pathogens.
4. There is an association between increased frequency of intercourse and the development of UTIs in young women.
5. The nonoxynol-9 in her spermicide increases her risk for recurrent UTIs.
6. Randomized, placebo-controlled studies demonstrate that cranberry juice decreases the rate of recurrences in patients with recurrent UTIs.

Physical examination reveals that she is alert, in no distress, and does not appear ill. Her temperature is 99°F, blood pressure is 120/82, pulse is 80 and regular, and respirations are 20. There is no CVA tenderness and no abdominal tenderness or masses.

Urine analysis reveals:

Specific gravity	1.020
Leukocyte esterase	2+
Blood	Trace+
Nitrite	+
Glucose	Negative
Protein	Trace+
Ketones	Negative

Appropriate additional tests or interventions at this time include:

7. Renal ultrasound
8. Voiding cystourethrogram
9. Vaginal culture for *Lactobacillus* species
10. Culture of male sexual partner

Appropriate treatment options after 3 to 7 days of antibiotic treatment for the acute infection include which of the following?

11. Daily prophylaxis with trimethoprim-sulfa for 6 months to 1 year
12. Postcoital prophylaxis with nitrofurantoin for 6 months to 1 year
13. Continuing acute antibiotic course for a minimum of 2 weeks
14. Trimethoprim-sulfamethoxazole double strength (320/1,600 mg) 2 tablets "prn" at onset of symptoms

Problem 49. An 18-year-old G-P0 female comes to the office complaining of irregular periods with occasional mild cramping occurring every 2 to 6 weeks and lasting for 7 to 10 days. She is sexually active with a single partner. She has not seen a physician for the past 2 years, but other than increased stress she denies health problems. On physical exam, she appears healthy. Her vital signs are: BP, 110/80; P 72; and RR, 18. She is a well-developed female with a normal general examination. Pelvic examination reveals a normal uterus and barely palpable ovaries. The patient is not bleeding at the time of the exam. Appropriate tests at this time include:

1. A serum pregnancy test
2. A complete blood count
3. A serum TSH level
4. A Pap smear
5. A pelvic ultrasound

The patient's lab results are normal except for hemoglobin of 11.2 g/dL. After talking with the patient, you learn that she desires contraception. Appropriate treatment actions might include which of the following?

6. Prescribing oral contraceptives
7. Provera intramuscular every 3 months
8. Prescribing clomiphene
9. Referring the patient for endometrial sampling
10. Prescribing nonsteroidal anti-inflammatory drugs
11. Prescribing iron sulfate orally

Problem 50. A 26-year-old female in good general health comes to the office complaining of vaginal itching and discharge for the past week. Her last menstrual period was 7 days ago, which was normal and on time. She is married and denies sexual contacts outside her marriage. She has never been pregnant and takes oral contraceptive pills. Which of the following statements are true about the patient's condition?

1. Frequent douching can cause vaginitis.
2. Cervicitis is a likely cause of this patient's vaginitis discharge.
3. Yeast infections are the most common cause of vaginitis.
4. Pregnancy is a risk factor for candidal vaginitis.
5. Bacterial vaginosis is considered a sexually transmitted disease.

Physical examination reveals a slender, healthy-appearing female. Her pelvic examination demonstrates a thick, white vaginal discharge that adheres to the vaginal wall. There is no cervical motion tenderness. The uterus and adnexa are normal size and nontender. Which of the following statements are true?

6. The discharge from this patient would most likely turn Nitrazine paper blue.
7. A wet mount will show numerous white blood cells.
8. A KOH "whiff test" would be positive.
9. The patient's blood glucose should be checked.

A wet mount demonstrates numerous epithelial cells. The KOH reveals numerous branching hyphae. Treatment options for this patient include:

10. A single dose of oral fluconazole (Diflucan) 150 mg
11. Metronidazole (Flagyl) 2 g as a single oral dose
12. Metronidazole (Flagyl) 500 mg twice a day for 7 days
13. Intravaginal clotrimazole
14. Ketoconazole (Nizoral) 200 mg twice a day orally for 7 days
15. Topical treatment metronidazole (MetroGel) for her partner

Chapter 9

Answer Key

Problem 1
1. T
2. F
3. F
4. F
5. T
6. T
7. T
8. F
9. T
10. T
11. F
12. T
13. T

Problem 2
1. F
2. T
3. T
4. T
5. F
6. F
7. T
8. F
9. F
10. F
11. F

Problem 3
1. F
2. T
3. F
4. F
5. F
6. T
7. F
8. F
9. F
10. T
11. T

Problem 4
1. T
2. F
3. F
4. F
5. T
6. F
7. T
8. T
9. T
10. T
11. T
12. F
13. F

Problem 5
1. T
2. T
3. F
4. T
5. F
6. F
7. T
8. T
9. T
10. T
11. F
12. F
13. T
14. T
15. F
16. T
17. F

Problem 6
1. F
2. F
3. T
4. T
5. T
6. F

7. F
8. T
9. T
10. T
11. F
12. T
13. F
14. T
15. F
16. F
17. F
18. T
19. T
20. T
21. F
22. T
23. T

Problem 7
1. T
2. F
3. F
4. T
5. F
6. F
7. T
8. F
9. F
10. T
11. F
12. T
13. F
14. T
15. T
16. F
17. F
18. T
19. F
20. T
21. T
22. F

Problem 8
1. T
2. T
3. T
4. F
5. T
6. F
7. F
8. T
9. F
10. T
11. T
12. T
13. T
14. T
15. F

Problem 9
1. T
2. F
3. T
4. F
5. T
6. T
7. T
8. T
9. T
10. T
11. T
12. T
13. F
14. T
15. T
16. F
17. T
18. T

Problem 10
1. F
2. T
3. F
4. F

5. T
6. T
7. T
8. T
9. F
10. F
11. F
12. T
13. T
14. T

Problem 11
1. T
2. F
3. F
4. F
5. F
6. T
7. F
8. T
9. T
10. T
11. F
12. T
13. T
14. T
15. F
16. T
17. T
18. F

Problem 12
1. F
2. F
3. F
4. T
5. T
6. T
7. T
8. T
9. T
10. T

11. T
12. F
13. T
14. F
15. F
16. F
17. F

Problem 13
1. T
2. F
3. F
4. T
5. T
6. F
7. T
8. T
9. T
10. T
11. F
12. T
13. T
14. T
15. F
16. T
17. F
18. T
19. T

Problem 14
1. T
2. F
3. T
4. T
5. F
6. F
7. T
8. T
9. T
10. T
11. F
12. T

13. T
14. T
15. F
16. F
17. T

Problem 15
1. T
2. T
3. T
4. F
5. F
6. T
7. T
8. T
9. F
10. F
11. F
12. T
13. T

Problem 16
1. T
2. F
3. F
4. F
5. T
6. F
7. T
8. T
9. F
10. F
11. F
12. T
13. F
14. F
15. T
16. T
17. T
18. T
19. T
20. T

Problem 17
1. F
2. T
3. T
4. F
5. F
6. T
7. T
8. T
9. F
10. F
11. T
12. T
13. T
14. F
15. F

Problem 18
1. T
2. T
3. T
4. F
5. F
6. F
7. T
8. F
9. F
10. F

Problem 19
1. T
2. T
3. F
4. F
5. T
6. F
7. T
8. F
9. F
10. T
11. T
12. T
13. F

Problem 20
1. F
2. T
3. F
4. T
5. T
6. T
7. F
8. T
9. T

Problem 21
1. T
2. T
3. F
4. F
5. T
6. T
7. T
8. T
9. T
10. T
11. T
12. T
13. F

Problem 22
1. F
2. T
3. T
4. F
5. F
6. F
7. F
8. F
9. T
10. T
11. T
12. F
13. F

Problem 23
1. F
2. F
3. F
4. T
5. T
6. T
7. T
8. F
9. T
10. T
11. T

Problem 24
1. F
2. F
3. F
4. T
5. T
6. T
7. T
8. T
9. T
10. F
11. F
12. T
13. T
14. F
15. F
16. F
17. T
18. T
19. T

Problem 25
1. T
2. T
3. F
4. T
5. T
6. F
7. T
8. T
9. F
10. T
11. F
12. T
13. F
14. F

Problem 26
1. F
2. T
3. T
4. F
5. T
6. F
7. F
8. T
9. T
10. F
11. F
12. T
13. T
14. F
15. F
16. T
17. F

Problem 27
1. T
2. T
3. F
4. T
5. T
6. T
7. F
8. F
9. T
10. F
11. F
12. F
13. T
14. T
15. F
16. T
17. F
18. T
19. F
20. T
21. T

Problem 28
1. T
2. F
3. F
4. T
5. T
6. F
7. F
8. F
9. F
10. F
11. F
12. T
13. F
14. T

Problem 29
1. T
2. T
3. T
4. F
5. F
6. F
7. F
8. T
9. T
10. F
11. T
12. T
13. F

Problem 30
1. F
2. F
3. T
4. T
5. T
6. T
7. T
8. T
9. F
10. T
11. F
12. F
13. F
14. F
15. F

Problem 31
1. T
2. F
3. T
4. T
5. T
6. F
7. T
8. T
9. T
10. T
11. T
12. T
13. F
14. F
15. F

Problem 32
1. F
2. T
3. T
4. F
5. T
6. T
7. T
8. T
9. T
10. F
11. F
12. F
13. T
14. T
15. T

Problem 33
1. T
2. F
3. F
4. F
5. T
6. T
7. F
8. F
9. T
10. T
11. T
12. T
13. F
14. F
15. F
16. F
17. F
18. F
19. T

Problem 34
1. F
2. F
3. T
4. T
5. F
6. F
7. F
8. F
9. F
10. T
11. T
12. F
13. T
14. F
15. T
16. F

Problem 35
1. T
2. T
3. T
4. F
5. F
6. T
7. T
8. F
9. F
10. F
11. T
12. T
13. F
14. F

Problem 36
1. T
2. F
3. F
4. F
5. F
6. F
7. F
8. F
9. F
10. T
11. F
12. F
13. T

Problem 37
1. T
2. F
3. F
4. F
5. F
6. F
7. F
8. F
9. F
10. F
11. T
12. F
13. F
14. T
15. F
16. F

Problem 38
1. F
2. F
3. T
4. T
5. F
6. T
7. F
8. F
9. T
10. T
11. T
12. F
13. F
14. T

Problem 39
1. T
2. F
3. F
4. F
5. F
6. F
7. F
8. T

9. F
10. F
11. F

Problem 40
1. F
2. F
3. F
4. F
5. T
6. F
7. F
8. T
9. T
10. T
11. F
12. T
13. F
14. T

Problem 41
1. T
2. T
3. T
4. F
5. T
6. F
7. T
8. T
9. F
10. F
11. F
12. T
13. F

Problem 42
1. T
2. T
3. T
4. F
5. F
6. F
7. T
8. T

Problem 43
1. T
2. T
3. F
4. F
5. F
6. T
7. T
8. F
9. T
10. T
11. T
12. T
13. F

Problem 44
1. T
2. F
3. F
4. F
5. F
6. F
7. F
8. F
9. T
10. T

Problem 45
1. T
2. T
3. T
4. T
5. F
6. T
7. F
8. F
9. T
10. T
11. F
12. F
13. T

Problem 46
1. T
2. T
3. F
4. F
5. T
6. F
7. F
8. T
9. T
10. F
11. F
12. F

Problem 47
1. T
2. T
3. T
4. T
5. T
6. F
7. F
8. F
9. T
10. T
11. T
12. F
13. T
14. F
15. F
16. T
17. T

Problem 48
1. F
2. T
3. F
4. T
5. T
6. F
7. F
8. F
9. F
10. F
11. T
12. T
13. F
14. T

Problem 49
1. T
2. T
3. T
4. T
5. F
6. T
7. T
8. F
9. F
10. T
11. T

Problem 50
1. T
2. F
3. F
4. T
5. F
6. F
7. F
8. F
9. F
10. T
11. F
12. F
13. T
14. F
15. F

Clinical Set Answers

Problem 1

Symptoms of acute angle closure glaucoma include conjunctivitis, eye pain, blurred vision, frontal headache, nausea, and vomiting. Colored halos around lights are a classic symptom of this entity. Acute angle glaucoma is much less common than open angle glaucoma. It occurs in less than 1 in 1,000 individuals and accounts for only 1% of all cases of glaucoma. It is more common in whites than in blacks or Asians. Cholinergic drugs may precipitate an acute attack, and these medications should be used cautiously in individuals with narrow angles. Although acute angle glaucoma is an important cause of red eye to recognize, there are many other more common causes of red eye that a family physician might encounter. These are summarized in Table 9.1.

Migraines are also associated with unilateral throbbing headaches, nausea, vomiting, fatigue, and photophobia. Visual disturbances include "zigzagging" lights, blurred vision, and visual field defects. Halos are *not* a characteristic of migraine. Visual disturbances typically precede a migraine. If the headache precedes the visual symptoms, this may indicate the presence of an arteriovenous malformation, mass lesion with cerebral edema, or seizure focus and neuroimaging should be considered.

Patients with acute angle glaucoma experience an acute rise in ocular pressure. The increased pressure causes extreme pain, headache, and can lead to a vagal response with nausea and vomiting. With very high pressures, corneal edema ensues, which causes blurred vision and colored halos around lights. The patient may also experience conjunctival injection and a fixed mid-dilated pupil. A dilated exam is contraindicated since it may exacerbate the attack in the involved eye and may even precipitate an attack in the at-risk contralateral eye.

Patients with pressures above 50 mmHg are at great risk of severe and permanent vision loss within hours. In this situation, immediate pressure reduction is indicated. This is done via a laser or surgical peripheral iridotomy. Usually, before the iridotomy can be performed, pressure reduction is necessary to relieve the corneal edema. This is done with topical beta-blocker, alpha agonist, or carbonic anhydrase inhibitor drops. Oral carbonic anhydrase inhibitors (acetazolamide) and osmotic diuretics are also helpful. Medical therapy is only temporizing, and after instituting medical therapy to reduce intraocular pressure the primary care physician should refer the patient to an ophthalmologist for urgent evaluation and definitive treatment. Ergotamine is not indicated for angle closure glaucoma.

The untreated contralateral eye in patients with acute angle closure glaucoma has about a 40% to 80% chance of developing an acute angle closure attack over the next 5 to 10 years.

A laser peripheral iridotomy is therefore indicated in the opposite eye.

Problem 2

The most likely diagnosis in a child with an acute episode of diarrhea, fever, and nausea is viral gastroenteritis. In children, the most common etiologic agent is rotavirus, whereas Norwalk virus is more common in adults. The Advisory Committee on Immunization Practices (ACIP) and the Centers for Disease Control and Prevention (CDC) recommend routine vaccination for rotavirus with a newly licensed vaccine. Children should receive the first dose of the vaccine by 12 weeks of age and should receive all doses of the vaccine by 32 weeks of age. In 1999, a different rotavirus vaccine was withdrawn from the market after it was found to be associated with a rare type of bowel obstruction called intussusception.

Table 9.2 summarizes some other causes of gastroenteritis. Viral infections affect the brush border of the epithelial cells that line the intestine, which can cause transient lactose intolerance. Most authorities recommend avoiding lactose in patients with acute gastroenteritis. A Sudan fat stain detects fat globules in the stool and is a sign of malabsorption. It is generally negative in acute gastroenteritis.

Checking a stool specimen for leukocytes is an invaluable test in a child with acute diarrhea. The absence of white blood cells suggests a noninflammatory diarrhea, whereas the presence of leukocytes is more consistent with tissue invasion as seen in a bacterial infection (e.g., salmonella or shigella) or an acute presentation of inflammatory bowel disease. Checking the stool for occult blood is also helpful for eliminating more serious causes of diarrhea. Although *Clostridium difficile* is a common cause of acute diarrhea, it is usually associated with recent antibiotic therapy. *Clostridium difficile* testing is recommended for patients with recent hospitalization, antibiotic use within the previous 6 weeks of onset of diarrhea, or residency in a long-term care facility. Clindamycin and cephalosporins are the most common antibiotics associated with *C. difficile* colitis, but nearly all antibiotics have been implicated. In this individual without risk factors, the yield for *C. difficile* testing appears low. Similarly, without travel or an exposure history, checking for ova and parasites would also likely be a low-yield test.

Other studies are usually of limited value in assessing acute gastroenteritis. Blood tests such as a CBC may be useful if there is rectal bleeding or suspicion of a bacterial infection. Electrolytes are useful in assessing the degree of dehydration or for detecting imbalances in patients with moderate to severe diarrhea. Abdominal x-rays are rarely helpful in patients with acute diarrhea.

Most often, acute gastroenteritis is a self-limited disease and appropriate management includes oral rehydration, altering diet, and monitoring for resolution of symptoms. Although it has been a common practice to rest the bowel in children with diarrhea by giving only clear fluids, most authorities believe this practice actually prolongs the diarrhea. As soon as an infant is rehydrated,

Table 9.1 Differential diagnosis of red eye

Disease	Description	Other
Blepharitis	Chronic lid margin erythema, scaling, loss of eyelashes	Associated with staphylococcal infection, seborrheic dermatitis
Hordeola/chalazion	Painful nodules on or along lids	Hordeola associated with staphylococcal infection; chalazion-sterile
Conjunctivitis	Burning, itching, discharge, lid edema	
• Viral	Clear, mucoid discharge	Associated with upper respiratory infection; very contagious
• hyperacute bacterial	Copious purulent discharge	Potentially sight threatening; associated with gonorrhea, STDs, neonates
• acute bacterial	Moderate purulent discharge	*H. influenza*, staphylococcal, *S. pneumoniae*
• inclusion conjunctivitis	Persistent watery discharge	Chlamydia; neonates and young adults Associated with STDs
• allergic	Itching, tearing	Associated with other allergy symptoms
Subconjunctival hemorrhage	Nonblanching red "spot," painless without visual changes or discharge	Associated with trauma, cough, or Valsalva (e.g., straining)
Corneal abrasion/ foreign body	Pain, "foreign body" sensation	Abrupt, associated with incident or work exposure
Iritis	Pain, photophobia, pupillary constriction, cloudy cornea, and anterior chamber	Associated with connective tissue diseases, ocular injury
Acute angle-closure glaucoma	Pain, tearing, dilated pupil, shallow anterior chamber, halos around lights	Ocular emergency, more common over age 50

he or she can either be started on full-strength formula or return to breast-feeding. In an older child, starting a low-residue bland diet is appropriate. Using antimotility drugs such as diphenoxylate (Lomotil) generally should be avoided. Antibiotic therapy is not indicated in acute viral gastroenteritis.

Problem 3

A minor may consent for testing and treatment for substance abuse, STDs, mental health problems, and contraceptive care. Laws regarding HIV testing and abortion vary from state to state. Discussions regarding these problems are considered confidential unless there is potential for harm to themselves or others. In addition, most states require notification regarding suspected abuse, notification of a gunshot or stab wound, or if there is a reasonable identified threat to another individual.

A pelvic exam is indicated if the patient requests one or if she presents with pelvic pain, vaginal discharge, history of sexual intercourse, or a menstrual disorder. Adolescence is a transitional phase from childhood to adulthood characterized by growth, hormonal changes, and sexual development. The Tanner stages are sexual maturity ratings from 1 to 5 that denote the level of sexual development. Tanner stages of secondary sex characteristics are summarized in Table 9.3. The person in Question 5 is in Tanner

stage 4. Although many variations occur, in general, the growth spurt heralds the beginning of puberty in girls followed by breast development (thelarche) and then the development of pubic hair. Menses or stage 4 follows at an average age of 12.5 years in U.S. girls. Stage 5 represents full sexual development.

Psychosocial topics should be discussed during an adolescent health maintenance visit and the acronym HEADSS (home, education, activities, drugs, safety, sexuality, suicide/depression) is helpful to remember to ensure taking a complete psychosocial history. Targeting these issues is important since alcohol, drugs, and sexual risk taking represent significant health risks for adolescents. Also, behaviors developed during these formative years frequently carry into adulthood. Depression is important since suicide is the third leading cause of death in adolescents. The number one cause of death in adolescents is unintentional injuries, with most injuries due to motor vehicle accidents. Advising adolescents to wear seat belts is therefore an important preventive health measure. Ninety-five percent of teenage pregnancies are unintended and about one-third of these end in abortion. Cholesterol tests are indicated only in adolescent patients with heart disease, diabetes, hypertension, and a strong family history of heart disease or hyperlipidemia. Cholesterol tests may be justified in morbidly obese adolescents. A sexually active adolescent should receive

Table 9.2 Causes of gastroenteritis

Agent	Pathogenesis	Clinical/Epidemiologic Features	Therapy
Bacillus cereus	Preformed toxin	Generally causes vomiting, may also produce diarrhea, classic association with fried rice	None
Staphylococcus aureus	Preformed toxin	Vomiting with some diarrhea, found in high-protein foods (meats, cream-filled cakes) also high sugar content (custards)	None
Clostridium difficile	Toxin production in colon	Fever, abdominal pain, diarrhea, toxic megacolon, association with previous antibiotic use	Metronidazole
Escherichia coli (4 main groups)			
Enterotoxigenic	Enterotoxin formation in small intestine	Voluminous watery diarrhea, fever generally absent, fecal/oral transmission	None
Enteroinvasive	Invasion of the colonic mucosa	Fever, bloody diarrhea, fecal/oral transmission	Antibiotics
Enteroadherent	Adherence to small intestinal mucosa	Diarrhea, can be prolonged, fecal/oral transmission	Antibiotics
Enterohemorrhagic (e.g., *E. coli* O157:H7)	Production of a cytotoxin (verotoxin) in colon	Causes hemorrhagic colitis, colitis can be followed by TTP/HUS*, from contaminated meats (especially ground meat)	Diarrhea—none Treatment of TTP/HUS is generally supportive
Campylobacter jejuni	Colonization (?invasion) of large and small bowel	Fever, watery diarrhea, abdominal pain	Antibiotics
Salmonella typhi	Invasion of small intestine can then (via bloodstream) disseminate systemically	Protracted illness with fever, headache, malaise, splenomegaly. Constipation is more common than diarrhea, fecal/oral transmission	Antibiotics
Salmonella (non-typhi)	Invasion of small and large intestine	Fever, diarrhea, animal reservoirs, also in eggs	Antibiotics
Shigella spp.	Invasion of colon	Fever, bloody diarrhea, fecal/oral spread	Antibiotics
Vibrio cholerae	Enterotoxin	Profuse watery diarrhea, fever is rare, fecal/oral spread (often via water contamination)	Doxycycline
Entamoeba histolytica	Invasion of colon mucosa	Diarrhea, often bloody, fecal/oral spread	Metronidazole
Giardia lamblia	Colonization of small intestine	Diarrhea, secondary to malabsorption, abdominal pain, waterborn ("beaver fever")	Metronidazole

Reproduced with permission from Young V, Kormas W, Goroll A. *Blueprints in Medicine*. 2nd ed. Maiden: Blackwell Science; 2001:135.

Table 9.3 Tanner stages of sexual maturity

Stage	Boys	Girls
1	Childlike penis No enlargement of testicles No pubic hair	No breast development No pubic hair
2	Penis unchanged Scrotum and testicles enlarge Small amount of fine long pubic hair	Breast buds Small amount of fine, long pubic hair
3	Penis elongates Continued growth of testicles and scrotum Coarse and curly pubic hair	Breasts enlarge, areolas enlarge Pubic hair coarse and curly
4	Penis increased in diameter Darkening of scrotum Adult hair texture over pubic area	Continued breast growth Adult hair texture over pubic area
5	Adult penis, scrotum Pubic hair extends to thighs	Adult breast contours Adult pubic hair extends to thighs

a Pap smear and be screened for chlamydia, gonorrhea, as well as for hepatitis B if not immune, hepatitis C, syphilis, and HIV. Immunizations for a 15-year-old would include hepatitis B series, dT, and possibly varicella or MMR if not previously immune.

Problem 4

Alcohol abuse and its related illnesses are among the most serious social and medical problems in the United States. An estimated 10% to 20% of Americans have a substance abuse problem and alcohol still remains the most commonly abused substance. Approximately 100,000 Americans die each year as a result of alcohol abuse.

Screening questionnaires such as the CAGE questions are more specific and sensitive than lab testing. The CAGE questionnaire is a self-reported instrument consisting of four questions:

1. Have you ever felt you ought to cut down on your drinking?
2. Have people annoyed you by criticizing your drinking?
3. Have you ever felt guilty about your drinking?
4. Have you ever needed an *eye* opener in the morning to get you going or to steady your nerves?

Two "yes" answers have a sensitivity of 75% and a specificity of 95%. Gamma–GTP is the most sensitive liver enzyme to alcohol abuse, although an elevated level is not specific. If the hepatocellular enzymes are elevated, the aspartate amino transferase (AST) is often more elevated than the alanine amino transferase (ALT), making this a useful but nonspecific marker of alcohol-induced hepatitis. Risk factors for alcohol abuse include male gender, family history of alcohol abuse, northern European descent, and younger age. Although the death rate for cirrhosis is higher in men than in women, women are more sensitive to alcohol-related liver disease. A common consequence of alcohol abuse is hypertension, and it is among the most common reversible causes of hypertension in middle-aged males. Screening for depression is appropriate since excessive alcohol intake may be a marker for psychologic problems such as depression or marital problems.

The symptoms of alcohol withdrawal are nonspecific but include autonomic hyperactivity developing within several hours to days after stopping alcohol. Symptoms may include sweating, tremor, tachycardia (pulse greater than 100), insomnia, nausea, and agitation. More severe symptoms include hallucinations and seizures. Alcohol withdrawal has a continuum of signs ranging from low-grade fever, tachycardia, and shakiness to profound hypertension, delirium, and seizures. The differential diagnosis for the symptom of alcohol abuse is extensive and includes the multiple causes of acute confusional states such as infection, hypoxemia, myocardial infarction, head trauma, and drug reactions. The decision to admit a patient is based on several factors, such as how toxic the patient appears, a previous history of withdrawal syndromes, and comorbidities. A scoring system known as the CIWA-A (Revised Clinical Institute Withdrawal Assessment for Alcohol Scale) is often used to assess patients and to follow therapy.

The goals of hospitalization are to control symptoms and to prevent complications. In addition to glucose, electrolytes, and a chemistry panel, other appropriate tests include a CXR, ECG, U/A, appropriate cultures or other x-rays in a febrile patient, and imaging if there is suspected trauma including a head CT if there is evidence of head trauma. Although many agents have been used for acute withdrawal, benzodiazepines are the only drugs repeatedly shown to be effective and are considered the drugs of choice. Evidence of increased autonomic activity as seen in this patient merits large doses of benzodiazepines at the onset of treatment. Typically, 75 to 100 mg of chlordiazepoxide (Librium) or 15 to 20 mg of diazepam is prescribed as initial doses. Lorazepam is also effective. Thiamine is indicated to replenish diminished stores and to avoid Wernicke's encephalopathy, a disorder related to thiamine deficiency. Although Wernicke's encephalopathy is not specific for alcoholism, it is by far the most common cause and probably reflects poor nutrition.

Alcoholic individuals are susceptible to hypomagnesemia and blood sugar fluctuations. Hypomagnesemia is associated with neuromuscular abnormalities such as tremor, fasciculations, spasticity, choreiform movements, anxiety, delirium, and seizures. It also predisposes individuals to cardiac dysrhythmias and replacement is indicated for patients with low serum levels. Beta-adrenergic agents have also been used to treat withdrawal symptoms such as tachycardia and hypertension and can be used in conjuction with benzodiazepines. Clonidine, a centrally acting alpha-adrenergic agent, can be used with benzodiazepines for resistant hypertension. Haloperidol can lower seizure thresholds and its use should be limited to those individuals with hallucinations, and it should be used in combination with benzodiazepines.

Problem 5

Allergic rhinitis (AR) is an inflammatory response of the membranes lining the nose to a variety of allergens. Runny nose, sneezing, nasal congestion, and itchy nose and eyes characterize typical symptoms. Approximately 15% of Americans are affected by symptoms of AR, making it the sixth most common chronic medical condition. Although AR is common, Table 9.4 lists other causes of chronic or recurrent nasal congestion to consider. AR frequently occurs in conjunction with other allergic diseases, including asthma. It is well described that treating AR can improve asthmatic symptoms. In addition, AR occurs more frequently in conjunction with otitis media and sinusitis. Most cases of perennial allergic rhinitis are due to indoor allergens such as house dust and mold. Seasonal pollution patterns are summarized in Table 9.5.

Table 9.4 Important causes of chronic or recurrent nasal congestion

Allergic
  Seasonal allergic rhinitis (pollens)
  Perennial allergic rhinitis (dusts, molds)

Vasomotor
  Idiopathic (vasomotor rhinitis)
  Abuse of nose drops
  Drugs (reserpine, guanethidine, prazosin, cocaine abuse)
  Psychologic stimulation (anger, sexual arousal)

Mechanical
  Polyps
  Tumor
  Deviated septum
  Crusting (as in atrophic rhinitis)
  Hypertrophied turbinates (chronic vasomotor rhinitis)
  Foreign body (usually in children)

Chronic inflammatory
  Sarcoidosis
  Wegener's granulomatosis
  Midline granuloma

Infectious
  Atrophic rhinitis (secondary Infection)

Hormonal
  Pregnancy
  Hypothyroidism

Table 9.5 Seasonal pollination patterns

Allergen	Typical Season
Tree pollens	Early spring
Grass pollens	Late spring/early summer
Ragweed	Late summer to first frost

Reproduced with permission from Marino B, Snead K, McMillan J. *Blueprints in Pediatrics*. 2nd ed. Malden: Blackwell Science; 2001:43.

The diagnosis of AR is made primarily by taking a thorough history and a focused physical examination. A variety of physical findings are seen with AR. These include facial pallor, mouth breathing, allergic shiners, allergic "salute," and a nasal (allergic) crease. Nasal polyps are an important finding but are seen in the minority of cases of AR. Additional diagnostic testing is sometimes useful. A complete blood count can determine the presence of eosinophilia, which can point to an allergic process. Similarly, nasal cytology can also demonstrate eosinophils. Skin testing for allergy is a time-proven method and can aid the evaluation of the atopic patient. Newer methods of in vitro testing for IgE have evolved and are currently an alternative way to predict atopy. One major drawback to in vitro testing is expense; however, these tests are convenient because they only require a single blood sample. Clinical correlation is important for assessing any positive test findings for whichever method is used.

Treatment of AR is best achieved with a stepwise approach. Initially, patients may try over-the-counter decongestants or first-generation antihistamines such as diphenhydramine (Benadryl). First-generation antihistamines are effective medications; however, they have many side effects such as drowsiness that limit their use. Patients often seek medical attention and receive a prescription for a second-generation antihistamine. These medications are effective and side effects are minimal. Second-generation antihistamines can be safely combined with a decongestant. They are also longer acting than the older first-generation antihistamines. Intranasal corticosteroids are quickly becoming a mainstay of therapy. These medications relieve all the symptoms of allergic rhinitis, including sneezing, runny nose, and nasal congestion. They are well tolerated, with the most common side effect being nasal irritation. Intranasal corticosteroids have been used in children with good results. The major concern with prescribing this medication to children is decelerated growth; however, this effect appears to be negligible.

Problem 6

Asthma is a common chronic disease characterized by reversible airway obstruction secondary to airway inflammation and bronchospasm. It affects roughly 5% of the population and, in children 4 years of age or younger, it is becoming more prevalent. Rates of hospitalization and death are highest among blacks and those between the ages of 5 and 24 years. A history of atopy is the most identifiable risk factor for the development of asthma. Patients who are exposed to allergens such as dust mites, cockroaches, or pollen or who have symptoms of postnasal drip or gastroesophageal reflux are more likely to develop asthma. Exposure to secondhand smoke, exercise, or cold air often increases frequency of asthma symptoms as well. Common symptoms of bronchospasm include wheezing, chest tightness, cough (especially at night), and difficulty breathing.

The child described is having an acute exacerbation of his asthma. Because an acute asthma attack is a potentially life-threatening event, prompt assessment is crucial. Pulse oximetry and peak flow are useful parameters in determining response to therapy. The use of inhaled short-acting bronchodilators such as albuterol is an important method for reversing the bronchospasms. Oral albuterol has similar efficacy to inhaled albuterol but a greater incidence of side effects, and therefore it is seldom used. A short course of systemic corticosteroids (3 to 10 days) has broad anti-inflammatory properties and thus hastens recovery. Inhaled steroids are not indicated in the treatment of an acute attack.

Unless there is concern about an acute process such as pneumonia or pneumothorax, a chest x-ray is seldom needed for evaluation in a known asthmatic with an acute attack. Although pulmonary function tests (PFTs) are useful for diagnosing asthma, they should not be performed when the individual is acutely ill. Unless there is suspicion for an underlying bacterial infection, antibiotics are not indicated for a simple exacerbation of asthma.

The National Asthma Education and Prevention Program published treatment guidelines to limit the frequency and severity of asthma exacerbations. These guidelines include classifying asthma as mild intermittent, mild persistent, moderate persistent, or severe persistent. Patients are then placed in a category and treated based on the severity of disease. Table 9.6 summarizes the National Heart, Lung, and Blood Institute's asthma guidelines. Paramount to this process is educating the patient and caregivers regarding the chronic course of the disease, the inflammatory nature of asthma, the use of preventive medications and acute care medications, and avoiding the triggers for asthma attacks.

Effective preventive medications include leukotriene inhibitors, inhaled corticosteroids, and long-acting beta-agonists. The advantage of leukotriene modifiers is their availability in pill form. Patients on inhaled corticosteroids who are not well controlled may benefit from the addition of a long-acting beta-2 agonist prior to increasing the steroid dose. Inhaled steroids are considered preventive therapy and thus are not appropriate treatment for acute exacerbations. All patients with asthma should receive annual flu shots.

Since this patient meets the criteria for mild persistent asthma (i.e., he has symptoms occurring more frequently than twice a week), he requires medications that provide more long-term control. Appropriate therapy includes daily use of inhaled corticosteroids at the lowest effective dose and/or a leukotriene inhibitor.

Problem 7

Increased distractibility, short attention span, and impulsivity characterize attention deficit hyperactivity disorder (ADHD). It is the most common behavioral syndrome in children. Prevalence among schoolchildren is 3% to 5% and is higher in boys than girls, although the number of cases seen in females is increasing. Symptoms begin in early childhood and persist to adulthood in 70% of cases. Family history is often positive, especially among male relatives.

The causes of ADHD are not well understood but there is strong evidence for a genetic predisposition. Evidence shows that neurotransmitter dysfunction involving dopamine and norepinephrine impairs inhibitory systems. The prefrontal lobes and basal ganglia appear to play a significant role in this disorder, as shown by neuroimaging in studies of patients with ADHD. New

criteria for ADHD require impairment of functioning in multiple settings. However, it is unlikely for a child to display the same level of dysfunction in all settings or within the same setting at all times. Symptoms are typically worsened in large groups, so often a physician may not observe the hyperactivity during a physical examination and must rely on parents' and teachers' reports.

ADHD occurs in all intellectual levels. Physical and neurologic examinations may reveal subtle deficiencies in behavior, language skills, and motor coordination. Laboratory tests such as thyroid tests and an EEG should be based on other clinical indications and are not necessary in most children with ADHD. It is suggested that lead levels and hematocrit screening be done on preschool children. Specific diagnostic tests are not available. Specifically, computer-based continuous performance tests (i.e., vigilance tests) are not reliable.

The two major forms of treatment are behavior modification programs and stimulant drugs such as methylphenidate (Ritalin), dextroamphetamine (Dexedrine), pemoline (Cylert), or a combination of amphetamine salts (Adderall). These agents act on dopamine and norepinephrine at the level of the synapse. Drug treatment is generally more effective than behavior modification, with 50% to 80% of children responding to stimulant therapy. However, response to the medications cannot be used as a test for ADHD since 10% to 30% of properly diagnosed children do not respond. Side effects include appetite suppression, weight loss, insomnia, stomachaches, headaches, fatigue, and jitteriness. Tics and dyskinesias can develop or worsen, but these effects are reversible. Stimulants do not lower seizure threshold and stimulant blood levels are not necessary. There is no evidence suggesting subsequent substance abuse is increased in those children treated with stimulants. It is recommended that treatment start with short-acting forms and long-acting medications be used once the optimal dose is found. Sometimes combinations of long- and short-acting forms are needed. In some instances, children need stimulants only on school days, but most require daily treatment if symptoms impair interaction with peers and family members.

Monitoring treatment is essential and ongoing input from teachers is helpful. Duration of treatment should be individualized and research has shown stimulants to also be helpful to adolescents and adults. Although stimulant medication is very effective in the treatment of ADHD, parents and children can benefit from referral to a mental health specialist for training in behavioral modification. Above all, it is the primary care physician's responsibility to explain to the parents and children that they did not cause this problem but that they are important for treatment success. Information sheets, books, and support groups can assist in this endeavor.

Problem 8

The differential diagnosis of a breast mass includes fibrocystic changes, fibroadenoma, breast cancer, and other inflammatory lesions such as traumatic fat necrosis or mastitis. Mastitis, which is an infection usually caused by staphylococci or anaerobic organisms, most commonly occurs in breast-feeding women and is associated with redness, tenderness, and increased warmth. The history and physical examination findings make this an unlikely cause of this patient's breast mass. Risk factors for breast cancer include age, genetic factors, and hormonal factors. Approximately one-fourth of breast cancers occur in women between the ages of 30 and 50. Family history of breast cancer in first-degree relatives increases the risk of breast cancer by two or three times. Hormonal risk factors include early menarche, late

Table 9.6 National Heart, Lung, and Blood Institute's asthma guidelines

Classification	Symptoms	Nighttime Symptoms	Lung Function	Long-Term Control	Quick Relief
Mild intermittent	Symptoms ≤2 times a week Asymptomatic and normal PEF between exacerbations Exacerbations brief (from a few hours to a few days), intensity may vary	≤2 times a month	FEV1 or PEF ≥80% predicted PEF variability <20%	No daily medication required	Short-acting β₂-agonist as needed for symptoms Use of short-acting β₂-agonist more than 2 times a week may indicate need to initiate long-term control therapy
Mild persistent	Symptoms >2 times a week but <1 time a day Exacerbations may affect activity	>2 times a month	FEV1 or PEF ≥80% predicted PEF variability 20–30%	One daily medication: Inhaled corticosteroid (low dose) or cromolyn or nedocromil Leukotriene modifier may be considered (exact position in therapy not fully established)	Short-acting β₂-agonist as needed for symptoms Use of short-acting β₂-agonist on a daily basis may indicated need for additional long-term control therapy
Moderate persistent	Daily symptoms Daily use of inhaled short-acting β₂-agonist Exacerbations affect activity Exacerbation ≥2 times a week; may last days	>1 time a week	FEV1 or PEF >60% to <80% predicted PEF variability >30%	Daily medication *Either* inhaled corticosteroid (medium dose) or inhaled corticosteroid (low-medium dose) and long-acting bronchodilator esp. for nighttime symptoms (either long-acting	Short-acting β₂-agonist as needed for symptoms Use a short-acting β₂-agonist on a daily basis indicates need for additional long-term control therapy

	Symptoms	Nighttime symptoms	FEV1 or PEF	Daily medications	Quick relief
				inhaled β$_2$-agonist, sustained-release theophylline, or leukotriene modifiers) *if needed:* High-dose inhaled corticosteroid *and* long-acting bronchodilator *Consider* referral to asthma specialist	
Severe persistent	Continual symptoms Limited physical activity Frequent exacerbations	Frequent	FEV1 or PEF ≤60% predicted PEF variability >30%	Daily medication Inhaled corticosteroid (high dose) *and* long-acting bronchodilator, esp. for nighttime symptoms (either long-acting inhaled β$_2$-agonist, sustained-release theophylline, or leukotriene modifiers) *and* corticosteroid tablets/syrup long term (make repeated attempts to reduce systemic steroids and maintain control with high-dose inhaled steroids) *Recommend* referral to asthma specialist	Short-acting β$_2$-agonist as needed for symptoms Use of short-acting β$_2$-agonist on a daily basis indicates need for additional long-term control therapy

FEV1, forced expiratory volume in 1 second; PEF, peak expiratory flow.

menopause, nulliparity, and first pregnancy after the age of 30. The most common cause of a breast lump that fluctuates in size in a young female with no family history of breast cancer is fibrocystic disease. Features of fibrocystic disease include breast pain, which usually varies with the menstrual cycle, and a greenish brown aspirate. Physical examination commonly demonstrates firm, tender lesions often in the upper outer quadrant, but can range from diffuse firmness to irregular patterns of firmness or a single nodule. On physical exam, it is difficult to differentiate a cyst from a solid mass. As a result, an ultrasound or aspiration should be done in patients suspected of having a cystic lesion. If the aspirate is bloody, the likelihood of a malignant lesion is greater and the fluid should be sent for cytology. Fluid aspirated from a cyst in a postmenopausal woman should also be sent for cytology; however, nonbloody aspirates in a menstruating woman do not require cytology.

Management of cystic lesions is as follows:

1. If the aspirate is nonbloody, discard the aspirate.
2. If the mass does not disappear after the aspiration, then send for cytology and evaluate for malignancy.
3. If the mass disappears after the aspiration, then follow up in 4 to 6 weeks for re-evaluation. Persistent cysts should be evaluated for malignancy.

Fibrocystic disease can often be treated with supportive measures such as loose clothing and avoiding foods rich in methylxanthines (tea, coffee, chocolate, and caffeinated beverages). Other options include vitamin A or E and increasing iodine intake. Pharmacologic management includes analgesics, oral contraceptives, and the synthetic androgens (e.g., danazol). Although danazol is approved by the FDA for treatment of fibrocystic disease, it is generally reserved for more severe cases unresponsive to conservative treatment. Some evidence suggests that primrose oil may be helpful for fibrocystic disease.

Any solid mass should be evaluated for malignancy even if the mammogram is normal or suggests that the lesion is benign. Mammography is helpful to rule out other nonpalpable masses, to establish a baseline, to help determine the size and the extent of the lesion, and to characterize a lesion as most likely benign or malignant to help in planning the surgical approach.

The American Cancer Society (ACS) recommends screening mammography starting at age 40 years. The ACS guidelines are summarized in Table 9.7 and highlight recent updates. However, if there is a strong family history of cancer, screening tests may be done earlier. In young patients, the breast tissue is dense and, as a result, mammography may not be indicated.

Problem 9

Child abuse is defined as inflicted injury to a child and can include bruises, fractures, soft tissue injuries, and internal injuries such as a splenic rupture or intracranial bleed. In addition to physical abuse, children may be sexually or emotionally abused or neglected. Neglect is a failure to provide a child's basic needs, such as nutrition, shelter, or supervision. In the United States, there are over 3 million cases of child abuse and neglect, including 2,000 to 4,000 deaths from abuse. The majority of deaths occur in children younger than 5 years of age.

Several signs and symptoms should alert a provider that a child might be in an abusive situation. Some signs of potential abuse include subnormal growth, such as weight less than the fifth percentile for age, and injuries such as a torn frenulum, bilateral black eyes, dental injury, or a significant central nervous system injury with a history of mild trauma. Skin injuries such as bites,

bruises in various stages of healing, burn marks, or injuries in normally protected areas such as the stomach should also be considered suspicious. Bruising on the shins in the absence of other signs is less suspicious. Other injuries such as rib fracture, complex injuries with a history of minor trauma, or any femur fracture in a child younger than 1 year old should also increase the index of suspicion for physical abuse. A single greenstick fracture with a consistent history in the absence of other signs of abuse is not indicative of abuse. Internal injuries to the gastrointestinal tract or GU tract or a history of genitally related complaints should also heighten the suspicion for abuse. Recent family crises such as financial problems or divorce, alcohol or drug use, or illness in the family are other common historical risk factors for abuse. A child who is mentally or physically impaired is also at increased risk.

When evaluating a child, the history can provide clues to the presence of abuse. Discrepant history, or when the story does not match the injury pattern, is a red flag for abuse. A parent who appears to be either overly aggressive or passive about his or her child's illness is another red flag. Failure to keep medical appointments or to bring the child in for routine health care visits such as immunization should heighten concerns about possible abuse or neglect. Abused children often exhibit aggressive behavior, have difficulty at school, and are at increased risk for substance abuse.

A key first step for managing child abuse is documentation since records often provide objective evidence of abuse. Detailed description of all injuries is important and drawings or photographs are often helpful. The physician's primary concern is the child's safety. A physician should not try to manage a case of abuse or neglect on his or her own. Child abuse must be reported to the appropriate governmental agencies (e.g., child protective services) that will arrange for protection of the children involved and pursue further investigation of the potential child abuse. Although a family conference may be helpful, initially a more appropriate action is to use a multidisciplinary approach that includes involvement of the appropriate agencies. Long-term treatment involves case management, social services, and a psychologic evaluation to identify and understand the reason for the abuse. Counseling for the individual and the family with an individual skilled in issues of abuse may need to be arranged. Psychiatric conditions such as depression and substance abuse should be treated.

Requesting previous medical records is important since there might be a history of previous injuries compatible with abuse. The presence of abuse in one child should always prompt an assessment of the other siblings and place the physician on alert for other kinds of abuse, such as spousal or elder abuse.

Problem 10

Colorectal cancer (CRC) is the second most common form of cancer in the United States, with about 150,000 cases annually. Lifetime risk is about 6% and CRC accounts for about 10% of all cancer deaths. The incidence increases dramatically after age 50 and is nearly equal in men and women. Annual fecal occult blood testing (FOBT) reduces the mortality of colon cancer by approximately 15% to 35% compared to an unscreened group. FOBT should be done with two slides prepared from each of three consecutive stool specimens. In order to avoid false positives, the individual should avoid nonsteroidal anti-inflammatory drugs (NSAIDs), red meat, horseradish, cantaloupe, or uncooked fresh vegetables such a broccoli, turnips, radishes, and cauliflower. High doses of vitamin C increase the risk of having a false negative. In addition to annual FOBT, which has low sensitivity in detecting cancer, for patients at normal risk most experts recommend an annual digital exam over

Table 9.7 ACS screening: What has changed and why

	Former Guidelines (1997)	Updated Guidelines and Information (May 2003)	Explanation
Women at average risk			
Mammography	Annually starting at age 40	No change from 1997 recommendation. There is a tremendous amount of additional, credible evidence of the benefit of mammography since 1997, especially regarding women in their 40s.	Women can feel confident about the benefits associated with regular screening mammography. However, mammography also has limitations: It will miss some cancers, and it sometimes leads to follow-up of findings that are not cancer, including biopsies.
CBE	Every 3 years for women 20 to 39; annually for women 40 or older	CBE should be part of a woman's periodic health examination, approximately every 3 years for women in their 20s and 30s and annually for women 40 or older.	CBE is a complement to regular mammography screening and an opportunity for women and their health care providers to discuss changes in their breasts, risk factors, and early detection testing.
BSE	Monthly starting at age 20	Women should report any breast change promptly to their health care provider. Beginning in their 20s, women should be told about the benefits and limitations of BSE. It is acceptable for women to choose not to do BSE or to do it occasionally.	Research has shown that BSE plays a small role in detecting breast cancer compared with self-awareness. However, doing BSE is one way for women to know how their breasts normally feel and to notice any changes.
Older women and women with serious health problems	Additional research is needed.	Continue annual mammography, regardless of age, as long as a woman does not have serious, chronic health problems. For women with serious health problems or short life expectancy, evaluate ongoing early detection testing.	There is a need to balance the potential benefits of ongoing screening mammography in women with limited longevity against the limitations. The survival benefit of a current mammogram may not be seen for several years.
Women known to be at increased risk			
Women known to be at increased risk	Women with a family history of breast cancer should discuss guidelines with their doctors.	Women known to be at increased risk may benefit from earlier initiation of early detection testing and/or the addition of breast ultrasound or MRI.	The evidence available is only sufficient to offer general guidance. This guidance will help women and their doctors make more informed decisions about screening.

age 40 (despite little evidence to support this practice) along with a screening flexible sigmoidoscopy every 5 years after age 50. Other screening methods the ACS considers acceptable include colonoscopy every 10 years or, as an alternative means of whole-bowel examination, a double-contrast barium enema (DCBE) every

5 years. However, DCBE is less sensitive than colonoscopy and there is no direct evidence that it is effective in reducing mortality rates. A six-slide Hemoccult test has a sensitivity that ranges from 30% to 70%, and negative FOBT does not exclude cancer. When mass screening programs are initiated, between 2% and 4% of individuals

older than age 50 are found to have a positive Hemoccult test. Although the patient has a possible explanation (e.g., hemorrhoid) for the positive occult blood slide, he should still be treated; since lesions may bleed intermittently, a single positive test requires further evaluation even if repeat FOBT testing is negative. A digital rectal examination is also not effective for ruling out colon cancer since less than 10% of colon cancers occur within 8 cm of the anal verge. Table 9.8 summarizes guidelines for colorectal cancer screening. In addition to the ACS, the U.S. Preventive Services Task Force (USP-STF) also supports periodic FOBT and found fair evidence that sigmoidoscopy alone or in combination with FOBT reduces mortality. Although there is no direct evidence that screening colonoscopy is effective in reducing colorectal cancer mortality, based on extrapolation from sigmoidoscopy studies, limited case–control evidence, and the ability of colonoscopy to inspect the proximal colon, the USPSTF also accepts colonoscopy as an alternative screening. The USPSTF found insufficient evidence that newer screening technologies (e.g., computed tomographic colography) are effective in improving health outcomes.

Approximately 5% to 10% of asymptomatic patients who screen positive for FOBT will have a CRC and another 20% to 40% will have polyps. A CBC can detect an anemia that might result from chronic blood loss. The best approach is to proceed directly to colonoscopy since this test can be both diagnostic and therapeutic. In places where colonoscopy is unavailable, sigmoidoscopy combined with an air contrast barium enema is an acceptable alternative. A CT scan of the abdomen is not part of the initial workup for an occult positive stool, although it may be helpful for evaluating patients with suspected metastatic disease. A CEA is not part of the initial evaluation, although in patients with CRC a preoperative CEA provides a baseline for postoperative monitoring and can help assess prognosis.

Several factors are associated with increased risk of CRC. Advancing age is an important risk factor, and a high-fat, low-fiber diet has been implicated in colon cancer. Family history is also a risk factor and having a first-degree relative with CRC increases the risk by two- to threefold. Other risk factors include a greater than 10-year history of ulcerative colitis, familial polyposis syndrome, Gardner's syndrome (polyps, osteomas, and soft tissue tumors), and a history of breast or gynecologic cancer or previous adenomatous polyp. Evidence suggests that aspirin and other NSAIDs appear to prevent polyp development and lower the risk of developing colon cancer.

Survival rates vary with the stage of the CRC. Tumors confined locally to the bowel wall (Duke's stage A) or pericolic fat (Duke's stage B) have about an 80% 5-year survival rate. A tumor with positive lymph nodes (Duke's stage C) has a much poorer prognosis, with 5-year survival rates falling to 30% to 65%. Tumors with widespread metastases (Duke's stage D) have about a 5% 5-year survival rate. Surgery is the primary treatment for CRC. However, patients with stage C CRC benefit from chemotherapy.

Follow-up is essential because the risk of a second CRC developing or a new polyp appearing is much greater than for the average individual. Yearly liver tests, CBC, and a follow-up colonoscopic evaluation at 6 months are appropriate. If the follow-up colonoscopy is normal, it should be repeated every 3 years with interim annual FOBT. If polyps are detected, colonoscopy should be repeated 6 to 12 months after resection.

Table 9.8 Guidelines for colorectal cancer screening

Risk Factor	Recommendation
None	Starting at age 50, annual FOBT, DRE: flexible sigmoidoscopy every 3–5 years
Ulcerative colitis	Colonoscopy after 8–10 years of disease, then surveillance colonoscopy every 1–2 years
Adenomatous polyps	Surveillance colonoscopy every 3–5 years after excision, every 1–3 years if multiple, large (>1 cm), villous, malignant (noninvasive)
Familial polyposis disorder (suspected)	Screening flexible sigmoidoscopy by age 20
Familial nonpolyposis disorder (suspected)	Screening colonoscopy or barium enema by age 35–40, then surveillance every 3–5 years
Positive family history	Screening as for average risks; consider barium enema or colonoscopy

DRE, digital rectal exam.
Reproduced with permission from Young V, Kormas W, Goroll A. *Blueprints in Medicine.* 2nd ed. Malden: Blackwell Science; 2001:192.

Problem 11

Congestive heart failure (CHF) affects an estimated 5 million Americans, and it is the number one cause of hospitalization in the elderly. The overall 5-year mortality is roughly 60% for men and 45% for women. CHF occurs when the heart is unable to adequately perfuse the tissues in the body. This may be the result of systolic or diastolic dysfunction. Systolic dysfunction is characterized by diminished left ventricular contractility, whereas diastolic dysfunction is characterized by diminished left ventricular filling due to poor compliance of the ventricular wall.

Heart failure is usually a sign of underlying heart disease, of which hypertension, coronary artery disease, and valvular dysfunction are the most common causes. In the United States, coronary artery disease is the most common cause of a dilated cardiomyopathy with systolic dysfunction. Other causes include congenital heart disease, infections, toxin exposure (alcohol, adriamycin), dilated cardiomyopathy, infiltrative heart disease (amyloid), constrictive pericarditis, renal failure, and thyroid disease. Severe anemia may result in high-output heart failure despite normal cardiac function. Lesser degrees of anemia can precipitate failure in patients with cardiac dysfunction.

Based on this patient's history of worsening dyspnea, lower extremity edema, and three-pillow orthopnea, CHF appears to be the likely diagnosis. Because the patient has tachypnea, JVD, bibasilar rales, an S3, and lower extremity edema, admission to the hospital is advisable.

The goal of the diagnostic evaluation is to identify the underlying pathophysiology of the heart failure and, if possible, to determine the triggering event. Some common precipitating causes of heart failure include myocardial ischemia, arrhythmias, valvular disease, uncontrolled hypertension, PE, pericardial disease, infections, anemia, dietary indiscretion, adverse drug effects, and nonadherence. Appropriate testing includes a CBC, a basic metabolic profile, pulse oximetry, CXR, ECG, and serial cardiac enzymes to rule out acute myocardial infarction. A chest x-ray is invaluable for the diagnosis of CHF. Characteristic findings include redistribution of blood flow, cardiomegaly, prominent interstitial markings, Kerley "B" lines, and perihilar haziness. CT scanning or a CT scan of the chest is unlikely to be helpful as an initial study in this patient, but rapid scanning is useful in the evaluation of a patient with a suspected PE. A CBC detects anemias that may contribute to debilitating CHF, whereas an ECG can help identify an arrhythmia or injury pattern. Acutely, the patient should receive intravenous furosemide and oxygen to reduce fluid volume and maximize oxygen delivery to tissues. A low-sodium diet, monitoring fluid intake and output, daily weights, and serial physical exams to determine response to therapy should be done as well. All patients with newly diagnosed CHF should have an echocardiogram to evaluate ejection fraction, chamber size, valvular function, wall motion, and left ventricular thickness.

Based on the test results, this patient likely has diastolic dysfunction as a cause of his CHF. Appropriate long-term management involves controlling his hypertension and educating the patient about his condition. A low Na^+ diet (less than 4 g per day) and antihypertensive medications are appropriate. The patient should remain active and monitor his daily weight because a weight increase is an early sign of fluid retention and possible CHF decompensation. Beta-blockers and ACE inhibitors should be considered in all patients with CHF. ACE inhibitors slow the progression of heart failure and decrease rates of hospitalization and mortality in those with CHF. Beta-blockers have also been shown in randomized controlled trials to reduce mortality in those with CHF and should be started at a very low dose and gradually increased. Table 9.9 summarizes medications used in the treatment of heart failure.

Digoxin is not indicated in patients with diastolic dysfunction and thus should be avoided. Lipitor is not indicated because this patient has an LDL less than 100 and no CAD or CAD equivalent.

Problem 12

Constipation is defined as having infrequent bowel movements or passing abnormally hard, dry stools that require straining at least 25% of the time. One useful objective definition is the passage of fewer than three stools per week. Although constipation is a common problem among older individuals, it is not a normal consequence of aging. Chronic constipation without a recent change in bowel movements is usually functional. Insufficient dietary fiber and poor fluid intake are the most common functional causes. Constipation is also associated with a sedentary lifestyle. A recent change in bowel habits in a previously normal individual increases the likelihood of an organic cause.

One of the most common reversible causes of constipation is a medication side effect. Opiates, agents with anticholinergic activity, and antacids containing aluminum or calcium are common causes of drug-induced constipation. Calcium channel blockers such as diltiazem and verapamil decrease gastric mobility and have constipation as a side effect. Tricyclic antidepressants and antipsychotic medications are also associated with

constipation, but the serotonin reuptake inhibitors are more likely to cause diarrhea.

In addition to abdominal or rectal pathology, neurologic impairment such as autonomic neuropathy, multiple sclerosis, or Parkinson's disease may present with constipation as an early finding. Therefore, careful neurologic examination is indicated.

Since diltiazem can cause constipation, it is reasonable to discontinue it and substitute a drug such as an ACE inhibitor, which is less commonly associated with constipation. Diuretics may cause hypokalemia and contribute to constipation. Clonidine is another antihypertensive agent associated with constipation. Other organic causes of constipation are gastrointestinal disorders, metabolic disorders, neurologic diseases, depression, cardiac disease, and immobility.

Metabolic causes include hypothyroidism, hypokalemia, and hypercalcemia. In this patient with an acute onset and mild fatigue, ruling out these conditions is appropriate. Ordering a CBC can identify an anemia, which would suggest a possible structural lesion such as a polyp or adenocarcinoma. The ACS recommends that starting at age 50 or older, an annual fecal occult blood test and a flexible sigmoidoscopy every 3 to 5 years is indicated for colon cancer screening. Therefore, checking three stool specimens for occult blood is justified to screen for the presence of a structural lesion even though the rectal exam did not reveal the presence of blood. When testing for occult blood, increasing the amount of fiber, avoiding horseradish and rare meats, and not taking vitamin C or aspirin can increase the sensitivity and specificity of the fecal occult blood testing.

One of the three tests in this individual is positive for occult blood. A single test out of three has the same clinical implication as a multiply positive test and repeating the testing is not indicated. Colonoscopy is an acceptable method to evaluate this patient. In a setting in which colonoscopy is unobtainable, a flexible sigmoidoscopy and an air contrast barium enema could be considered as an alternative method of evaluation. A CT scan is not indicated for the routine evaluation of a heme positive stool. Although a CEA may be elevated in patients with colon cancer, it is used primarily for monitoring treatment and not for diagnosis.

Stopping the diltiazem and increasing the dietary fiber improved the patient's condition and should be continued. Bloating and gas is a common side effect of increased fiber for the first few weeks of a high-fiber diet, and the patient should be counseled that this will improve with time and to maintain her fiber intake. Bisacodyl is a laxative that stimulates the colon and should be avoided since chronic use can lead to constipation and degeneration of myoneuronal plexuses. Although stool softeners (docusate) are commonly used, their efficiency is questioned and long-term use has been associated with hepatotoxicity and skin rashes. Hyperosmia agents such as lactulose are used for refractory cases or in individuals who cannot or will not use a bulking agent. These agents can cause bloating and flatulence, which tends to lessen over time.

Problem 13

Chronic obstructive pulmonary disease (COPD) affects 14 million Americans and is usually diagnosed between ages 55 and 65. Cigarette smoking (usually more than 20 pack-years) causes approximately 90% of all cases. COPD is a chronic disease with intermittent acute exacerbations defined by increased sputum production, more purulent sputum, and worsening dyspnea. Unlike asthma, the airflow obstruction in COPD is not easily reversible by

Table 9.9 Medications used in the treatment of heart failure

Agent	Usual Initial Dose	Target Dose[a]	Comments
Diuretics			
Furosemide	20–200 mg IV (intermittent therapy) 5–10 mg/hr (continuous infusion) 20 mg qd–240 mg bid PO	Titrate to clinical response	May cause metabolic alkalosis. When used with ACE inhibitors, may cause deterioration in renal function.
Bumetanide	0.5–3.0 mg IV 0.5 mg qd–10 mg qd PO	Titrate to clinical response	Same as furosemide.
Ethacrynic acid	5–100 mg IV (0.5–1.0 mg/kg) 50 mg qd–200 mg bid PO	Titrate to clinical response	Beware of ototoxicity.
Metolazone	2.5–10 mg qd PO	Titrate to clinical response	Enhanced sodium excretion when combined with loop diuretics.
Inotropic/vasopressor agents			
Dobutamine	2.5–20 μg/kg/min IV	Titrate to clinical response	Increases in contractility and stroke volume do not lead to increased myocardial oxygen consumption because of reduction in afterload and filling pressures. Major concerns relate to tachycardia and arrhythmogenesis.
Milrinone	Initial 50 μg/kg bolus over 10 min, followed by continuous infusion at 0.25–1.0 μg/kg/min	Titrate to clinical response	Dose reduction necessary in presence of renal dysfunction. Greater vasodilatory potency than dobutamine, which may cause more profound reductions in filling pressures and BP. Major concerns related to tachycardia and arrhythmogenesis.
Dopamine	1–20 μg/kg/min	Titrate to clinical response	Dopaminergic doses (≤2 μg/kg/min promote renal and splanchnic vasodilation. Doses of 2–10 μg/kg/min are primarily inotropic. At 10–20 μg/kg/min, vasoconstriction predominates.
Norepinephrine	2–12 μg/min	Titrate to clinical response	May reduce cardiac output because of increased afterload.

Table 9.9 (continued)

Agent	Usual Initial Dose	Target Dose[a]	Comments
Digoxin	0.125–0.375 mg	Titrate to clinical response	Narrow therapeutic toxic ratio. Serum level increased by many medications. Dose adjustment necessary in renal dysfunction.
Vasodilators			
Nitroglycerin	0.3–0.6 mg SL 0.2–10 µg/kg/min IV	Titrate to clinical response	Continuous therapy for ≥24 hours leads to tolerance.
Nitroprusside	0.2–10 µg/kg/min	Titrate to clinical response	Is light sensitive. Must be carefully titrated to BP.
Hydralazine	10–75 mg qid PO	Titrate to clinical response	Used in combination with oral nitrates in ACE inhibitor-intolerant patients. Can cause tachycardia and lupus-like syndrome.
ACE inhibitors			
Enalapril	2.5–10 mg bid	10–20 mg bid	Reduction in dose or increase in dosing interval may be necessary in renal failure. Cough relatively frequent (about 5%) side effect.
Captopril	6.25–50 mg bid	50 mg tid	
Lisinopril	5–20 mg qd	20–35 mg bid	
Quinapril	5–20 mg bid	Not established	
Ramipril	1.25–5 mg bid	5 mg bid	
Angiotensin II (AT$_1$ type) receptor antagonists			
Losartan	25–50 mg qd PO	Not established	Currently not approved by FDA for use in heart failure. Used only in patients intolerant to ACE inhibitors.
Valsartan	80–160 mg qd PO	Not established	
β-Blocking agents			
Carvedilol	3.125–25 mg bid	25–50 mg bid	Not for use in acute heart failure.
Metoprolol	6.25–50 mg bid	200 mg qd	Indicated in patients with stable NYHA class II–III heart failure resulting from systolic dysfunction.
Bisoprolol	1.25–5 mg qd	10 mg qd	
Aldosterase antagonists			
Spironolactone	12.5–25 mg qd	25 mg qd	Recent data indicating incremental benefit.

[a]Dose shown to be beneficial in randomized trials. This dose often is not achievable acutely in the hospital, but it should be the goal in patients with chronic heart failure unless they cannot tolerate it.

bronchodilators. Alpha-1-antitrypsin deficiency and cystic fibrosis are uncommon but important causes of COPD.

Although in early COPD the physical examination may be normal, patients with more advanced COPD often have a barrel-shaped chest and a prolonged expiratory phase. In patients with an acute exacerbation, appropriate tests include a complete blood count, chest x-ray, and pulse oximetry. Indications for an arterial blood gas include reduced pO_2 on pulse oximetry; to initially assess a moderately to severely symptomatic patient; acute decompensation; the presence of cor pulmonale, polycythemia, or arrhythmias; or preoperative evaluation. Routine screening of patients with COPD by using CT of the chest has not been shown to be cost-effective and would be appropriate only if initial chest x-ray showed an abnormality that required further study. In patients with COPD, arterial blood gas analysis typically shows CO_2 retention and mild hypoxia, whereas CXR often demonstrates a flattened diaphragm and hyperinflation. Pulmonary function tests are useful in diagnosing and monitoring COPD. Typical results reveal a decrease in FEV1 (normal, 80% of predicted value) and in the FEV1/FVC ratio (normal, greater than 75%). The American Thoracic Society uses a staging system for the severity of COPD based on FEV1: stage I, greater than 50% (mild); stage II, 35% to 45% (moderate); and stage III, less than 35% (severe).

The goals for treating COPD are to prevent progression, minimize exacerbations, prevent and treat complications, and maintain functional capacity. Smoking cessation is an essential component of treatment and is the most important element in preventing disease progression. Annual influenza immunization and pneumococcal vaccination are indicated. Many patients with moderate to severe COPD have an asthmatic component and may benefit from bronchodilators such as ipratropium bromide and beta-adrenergic agonists. Corticosteroids are used in patients who do not respond adequately to bronchodilators or during acute exacerbations. For acute episodes, oral prednisone is commonly used. Intravenous steroids for a short duration are useful for patients with severe exacerbations requiring inpatient management. For long-term use in patients with more severe disease with symptoms uncontrolled by bronchodilators, adding inhaled corticosteroids (ICS) or administering a 2- to 4-week trial of prednisone can be given to determine if there is a significant response. ICS have much fewer side effects but are less effective than oral steroids. If the FEV1 improves by 20% to 25%, then the dose should be tapered to the lowest dose that maintains the improvement. Steroids should not be continued in those individuals whose FEV1 does not improve. The Global Initiative for Chronic Obstructive Pulmonary Disease outlined a rationale for treatment that is summarized in Table 9.10.

In patients with resting hypoxia (88%), home oxygen has been shown to prolong survival, to reduce the rate of hospitalization, and to improve quality of life. Because the patient in this case is not hypoxic, continuous home oxygen therapy is not indicated. Appropriate intervention in patients suffering from an exacerbation includes antibiotics, anticholinergics, beta-agonists, and, if moderately severe, oral corticosteroids.

Table 9.10 Summary of the GOLD guidelines

			Therapy at Each Stage of COPD		
New	**0: At Risk**	**I: Mild**	**II: Moderate**	**III: Severe**	**IV: Very Severe**
Characteristics	• Chronic symptoms • Exposure to risk factors • Normal spirometry	• FEV1/FVC <70% • FEV1 ≥80% • With or without symptoms	• FEV1/FVC <70% • 50% ≤FEV+ < 80% • With or without symptoms	• FEV1/FVC <70% • 30% FEV1 < 50% • With or without symptoms	• FEV1/FVC <70% • FEV1 <30% or • FEV1 <50% predicted plus chronic respiratory failure
	Avoidance of risk factor(s); influenza vaccination				
		Add short-acting bronchodilator when needed			
			Add regular treatment with one or more long-acting bronchodilators Add rehabilitation		
				Add inhaled glucocorticosteroids if repeated exacerbations	
					Add long-term oxygen if chronic respiratory failure Consider surgical treatments

Problem 14

The cause of chest pain ranges from benign musculoskeletal pain to a life-threatening process. Thus, stratifying individuals with complaints of chest pain into higher and lower risk of coronary artery disease (CAD) is essential. Absolute risk factors for CAD include a family history, smoking, diabetes, elevated cholesterol, low HDL (less than 35), being male, and age (male greater than 45, female greater than 55). Although weight loss and stress reduction are important in patients with CAD, obesity in the absence of other associated risk factors and a stressful lifestyle are not absolute risk factors.

The patient's history, risk factors, and ECG findings are consistent with the clinical diagnosis of an acute myocardial infarction (MI). Since the pathophysiology of an acute MI involves an acute disruption of oxygen delivery to heart muscle, therapy includes reducing the oxygen demand of the myocardium, maximizing oxygen delivery, attenuating further disruption of oxygen delivery, and re-establishing normal blood flow. Intravenous beta-blockade, nitro paste, and morphine function to reduce oxygen demand. Chewing an aspirin is a simple and effective treatment for acute MI because it inhibits the propagation of thrombus formation, which is the cause for the initial disruption of blood flow. Oxygen therapy via nasal cannula maximizes oxygen delivery to the myocardium.

Intravenous administration of a thrombolytic such as tissue plasminogen activator (T-PA) or acute cardiac catheterization can be used to lyse a thrombus. Either intervention is appropriate in this case and often depends on the availability of local resources. Some studies show a better outcome with early catheterization versus thrombolysis in settings in which cardiac catheterization is readily available 24 hours a day. The use of atropine or calcium channel blockers in a patient with normal sinus rhythm is not appropriate initial treatment for acute MI.

Post-myocardial infarction in patients who do not undergo acute cardiac catheterization needs to be stratified to identify those at high risk for future cardiac events since these patients may benefit from coronary revascularization. Those with diminished left ventricular ejection fraction (less than 45%), recurrent chest pain, arrhythmias, or a positive submaximal stress test prior to discharge are considered to be at high risk and should undergo cardiac catheterization.

Risk factor modification is essential for patients who have had an MI. Thus, smoking cessation, decreasing LDL to less than 100 mg/dL, control of hypertension, and tightly regulated blood sugars are all essential. Since this patient's LDL is greater than 100 on her current dose of fluvastatin, it should be increased, or additional therapy, such as niacin, should be provided. Aspirin, beta-blockers, and ACE inhibitors have all been shown to provide significant benefit to patients who have suffered an MI and are indicated in post-MI patients without contraindications who can tolerate the medication. An individualized exercise program should also be initiated in all post-MI patients because it can decrease mortality. This patient has no indication for the use of coumadin (e.g., atrial fibrillation). See Table 9.11.

Problem 15

Depression is second only to hypertension as the most common diagnosis encountered in primary care practices. Table 9.12 lists the criteria for major depression. It is more common in women (20% to 25% lifetime occurrence) compared to men (7% to 12% lifetime occurrence). Often, depressed patients present with physical complaints and may not consider that their physical problems can be related to depression or a psychological condition. It is important to consider organic causes of depression. Chronic fatigue and a depressed mood are common nonspecific symptoms associated with a number of conditions, such as fibromyalgia, cancer, heart disease, hypothyroidism, irritable bowel syndrome, sleep apnea, rheumatoid arthritis, other endocrinopathies, chronic fatigue syndrome, menopause, anxiety, anemia, renal failure, alcoholism, as well as depression. In some medical illnesses, such as pancreatic cancer or HIV, depression may even dominate the early clinical picture. Other psychologic conditions, such as substance abuse or domestic violence, may also mimic depression.

The patient's history and physical exam should direct the laboratory evaluation. If depression seems likely in a patient with an otherwise completely normal history and physical, there is no need to order extensive laboratory tests. However, testing such as a CBC, chemistry panel, and TSH is useful in screening for organic disease, and in this patient with symptoms such as dry skin and muscle aches, a basic laboratory evaluation would be helpful in ruling out an underlying organic disease. An FSH and LH are not indicated. Lipid screening is recommended for general health maintenance, and the patient's obesity, lack of exercise, and alcohol intake place her at higher risk for dyslipidemia.

Physicians should educate patients that certain drugs and substances are associated with depression. These include alcohol, benzodiazepines, corticosteroids, oral contraceptives, antihypertensives (especially beta-blockers, reserpine, and clonidine), neuroleptics, sedative–hypnotics, marijuana, amphetamines, cocaine, and opiates. It is important for this patient to eliminate or at least reduce her alcohol intake. It appears that this patient also suffers from comorbid anxiety. Long-term treatment with benzodiazepines is contraindicated since it may worsen the patient's depression. Most antidepressant therapy generally takes between 2 and 6 weeks to see a response. Therefore, it may occasionally be helpful in initial treatment of an anxious depressed patient to use benzodiazepines on a short-term basis only until the patient begins to respond to the antidepressant therapy. Anxiety coexists with depression approximately 50% of the time.

Fibromyalgia is often associated with depression and insomnia. In this patient, fibromyalgia is unlikely because the complaints involve both proximal and distal musculature. However, because of the subjective muscle tenderness, checking a CPK is reasonable to exclude a myopathy. Without subjective or objective complaints of joint pain, rheumatoid arthritis is unlikely in the patient.

Often, there is resistance to treating depression. Patients believe many of the antidepressants are ineffective and fear the side effects. Cost is also a factor. It is imperative for the physician to take the time to listen to the patient's complaints and educate the patient regarding depression and its treatment. The different classes of antidepressants are roughly equivalent in efficacy and an individual medication is effective in about 60% to 80% of patients, although it may take 6 to 8 weeks at full dose to see the impact of pharmacologic treatment. An individual who does not respond to one class of medications may respond to a different class. The initial choice may depend on comorbidities and also on symptoms. For example, a more energizing antidepressant such as bupropion is useful in patients with excessive sleepiness, whereas a sedating antidepressant such as a TCA or trazadone should be considered in a patient with difficulty sleeping. In this patient, thyroid supplementation is not indicated unless there is laboratory evidence of hypothyroidism. Thyroid medication should not be used for weight loss or to give patients extra energy. Overtreatment can result in cardiac arrhythmias and induce

Table 9.11 AHA/ACC secondary prevention for patients with coronary and other vascular disease

Goals	Intervention Recommendations
Smoking: Goal Complete cessation	Assess tobacco use. Strongly encourage patient and family to stop smoking and to avoid secondhand smoke. Provide counseling, pharmacological therapy, including nicotine replacement and buproprion, and formal smoking cessation programs as appropriate.
BP control Goal <140/90 mmHg or <130/85 mmHg if heart failure or renal insufficiency <130/80 mmHg if diabetes	Initiate lifestyle modification (weight control, physical activity, alcohol moderation, moderate sodium restriction, and emphasis on fruits, vegetables, and low-fat dairy products) in all patients wit blood pressure ≥130 mmHg systolic or 80 mmHg diastolic. Add blood pressure medication, individualized to other patient requirements and characteristics (i.e., age, race, need for drugs with specific benefits) *if* blood pressure is not <140 mmHg systolic or 90 mmHg diastolic *or* if blood pressure is not <130 mmHg systolic or 85 mmHg diastolic for individuals with heart failure or renal insufficiency (<80 mmHg diastolic for individuals wit diabetes).

Lipid management
Primary goal
LDL <100 mg/dL

Start dietary therapy in all patients (<7% saturated fat and <200 mg/day cholesterol) and promote physical activity and weight management. Encourage increased consumption of omega-3 fatty acids. Assess fasting lipid profile in all patients, therapy on discharge. Add drug therapy according to the following guide:

LDL <100 mg/dL (baseline or on-treatment)	LDL 100–129 mg/dL (baseline or on-treatment)	LDL ≥ 130 mg/dL (baseline or on-treatment)
Further LDL-lowering therapy not required Consider fibrate or niacin (if low HDL or high TG)	Therapeutic options Intensity LDL-lowering therapy (stalin or resin Fibrate or niacin (if low HDL or high TG) Consider combined drug therapy (stalin + fibrate or niacin) (if low HDL or high TG)	Intensity LDL-lowering therapy (statin or resin) Add or increase drug therapy with lifestyle therapies

Secondary goal If TG ≥200 mg/dL, then non-HDL[b] should be <130 mg/dL	If TG ≥150 mg/dL or HDL <40 mg/dL: Emphasize weight management and physical activity. Advise smoking cessation. If TG 200–499 mg/dL: Consider fibrate or niacin *after* LDL-lowering therapy[a] If TG ≥500 mg/dL: Consider fibrate or niacin *before* LDL-lowering therapy[a] Consider omega-3 fatty acids as adjunct for high TG
Physical activity Minimum goal 30 minutes 3 to 4 days per week Optimal daily	Assess risk, preferably with exercise test, to guide prescription. Encourage minimum of 30 to 60 minutes of activity, preferably daily, or at least 3 or 4 times weekly (walking, jogging, cycling, or other aerobic activity) supplemented by an increase in daily lifestyle activities (e.g., walking breaks at work, gardening, household work). Advise medically supervised programs for moderate- to high-risk patients.
Weight management Goal BMI 18.5–24.9 kg/m²	Calculate BMI and measure waist circumference as part of evaluation. Monitor response of BMI and waist circumference to therapy. Start weight management and physical activity as appropriate. Desirable BMI range is 18.6–24.9 kg/m². When BMI ≥25 kg/m², goal for waist circumference is ≤40 inches in men and ≤35 inches in women.

Table 9.11 (continued)

Goals	Intervention Recommendations
Diabetes management Goal HbA1$_c$ <7%	Appropriate hypoglycemic therapy to achieve near-normal fasting plasma glucose, as indicated by HbA1$_c$. Treatment of other risks (e.g., physical activity, weight management, blood pressure, and cholesterol management).
Antiplatelet agents/ anticoagulants	Start and continue indefinitely aspirin 75 to 325 mg/day if not contraindicated. Consider clopidogrel 75 mg/day or warfarin if aspirin contraindicated. Manage warfarin to international normalized ration = 2.0 to 3.0 in post-MI patients when clinically indicated or for those not able to take aspirin or clopidogrel.
ACE inhibitors	Treat all patients indefinitely post MI; start early in stable high-risk patients (anterior MI, previous MI, Killip class II [S$_3$ gallop, rates, radiographic CHF]]. Consider chronic therapy for all other patients with coronary or other vascular disease unless contraindicated.
β-Blockers	Start in all post-MI and acute ischemic syndrome patients. Continue indefinitely. Observe usual contraindications. Use as needed to manage angina, rhythm, or blood pressure in all other patients.

BP, blood pressure; TG, triglycorides; BMI, body mass index; HbA1$_c$, major fraction of adult hemoglobin; MI, myocardial infarction; CHF, congestive heart failure.

a The use of resin is relatively contraindicated when TG >200 mg/dL
b Non-HDL cholesterol, total cholesterol minus HDL cholesterol.

Table 9.12 Criteria for major depressive episode[a]

Mood: depressed mood most of the day, nearly every day

Sleep: insomnia or hypersomnia

Interest: marked decrease in interest and pleasure in most activities

Guilt: feelings of worthlessness or inappropriate guilt

Energy: fatigue or low energy nearly every day

Concentration: decreased concentration or increased indecisiveness.

Appetite: increased or decreased appetite or weight gain or loss

Psychomotor: psychomotor agitation or retardation

Suicidality: recurrent thoughts of death, suicidal ideation, suicidal plan, suicide attempt

[a]General criteria for a major depressive episode require five or more of the above symptoms to be present for at least 2 weeks; one symptom must be *depressed mood* or *loss of interest of pleasure*. These symptoms must be a change from prior functioning and cannot be due to a medical condition, cannot be substance induced, and cannot be due to bereavement. The symptoms must also cause *distress* or *impairment*.
Reproduced with permission from *Diagnostic and Statistical Manual of Mental Disorders*. 4th ed. Washington, DC: American Psychiatric Association; 1994:327.

osteoporosis. Although the patient's cholesterol is elevated, therapeutic lifestyle changes such as diet and exercise should be initiated before considering the use of pharmacologic therapy. Exercise may also help depression. A lipid profile should be rechecked 6 months after initiating lifestyle changes. Prempro is not indicated in this patient since she is not menopausal. Also, in light of recent studies, Prempro may actually increase her risk for cardiovascular disease. Addressing the patient's alcohol intake is important. People often use alcohol to self-medicate or to calm their nerves. Alcohol can aggravate depression. Although many patients use alcohol to fall asleep, it disturbs their sleep cycle and often causes early morning awakening.

Problem 16
Although the HbA1c is the most important predictor of microvascular complications and of long-term control, it is not part of the diagnostic criteria. The most common way to diagnose diabetes is with a fasting blood sugar greater than 126 mg/dL on two separate occasions. Other criteria include a random plasma glucose greater than 200 mg/dL and classic diabetes symptoms such as polyuria, polydipsia, and polyphagia or a 2-hour postprandial glucose of greater than 200 mg/dL. A glucose tolerance test is rarely indicated in a nonpregnant adult patient. African Americans, Hispanics, Native Americans, and Pacific Islanders are all at increased risk for developing type 2 DM. Other risk factors include a family history of DM, obesity (20% over ideal body weight or a BMI greater than 27 kg/m^2), age older than 45 years, hypertension (greater than 140/90), and a history of gestational DM. Patients with type 2 DM usually have insulin resistance accompanied by a beta cell defect that progresses over time. Initially, insulin levels may be high or normal in type 2 DM, but as the beta cell begins to fail it can no longer produce enough insulin to overcome insulin resistance. Depending on how long a patient has had type 2 DM, insulin

levels can be high, normal, or low. In this individual with a 10-year history of type 2 DM and worsening symptoms despite maximal sulfonylurea therapy, it is unlikely that the insulin level would be elevated. However, most individuals produce sufficient insulin to avoid diabetic ketoacidosis, unless there is a severe underlying stress such as a severe infection.

The initial laboratory evaluation for a patient with type 2 DM should include fasting plasma glucose, glycosylated hemoglobin, fasting lipid profile, serum creatinine, urinalysis and urine for microalbuminuria if the urinalysis is negative for protein, thyroid function tests, and an electrocardiogram. The patient's neurologic symptoms seem consistent with a peripheral neuropathy most likely due to diabetes, and at this time an MRI is not indicated. Likewise, a chest x-ray is not recommended in the initial evaluation for a patient diagnosed with diabetes unless there is another indication. Fasting insulin levels are not recommended by the American Diabetes Association (ADA) as a routine part of the initial evaluation for patients with diabetes.

The ADA recommends a goal of less than 7% for HbA1c. Other organizations target levels less than 6.5%. The American Academy of Family Physicians recommends that glycemic targets be individualized incorporating factors such as age, comorbidities, and the risk of hypoglycemia. Normalizing the HbA1c provides primary and secondary prevention benefits for the microvascular complications of neuropathy, nephropathy, and retinopathy. An annual dilated eye examination is recommended and patients with diabetic retinopathy should be followed by an ophthalmologist. There is no advantage to switching from a sulfonylurea to metformin. Instead, combination therapy is indicated. Metformin can lower the HbA1c by approximately 1.5% to 2.0%. Sulfonylureas are insulin secretagogues and work well in combination with insulin sensitizing agents such as metformin or glitazones. Adding bedtime insulin to daytime sulfonylureas is an effective strategy, but it requires long-acting insulin such as glargine or NPH insulin to avoid hypoglycemic episodes. Since cardiovascular disease accounts for the majority of excess mortality in individuals with type 2 DM, it is critically important to address other cardiovascular risk factors, such as hypertension, smoking, and hyperlipidemia. The ADA recommends a target blood pressure of 130/80. Adding an ACE inhibitor to improve the blood pressure is a good option since ACE inhibitors offer a renal protective effect if microalbuminuria is present. If a patient cannot tolerate an ACE inhibitor, an angiotensin receptor blocker is a good alternative. The recent NCEP guidelines established type 2 DM as a coronary artery disease risk equivalent with an LDL-C target goal of less than 100 mg/dL. If there are no contraindications, a statin is the drug of choice. Aspirin prophylaxis, annual flu vaccine, and pneumococcal vaccination are also recommended for type 2 DM patients.

Problem 17

Failure to thrive (FTT) is a term used to describe inadequate growth in infants and young children. It is frequently accompanied by retarded social and motor achievements and many of these children remain behind in growth and intelligence. Although strict criteria for diagnosis of FTT have yet to be defined, most practitioners are concerned about FTT when the patient's weight or height or weight for length is below the fifth percentile on the growth chart or the child has dropped two major percentile curves over a 6-month period.

A child with intrauterine growth retardation (IUGR) would be expected to be small in stature at 6 months of age. Although infants with IUGR have normal growth velocities, 50% are below average in height at 3 years of age, and many of these children do not obtain their full genetic height or intellectual potential. Children of small parents may be growing normally, but along lower percentiles on standardized growth charts. A correction of the growth chart for mid-parental height will show that these children are growing within their genetic limits. Although even FTT children will develop a pubertal growth spurt, it will not correct for their previous deficiency in height. It is important to intervene before puberty, when there is still opportunity to affect final adult height. Although most cases of FTT are caused by psychosocial deprivation or inadequate caloric provision, there is still a substantial list of organic causes that must be considered. The most common organic causes are gastroesophageal reflux disease, chronic diarrhea, malabsorption secondary to celiac disease, and chronic infections (especially urinary tract infections). Although hypothyroidism is a potential organic cause, its incidence in the FTT population is low.

Workup in infants and children with FTT is best targeted based on likely etiologies obtained through the history and physical examination. Nevertheless, FTT often presents without a clear diagnosis, and what constitutes reasonable baseline laboratory testing is controversial. There is general agreement that a CBC (possibly with serum ferritin), sedimentation rate, urine analysis and culture, and basic metabolic profile are appropriate. A karyotype would not be indicated in this male infant but would be a consideration in a female infant in whom Turner syndrome may initially present as slow growth without other physical examination abnormalities. Although organic acidemia is a cause of FTT, urine assay for organic acids is not indicated in this infant. Children with organic acidemia typically have feeding difficulty and lethargy within the first week of life, and by 6 months they would show developmental delays. Further testing would only be indicated in this child if the basic metabolic profile detected a metabolic acidosis. Baseline laboratory testing is not mandated in every case of FTT. A history of inappropriate nutritional restriction in a medically stable child would allow for a strategy of nutritional correction and follow-up weights and height checks without obtaining baseline labs.

The mainstays of management are identification and addressing of any underlying etiologies. A multidisciplinary approach with input from dietitians, social workers, psychiatrists, psychologists, and social workers is useful. Lactation evaluation would be indicated in this case. Growth hormone use is indicated only for cases of proven growth hormone deficiency, growth failure secondary to renal failure, or Turner and Prader–Willi syndromes. Although growth hormone may initially improve growth velocity in genetically short children, there is controversy as to any effect on final adult height in this setting, and at this time it is not recommended for these children. The indications for hospitalization in FTT are (a) failure of outpatient management, (b) severe malnutrition or dehydration, (c) suspected child abuse, and (d) extreme parental anxiety for child care that in the short term will interfere with therapeutic plan and establishment of nurturing parent–child relationship. This infant and family meet none of these criteria.

Problem 18

Oral contraceptives (OCPs) are among the safest and most effective of reversible contraceptives. Combined oral contraceptive pills have several mechanisms of action. They work by inhibiting ovulation by suppressing pituitary and hypothalamic action, altering the endometrial lining, and by inducing changes in the cervical mucus that inhibit the motility of sperm. OCPs have a theoretical effectiveness that is greater than 99%, although in typical use their effectiveness is approximately 95%. Severe complications from oral contraceptives, particularly newer low-dose formulations, are rare. These complications are primarily cardiovascular and include thrombophlebitis, pulmonary embolus, cerebrovascular accident, myocardial infarction, hypertension, migraine headache, depression, and hypertension. Other problems include an increased risk of hepatic adenomas and gallbladder disease. Individuals older than the age of 35 who smoke are at the greatest risk for ill effects. Because of this increased risk, smoking after 35 is considered an absolute contraindication to subscribing oral contraceptives. Other absolute contraindications include a history of thrombophlebitis, cerebral vascular disease, significantly impaired liver function, known or suspected estrogen responsive cancers (e.g., breast cancer), pregnancy, or undiagnosed vaginal bleeding. Common but less serious OCP side effects include nausea, fluid retention, weight gain, and breast tenderness. Although many women fear that oral contraceptives might increase the risk of breast cancer, no association with oral contraceptives and an increased risk of breast cancer has been established. The use of oral contraceptives actually decreases the risk of endometrial carcinoma and ovarian cancer. Other noncontraceptive benefits of oral OCPs include a decrease in menstrual bleeding, dysmenorrhea, and anemia.

Spotting between periods is a common side effect of oral contraceptives. The same pill should be continued for 3 months to determine if the spotting resolves before switching to a different contraceptive formulation. Since the patient has not missed a pill or taken a new medicine that might interfere with the metabolism of the pill, there is no need to use a backup method. The spotting is mild, so reassuring the patient and continuing the pill is appropriate. If spotting persists after 3 months, changing to a pill containing a higher dose of estrogen or containing a different progesterone is reasonable. If the patient's spotting is because of missed pills, a backup barrier method is important to reduce the risk of an unwanted pregnancy. If the patient misses 3 consecutive days of pills, then stopping the pill, having a menstrual period, and starting a new pill pack the following Sunday would be appropriate advice.

Problem 19

Febrile seizures are a common problem, affecting between 2% and 5% of children younger than 6 years of age. On average, approximately 30% suffer a reoccurrence. The risk increases to 50% if the first seizure occurs before 1 year of age. Most children with a simple seizure need minimal evaluation. Simple febrile seizures are characterized by being nonfocal, a solitary event lasting less than 15 minutes, and having a normal neurologic exam before and after the seizures. Atypical characteristics, such as extended duration, focal seizures, repetitive seizures, and neurologic findings, mandate more extensive testing. Children with a first-time atypical seizure should undergo a lumbar puncture to rule out meningitis. Children with a focal seizure or neurologic findings should undergo CT scanning to rule out a structural disorder. An EEG is not indicated in this patient at this time since with a history of simple febrile seizure and a normal neurologic examination, an EEG is unlikely to be predictive of reoccurrence or the development of epilepsy. The risk of epilepsy in an otherwise normal child is approximately 1%. Factors that increase the likelihood for future seizures include a family history of a seizure disorder, history of either developmental or neurologic abnormalities, or atypical febrile seizures. Intermittent phenobarbital therapy is not

effective. Continuous administration of either phenobarbital or primidone is effective but not indicated in this child with a history of a single simple febrile seizure.

Absolute contraindications to pertussis vaccination are an immediate anaphylactic reaction or evidence of encephalopathy within 7 days of vaccination. Relative contraindications include convulsions within 3 days of vaccination; persistent, severe, or inconsolable crying for more than 3 hours within 2 days of vaccination; a shock-like state within 2 days of vaccination; or fever of 104.9°F unexplained by another cause within 2 days of vaccination. These "relative" contraindications were considered absolute contraindications before the introduction of the new acellular pertussis vaccine, which has a much lower incidence of local and systemic reactions. Children over age 6 months should receive influenza vaccine. Children at high risk for severe complications from influenza include children with chronic lung or congenital heart disease, sickle cell disease, and those receiving immunosuppressive therapy. Other high risk groups include children with diabetes mellitus, chronic renal failure, chronic aspirin therapy, children in contact with other high-risk individuals, and children living in institutions, colleges, or attending day care.

Heart murmurs are very common in children and are usually innocent. Features that suggest the need for further evaluation include diastolic murmurs, loud murmurs, pansystolic murmurs, the presence of a thrill, continuous murmurs, or other associated cardiac findings such as abnormal splitting or asymmetric pulses. A family history of congenital heart disease also increases the risk that a murmur is pathologic. Although a family history of atherosclerosis may merit early lipid testing, it does not increase the risk that a murmur is pathologic.

Problem 20

Normal body temperature is 98.6°F or 37°C. Fever is defined as a temperature greater or equal to 100.4°F or 38°C using rectal temperature measurements. The majority of pediatric patients presenting with fever will have an obvious source for the temperature elevation, such as a viral upper respiratory infection, otitis media, or gastroenteritis. In children without an apparent source for fever, further evaluation is needed, and in performing this evaluation an age-dependent approach is often employed. The sources of fever, organisms causing infections, and the host immune response to infection can vary by age. When fever persists for longer than 14 days in a child, it is defined as a fever of unknown origin (FUO). When the fever persists and is classified as a FUO, then additional diseases, such as occult infections, malignancies, or connective tissue diseases, need to be considered.

The approach to the child with fever varies by age group. For example, clinical assessment of infants between birth and 3 months of age cannot reliably distinguish those with serious infections from those with less serious causes for fever. Thus, the approach to infants in this age category often involves a full septic workup that entails a complete blood count (CBC), blood cultures, chest x-ray, urinalysis, urine culture, and lumbar puncture. For neonates (age birth to 1 month) and ill-appearing infants 1 to 3 months of age, hospitalization and empiric parenteral antibiotic coverage is provided to cover the most common bacterial pathogens until culture results are available. Infants 1 to 3 months of age who appear well, have normal laboratory studies, and have a white blood cell count between 5,000 and 15,000 may be discharged with a follow-up visit in 24 hours. Empiric parenteral antibiotic coverage (ceftriaxone IM) is commonly provided pending follow-up and culture results. Figure 9-1 summarizes the approach to infants 1 to 3 months of age.

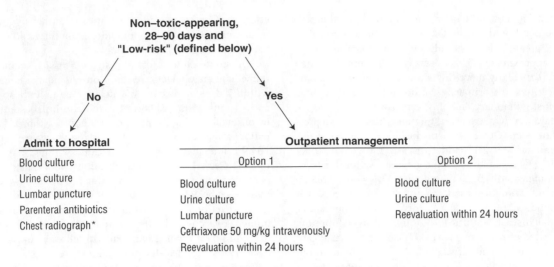

Non–toxic-appearing,
28–90 days and
"Low-risk" (defined below)

No → **Admit to hospital**

Yes → **Outpatient management**

Admit to hospital

Blood culture
Urine culture
Lumbar puncture
Parenteral antibiotics
Chest radiograph*

Outpatient management

Option 1

Blood culture
Urine culture
Lumbar puncture
Ceftriaxone 50 mg/kg intravenously
Reevaluation within 24 hours

Option 2

Blood culture
Urine culture
Reevaluation within 24 hours

*Chest radiograph if signs of pneumonia; respiratory distress, abnormal breath sounds, tachypnea, pulse oximetry <95%.

Follow-up of low-risk infants treated as outpatients with positive culture results:

Blood culture positive (pathogen): Admit for sepsis evaluation and parenteral antibiotic therapy pending results
Urine culture positive (pathogen): Persistent fever: Admit for sepsis evaluation and parenteral antibiotic therapy pending results
Outpatient antibiotics if afebrile and well

Low-risk criteria for febrile infants:

Clinical criteria:
    Previously healthy, term infant with uncomplicated nursery stay
    Nontoxic clinical appearance
    No focal bacterial infaction on examination (except otitis media)
Laboratory criteria:
    WEC count: 5–15,000/mm^3, <1,500 bands/mm^3, or band/neutrophil ratio <0.2
    Negative Gram stain of unspun urine (preferred), or negative urine leukocyte esterase and nitrite, or <5 WBCs/hpf
    When diarrhea present: <5 WBCs/hpf in stool
    CSF: <8 WBCs/mm^3 and negative Gram stain (option 1 only)

Figure 9-1. Algorithm for the management of a previously healthy infant (birth to 90 days) with FWS with a temperature of 38.0°C (100.4°F) or greater. From Baraff. Ann Emerg Med. 2000;36(6):602–614.

Children between the ages of 3 months and 3 years are more likely to have an identifiable source of fever and the clinical assessment is more reliable in establishing the severity of illness. Children without a source for their fever can be managed based on their clinical appearance and height of the temperature. Toxic-appearing children should be admitted to the hospital for an evaluation including CBC, blood cultures, urinalysis, urine culture, and chest x-ray. If the child has clinical signs of meningitis or appears seriously ill, then lumbar puncture may be warranted. The decision to perform a lumbar puncture is based on the physician's judgment and would be considered appropriate testing in the case presented because of the irritability, high fever, and no source identified with a thorough clinical evaluation. Empiric parenteral antibiotic coverage is usually provided pending culture results. Well-appearing children without a source for fever and a temperature less than 102°F (39°C) may be followed clinically. Children with temperatures above 102°F (39°C) have a 5% risk for occult bacteremia. Thus, the approach to these children often includes obtaining a CBC, urine analysis, and blood cultures in those whose WBC is greater than 15,000. A chest x-ray should be obtained in those with respiratory symptoms. Children in whom cultures are obtained are provided with empiric parenteral antibiotic coverage such as ceftriaxone. Oral amoxicillin would not provide sufficient antibiotic coverage in this situation. Children between 3 months and 3 years of age with temperatures above 102°F should have follow-up the next day. The decision to hospitalize or discharge the patient with close follow-up is based on the physician's judgment regarding the severity of the illness, the appearance of the child, and the reliability of the parents, and thus either of these two choices may be appropriate in the case presented.

In children older than age 3, occult bacteremia is significantly less common and clinical evaluation including a thorough history and physical examination can usually identify the source for fever. Laboratory evaluation in these older children is dictated by the clinical findings.

Studies such as the abdominal CT scan or gallium scan would not be routinely indicated for children presenting with an acute fever and no identifiable source. Use of these tests would be reserved for those with clinically suspected abdominal sources or FUO.

Problem 21

Gallbladder disease affects over 20 million Americans and more than 500,000 cholecystectomies are performed each year. Risk factors for developing gallstones include increasing age, obesity, female gender, pregnancy, and ethnicity. Gallstones can be classified as cholesterol, pigmented, or mixed stones depending on their chemical composition.

Only about one-third of patients with gallstones experience symptoms. Biliary colic is a dull pain often located in the right upper quadrant or midepigastric area. It is usually sudden in onset, builds to a maximum within 1 hour, and may last up to 3 hours. It is often accompanied by nausea and vomiting. Although classically fatty food intolerance, belching, and bloating have been attributed to chronic gallbladder disease, the association has never been proven. The pain of biliary colic is due to spasm of the cystic duct from obstruction by a stone. Acute cholecystitis occurs when a stone becomes impacted in the cystic duct and inflammation develops behind the obstruction. The pain of acute cholecystitis may be similar to biliary colic but is highly variable. Usually it last more than 6 hours and is associated with a low-grade fever.

The diagnosis of gallstones can be established by ultrasound testing, which is approximately 95% sensitive and specific for stones greater than 2 mm. It is not a good test for stones in the common bile duct. Prior to having the ultrasound, the patient should fast for about 8 hours so that the gallbladder is filled with bile, allowing for better visualization of stones. Often, liver function tests are normal in patients with biliary colic. However, with complications such as acute cholecystitis, cholangitis, and pancreatitis, blood tests are usually abnormal. Although ultrasound is excellent for detecting gallstones, it is less sensitive in detecting stones in the common bile duct. Approximately 15% of patients with gallstones have common bile duct stones and the best test for diagnosing stones in the common bile duct is an endoscopic retrograde cholangiopancreatography (ERCP). An ERCP is more than 90% sensitive and may allow for a therapeutic sphincterotomy to be performed at the same time.

Patients with gallstones may be asymptomatic, have one episode of biliary colic, multiple episodes of biliary pain, or suffer complications requiring hospitalization. After the first episode of biliary colic, there is a 40% to 50% chance of recurrent episodes of pain with a 1% or 2% risk of developing one of the biliary complications. Most people with recurrent attacks of biliary colic and gallstones should be advised to have surgery provided they are reasonable surgical candidates. A laparoscopic cholecystectomy provides the benefit of being less invasive than open procedures but has a higher rate of bile duct injury. If the patient decides against surgical management or is a poor surgical risk, medical therapy (e.g., ursodiol) or extracorporeal shock wave lithotripsy may be done. Ursodiol (Actigall) is 30% to 90% effective in clearing stones. However, 12 to 24 months of therapy is often necessary. The effects of therapy should be monitored with a gallbladder ultrasound every 6 months. After treatment, there is a 50% chance of recurrent stones. Results are best in patients with stones that are less than 2 cm and do not contain calcium. Lithotripsy is approximately 70% to 90% effective in clearing stones, but the recurrence rate is approximately 70%.

Problem 22

Giant cell arteritis (GCA) is an inflammatory disease of large and medium size arteries that occurs almost exclusively in patients older than age 55. It is very rare in black patients. The incidence of GCA increases rapidly with advancing age and occurs equally among the sexes. The arteries of many organ systems, including renal, hepatic, mesenteric, coronary, and, rarely, intracranial, may be involved. Inflammation of the posterior ciliary arteries usually occurs with ocular involvement.

Patients with GCA may experience malaise, weight loss, fever, scalp pain or tenderness, pain and tenderness of the muscles and joints (polymyalgia rheumatica), tenderness over the temporal arteries, ear pain, and jaw claudication. The tenderness experienced when this patient brushes her hair along with her visual symptoms make cataracts an unlikely cause of her symptoms and merit an urgent evaluation by an ophthalmologist. Ocular symptoms also include amaurosis fugax, sudden visual loss (partial or complete), and diplopia.

It is important to initiate treatment if the diagnosis of GCA is suspected. If there is a loss of vision from arteritis-related ischemic optic neuropathy in one eye, about 65% of untreated patients lose vision in the second eye, usually within 10 days. Compressive mass lesions generally result in slow progressive loss of vision. Therefore, in this case imaging is not warranted. Loss of vision in the involved eye is usually permanent. Treatment is instituted to protect the opposite eye (or the remaining vision in the involved eye) and to prevent systemic vascular complications.

GCA may be suspected on the basis of clinical symptoms and signs and abnormal laboratory studies. To establish a diagnosis unequivocally, a temporal artery biopsy is necessary. When a diagnosis of GCA is suspected, a Westergren erythrocyte sedimentation rate (ESR) should be obtained since it is elevated (more than 50 mm per hour) in approximately 90% of patients. A patient with ischemic optic neuropathy with a normal ESR and without signs or symptoms suggesting GCA probably does not need a biopsy. However, the presence of signs or symptoms along with either an abnormal or equivocal ESR merits a temporal artery biopsy.

Once the diagnosis of GCA is considered, therapy should be instituted immediately. A dosage of 80 to 100 mg of prednisone orally daily, with consideration of intravenous corticosteroid therapy for the first 48 hours, is indicated. An involved temporal artery remains positive histopathologically for 1 or 2 weeks after institution of corticosteroids. Therefore, therapy should not be withheld pending the results of a biopsy. Instead, treatment should be initiated and a biopsy scheduled as soon as possible. Patients should be monitored and the dose of prednisone slowly lowered with each decrease in ESR or improvement of symptoms. Patients require treatment for at least 3 to 6 months but frequently need steroids for up to 1 year or more.

Since 5% to 10% of biopsies can be false negatives, the clinician should consider biopsy of the opposite artery if steroid therapy results in dramatic improvement and the biopsy is negative.

Problem 23

Human immunodeficiency virus (HIV) is an RNA retrovirus that causes acquired immunodeficiency syndrome (AIDS). The spectrum of disease includes primary infection with or without acute HIV syndrome (a mononucleosis-like illness), asymptomatic infections, and advanced disease. The hallmark of HIV disease is an immunodeficiency resulting from a progressive quantitative and qualitative deficiency of helper T lymphocytes. These cells are defined phenotypically by the expression on the cell surface of the CD4 molecule, which serves as a cellular receptor for HIV. The CDC surveillance definition of AIDS requires one of the following: a CD4 count below 200/mm with laboratory evidence of HIV-1 infection, the presence of an AIDS-indicator disease such as pulmonary tuberculosis, recurrent pneumonia, or invasive cervical cancer in a patient with laboratory evidence of HIV and no other reason for immune impairment. The decision of when to initiate antiretroviral therapy is controversial. The previous consensus was that therapy should not be initiated until the CD4 level fell to less than 500 or until the patient developed an AIDS-defining illness. Some now advocate treatment at the initial diagnosis regardless of CD4 count, whereas others use the viral load to guide initiation of therapy. Table 9.13 lists the antiviral agents and their side effects. Patients with CD4 T cell counts below 200 are at high risk for infection with opportunistic organisms such as candida and *Pneumocystis carinii*. Adherent white patches, which bleed with removal in the setting of HIV, indicate oral thrush. Topical agents

Table 9.13 Antiviral agents

Drug	Trade Name	Class	Side Effects
Zidovudine (AZT, ZDV)	Retrovir	NRTI	Leukopenia, anemia, lactic acidosis with hepatic steatosis (rare but can be fatal)
Zalcitabine (ddC)	Hivid	NRTI	Neuropathy, pancreatitis (less than with didanosine), lactic acidosis with hepatic steatosis (rare but can be fatal).
Dicanosine (ddl)	Videx	NRTI	Pancreatitis, neuropathy, lactic acidosis with hepatic steatosis (rare, but can be fatal).
Lamivudine (3TC)	Epivir	NRTI	Minimal toxicity, lactic acidosis with hepatic steatosis (rare, but can be fatal)
Stavudine (d4T)	Zerit	NRTI	Neuropathy, pancreatitis, lactic acidosis with hepatic steatosis (rare, but can be fatal).
Abacavir	Ziagen	NRTI	Hypersensitivity reaction (may be fatal)
Tenofovir	Viread	NRTI	Asthenia, headache, GI upset, lactic acidosis with hepatic steatosis (rare, but can be fatal)
Delavirdine	Rescriptor	NNRTI	Rash, increased transaminase levels
Efavirenz	Sustiva	NNRTI	Rash, nervous system symptoms (headache, dizziness, insomnia, impaired concentration), increased transaminase levels.
Nevirapine	Viramune	NNRTI	Rash (generally most severe with initiation of treatment), hepatitis
Amprenavir	Agenerase	PI	GI upset, rash, fat redistribution, lipid abnormalities
Indinavir	Crixivan	PI	Nephrolithiasis (esp. in setting of poor water intake), rash, fat redistribution, lipid abnormalities
Nelfinavir	Viracept	PI	Diarrhea, rash, fat redistribution, lipid abnormalities
Ritonavir	Norvir	PI	GI upset, rash, fat redistribution, lipid abnormalities
Saquinavir	Invirase, Fortovase	PI	GI upset, rash, fat redistribution, lipid abnormalities
Lopinavir plus ritonavir	Kaletra	PI	GI upset, rash, fat redistribution, lipid abnormalities

NRTI, nucleoside/nucleotide reverse transcriptase inhibitor; NNRTI, nonnucleoside reverse transcriptase inhibitor; PI, protease inhibitor.

such as clotrimazole or fluconazole are effective for treating mucosal candidiasis. Amphotericin is a highly toxic medication, which is not indicated for the treatment of localized thrush. Prophylactic treatment with fluconazole is not recommended because although fluconazole is very effective for acute candidiasis, chronic therapy increases the risk of developing resistance and of drug interactions. This applies even when the CD4 cell count is low.

The most common opportunistic infection seen in HIV is *Pneumocystis carinii* pneumonia (PCP), occurring in up to 80% of individuals during the course of their disease. Although patients with PCP have classic pneumonia symptoms such as dyspnea, fever, and cough along with tachypnea, tachycardia, and sometimes cyanosis, lung auscultation usually reveals few abnormalities. The initial diagnostic study of choice is the chest x-ray. The chest x-ray classically demonstrates bilateral diffuse infiltrates, but many other patterns have been associated with PCP, including nodular densities, cavitary lesions, upper lobe infiltrates, and pneumothorax. Early in the course, a chest x-ray may be normal. Evaluation of arterial blood gases typically reveals hypoxemia and an increase in alveolar or arterial oxygen gradient. Although the sputum of some patients may demonstrate the organism with special stains such as methenamine silver or immunofluorescence, the mainstay of diagnosis is the staining of specimens obtained by fiber-optic bronchoscopy with bronchoalveolar lavage.

The treatment of choice is trimethoprim-sulfamethoxazole (TMP-SMZ). Patients with oxygen level less than 70 mmHg may also benefit from prednisone. The recommendations for starting prophylactic TMP-SMZ include CD4 cell counts of less than 200, a history of PCP, or oropharyngeal candidiasis. A summary of primary prophylaxis in HIV patients for opportunistic infections is listed in Table 9.14. As a result, this patient would qualify for prophylaxis with TMP-SMZ. One double-strength tablet is the recommended dose; however, one single-strength tablet may be substituted if the patient is unable to tolerate the higher dose. In those patients with non-life-threatening reactions such as fever and rash, TMP-SMZ may be restarted at a lower dose after the side effects have resolved. If TMP-SMZ cannot be tolerated, dapsone may be used as an alternative drug. Other alternative drugs include pyrimethamine, pentamidine, and atovaquone. Patients responding to antiretroviral therapy may discontinue TMP-SMZ if their CD4 count remains greater than 200/mm^3 for 3 to 6 months. TMP-SMZ also protects against toxoplasmosis encephalitis. Patients with a CD4 count of less than 100 should be started on one double-strength TMP-SMZ for prophylaxis against toxoplasmosis encephalitis. An alternative to TMP-SMZ prophylaxis is dapsone-pyrimethamine. Pentamidine does not protect against toxoplasmosis encephalitis.

Problem 24

The clinical presentation of hypercalcemia can range from an incidental finding on an automated chemistry panel to confusion and severe dehydration. Common symptoms of mild hypercalcemia are often subtle and nonspecific. They include fatigue, weakness, depression, hypertension, polyuria, and mild gastrointestinal symptoms such as constipation. A review of medications is important since several commonly used drugs, such as excessive calcium carbonate intake, hydrochlorothiazide, lithium, or excessive vitamin D or A intake, can cause hypercalcemia. Oral contraceptives do not increase serum calcium levels and furosemide is sometimes used in the treatment of hypercalcemia since it can increase renal calcium excretion.

Reviewing previous lab work is important since it may provide clues to the cause of an elevated calcium level. Hyperparathyroidism, which is the most common cause of hypercalcemia in a young, otherwise healthy individual, can cause hypophosphatemia and bicarbonate wasting. An anemia, particularly in a middle-aged or older individual, raises the possibility of multiple myeloma. Hypercalcemia secondary to hyperparathyroidism may be associated with a familial disorder such as the autosomal dominant syndromes of multiple endocrine neoplasia (MEN) types 1 and 2. In MEN 1, parathyroid hyperplasia occurs in combination with adenomas of the pituitary and pancreas. In MEN 2, parathyroid hyperplasia may occur with medullary cancer of the thyroid and bilateral adrenal pheochromocytoma. Familial hypocalciuric hypercalcemia may also cause hypercalcemia. Table 9.15 summarizes the causes of hypercalcemia.

After hypercalcemia is confirmed on repeat testing, an immunoradiometric assay of intact parathyroid hormone (iPTH) is a critical test since hyperparathyroidism from either an adenoma or hyperplasia is the most likely cause for this patient's hypercalcemia. The differential diagnosis includes other causes such as medications, tumors, multiple myeloma, granulomatous disease, hyperthyroidism, and other endocrine disorders. Generally, a history and physical along with a limited lab workup (CBC, chemistry panel, and chest x-ray) are sufficient to suggest the diagnosis. Fasting hypophosphatemia, low serum bicarbonate,

Table 9.14 Primary prophylaxis against opportunistic infections

Infection	Indications	Primary tx	Secondary
PCP[a]	CD4 cells <200/mm^3	Bactrim	Dapsone
Toxoplasmosis	CD4 cells < 100/mm^3	Bactrim	Dapsone
MAC[b]	CD4 cells < 50/mm^3	Clarithromycin	Rifabutin
TB	PPD >5mm	INH w/pyridoxine	Rifampin
VZV	exposure	VZIG	Acyclovir

[a]In neonates, PCP prophylaxis treatment (Bactrim or Dapsone) begins when zidovudine therapy is stopped or the child reaches age six weeks, and continued until the child is found to be HIV-free or for at least one year.
[b]MAC (Mycobacterium avium complex), VZV (Varicella zoster virus).

Table 9.15 Causes of hypercalcemia

Parathyroid related: Parathyroid adenoma; sporadic, familial (multiple endocrine neoplasia types I and II); parathyroid carcinoma

Malignancy related: Tumor metastases to bone; humoral hypercalcemia of malignancy

Vitamin D related: Vitamin D intoxication; excessive production of vitamin D in granulomatous disorders (e.g., TB, sarcoidosis)

Associated with high bone turnover: Thyrotoxicosis; hypoadrenalism; immobilization with increased bone turnover (e.g., Paget)

Drug related: Thiazide diuretics, lithium, theophylline toxicity, estrogens, antiestrogens

Associated with renal failure: Acute renal failure with rhabdomyolysis; secondary hyperparathyroidism in chronic renal failure; aluminum toxicity

Ingestions: Excessive calcium carbonate ingestion (milk alkali syndrome), vitamin A toxicity

Other: Familial hypocalciuric hypercalcemia

Reproduced with permission from Gandi M, Bacon O, Caughey A. *Blueprints Clinical Cases in Medicine.* Malden: Blackwell Science; 2002:61.

elevated serum chloride, and an elevated serum alkaline phosphatase level are commonly seen in hyperparathyroidism. Hypercalcemia is seen in 10% to 20% of patients with sarcoidosis, and in an African American female a chest x-ray is helpful to exclude that diagnosis.

More extensive testing should be directed by the history, physical, and initial laboratory findings. Findings such as lymphadenopathy or a breast mass increase the suspicion of an underlying malignancy. Cancer detection studies should also be considered in patients with unexplained hypercalcemia and suppressed iPTH levels. However, until the iPTH is available, a mammogram at age 32 with a normal exam is not indicated. Likewise, a CT of the head for a patient with mild headaches and a normal physical examination is not indicated. Although the patient's blood pressure elevation may be secondary to the hypercalcemia, in light of her relatively rapid resting pulse, a serum TSH would be helpful for excluding hyperthyroidism.

Factors that favor surgery are younger age (younger than 50), pancreatitis, the patient's desire for surgical treatment, marked elevation of calcium (greater than 12.5 mg/dL), declining renal function, hypertension, calcium kidney stones, and reduced bone mass. Nonadherence to follow-up also favors surgical management. Hydrochlorothiazide increases calcium levels and intolerance to this agent is not an indication for surgery. Biphosphonates and calcitonin have not proved useful on a long-term basis for hyperparathyroidism. Medical management includes limiting dietary calcium and maintaining a fluid intake of at least 2 liters a day. Furosemide in combination with sufficient fluid intake to avoid dehydration and oral phosphate therapy has also been used to medically treat hyperparathyroidism.

Problem 25

Hypertension affects 43 million Americans and is often referred to as the "silent killer" because it is generally an asymptomatic chronic disease and usually only becomes symptomatic once there is end-organ damage. Hypertension is one of the most important modifiable risk factors for development of cardiovascular disease, yet it is often unrecognized or uncontrolled. Only 69% of adult hypertensives are aware of their hypertension, and of these, only 39% are controlled.

Hypertension is usually diagnosed during a routine office visit screening. The history in the patient with hypertension should focus on assessing the patient for evidence of end-organ damage, additional risk factors for cardiovascular disease, and for secondary causes for the hypertension. The physical examination should focus on the cardiovascular system, including funduscopic examination, taking the blood pressure in both arms, and palpation of the extremities for peripheral pulses and edema. The physical examination is often normal, other than the finding of elevated blood pressure.

Hypertension is staged according to Table 9.16. Once the diagnosis of hypertension is confirmed by three readings of greater than 140/90 mmHg, an evaluation to detect end-organ damage, to identify additional cardiovascular risk factors, to exclude secondary causes, and to assist in choice of medications is indicated. A CBC is recommended as a baseline for future evaluation in the event of medication-induced neutropenia or agranulocytosis. A fasting serum glucose, K+, serum creatinine, urinalysis, total cholesterol, and HDL are recommended for newly diagnosed hypertensives. Serum glucose screens for diabetes mellitus and unprovoked hypokalemia (less than 3.5 mEq/L) may indicate a high-aldosterone state, an elevated creatinine may indicate renal insufficiency, and proteinuria or microalbuminuria may indicate renal end-organ damage. The potassium level of a patient should be checked before instituting diuretic therapy. Two other recommended tests are serum calcium (with albumin) and uric acid since hypercalcemia or hyperuricemia may preclude the use of thiazide diuretics. Hypercalcemia may also indicate hypertension secondary to hyperparathyroidism. An ECG is helpful in assessing for prior myocardial infarction, heart block, or left ventricular hypertrophy. A plain chest x-ray is also helpful to assess for cardiomegaly and to rule out the remote possibility of coarctation of the aorta.

Table 9.16 Staging of hypertension

	Systolic BP (mmHg)		Diastolic BP (mmHg)
Optimal	<120	*and*	<80
Normal	<130	*and*	<85
High-normal	130–139	*or*	85–89
Stage 1 hypertension	140–159	*or*	90–99
Stage 2 hypertension	160–179	*or*	100–109
Stage 3 hypertension	>180	*or*	≥110

Hypertension (HTN) can be either primary (essential) or secondary. Primary hypertension accounts for approximately 95% of all cases of HTN. Primary hypertension is a multifactorial process that can result from a variety of interrelated mechanisms. Secondary causes of hypertension comprise only 5% of all adult hypertensives. The most common secondary cause for hypertension is renal parenchymal disease, followed by renovascular disease, exogenous drugs or medications, and endocrine diseases. The history, physical examination, and initial laboratory may suggest a cause and help direct any further evaluation. Features of the history suggestive of secondary causes include malignant or accelerated hypertension, early or late onset of HTN (younger than 20 and older than 50 years of age), an associated history of tachycardia, sweating, headache, a history or a family history of renal disease, resistant hypertension in a compliant patient, history of drug or alcohol abuse, use of medications (e.g., oral contraceptives, estrogens, corticosteroids, and NSAIDs), or history of hirsutism or easy bruising.

The patient presented is a younger woman with stage 2 hypertension and no significant personal or family history of hypertension. The next appropriate step would be to evaluate for secondary causes. With a normal urinalysis, BUN, and creatinine, renal parenchymal disease is unlikely and attention should be focused on renovascular and endocrine causes. Renal magnetic resonance angiography can noninvasively evaluate the renal arteries. Other tests that can assess for renovascular disease include a captopril renal scan and a renal artery duplex ultrasound scan. Arteriography is the definitive test but is invasive. Endocrine causes focus on evaluating the adrenal glands for pheochromocytoma, Cushing's syndrome, and primary aldosteronism. Tests useful to screen for these diseases include a urine for VMA and metanephrines, dexamethasone suppression test, and plasma aldosterone:renin ratio. Urine testing for VMA and metanephrines is 99% specific and 84% to 96% sensitive for detecting pheochromocytomas. A normal overnight dexamethasone suppression test excludes Cushing's disease with a negative predictive value of 98%.

A plasma aldosterone:renin ratio of over 20:1 along with a significantly elevated aldosterone level is considered positive and should be further evaluated by checking aldosterone levels after sodium loading. Although hyperparathyroidism is associated with concomitant hypertension, a parathyroid scan is not recommended as a screening tool for this disorder. The serum calcium screens for hyperparathyroidism followed by a parathyroid hormone level if the calcium level is elevated. Thyroid disease is an uncommon underlying cause of hypertension but can be evaluated by checking a serum TSH. A thyroid ultrasound would serve no role in screening.

The treatment target for uncomplicated hypertension is generally accepted at a BP less than 140/90, whereas a target of 130/85 is appropriate in patients with renal failure, heart failure, or diabetes. Patients with proteinuria or microabuminuria may benefit from blood pressure reduction to less than 125/75. Even though there is a reduction in BP from her lifestyle modifications, her BP is still above the recommended level. Preferred initial agents include beta-blockers, ACE inhibitors, and diuretics because of their proven beneficial effect on morbidity and mortality. The choice of agent may also be influenced by coexisting medical conditions. For example, an ACE inhibitor may be preferred in the setting of diabetes and a beta-blocker in patients with coexisting CAD or compensated heart failure because of their mortality benefit in this setting.

Problem 26

Symptoms of hypothyroidism can mimic many other diseases. Initial complaints include fatigue, dry skin, heavy menstrual periods, weight gain, and cold intolerance. If untreated, patients can go on to develop coarse hair, hoarseness, constipation, increasing weight gain, and significantly impaired mental activity. The skin can become doughy, the face puffy, and the tongue enlarged. Muscle weakness, arthralgias, and heavy periods experienced by this patient can also be seen in hypothyroidism.

The most sensitive screening test for primary hypothyroidism is a TSH. In this patient, a CBC is indicated because of the patient's fatigue and heavy menstrual periods. In the absence of more specific symptoms suggesting connective tissue disease, an ANA is unlikely to be helpful as part of the initial workup. Estrogen levels vary throughout menses and are not indicated in this patient. Hyperlipidemia is a common consequence of hypothyroidism and the lipid profile is indicated in this patient both for screening and because of her probable hypothyroidism. A dexamethasone suppression test is not generally necessary in a typical clinical setting to diagnose depression. In the patient presented, her depressive symptoms appear to be secondary or reactive to her underlying physical disease. Lyme disease titers are not indicated in the absence of a history of a deer tick bite or of erythema migrans.

The most common cause of primary hypothyroidism is Hashimoto's thyroiditis, which occurs more frequently in women than men. Secondary hypothyroidism is a common consequence of thyroid surgery and radiation therapy. Iodine is a constituent of thyroid hormone and geographic areas that lack iodine have an increased rate of endemic hypothyroidism and goiter. Most developed nations provide iodine as a dietary supplement. Hashimoto's thyroiditis is an autoimmune disorder resulting in damage to the thyroid gland. Antimicrosomal antibodies serve as a laboratory marker for the illness. Postpartum thyroiditis is a variant of Hashimoto's, affecting 5% of women after delivery. Antibody production peaks at 3 to 4 months and then declines. Most patients spontaneously return to euthyroid status but tend to relapse with subsequent pregnancies.

Medications such as lithium, interferon, and iodine can cause hypothyroidism. Ibuprofen is not known to cause hypothyroidism. Patients with hypothyroidism often have coarse dry hair, peeling skin, and nails that are thin and brittle. Thinning of the outer third of the eyebrows is common. Levothyroxine is the preferred form of replacement therapy. The starting dose for thyroid hormone replacement depends on age, the presence of chronic illness, severity and duration of symptoms, and pretreatment TSH level. In patients older than 50 years or in younger patients with known or suspected cardiac disease, therapy should be initiated with lower doses. The onset of improvement is gradual and it takes about 2 to 4 weeks to notice improvement. One should allow 4 to 6 weeks between dose adjustments because it can take that long for a given dose to become fully effective.

Problem 27

A painful, swollen, and red joint merits prompt evaluation since it may be associated with significant morbidity. The most common causes of an acute painful, swollen joint are infection, trauma, or a crystalline arthropathy. A complete blood cell count and an ESR may be abnormal in those with septic arthritis or gout. Arthrocentesis with gross examination, microscopic examination, and culture of joint fluid is essential for evaluating a single "hot joint." A Gram stain and culture is indicated to rule out infection and examining the fluid for crystals can diagnose a crystalline arthropathy. Table 9.17 provides guidelines for interpreting the WBC count in the joint fluid. A rapid strep test would be appropriate if an individual has a history of a sore throat, has a known exposure to someone with strep pharyngitis, or has a migratory polyarthritis. MRI and rheumatoid factor are less useful in the acute setting but may be appropriate if the basic workup is nondiagnostic.

The presence of negatively birefringent crystals in the joint fluid confirms the diagnosis of gout. The presence of calcium pyrophosphate crystals, which are positively birefringent, can confirm the diagnosis of pseudogout. Acute management includes NSAIDs such as indomethacin given at the high end of the normal dosage range for a few days and then tapered. Colchicine is also useful for treating acute gout and can be given at a dose of 0.6 mg by mouth every hour until pain is relieved, nausea or diarrhea develop, or a maximal dose of 5 mg is reached. Although corticosteroids given as an intra-articular administration, by mouth, or intravenously typically provide excellent pain relief, they should be reserved for those individuals whose pain is unrelieved by or who are unable to take NSAIDs or colchicine. Bed rest for the first day or two should be encouraged because early activity may precipitate another attack. Allopurinol, which inhibits the formation of uric acid, is not useful in the acute setting since acutely lowering

serum uric acid may prolong or precipitate another attack. Allopurinol is used to prevent attacks in those who have repeated occurrences. Thiazide diuretics should be avoided in individuals with gout because they inhibit renal excretion of uric acid, thus increasing serum levels. Other drugs that increase uric acid levels include cyclosporine, niacin, furosemide, and low-dose aspirin.

Reversible causes contributing to an elevated serum uric acid include frequent alcohol consumption, obesity, and a high-purine diet. After their first episode of acute gout, patients should be educated to avoid alcohol, to lose weight if appropriate, and to avoid foods high in purine. For recurrent attacks, prophylactic medications such as colchicine at a dose of 0.6 mg twice daily, uricosuric medications such as probenecid at a dose of 500 mg PO bid, or allopurinol at a dose of 100 mg PO qid are helpful. Uricosuric medications are ineffective in patients with renal insufficiency and should not be used in patients with uric acid kidney stones, chronic tophaceous gout, and in patients with increased urinary uric acid levels. Allopurinol may cause exfoliative dermatitis. Low-dose daily use of NSAIDs may also help prevent future attacks of gout but, because this patient has had only one episode, are not indicated in this case.

Gout is a metabolic disease characterized by overproduction or undersecretion of uric acid. Roughly 90% of those with primary gout are men, and it is uncommon in those younger than the age of 30. Uric acid kidney stones develop in 5% to 10% of those who suffer from gout and usually occur in people with elevated serum uric acid. Rapid breakdown of cells, as occurs with treatment of lymphoma or leukemia, will often lead to elevated uric acid and a resultant attack of gout. In these patients, allopurinol may be used as prophylaxis for those undergoing chemotherapy.

Problem 28

Approximately three-fourths of all adults experience back pain some time during their lifetime. Many structures in the back, such as muscles, facet joints, ligaments, nerve roots, vertebral bones, and intervertebral discs, are pain sensitive. Most back pain occurs from a strain injury or from degeneration involving one of the pain-sensitive structures. Although an exact diagnosis is often difficult to establish, only a small fraction (less than 5%) of patients have a serious underlying cause, such as malignancy, infection, fracture, or referred pain from a visceral structure near the spine. Mechanical back pain accounts for the vast majority of back pain cases and is typically relieved by rest. Pain that worsens at night increases the likelihood of a serious cause such as neoplasm. Spinal stenosis, which occurs predominantly in elderly individuals with chronic degenerative joint disease and disc degeneration, is an important cause of lower back and lower extremity pain and presents with symptoms such as numbness and weakness. The characteristic symptom is pain that is worsened by standing, walking, or other activities that cause lumbar extension.

True sciatica, which is pain that radiates from the back down the side of the leg, past the knee, is a sign of nerve root irritation, often due to a herniated disc. The pain may be accompanied by numbness and usually involves injury at the L5–S1 level (the most common level for disc injury). Weakness in dorsiflexing the foot and a decreased ankle reflex are consistent with S1 nerve root irritation and an L5–S1 disc herniation. Quadricep weakness is associated with an L4–L5 herniation. Lumbosacral (L-S) spine films are usually not helpful in making the diagnosis. By middle age, many individuals have narrowing between vertebrae and radiologic evidence of osteoarthritis. L-S spine films are most helpful after trauma or when there are "red flags" suggesting a

Table 9.17 General guidelines for interpreting leukocyte count

WBC Count (cells/mm³)	Interpretation
<200	Normal fluid
<2,000	Noninflammatory (e.g., osteoarthritis)
2,000–50,000	Mild to moderate inflammation (rheumatologic, crystalline)
50,000–100,000	Severe inflammation (sepsis or gout)
>100,000	Sepsis until proven otherwise

systemic illness. Red flags include a history of cancer, severe nighttime pain, weight loss, fever, age older than 50 years or younger than 20, history of osteoporosis, chronic steroid usage, immunosuppression, intravenous substance abuse, a significant neurologic deficit, or pain that fails to improve after 4 to 6 weeks of therapy. Likewise, urgent CT and MRI scanning should be reserved for patients with significant neurologic impairment or for suspected serious causes of low back pain. Similar to plain films, MRI often reveals abnormalities in pain-free individuals. Since the patient's symptoms are fairly mild and no red flags exist, a trial of therapy for 4 to 6 weeks is indicated before obtaining an MRI. Individuals with symptoms such as saddle anesthesia, bowel dysfunction, and severe or progressive neurologic deficit will require MRI evaluation consultation with either an orthopedist or neurosurgeon. Table 9.18 provides a summary of clinical manifestations of back pain.

Table 9.18 Clinical manifestations of back pain

Type	Onset	Trigger	Symptoms
Muscular	Acute	Heavy lifting	Lateralized back pain, pain in buttock, posterior upper thigh
Disk herniation	Recurrent	Trivial stress	Nerve root L5, S1 impingements, frequent sciatica
Spinal stenosis	Old age or congenital	OA* or congenital	Pseudoclaudication*
Spondylolisthesis+	Chronic	OA, spondylolysis	Nerve root L5, S1 impingement hyperextension activities
Compression fx	Acute	Osteoporosis	Pain limited in middle to lower spine Steroid use or myeloma
Neoplasms	Insidious	Neoplasms^	Night pain, not relieved w/supine position
Cauda equina syndrome	Old age	Massive disk herniation	Overflow incontinence (90%) saddle anesthesia$ (75%) decreased anal sphincter tone
Osteomyelitis	Acute	Back procedure	Fever, spinal tenderness
Inflammatory diskitis	Young age	S. aureus	Refusal to walk, fever, signs of sepsis; disk space narrowing, sclerosis per radiographic
Ankylosing spondylitis	Young age	HLA-B27	Morning spinal stiffness, history of inflammatory bowel dz sacroiliitis, chest expansion less than 2.5 cm, "bamboo-spine" in radiographic
Spondylolysis	>10y	Hyperextension	Back, buttock pain with lordosis w/activity, tight hamstrings
Scheuermann disease	Young age	Fatigue	Round back; vertebral wedging, end plate irregularity per radiographic

*OA (osteoarthritis); pseudoclaudication is pain in the lower extremity worsened by walking and relieved by sitting down that mimicks vascular insufficiency.
+Spondylolisthesis is forward subluxation of a vertebral body, usually in L4–5 or L5–S1.
^Neoplasms include primary (i.e., multiple myeloma, spinal cord tumor) or metastatic to the spine (i.e., breast, lung, prostate, gastrointestinal, genitourinary neoplasms)
$Saddle anesthesia is reduction in sensation over the buttocks, upper posterior thighs, and perineum

Strict bed rest should be generally limited to only a few days. Patients with sciatica may require slightly longer periods of up to 1 week. However, prolonged periods of bed rest have not proven beneficial and may result in deconditioning, loss of muscle, constipation, and demineralization of bone. Ninety percent of patients with lower back pain improve spontaneously in about 6 to 8 weeks. Medications such as acetaminophen or NSAIDs, which provide symptomatic relief aid, are considered first-line agents. Opiates can cause sedation, constipation, and nausea but may be of help in pain unrelieved by first-line therapies. Oral steroids have not been shown to improve recovery time. Muscle relaxants are not considered first-line therapy but may occasionally be of use in some patients. Manipulation can improve recovery time but should not be used in patients with a radiculopathy or fracture. It is important to return patients to work as soon as possible. Only about one-half of those individuals who have not returned to work by 6 months will ever return to work.

Problem 29

Secondary amenorrhea is the absence of menses for more than 3 months or for the equivalent of three menstrual cycles in a patient who previously had normal menstrual cycles. The leading cause of secondary amenorrhea is pregnancy, and a pregnancy test should be obtained even though it seems unlikely that this patient is pregnant. Other causes of secondary amenorrhea can be divided into hypothalamic, pituitary, ovarian, and uterine etiologies. Serum TSH and prolactin levels should be checked to rule out hypothyroidism and hyperprolactinemia, both of which can cause amenorrhea. Although adrenal disorders can cause abnormal menses, there is no feature in the history and physical to suggest this as a cause, and routine screening with a morning cortisol level is not indicated. Likewise, with a normal gynecologic exam, an ultrasound would also not be considered part of the initial evaluation. Serum estrogen levels are variable and the patient's estrogen production and uterine responsiveness are better assessed by a progesterone challenge. A progesterone challenge can be administered by giving a patient 100 mg of medroxyprogesterone intramuscularly or by giving oral medroxyprogesterone for 7 to 10 days. Low-dose contraceptive pills contain both estrogen and progesterone and do not constitute a progesterone challenge.

Patients with withdrawal bleeding usually have mild hypothalamic dysfunction from conditions such as stress, excessive exercise, excessive weight loss, or polycystic ovarian disease. Clinical features of polycystic ovarian disease (PCO) include menstrual irregularity, increased body weight, and hirsutism. A persistently elevated LH with a LH-to-FSH ratio of greater than 3:1 is consistent with PCO.

Patients who fail to bleed can be given a trial of estrogen and progesterone to assess uterine function. No bleeding confirms uterine disease such as Asherman's syndrome, which is amenorrhea secondary to a scarred uterine lining following a procedure such as a D&C. Bleeding after combined estrogen and progesterone suggests a normal uterus and increases the likelihood of more serious hypothalamic dysfunction, pituitary disease, or ovarian failure. A high FSH suggests ovarian failure, whereas a low or low-normal level is consistent with pituitary disease or hypothalamic dysfunction. Figure 9-2 outlines the testing of a patient with secondary amenorrhea. Among patients who are not pregnant, hypothalamic dysfunction accounts for approximately 30% of cases of amenorrhea, PCO for 30%, pituitary disease (mostly prolactinomas) for 15%, ovarian failure for 12%, and uterine problems for approximately 5%. Patients with PCO will usually experience withdrawal bleeding after administering progesterone.

Problem 30

Cluster and migraine headaches differ in presentation. Cluster headaches are classically multiple episodes of unilateral orbital headache pain that last between 30 to 90 minutes and occur daily over weeks to months. Cluster headaches are more common in men and may be accompanied by conjunctival irritation, tearing, and sweating. Common migraine accounts for approximately 85% of all migraine headaches and is characterized by a throbbing pain and nausea often accompanied by vomiting, pallor, and sensitivity to light and noise. Classic migraine is characterized by a preceding aura such as flashing lights or neurologic symptoms and has symptoms similar to common migraine. Migraine headaches are more common in women (3:1) and usually begin between the ages of 15 and 45. They are often unilateral and last between 4 and 72 hours. A family history is present in more than 80% of patients. Possible triggers for migraine include irregular sleep patterns, alcohol, humidity, hunger, and food such as chocolate, aged cheese, nuts, and red wine. Headaches can also be induced by many medications, including oral contraceptive pills, cimetidine, atenolol, indomethacin, nifedipine, and nitrates.

Although the severity of pain of an acute headache helps to identify individuals with serious pathology, it is of little value in chronic or recurrent headaches. New-onset headaches demand prompt attention, especially when accompanied by a fever, neck stiffness, or neurologic deficits. A headache with stiff neck and fever suggests acute meningitis, whereas fever with a frontal or periorbital headache are signs of sinusitis. Headaches worsened with cough or bending over can be due to sinusitis or to an intracranial mass. Acute headache, stiff neck, gait ataxia, and profuse nausea with vomiting suggest a cerebellar hemorrhage. A severe headache that reaches maximum intensity rapidly suggests a possible ruptured cerebral aneurysm. An acute headache in a patient older than 50 with tenderness over the temples suggests temporal arteritis.

Tension headaches may produce dull and steady pain, often described as band-like. They can last days to months and often are caused by anxiety, depression, and situational stress. Tension headaches typically do not awaken a patient from sleep and usually are not associated with vomiting or neurologic symptoms. Tension headaches can be caused by cervical strain and TMJ disorder. Diagnostic testing is unnecessary for low-risk patients with chronic or recurring headaches. Low-risk patients are characterized by a prior history or family history of headache and have none of the worrisome signs such as fever, stiff neck, hypertension, abrupt onset, confusion or drowsiness, localized headache pain, or a headache that began with exertion. There are also no focal findings on the neurologic examination.

Treatment of tension headache includes stress reduction using techniques such as relaxation exercises, biofeedback, and deep breathing exercises. NSAIDs or acetaminophen help alleviate symptoms. Low-dose tricyclic antidepressants such as amitriptyline are sometimes used to reduce the number and severity of chronic tension headaches.

Primary treatment of migraine headaches involves avoiding triggers. If headache is present, withdrawing from stressful environments and resting may be beneficial. Specific abortive therapies include triptans, dihydroergotamine, and ergotamine. In general, the triptans produce a good response (mild or no headache) in 60% to 70% of patients when given as an oral tablet, and pain-free status is achieved in between 25% and 40% of patients. Central nervous system symptoms such as somnolence, fatigue, weakness, and dizziness are the most common and troublesome side effects.

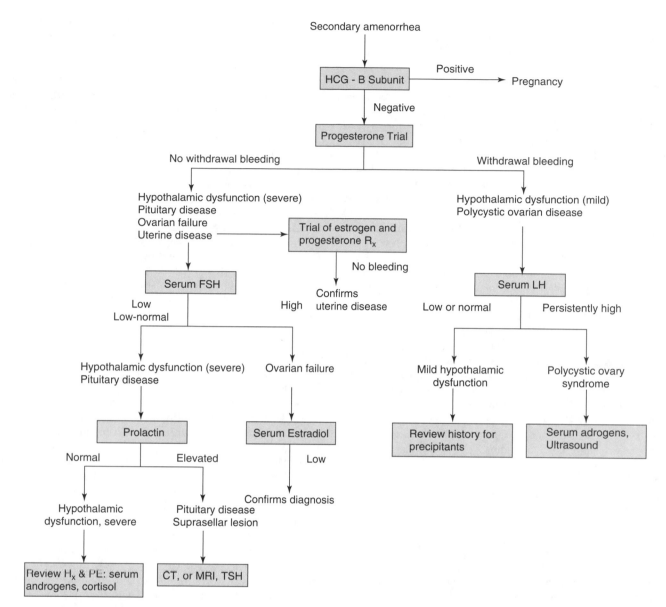

Figure 9-2. *Initial testing of the patient with secondary amenorrhea.*

Chest pain occurs in a significant number of patients after using a triptan, but it is thought to be related to stimulation of the esophageal receptors, which causes esophageal spasm. However, in a patient presenting with chest pain, cardiac chest pain must also be considered. Overuse of triptans can produce rebound withdrawal headaches, and triptan use should be limited to no more than 3 days per week and in general no more than two or three doses of a triptan per day.

Ergotamines are contraindicated in patients with coronary artery disease and peripheral vascular disease. NSAIDs, acetaminophen, antiemetics, narcotics, and caffeine are also commonly prescribed for patients with migraine headaches and are often helpful. However, care must be used with mild analgesics since their limited duration of effectiveness can result in rebound symptoms. Use of narcotics should be limited to patients who have only occasional severe headaches or are refractory to other non-narcotic therapies. If narcotics are used more frequently, the likelihood of habituation and development of a rebound withdrawal headache is high.

Problem 31

An estimated 97 million adults in the United States are overweight or obese. Overweight is defined as a body mass index (BMI) of 25 to 29.9 kg/m² and obesity as a BMI ≥30. Although obesity appears to have a genetic component, it is a complex multifactorial chronic disease that involves social, behavior, cultural, physiologic, metabolic, and genetic factors. Patients with obesity have a substantially increased risk of sleep apnea as well as an increase in morbidity from hypertension, dyslipidemia, type 2 diabetes, coronary heart disease, stroke, gallbladder disease, osteoarthritis, respiratory problems, and endometrial breast, prostate, and colon cancer. There is strong evidence that weight loss reduces blood pressure and reduces the risk for developing diabetes and cardiovascular disease. Obesity lowers the risk of osteoporosis rather than increasing it. The presence of excess abdominal fat out of proportion to total body fat is an independent predictor of risk factors and morbidity. High risk is defined as waist circumference greater than 40 inches in men and greater than 35 inches in women or a waist:hip ratio of greater than 0.85 in women and greater than 1.0 in men. Rapid weight loss from low-calorie diets increases the risk of gallstones. Experts recommend at least an 800-calorie per day intake to avoid cholecystitis and the risk of sudden death associated with very low-calorie diets. Obese individuals are at risk for hyperlipidemia and diabetes and should be screened for these disorders. The National Institutes of Health guidelines recommend an initial goal for overweight patients of a 10% reduction in body weight over a 6-month period. Weight should be lost at approximately 1 or 2 lbs per week, based on a caloric deficit between 500 and 1,000 kcal/day. Since 1 lb of weight loss equals a 3,500-calorie deficit, this should result in a loss of between 26 to 52 lbs. However, the average weight loss observed over this time is between 20 and 25 lbs, partially because energy requirements decrease as weight is lost. Recommending an increase in exercise is important and should be tailored to the patient's current fitness levels. A goal of moderate levels of physical activity for 30 to 45 minutes, 3 to 5 days per week, should be encouraged. Although there is no evidence to support an exact follow-up regimen, most patients on a weight-loss regime should be seen in the office within 2 to 4 weeks of starting treatment in order to monitor treatment effectiveness and to motivate the patient. Weight-loss drugs may be useful as an adjunct to diet and exercise for patients with a BMI over 30 or in patients with a BMI over 27 and a concomitant obesity-related risk factor or disease. However, most authorities recommend a trial of a low-calorie diet, increased physical activity, and behavior therapy before considering pharmacotherapy. Bariatric surgery is generally reserved for individuals with a BMI greater than 40 or for those with a BMI between 35 and 40 if there are significant comorbidities related to obesity.

Problem 32

In the United States, more than 150,000 hip fractures occur annually in women older than the age of 65. Fractures occur more commonly in women because of the increased prevalence of osteoporosis in females. In addition to gender and advanced age, other risk factors for osteoporosis include a positive family history, sedentary lifestyle, white and Asian background, a history of inadequate calcium intake, smoking, and low body weight. Medical conditions including Cushing's syndrome, exogenous steroid therapy, hyperthyroidism, hypogonadism, and hyperparathyroidism are also associated with osteoporosis.

There is a 15% to 20% 6-month mortality in trochanteric fractures and 10% in femoral neck fractures. Normal mental status and good nutritional state are the best indicators of a good recovery. Patients should be up as soon as possible after surgery, and generally the earlier the patient can begin ambulation, the better the long-term prognosis. Recent studies show that geriatric patients benefit from rehabilitation after a hip fracture and that receiving PT improves outcomes. Although the skill of the surgeon would appear to benefit the patient, there is no evidence documenting this as a predictor of a good outcome.

There are numerous complications of hip fractures, but deep venous thrombosis of the lower extremity and pulmonary embolus are among the more serious and life-threatening complications. Edema is common after surgery and there may even be some asymmetry between the lower extremities from the surgery. However, asymmetric leg swelling suggests the possibility of deep vein thrombosis, and venous duplex scanning is a noninvasive means of testing. If duplex scanning is negative, the physical exam is otherwise normal, and there are no pulmonary or cardiovascular symptoms, then the most likely cause for the leg swelling is venous

insufficiency. Ted hose would be appropriate along with daily weights to monitor fluid balance. Furosemide and a chest radiograph would not be indicated at this time.

A DEXA scan is considered by most experts to represent the best combination of sensitivity, technical simplicity, cost, and reproducibility for the diagnosis of osteoporosis. The diagnostic criterion for osteoporosis is a T score below -2.5. The T score is the comparison of the patient's bone density with that of young healthy adults and is reported in standard deviations from the mean. Osteopenia is defined as a T score between -1.0 and -2.5. The Z score compares a patient's bone density to that of age-matched controls and the finding of a Z score below -1.5 suggests a secondary cause of osteoporosis.

Treatment includes weight-bearing exercise, a daily calcium intake of 1500 mg, adequate vitamin D intake (800 IU), and correcting any underlying causes for osteoporosis. The goal of treating osteoporosis is to reduce the risk for fracture. Fall prevention including attention to the home environment is an essential component of treating osteoporosis. A safety check to eliminate slippery surfaces, obstacle-laden paths, inadequate lighting, and bathroom hazards are examples of items that are part of a safety check. Medications including estrogen, calcitonin, bisphosphonates (Fosamax), and SERMS (Evista) are all effective in reducing fracture risk.

Problem 33

Acute otitis media (AOM) is among the most common pediatric ailments. Most cases occur between 6 months and 3 years of age, with a peak incidence between 6 and 18 months. Most cases of AOM are preceded by a viral upper respiratory tract infection (URI). URIs cause swelling that hinders middle ear drainage and impairs the clearance of bacterial pathogens from the middle ear. Although the majority of cases of AOM are thought to be bacterial, it appears that approximately 25% do not have a bacterial etiology. The most common bacterial pathogen is *Streptococcus pneumoniae*, followed by *Haemophilus influenzae* and *Moraxella catarrhalis*. Risk factors for AOM include attending day care and exposure to secondhand smoke. Polynesians, Native Americans, and Eskimos are also at increased risk. Low birth rate and a family history of allergies or asthma are not associated with an increased risk.

History and physical examination in this case are consistent with AOM. Although it is not possible to make an exact etiologic diagnosis without tympanocentesis, this procedure is reserved for cases in which a child appears "toxic" or is not responding to antibiotics. Other indications for tympanocentesis include suspected AOM in a newborn, AOM in an immunocompromised host, or patients with a suppurative complication.

The management of AOM is somewhat controversial and some experts recommend watchful waiting as a treatment option since 60% of children resolve their symptoms without an antibiotic. Clinical indications that favor watchful waiting include age older than 6 months, mild disease or uncertain diagnosis, and reliable parents. Appropriate pain medication should be offered regardless of whether antibiotics are given. These include oral pain relievers such as ibuprofen, acetaminophen, and topical pain relievers such as Auralgan.

If an antibiotic is used, the agent chosen should be the one with the narrowest spectrum likely to be effective. In patients not allergic to penicillin, amoxicillin at a dose of 40 mg/kg/day is a good choice for patients not at risk for a drug-resistant organism. Risk factors for infection with a resistant organism include attending day care, having a sibling who attends day care, or having received a course of antibiotics within the past 3 months. In these instances, either high-dose amoxicillin (80 to 90 mg/kg/day) or second-line agents such as amoxicillin-clavulanate or a second-generation cephalosporin are recommended. TMP-SMZ is used less often as a first-line agent because of its risk for serious skin reactions and increasing resistance to this antibiotic. However, it is acceptable as a first-line agent in a penicillin-allergic patient. Cefazolin and erythromycin are not active against *H. influenzae* and are not good agents for treating otitis media. Ceftriaxone given intramuscularly for 1 to 3 days is also an effective treatment for otitis media but is generally reserved for patients who cannot tolerate oral medications, are toxic, or are unlikely to be compliant with oral medications.

The follow-up examination demonstrates resolution of the acute infection but persistent fluid. This is not unexpected since 70% of children have fluid present at 2 weeks, 50% at 1 month, and 10% at 3 months. Additional antibiotics are not helpful and studies indicate that decongestants, antihistamines, or inhaled steroids do not hasten the resolution of an effusion. Scheduling a repeat examination in 8 weeks is appropriate. If the fluid is still present, a hearing evaluation is indicated. Those with effusion and impaired hearing should be referred to an otolaryngologist for possible myringotomy with tympanostomy tube placement. A child with an effusion that persists beyond 6 months should also be referred for evaluation.

Problem 34

Parkinson's disease (PD) is a progressive, degenerative neurologic disorder involving the substantia nigra. The disease is characterized by bradykinesia, rigidity, gait abnormalities, postural instability, and resting tremor. An intention tremor is more compatible with benign essential tremor, whereas a resting tremor is consistent with PD and is often the presenting sign. In the initial stages of PD the tremor is typically a unilateral pill-rolling tremor that eventually becomes bilateral as the disease progresses. However, a unilateral tremor that persists for more than 3 years suggests a diagnosis other than PD. A history of multiple strokes, a poor response to levodopa, cerebellar signs, and a Babinski sign also point to a diagnosis other than PD. Dementia occurs in up to 30% of PD patients but is a late sign of the disease. Depression is present in approximately 50% of patients, often due to the physical limitations the disease places on the individual. Dysautonomic manifestations including the clinical symptoms of constipation, incontinence, sexual dysfunction, and seborrhea are common clinical findings. Sensory loss in the lower extremities is not usually associated with PD. The onset of PD is usually between the ages of 50 and 70, with a peak age of 60. Onset younger than the age of 40 is rare (less than 5% of cases). Genetic factors do not appear to play a major role in a typical PD patient presenting after age 50, so the patient's children are not at increased risk. Although some studies suggest selegiline may slow the rate of progression of symptoms and delay the need for levodopa, there is no evidence that Sinemet delays the progression of the disease.

The decision to start carbidopa–levodopa depends on the patient's symptoms and age. Most experts recommend delaying the start of carbidopa–levodopa until symptoms significantly impair the patient's activity or job performance in order to avoid potential tolerance and side effects. Sinemet can improve all major symptoms of the disease; however, the rigidity and bradykinesia generally respond better than the tremor. Anticholinergics (e.g., diphenhydramine) are helpful for tremor, especially in younger patients. Side effects such as confusion, delirium, and constipation may limit their role in older patients.

The most common side effect of levodopa is nausea. Other side effects include dyskinesia and hallucinations. Taking the drug with a light meal may reduce nausea. However, taking the medicine with a heavy meal or a meal with a large amount of protein should be avoided since protein can interfere with L-dopa absorption. Carbidopa is combined with levodopa because it blocks the peripheral conversion of L-dopa to dopamine, which allows the use of smaller doses of L-dopa and helps to minimize side effects. Holidays from Sinemet are generally not recommended since there is no evidence of long-lasting improvement from a drug holiday and the drug holiday may be dangerous. If the dose of levodopa approaches 600 to 800 mg per day, a dopamine agonist such as ropinirole or pergolide may be helpful. Table 9.19 summarizes medications useful for PD.

Problem 35

J.S. most likely has polymyalgia rheumatica (PMR), a condition characterized by pain and stiffness in the neck, shoulder girdle, and the hip girdle. It occurs almost exclusively in persons older than age 50 and affects women about twice as often as men. Although PMR can present abruptly, more commonly the onset is gradual over weeks to months. Fatigue, depression, mild weight loss, and low-grade fever often accompany it. Examination, as in this patient, usually reveals few physical findings. Mild tenderness in the muscles of the hip may be the only finding. Muscle strength is normal, even in patients who complain of weakness.

Almost all patients with PMR have an elevated erythrocyte sedimentation rate (ESR), typically over 80 mg/hour. A mild anemia is also common. Since hypothyroidism can mimic PMR, obtaining a TSH is helpful to exclude this disorder. A uric acid level is not likely to be helpful. Although the patient has a history of cramping and fatigue, *B. burgdorferi* titers are unlikely to be of benefit unless there is a history of a tick bite or a rash consistent with erythema migrans. Erythema migrans is an expanding red papule or macule that develops central clearing.

Naprosyn or other NSAIDs can improve the symptoms of PMR, but most patients require steroids. Usually, patients respond rapidly (within a few days) to low-dose steroids (prednisone 15 to 20 mg per day). A rapid response to steroids helps confirm the diagnosis. Benemid, which is a treatment for gout, and doxycycline, which is an effective treatment for Lyme disease, would not be likely to benefit this patient.

The good response to prednisone helps confirm the diagnosis of PMR. Patients with PMR are at risk for temporal arteritis. Usually, manifestations of each illness occur within a few months of one another; however, the interval can be up to several years. Headache is the most common symptom of temporal arteritis and is usually frontal or over the temples. There may be an associated scalp tenderness in the temporal area, and the temporal artery may be tender and swollen with palpable nodules. Chewing may precipitate claudication in the jaw muscles. Temporal arteritis can cause visual loss from an ischemic optic neuropathy and the patient should be started promptly on high-dose prednisone (60 to 100 mg per day). Symptoms of temporal arteritis should prompt consideration of a temporal artery biopsy since this is the only means of confirming the diagnosis of temporal arteritis. Usually, the ESR will be markedly elevated. A cerebral angiogram is an invasive procedure that is not as reliable diagnostically as a temporal artery biopsy. It may occasionally be helpful in a patient with suspected temporal arteritis in choosing a biopsy site if an initial biopsy was negative. Ergotamines, which are vasoconstrictors, are useful for migraine headaches. They are not indicated in this

Table 9.19 Summary of anti-Parkinson medications

Agent	Benefits	Drawbacks
Dopamine precursor + peripheral decarboxylase inhibitor		
Carbidopa/levodopa	• Most effective therapy for motor symptoms • Improves disability • Virtually all patients will require it at some time • Immediate and controlled-release formulations available • CR as effective as IR • CR more convenient • Generic formulation available (less expensive)	• Motor complications • Does not treat all features • Does not stop disease progression • Sedation • Titration required • No difference between IR and CR in forestalling development of dyskinesias/motor fluctuations
Levodopa/carbidopa/ entacapone + (COMT inhibitor)	• Combination in 1 pill • Prolongs levodopa half-life • Reduces "off" time • Helps smooth the clinical response • May delay dyskinesias	• Requires titration because levodopa/carbidopa • COMT inhibitor + levodopa side effects
Dopamine agonists (non-ergot)		
Pramipexole	• Delays motor complications as monotherapy • Effective monotherapy in early disease or as adjunct to levodopa in advanced disease • Levodopa-sparing • Possibly Neuroprotective • Fewer motor SEs than levodopa	• Less effective than levodopa for motor symptoms • Neuropsychiatric SEs • Sedation • Does not treat all features • Neuroprotective effects not proven • Titration required
Ropinirole	• Delays motor complications as monotherapy • Effective as monotherapy in early disease or as adjunct to levodopa in advanced disease • Levodopa-sparing • Possibly Neuroprotective • Fewer motor SEs than levodopa	• Less effective than levodopa for motor symptoms • Neuropsychiatric side effects • Sedation • Does not treat all features • Neuroprotective effect controversial • Titration required
Dopamine agonists		
Bromocriptine	• Usually as an adjunct to levodopa	• Nausea, vomiting, orthostatic hypotension, confusion, anorexia, hallucinations, erythromelalgia, and rarely retroperitoneal fibrosis
Pergolide	• Long half-life • Used as an adjunct • Reduces required doses of levodopa	• Same side effects as bromocriptine • Heart valve fibrosis, rare
COMT inhibitors		
Entacapone	• No titration required • Decreased "off" time • Increased "on" time	• Only adjunctive therapy • Dopaminergic effects (esp. dyskinesias) • Urine discoloration

Table 9.19 (continued)

Agent	Benefits	Drawbacks
	• May reduce risk for motor complications if used with levodopa initially	• Diarrhea
Tolcapone	• No titration required • Easy to administer • Decreased "off" time • Increased "on" time • May reduce risk for motor complications if used with levodopa initially	• Only adjunctive therapy • Dopaminergic effects (esp. dyskinesias) • Urine discoloration • Requires hepatic function monitoring • 10% explosive diarrhea
MAO-B inhibitors Rasagiline	• No amphetamine-like metabolites • May delay the need for levodopa • Effective as monotherapy in early disease • Adjunct to levodopa in advanced disease • Possibly Neuroprotective	• Less effective than levodopa for motor symptoms • Does not treat all features • Neuroprotective effect not proven • Titration required
Selegiline	• Modest symptomatic effect • Adjunct to levodopa • Increases "on" time	• Only mildly effective • Amphetamine-like metabolites
Others Trihexyphenidyl (anticholinergic)	• Most effective against tremor • Best used in younger patients with tremor only	• Limited usefulness • Moderately effective • Cognitive side effects • Peripheral anticholinergic side effects • Avoid in elderly • Possible withdrawal effects
Amantadine (antiviral with dopaminergic effect)	• Mild benefit in early PD • May have antidyskinetic effect	• Limited effectiveness • Potential worsening of PD when withdrawn • Cognitive side effects • Tolerance may develop
Apomorphine (parenteral dopamine agonist)	• Rescue therapy for severe "off" episodes • Rapid and short-acting	• Only rescue therapy • Parenteral drug • Emetic side effects

Source: Olanow et al. (2001) and Hauser et al. (2003).

patient and may actually be harmful if there were underlying cardiac or peripheral vascular disease.

Problem 36

Pneumonia still remains an important cause of mortality (the sixth leading cause of death) and morbidity. Unfortunately, it is difficult to differentiate between bronchitis and pneumonia solely on a clinical basis. The Infectious Disease Society of America (IDSA) recommends a chest x-ray to confirm suspected cases of pneumonia. In addition to identifying infiltrates, a chest x-ray can determine the extent of the pneumonia, detect the presence of a pleural effusion or mass, and identify conditions such as congestive heart failure that might mimic pneumonia. A Gram stain is helpful in identifying the etiologic cause and in directing therapy but cannot

determine if a patient has pneumonia. A chest x-ray (CXR) can provide clues to the etiology of the pneumonia, such as an apical infiltrate as seen in TB or abscess formation as seen in necrotizing staphylococcal pneumonia. However, a CXR cannot accurately distinguish between bacterial pneumonia and pneumonia due to an atypical organism, such as mycoplasma or Legionella.

Several tests are helpful in evaluating patients with pneumonia. An arterial blood gas (ABG) is indicated in patients with suspected acid–base imbalance or hypoxia. However, in a healthy patient with a pulse oximeter reading of greater than 92% and a respiratory rate of 20, an ABG is unlikely to provide additional significant information.

A sexual history is important to the care of patients with pneumonia. Many patients hospitalized with pneumonia, particularly in the age range of 15 to 54, are HIV positive. Other factors such as travel history, pet exposure, and geographical setting (hospital vs. community) can all provide clues to the type of organism causing the pneumonia.

The most common identifiable etiologic agent causing pneumonia is *Streptococcal pneumoniae*. However, even aggressive efforts to identify the etiology often fail. Therefore, both the American Thoracic Society (ATS) and IDSA make recommendations regarding empiric therapy. ATS recommendations for treatment based on different groups (e.g., healthy outpatient vs inpatient) are summarized in Table 9.20. In this case, the Gram stain appears most consistent with atypical pneumonia. It is a good quality smear (less than 10 epithelial cells and greater than 20 white blood cells per high power field) yet no organism is identified. Unfortunately, there is no good single test for mycoplasma pneumonia. A single elevated IgM antibody titer supports the diagnosis in a symptomatic person but is not diagnostic. The only accurate way to diagnose mycoplasma is by observing a fourfold increase in antibody titers in paired sera.

Unfortunately, this provides a retrospective diagnosis that is useful for defining the epidemiology of pneumonia but not helpful for diagnosing an individual. A positive urinary antigen in the appropriate clinical setting is diagnostic for Legionella but is only 70% sensitive. Since an accurate diagnosis of the etiologic agent of pneumonia is often elusive, empiric therapy is commonly indicated. For outpatient management in younger individuals without comorbidities, doxycycline or an extended spectrum macrolide such as azithromycin is recommended. For older individuals or those with comorbidities, a fluoroquinolone with streptococcal activity is recommended.

The Pneumonia Outcomes Research Team (PORT) developed a prediction model to assess a patient's mortality risk. Generally, patients younger than 50 years without a history of neoplastic disease, congestive heart failure, cerebrovascular disease, renal or liver impairment and no marked abnormalities on physical exam, such as altered mental status, pulse greater than 125, respirations greater than 30, systolic blood pressure less than 90, or temperature less than 35°C or greater than 40°C, can be safely managed as an outpatient.

Table 9.20 American Thoracic Society's classification of community acquired pneumonias

	Major Pathogens	Miscellaneous Pathogens	Empiric Therapy
Group I: Outpatient, no cardiopulmonary disease, no modifying factors*	S. pneumoniae M. pneumoniae C. pneumoniae H. infleunzae Respiratory viruses	Legionello spp. M. tuberculosis Endemic fungi	Advanced-generation macrolide† (e.g., azithromycin or clarithromycin) or Doxycycline‡
Group II: Outpatient, with cardiopulmonary disease and/or modifying factors*	S. pneumoniae (including DRSP) M. pneumoniae C. pneumoniae Mixed infection (bacteria plus atypical pathogen of virus) H. Influenzae Enteric gram-negative organisms Respiratory viruses	M. catarrhalis Legionella spp. M. tuberculosis Aspiration (anaerobes) Endemic fungi	Beta-lactam (oral cefpodoxime, cefuroxime, high-dose amoxicillin, amoxicillin/clavulanate) or parenteral ceftriaxone followed by oral cefpodoxime plus Macrolide or doxycycline or Anti-pneumococcal fluoroquinolonel (used alone)
Group IIIa: Inpatient, not requiring ICU admission, with cardiopulmonary disease and/or modifying factors*	S. pneumoniae (including DRSP) H. influenzae M. pneumoniae C. pneumoniae Mixed infection (bacteria plus atypical pathogen or virus) Enteric gram-negative organisms Respiratory viruses Aspiration (anaerobes) Viruses Legionella, spp.	M. tuberculosis Endemic fungi Pneumocystis carinii	Intravenous beta-lactam (cefotaxime, ceftriaxime, ampicillin/sulbactam, high-dose ampicillin) plus Intravenous of oral macrolide or doxycline or Intravenous anti-pneumococcal fluoroquinolone alone

Table 9.20 (continued)

	Major Pathogens	Miscellaneous Pathogens	Empiric Therapy
Group IIIb: Inpatient, not requiring ICU admission, *no* cardiopulmonary disease and/or modifying factors*	S. pneumoniae H. Influenzae M. pneumoniae C. pneumoniae Mixed infection (bacteria plus atypical pathogen of virus) Respiratory viruses Legionella. spp.	M. tuberculosis Endemic fungi Pneumocystis carinii	Intravenous azithromycin alone *If* macrolide allergic or intolerant; doxycycline *and* beta-lactam *or* Antipneumococcal fluoro-quinolone (used alone)
Group IVa: Inpatient, severe, requiring ICU admission, no risk for Pseudomonas aerigompsa	S. pneumoniae (including DRSP) Legionella spp. H. Influenzae Enteric gram-negative organisms S. aureus M. pneumoniae Respiratory viruses	C. pneumoniae M. tuberculosis Endemic fungi	Intravenous beta-lactam (e.g. cefotaxime, ceftriaxone) *plus either* Intervenous macrolide (azithromycin) *or* Intravenous fluoroquinolone
Group IV: Inpatient severe, requiring ICU admission *with* risk for Psuedomonas aeruginosa	Same as group IVa *plus* P. aeruginosa	C. pnuemoniae M. tuberculosis Endemic fungi	Selected intravenous anti-pseudomonal beta-lactam** (cefepline, imipenem, meropenem, piperacillin/tazobactam) *plus* Intravenous antipseudomonal quinolone (e.g., ciprofloxacin) *or* Selected Intravemous anti-pseudomonal beta-lactam as above *plus* Intravenous aminoglycoside *plus either* Intravenous anti-pneumococ-cal macrolide

DRSP, drug resistant *Streptococcus pneumoniae*

*Modifying factors are risk for DRSP (e.g., alcoholism, age >65 years, beta-lactam therapy with 3 months, multiple medical comorbidities, exposure to children in a day care center) and risk for gram-negative organisms (e.g., nursing home resident, multiple recent antiobiotic therapy underlying cardiopulmonary disease).

Erythromycin is not active against *H. Influenzae* and is often less well tolerated.

Many isolates of *S. pneumoniae* are resistant to tetracyclines, so generally reserve for patients allergic to or intolerant of macrolides.

For example moxifloxacin, gatifloxacin, sparfloxacin, levoflaxacin.

Several anti-pseudomonal beta-lactams (e.g., cefepime, piperacillin/taxobactam, imipenen, meropenem) are also effective against DRSO but are not recommended for use if the patient does not have risks for *P. aeruginosa*.

Risks for *P. aeruginosa* infection include chronic or prolonged (i.e., >7 days within last month) broad-spectrum antibiotic use, bronchiectasis, malnutrition, therapies associated with neutrophil dysfunction (e.g., ≥10 mg of prednisone per day).

**For beta lactam allergic patients replace listed beta-lactam with aztreonam and combine with aminoglycoside and anti-pneumococcal fluoroquinolone.

A good quality Gram stain can help guide therapy. The presence of a single predominant organism on Gram stain suggests the etiology of pneumonia. In the described case, either doxycycline or an extended spectrum macrolide are acceptable antibiotic choices. High-dose amoxicillin is useful for treating *S. pneumoniae* but is not effective for atypical organisms and is a suboptimal choice in this patient. Similarly, amoxicillin and clavulanate is not indicated.

Problem 37

Pharyngitis is an inflammation of the pharynx most often caused by infection. Viruses including rhinovirus, adenovirus, parainfluenza virus, and coxsackie virus are the most common infectious cause of pharyngitis. The most common bacterial cause of pharyngitis is group A beta hemolytic strep. *Neisseria gonorrhoeae*, *Corynebacterium diphtheriae*, *H. influenzae*, and *B. catarrhalis* are much less common bacterial causes of pharyngitis. Allergies, inhalation of irritant gases, GERD, smoking, and sleep apnea are among the noninfectious causes of pharyngitis.

Group A strep should be treated with antibiotics to prevent the rheumatic sequelae, to reduce the spread of infection, and to reduce the likelihood of local complications such as peritonsillar abscess. Treatment only modestly reduces the intensity or duration of symptoms. Approximately 10% to 15% of all school-age children will visit a physician each year with pharyngitis. Only 15% to 25% of these infections will be caused by group A strep. The greatest incidence occurs between the ages of 5 and 15 years. Infection with strep is rare in children younger than age 3, and males and females have equal incidence. Symptoms include sore throat, enlarged tonsils with erythema and exudates, petechiae on the soft palate, and a fever over 101°F. There is usually no significant cough, hoarseness, or lower respiratory symptoms. Rhinorrhea, conjunctivitis, and diarrhea decrease the likelihood of a strep infection, and vesicular lesions suggest a viral cause. However, no constellations of symptoms or physical examination findings are pathognomonic for a strep infection. Scarlatina (the rash of strep throat) results from infection with a toxigenic strain of strep pyogenes. Although the characteristic rash may suggest the presence of a strep infection, the rash does not increase the risk of complications and requires no alteration of therapy.

Rapid strep testing has a 5% to 10% false-negative rate so that strep cultures may need to be performed in cases in which the clinical presentation suggests a high likelihood of a strep infection and the rapid strep test is negative. Antibiotic resistance has not been an issue with group A streptococcus. Penicillin is the drug of choice and must be given for a full 10 days. Symptoms will abate whether treated with antibiotics or not. Erythromycin is the drug of choice for penicillin-allergic patients. Although symptoms may last for 5 to 7 days, patients are only contagious until they have received 24 hours of antibiotic therapy. Family members do not require treatment unless they have a positive strep test. Complications include rheumatic fever, post-streptococcal glomerulonephritis (PSGN), peritonsillar abscess, otitis media, sinusitis, and pneumonia. The risk of PSGN is not decreased by antibiotic treatment.

Problem 38

At least one surgical complication occurs in 17% of patients undergoing surgery. Surgical morbidity and mortality generally fall into one of three categories: cardiac, respiratory, and infectious complications. Identifying patients at increased risk is key to preoperative assessment. Healthy elderly patients have complication rates comparable to those of healthy younger patients, although older individuals often have diseases such as pulmonary and cardiac disease, malnutrition, and diabetes mellitus that are associated with an increased risk for surgical complications. The type of surgery contributes to the risk of complications. For example, abdominal and thoracic surgery increases the risk for pulmonary complications.

Ideally, the patient should be evaluated several weeks in advance of elective surgery. Several guidelines for preoperative evaluation have been published, and Figure 9-3 summarizes the ACC/AHA recommendations for preoperative cardiac evaluation. The history and physical examination form the cornerstone of the preoperative evaluation. Medications, including over-the-counter medications, must be noted. Aspirin and nonsteroidal anti-inflammatory medications should be discontinued 1 week prior to surgery to avoid excessive bleeding.

The patient's functional capacity or ability to exercise can be estimated by using an activity index or through formal exercise testing in which results are expressed in metabolic equivalents (METs). One MET is equivalent to an awake patient sitting quietly. Persons with poor functional capacity are limited to activities such as personal care or walking slowly on level ground. Moderate functional capacity (4 to 6 METs) generally means the person can climb two flights of stairs, walk four or more blocks easily, and participate in moderately active recreational sports such as golfing.

In general, asymptomatic patients with good exercise tolerance do not merit further cardiac evaluation unless they are facing high-risk procedures such as vascular surgery, a surgery associated with significant blood loss, or an emergent procedure. Patients with major clinical indicators that suggest increased risk, such as decompensated CHF, unstable angina, arrhythmia, or valvular disease, need further evaluation unless they have been recently tested. Patients with intermediate clinical predictors, such as compensated CHF, diabetes mellitus, or prior history of angina or MI, warrant testing if they have poor functional capacity or are undergoing a high-risk procedure. Patients with minor clinical predictors, such as uncontrolled hypertension, abnormal rhythm, or history of stroke, warrant testing if they have limited functional capacity and are undergoing a high-risk procedure. A person with a normal stress test within 2 years or coronary bypass within 5 years and no interim change in symptoms or functional capacity generally requires no further testing. Assessing left ventricular function is not routinely indicated for the preoperative evaluation of patients with or without cardiac disease. This patient has intermediate clinical predictors with a recent normal stress test, good functional capacity, and is not undergoing a high-risk procedure. She would not require any further preoperative cardiac testing other than an ECG for comparison postoperatively should unexpected complications arise.

Preoperative laboratory studies once routinely included ordering CBC, chemistry profiles, urine analyses, PT, PTT, ECG, and chest x-rays. Studies demonstrated that if these tests were ordered without a clear indication, the results rarely altered management. Guidelines recommend selective ordering based on patient-specific indications and few routine tests. A CBC is useful in detecting unsuspected anemia and providing baseline for postoperative comparison, particularly for surgeries with potential hemorrhagic complications. Renal and liver testing should be reserved for those with surgical or preoperative medical conditions or medication use that might affect these organs. The patient presented is on lisinopril, which may increase potassium and affect renal function. Coagulation times are not performed routinely in healthy individuals since the results rarely affect management. Examples of indications for coagulation studies would include anticoagulation therapy, patients with family or personal history suggesting bleeding disorders, and liver disease.

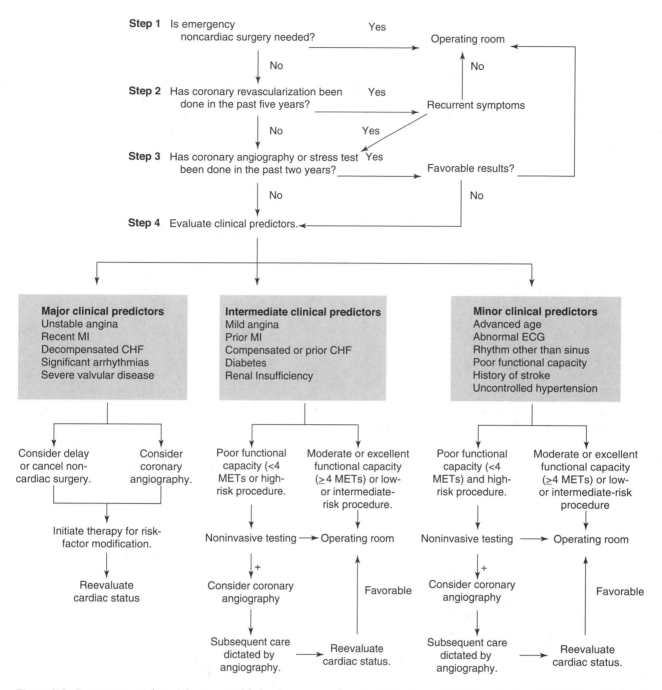

Figure 9-3. Preoperative cardiac evaluation. Modified with permission from Eagle KA, Berger PB, Calkins H, et al. ACC/AHA guideline update for perioperative cardiovascular evaluation for noncardiac surgery–Executive summary. J Am Coll Cardiol. *2002;39:542–553. © 2002, American College of Cardiology Foundation.*

The risk of DVT is 15% or more for general surgery patients and as high as 60% to 70% for orthopedic surgery. Risk factors include obesity, orthopedic surgery, stroke, heritable coagulopathies, and prolonged surgical time. For lower risk patients, such as this patient, compression stockings and subcutaneous unfractionated heparin or low–molecular-weight heparin are sufficient prophylaxis. Higher risk patients require low–molecular-weight heparin or coumadin along with pneumatic compression stockings. Beta-blockers reduce perioperative cardiovascular risk and should be continued in patients receiving them and considered for others at risk. Instruction in incentive spirometry and deep-breathing exercises can decrease pulmonary complications, particularly in obese patients, those with underlying lung disease, and those undergoing abdominal or thoracic procedures. Finally, antibiotic prophylaxis should be considered in those with potentially contaminated surgery, implantation of prosthetic devices, and for patients at risk for endocarditis.

Problem 39

Pressure ulcers are a common problem in elderly patients, particularly in those with limited mobility. Four major mechanisms are involved in the formation of pressure ulcers: moisture, shearing forces, traction, and pressure. Studies demonstrate that ischemic changes can occur in a little as 2 hours of external pressure. This finding supports the clinical recommendation that patients should be repositioned every 2 hours. Moisture is also a risk factor, and urine and/or stool incontinence predispose patients to ulcer formation. Aging patients are more at risk for pressure ulcers since there may be decreased blood supply, decreased subcutaneous fat, and thinning of the skin. Other factors increasing risk of ulcers include malnutrition, anemia, renal insufficiency, dehydration, nutritional and vitamin deficiencies, sedation, and major surgery. Although poor nutrition places individuals at risk, at this time there is no evidence that supplemental zinc reduces the risk of pressure ulcers. The patient should be provided with an adequate diet with 30 to 40 kcal/kg per day to help prevent malnutrition and increased risk for ulcer development. Coumadin is not associated as a risk factor for developing an ulcer.

A stage 1 pressure ulcer is an acute inflammation that is typically seen as swelling and redness over a pressure point. The skin is intact and the redness does not blanche. Most ulcers develop over a bony prominence such as the sacrum, ischial tuberosity, greater trochanter, and the heel. In a stage 2 ulcer, the skin is no longer intact and there is a shallow blister or crater in the skin. Stage 3 ulcers involve the subcutaneous layer, often with a necrotic base. A stage 4 ulcer penetrates to the deep fascia and may also involve muscles or bone. Stage 4 ulcers can lead to sepsis and osteomyelitis. Wound cultures are indicated in the presence of local or systemic infection. This patient has a stage 3 ulcer with no signs of local or systemic infection; thus, a wound culture and antibiotic therapy would not be indicated. Wet to dry dressings may be helpful in this patient to provide mechanical debridement. Whirlpools and irrigation may also be beneficial. Topical agents such as povidone–iodine are toxic and have been shown to delay wound healing. Pressure ulcers are contaminated with bacteria, but unless infection is present, antibiotics are not indicated. Signs of infection include increased pain, foul odor, increased redness, excessive draining, and a worsening wound in the face of appropriate local treatment.

Problem 40

This patient has a massive pulmonary embolism (PE). Massive PE is defined as pulmonary embolism with severe hemodynamic compromise, such as hypotension, shock, severe hypoxemic respiratory failure, or acute right-sided heart dysfunction. Internal jugular venous distension, right ventricular heave, and loud P2 are indicative of right ventricular dysfunction from pulmonary hypertension. Increased pulmonary vascular resistance from obstruction increases the pulmonary artery pressure, and secondarily the pressure in the right atrium and ventricle rises, resulting in right ventricular overload. ECG findings are abnormal in approximately 75% to 90% of cases, most often tachycardia with nonspecific ST segment and T wave changes. The triad of S wave greater than 1.5 mm in lead I and Q wave and inverted T wave in lead III (S1Q3T3) is consistent with PE and is present in about one-half of patients. The arterial blood gas is less than 60 mmHg in most cases and is less than 80 mmHg in 96% of patients. However, arterial blood gases are not diagnostic and a PE can be present in someone with a normal O_2. A chest x-ray may be entirely normal but most often shows atelectasis, which is seen in 60% to 70% of patients. Other x-ray findings include increased lung lucency in the area of the embolus, an abrupt cutoff of a blood vessel, a wedge-shaped pleural-based infiltrate, and a pleural effusion, which if sampled is often hemorrhagic.

In critically ill patients who are unable to leave the ICU, transthoracic or transesophageal echocardiography and pulmonary artery catheterization are recommended. Right ventricular overload and pulmonary hypertension can be detected by TTE, and TEE can sometimes visualize a clot in the main pulmonary arteries. Pulmonary artery (Swan–Ganz) catheterization can demonstrate the hemodynamic pattern consistent with PE: increased right atrial pressure, mean pulmonary artery pressure of 25 to 40 mmHg, low cardiac index, normal pulmonary artery wedge pressure, and five- to 15-fold increase in pulmonary vascular resistance.

Only 40% of patients with PE have a high-probability lung scan. Helical CT scans can detect emboli in segmental or larger pulmonary arteries with a sensitivity of 90%. It is less sensitive for an embolus in the smaller segmental and subsegmental arteries. A normal helical CT as well as a low-probability lung scan markedly reduce the probability of PE but do not exclude the diagnosis. Although pulmonary angiography is considered the reference standard, it is invasive, technically difficult, and may cause arrhythmias, cardiac perforation, cardiac arrest, and hypersensitivity to contrast dyes.

Normal compression ultrasonography of the legs also cannot exclude the diagnosis of PE. Between 20% and 40% of patients with suspected PE but normal compression ultrasonography have PE by angiography. Compression ultrasonography is best used in conjunction with pretest probability and D-dimer assays. The diagnosis of PE can be safely excluded in patients with nondiagnostic lung scans and low to moderate pretest probabilities if the presenting compression ultrasonography test is normal and the D-dimer test is negative. The D-dimer can be elevated following surgery or in patients with an underlying malignancy or vasculitis, so a positive D-dimer test is not diagnostic of DVT or PE.

Low–molecular-weight heparin (LMWH) is now preferred over unfractionated heparin for venous thrombosis prophylaxis as well as treatment of venous thrombosis or PE. LMWH does not require an IV drip or PTT monitoring, has a decreased risk of DVT recurrence in some studies, appears to carry an equivalent or lower risk of hemorrhage, and although immune-mediated thrombocytopenia occurs, it is less common. Heparin-induced thrombocytopenia manifests as a dramatic drop in platelets 1 to 20 days after initiating therapy. Switching from unfractionated heparin to LMWH is not effective and discontinuation of heparin is recommended if the platelet count is below 75,000. In cases of massive PE, thrombolytic therapy is more effective in achieving early lysis of thromboembolism and should be considered in patients who are at high risk for dying and in whom the more rapid resolution of a thrombus may be lifesaving. Such patients are hemodynamically unstable despite heparin therapy (e.g., hypotensive or severe respiratory failure). Thrombolytics are absolutely contraindicated in patients who have had major surgery in the past 10 days, active internal bleeding, and stroke within the past 3 months. Along with recent organ biopsy, puncture of a noncompressible vessel, liver or renal disease, severe arterial hypertension, and severe diabetic retinopathy, recent GI bleeding is a relative contraindication to thrombolytic use. IVC filters are indicated for patients at high risk for death if they have a recurrent thromboembolism, such as patients with mild to moderate RV dysfunction plus (a) underlying cardiopulmonary disease, (b) mean PA pressure greater than 30 mmHg, (c) systolic PA pressure greater than 50 mmHg, (d) HR greater than 120, (e) PaO_2:FIO_2 less than 250, and (f) age older than 65. IVC filters should also be considered in patients with recurrent thromboembolism despite adequate medical therapy.

Problem 41

RSV is the most common cause of lower respiratory tract infection in children and accounts for 50% to 95% of cases of bronchiolitis.

Other agents that cause bronchiolitis include parainfluenza virus, influenza A and B, adenovirus, and mycoplasma pneumonia. Hospitalization for RSV bronchiolitis is 5 to 10 times more likely in infants of low-income families and 1.5 to 2 times more likely in male infants. RSV is spread through direct contact with nasal secretions, thus making hand washing important for infection control. Chest radiographs may include all of those features noted, but 10% of patients may have normal radiographs. Rapid RSV enzyme-linked immunosorbent assay and direct fluorescent assays can provide a diagnosis with 85% to 90% sensitivity and specificity. Its sensitivity largely relies on adequate sampling of nasal aspirates. The proper method to obtain the sample is by instilling and then aspirating 5 mL of isotonic saline into the nasopharyngeal passages. The initial oxygen saturation is the best outpatient assessment tool. A saturation of less than 95% correlates with more severe disease. Other indicators of severe disease include an ill appearance, a history of prematurity, atelectasis on chest x-ray, a respiratory rate greater than 70 per minute, and age younger than 3 months.

The mainstay of treatment includes oxygenation, humidification, and hydration. The use of bronchodilators remains controversial. Some studies show that beta-adrenergic agents may cause a mild, short-term decrease in respirations. Infants with a strong family history of asthma or previous episodes of wheezing are most likely to respond. However, studies with racemic epinephrine show decreases in both the respiratory rate and improved oxygenation. Although commonly used, clinical trials do not support the use of corticosteroids. Antibiotics are rarely indicated because secondary bacterial infections occur in less than 2% of cases.

Prevention of RSV infection may be indicated for children younger than 2 years of age with chronic lung disease. Preventive therapy may be provided in the form of RSV-IVIG or with palivizumab, a humanized mouse monoclonal antibody. Both of these are administered intramuscularly once per month during the RSV season. They may also be beneficial to premature infants and children with heart disease, but therapy is not currently indicated for these groups. After administration of these products, MMR and varicella vaccination should be delayed until 9 months after the last injection.

Therapies specific for RSV include the antiviral ribavirin. Ribavirin is potentially toxic, teratogenic, expensive, and, because of conflicting data regarding its effectiveness, is only recommended on an individualized basis in patients with congenital heart disease, bronchopulmonary dysplasia, and cystic fibrosis. It should also be considered for others at risk of severe or complicated disease, such as infants whose oxygen saturations are less than 65%.

Although the cause remains unclear, the development of RSV infection in early infancy has been implicated as a predisposing factor for chronic lung disease in patients who have a genetic predisposition toward airway hyper-reactivity. Reinfection with RSV is common, although subsequent infections tend to be milder.

Problem 42

Although different groups offer varying recommendations, the U.S. Preventive Services Task Force recommendations are among the most widely accepted set of recommendations. Screening tests are used to detect a condition before symptoms occur. Several factors are important when considering the appropriateness of a screening test. First, the condition should be common and associated with significant morbidity or mortality. For example, seborrhea is a common condition that does not cause sufficient morbidity to merit

screening, whereas a hepatoma is a serious condition that is not sufficiently common to merit screening in the general population. An effective screening test should be sufficiently accurate, cost-effective, acceptable to patients and physicians, and have few side effects. Finally, screening for a condition requires that treatment must be available and that early treatment is superior to treatment started after a patient becomes symptomatic.

In the patient described, annual fecal occult blood (FOB) testing is recommended to screen for colorectal cancer. Both the American Cancer Society and the U.S. Preventive Services Task Force recommend flexible sigmoidoscopy every 5 years starting at age 50. Patients with a strong family history of colon cancer may merit screening at an earlier age (10 years younger than the index case) and with colonoscopy rather than sigmoidoscopy.

Preventive cardiology receives significant attention because of the burden of disease and because of the opportunity to ameliorate risk factors. Measuring blood pressure to detect hypertension at 1- or 2-year intervals along with cholesterol screening at 5-year intervals are recommended. For those without risk factors for heart disease, initial cholesterol screening should begin at age 45 in women and age 35 in men. Screening should occur earlier in those with risk factors, such as diabetes or a significant family history of heart disease or hypercholesterolemia. The fact that this patient smokes places her at a higher risk for heart disease than the average individual and smoking cessation should be a high priority in this individual. An ECG is important for detecting heart disease in a symptomatic individual, but it is not recommended as a routine screening exam. A chest x-ray and pulse oximeter reading are also not indicated in an asymptomatic individual—even one with a smoking history.

Mammography is recommended every 1 or 2 years beginning at age 40. Mammograms should be continued in women up to age 70 and beyond, depending on the presence of comorbid conditions that may limit life expectancy. Pap smears are one of the most effective screening tests. PAP smears should be performed at least every 3 years for sexually active individuals. More frequent testing is indicated in higher risk individuals. Unfortunately, other than cervical, colorectal, and breast cancer, few other common cancers have screening procedures that meet the screening criteria. For example, some tests have low sensitivity (e.g., CA125 for ovarian cancer), or in other cancers early treatment may not be effective.

Problem 43

Herpes zoster (shingles) is a common viral eruption that is due to the reactivation of the varicella-zoster virus (VZV). Varicella, which is the virus that causes chickenpox, usually affects children and then lies dormant in a nerve ganglion until reactivation occurs. It has been suggested that all people who have had chickenpox harbor latent virus and that about one-half of individuals who live to age 85 will have an attack of zoster. Pain usually precedes the rash by 48 hours or more followed by the appearance of grouped vesicles on an erythematous base in a dermatomal distribution. More than one-half of patients have involvement of one or more thoracic dermatomes. The next most common area is the face, followed by the cervical and lumbar dermatomes. Shingles is communicable by direct contact with the rash, which is in contrast to chickenpox, which has an airborne means of spread. Approximately one in eight patients have a complication, of which the most common is postherpetic neuralgia. Postherpetic neuralgia occurs most commonly in patients older than age 50. Most often, the diagnosis of shingles can be made clinically by the characteristic dermatomal pattern and appearance. However, other vesicular rashes such as poison ivy can occur unilaterally and may at times be confused with zoster. A Tzank smear, which demonstrates the presence of multinucleated giant cells, strongly supports the diagnosis. Dermatomal zoster as seen in this case does not imply the presence of an underlying malignancy. However, generalized disease does raise the suspicion of underlying immunosuppression from diseases such as lymphoma or HIV.

The goal of therapy is to relieve pain, dry the vesicles, and prevent complications. If mild analgesics such as acetaminophen or aspirin are ineffective, then stronger pain medication such as codeine is indicated. Calamine lotion or wet compresses of Burow's solution are topical agents that may help provide some relief of symptoms and, if started within 48 hours, may help dry the lesions. Antiviral medication such as acyclovir can reduce the incidence of postherpetic neuralgia and also may alleviate the need for stronger pain medications. Since VZV is less sensitive to acyclovir than herpes simplex virus, high-dose therapy is recommended (e.g., acyclovir 800 mg 5 times a day instead of 200 mg). There is evidence that the incidence of postherpetic neuralgia may be reduced by the early use of systemic steroids. If not contraindicated, a tapering 3-week course of steroids starting at 60mg/day should be considered in conjunction with antiviral therapy, particularly in patients older than age 50 who have a large number of lesions.

Tricyclic antidepressants are considered an effective therapy for postherpetic neuralgia and provide significant relief to about one-half of patients. The anticonvulsant gabapentin and topical capsaicin ointment are also effective, although capsaicin may produce a burning sensation. Regional nerve blocks may occasionally be needed for chronic pain. Vitamin B12 shots, although used by some physicians, are no more effective than placebo.

Problem 44

Upper respiratory infections (URIs) are among the most common illnesses encountered by a family physician. On average, children contract between six and eight colds annually compared to one or two per year in adults. The term rhinosinusitis is now preferred over the term sinusitis to describe an inflammatory process that occurs within the sinus cavity and nasal passages and is most commonly due to infection. Acute bacterial rhinosinusitis is the term used when the condition results from a bacterial infection. In children, approximately 5% to 10% of URIs develop into an acute bacterial rhinosinusitis, compared with approximately 0.5% to 2% in adults. Risk factors for developing bacterial infections include cystic fibrosis, allergies, diabetes, chronic dental disease, and immunosuppression.

Signs of sinusitis include fever, nasal discharge, cough, and sinus tenderness. Younger children may have mouth breathing, feeding problems, snoring, and halitosis. An acute bacterial infection is more likely when the patient experiences double sickening or a period when the URI seems to be resolving and then symptoms worsen. A purulent discharge lasting more than 5 to 7 days and maxillary pain are also associated with an increased likelihood of bacterial infection. However, clinical evaluation is unreliable in accurately distinguishing a bacterial from a viral infection. Sinus aspiration and cultures are the gold standards, but the procedure is invasive, expensive, and not practical in the primary care setting. Transillumination is of limited value and plain radiographs are not recommended for the routine diagnosis of sinusitis because of the poor sensitivity and specificity of these tests. Although CT scans are more sensitive tests for sinusitis, their use

should be reserved to define the anatomy in patients with chronic sinus disease, for those patients with an acute presentation unresponsive to therapy, or in cases with a suspected complication such as an orbital cellulitis or brain abscess.

The patient in this case does not merit antibiotic treatment. Most cases of upper respiratory viral infection are complicated by purulent discharge and sinus involvement. Initial therapy should be aimed at controlling symptoms and promoting sinus drainage, and most authorities recommend waiting for 7 days before initiating antibiotic treatment in uncomplicated cases. Antihistamines are generally not recommended except in cases in which allergies are believed to be playing an important role since they can dry secretions and hinder drainage. Topical decongestants may be helpful in relieving symptoms and promoting drainage by reducing blockage of the osteomeatal complex. However, their use should be limited to 3 days since overuse of topical decongestants can lead to rebound congestion and rhinitis medicamentosa. Saline nasal sprays are safe and may help liquefy and clear secretions. Expectorants such as guaifenesin are of questionable benefit despite their widespread use.

Problem 45

Some patients self-medicate with alcohol to help sleep. Although alcohol may help some people fall asleep, it disturbs sleep architecture and can worsen sleep disorders.

As people age, sleep architecture changes and elderly individuals tend to take longer to fall asleep, spend less time in deep sleep (stage 3 and stage 4), and experience more nocturnal awakenings. Older people are also more likely to have illnesses that interfere with sleep. Examples of medical conditions that interfere with sleep include congestive heart failure, gastroesophageal reflux, respiratory diseases (e.g., asthma), painful arthritis, Parkinson's disease, Alzheimer's disease, and endocrine disorders. Sleep apnea, which is defined as five or more episodes of apnea or hypo-apnea per hour, is also more common in the elderly.

Hypnagogic hallucinations, which are hallucinations that occur soon after falling asleep or upon awakening, are associated with narcolepsy. Other narcolepsy symptoms include cataplexy, which is abrupt loss of muscle strength following excitement or fear; sleep paralysis, which is global paralysis occurring at transitions between wakefulness and sleep; restless and disturbed sleep; and the sudden onset of daytime sleepiness.

Sleep apnea is the absence of breathing for at least 10 seconds while sleeping. It may result from obstruction of the upper airway (obstructive sleep apnea), failure of respiratory drive (central sleep apnea), or a combination of the two. Obstructive sleep apnea is estimated to affect 2% to 4% of middle-aged individuals. Symptoms include loud snoring, a disturbed or restless sleep, daytime sleepiness, and occasional reports from a bed partner that there is an irregular breathing or gasping episode. More than 20 episodes per hour correlates with an increased risk of complications and poor outcomes. Complications include hypercapnia from hypoventilation and hypoxemia. If severe and chronic, sleep apnea can result in pulmonary hypertension and cor pulmonale. Other complications include systemic hypertension, cardiac arrhythmias, and increased cardiovascular morbidity and mortality.

The patient's symptoms suggest the need for a formal sleep study. Empiric treatment with oxygen is not recommended because clinical evaluation alone lacks sufficient sensitivity and specificity. Likewise, periodic oximetry monitoring overnight is insufficient to make the diagnosis of sleep apnea. Although few routine studies are beneficial, a TSH to detect hypothyroidism is useful. Since obesity can contribute to obstruction and may help improve blood pressure, weight loss is recommended. Surgical approaches should be considered in patients with severe symptoms but only after more conservative measures have been tried. The most important drug intervention is to avoid sedative medications that might suppress respiration. The tricyclic antidepressant, protriptyline, which reduces REM sleep during which upper airway muscles are most relaxed, may provide some benefit. Theophylline is not indicated in obstructive apnea. Mechanical measures such as nasal continuous positive airway pressure are indicated for more severe cases of sleep apnea.

The clinical history and clinical examination (loud S2, hypertension, and obesity) suggest the described patient has sleep apnea. Changes in sleep position to the side instead of the back may also improve apnea. Commercial devices that attach to the back of the patient's garment to foster "side sleeping" are available.

Problem 46

Tobacco use remains the leading cause of preventable death in the United States. Approximately one-half of all regular smokers die prematurely of a tobacco-related disease, accounting for about one in five deaths. The age-related decline in FEV1 is much greater in smokers than in nonsmokers, and 90% of all adults with chronic COPD smoke. However, 2 years after smoking cessation the rate of decline in FEV1 improves to a rate parallel to that of nonsmokers. Other nonpulmonary-related diseases associated with smoking include atherosclerosis, osteoporosis, lower birth weight babies and oral, esophageal, bladder, cervical, laryngeal, and pancreatic malignancies. Secondhand smoke is also a health hazard, and there is a higher risk of asthma, respiratory infections, and lung cancer in household members of smokers.

Smoking cessation before age 35 eliminates much of the excess mortality and translates to about 7 more years of life when compared with continuing smokers. Smokers who quit after age 65 still show significant improvement in overall survival compared with nonsmokers. Individuals who stop smoking gain an average of 5 to 10 lbs, making this a concern for smokers contemplating quitting. Smoking cessation counseling should address this issue and include advice about diet and exercise. Even a brief counseling intervention of 3 minutes or less doubles the quit rate when compared with no intervention. However, most clinicians combine drug therapy with counseling. The FDA has approved bupropion and four nicotine replacement products (nicotine gum, transdermal patches, a nasal spray, and a vapor inhaler). In randomized trials, nicotine replacement therapy doubles the long-term (1-year) quit rates compared to placebo. Most trials yield smoking cessation rates between 40% and 60% at the end of drug therapy and 22% to 30% quit rates at 1 year. Nortriptyline and clonidine have also been found to improve quit rates but are not FDA approved for this indication. Although nicotine affects the cardiovascular system, nicotine replacement therapy is safe for patients with stable cardiovascular disease. Although the safety of nicotine replacement in patients with unstable angina or a recent myocardial infarction has not been studied, many experts believe the risk of nicotine replacement is lower than that of continued smoking.

The Public Health Service guidelines recommend using the four A's as a strategy to stop smoking: asking about smoking, advice to quit smoking and assessing readiness to quit, assisting patients to quit and offering pharmacologic therapy to help, and arranging follow-up. Part of the quitting strategy involves setting a quit date and scheduling a follow-up visit within 2 to 4 weeks after the quit date.

Picking a quit date results in an increased likelihood of smoking cessation compared with a gradual reduction in smoking.

As noted previously, nicotine replacement therapy increases the quit rate and should be offered to this patient. Bupropion, an antidepressant with dopaminergic and noradrenergic activity, doubles quit rates when combined with counseling compared to placebo. Buproprion lowers the seizure threshold and is contraindicated for patients with seizures or those at risk for seizures. Although many clinicians combine bupropion with nicotine replacement therapy, a trial showed that treatment with both did not lead to significantly improved quit rates (36% versus 30%). If used, bupropion is prescribed at 150 mg per day for 3 days, with an increase to 150 mg twice a day. Typically, it is continued for 7 to 12 weeks, although some individuals may require longer duration of therapy. Since bupropion raises the seizure threshold, it should not be used in this patient, who has a history of seizures. Nortriptyline has also been shown to be effective at doses of 75 to 100 mg daily. However, it should be started 10 to 28 days before the quit date. Nicotine withdrawal symptoms can include irritability, agitation, insomnia, anxiety, depressed mood, restlessness, and increased appetite. Symptoms begin as early as a few hours after the last cigarette, peak at 2 or 3 days, and generally resolve over a few weeks. Benzodiazepines are not recommended for treating tobacco withdrawal symptoms.

Problem 47

Dysuria is the sensation of discomfort with or after urination. There are multiple causes, depending on the patient's age and sexual activity. A penile discharge is usually a consequence of urethral inflammation or infection and may be the presenting sign of a sexually transmitted disease, particularly in a younger sexually active male with either a new or multiple sexual partners. Numerous bacteria and nonbacterial organisms can cause urethritis. A convenient way to group infections is to divide them into gonococcal (GC) and nongonococcal (NGU) etiologies. In men, gonorrhea causes a urethritis that typically presents with a 2- to 4-day history of dysuria and a purulent discharge, whereas NGU typically has a more indolent course and produces a scant mucoid discharge. However, symptoms for both infections can vary and there is overlap in the presentation. *Chlamydia trachomatis*, *Ureaplasma urealyticum*, and *Mycoplasma genitalium* are common causes of NGU. Trichomonas, which is a common cause of vaginitis in women, can also cause urethritis in men. Although candida may cause an external infection or balanitis, it does not cause urethritis. *Haemophilus ducreyi*, which causes chancroid, is characterized by one or more painful genital ulcers often accompanied by painful inguinal lymphadenopathy. Primary syphilis can cause a chancre to appear on the penis that begins as a reddened papule that ulcerates before healing with 2 to 4 weeks. Both do not cause urethritis. Other causes of urethritis include Reiter's syndrome, prostatitis, and, rarely, a urethral malignancy. Occasionally, a herpes infection or human papillomavirus can infect the urethra and cause a discharge.

The Gram stain finding of gram-negative intracellular diplococci suggests the presence of GC. A culture or testing with DNA amplification testing is appropriate to confirm the diagnosis. Culture has the advantage of being able to identify resistant strains. Testing for chlamydia with either DNA amplification testing or direct fluorescent antibody staining of a urethral smear is also appropriate because of the overlap in clinical presentation and because mixed infections occur in up to 40% of patients with GC urethritis. Patients with one STD are at risk for additional STDs, and obtaining an RPR to screen for syphilis is appropriate. In a healthy

Table 9.21 Clinical syndromes seen in sexually transmitted diseases

Clinical Syndrome	Common Etiologies	Clinical Findings	Laboratory Findings	Treatment
Urethritis (male)	*Neisseria gonorrhoeae, Chlamydia trachomatis, Ureaplasma urealyticum*	Dysuria, urethral discharge, fever, arthritis, Reiter's syndrome	Gram-negative diplo-cocci inside PMNs (*N. gonorrhoeae*); PMNs without organisms (NGU)	Third-generation cephalosporin *or* quinolone (*N. gonorrhoeae*); doxycycline *or* azithromycin *or* quinolone (NGU)*
Urethritis (female)	*N. gonorrhoeae, C. trachomatis, E. coli.*	Dysuria (without frequency and urgency), ± cervicitis	Pyuria	Third-generation cephalosporin *or* quinolone (*N. gonorrhoeae*); doxycycline *or* azithromycin *or* quinolone (NGU)*
Epididymitis	*C. trachomatis, N. gonorrhoeae,* Enterobacteriaceae	Testicular pain and tenderness (usually unilateral)	None specific	Third-generation cephalosporin (*N. gonorrhoeae*), *plus* doxycycline (*C. trachomatis*), quinolone (Enterobacteriaceae).
Vulvovaginitis	*Trichomonas vaginalis, Candida albicans*	Vulvar itching, "cottage cheese" discharge (candidiasis), vulvar, itching, purulent, malodorous discharge, mucosa visibly inflamed (*T. vaginalis*)	PMNs, budding yeast on KOH prep or Gram's stain (candidiasis), PMNs with motile organisms seen (trichomoniasis)	Intravaginal azoles (e.g., clotrimazole miconazole), (candidiasis); metronidazole (trichomoniasis)
Bacterial vaginosis	*Gardnerella vagrinalis, Mycoplasma hominis,* anaerobic bacteria	Malodorous, thin discharge (clear to white)	"Clue cells" on wet prep, replacement of Lactobacilli with mixed organisms of Gram's stain, few PMNs	Metronidazole (either orally or intravaginally)
Pelvic inflammatory disease	*C. trachomatis, N. gonorrhoeae*	Abdominal pain, purulent vaginal discharge cervicitis (purulent); nausea/vomiting, fever, cervical motion tenderness	Elevated WBC, PMNs in vaginal discharge gram-negative diplococci seen within PMNs (*N. gonorrhoeae*)	Inpatient: Third-generation cephalosporin or clindamycin and gentamicin *or* ampicillin/sulbactam *plus* doxycycline Outpatient: Third-generation cephalosporin × 1 *plus* doxycycline, *or* quinolone *plus* metronidazole*
Genital ulcers	Herpes simplex virus (HSV); *Treponema pallidum* (syphilis) *Haemophilus ducreyi* (chancroid)	Painful ulcers (HSV, chancroid); painless ulcers (syphilis); painful ulcers and inguinal adenopathy with overlying erythema (chancroid)	Multinucleated giant cells/positive DFA/viral culture (HSV); spirochetes seen on darkfield microscopy (syphilis); isolation of *H. ducreyi* from lesion or lymph node aspirate	Acyclovir (HSV); benzathine penicillin G (syphilis); single IM dose for early disease, three doses for late disease (neurosyphilis requires intravenous therapy), doxycycline for penicillin allergy; ceftriaxone or azithromycin (chancroid)

Table 9.21 (continued)

Clinical Syndrome	Common Etiologies	Clinical Findings	Laboratory Findings	Treatment
Genital warts	Human papilloma virus	Visible papillomas, associated with the development of epithelial cancers	Molecular typing is available, but not usually needed to make the diagnosis	Local wart removal (cryosurgery, laser surgery, podophyllin)
Hepatitis	Hepatitis B virus, possibly hepatitis C virus, hepatitis A (fecal–oral contact)	Fever, hepatomegaly, abdominal pain	Elevated liver transaminases; serologic testing available	None available

PMN, polymorphonuclear lymphocyte; NGU, non-gonococcal urethritis.

*When treating presumed *Neisseria gonorrhoeae* infection, empric treatment for *Chlamydia trachomatis* is also added unless ruled out by definitive (e.g., DNA) tesing.

young male with localized urethritis, a CBC is unlikely to be abnormal and is not indicated. Reiter's syndrome presents with urethritis accompanied by musculoskeletal symptoms, conjuctivitis and iritis, fever, and skin manifestations such as circinate balanitis and keratoderma blennorrhagicum. If clinically suspected, patients can be checked for the presence of the HLA-B27 histocompatibility antigen, which is associated with the disorder. However, the presence of HLA-B27 is not diagnostic for Reiter's syndrome.

Although penicillin and its derivatives were considered first-line treatment for GC urethritis for many years, the increase in resistance of gonococcal isolates to penicillin and tetracycline makes these agents inappropriate for empiric treatment. Oral alternatives to the penicillins include cefixime, ciprofloxacin, or ofloxacin. Because up to 40% of patients with GC have a concomitant chlamydia infection, this patient should also be treated with azithromycin 1 g orally once or doxycycline 100 mg bid for 1 week. Since this patient most likely has GC, recommending that the partner be treated is appropriate.

A more comprehensive summary of clinical syndromes seen in STDs is listed in Table 9.21.

Problem 48

Recurrent UTIs are defined as more than three episodes in 12 months. Recurrent UTIs in women are usually secondary to altered vaginal flora and not structural abnormalities of the urinary tract. Spermicides with nonoxynol-9 are known to kill vaginal *Lactobacillus* species but not coliforms such as *E. coli*. There is an association between the frequency of sexual intercourse and the number of recent partners with UTIs even though UTI is not classified as a sexually transmitted disease. *Escherichia coli* causes the vast majority of recurrent UTIs. The second most likely pathogen in women of college age is *Staphylococcus saprophyticus*. It causes more than 20% of cystitis episodes in this age group but decreases in incidence in older age groups. Other common organisms are *Klebsiella* and *Proteus* species. In women with recurrent UTIs, these

organisms from the perineal region gain entrance to the urethra often during intercourse.

Cranberry juice has been touted as a dietary measure to decrease UTIs and was shown to be effective in several poorer quality studies. However, good quality placebo-controlled randomized trials are lacking. A recent Cochrane database analysis reported that there was insufficient evidence to take a position for or against the recommendation of cranberry juice for UTIs.

The yield of imaging studies and cystoscopies in women with recurrent cystitis is poor. The overwhelming majority of these women have altered vaginal flora, not anatomic abnormalities. Despite the known incidence of vaginal flora alteration in this setting, vaginal culture for coliforms or *Lactobacillus* species is not recommended as part of clinical practice.

Even in women with recurrent postcoital UTIs, the organism is not usually identifiable on their sexual partner and culturing the partner is not indicated.

A number of nonpharmacologic and pharmacologic interventions have been recommended for recurrent UTIs. Although never tested in controlled studies, voiding after intercourse continues to be recommended, especially for women with postcoital UTIs. Atrophic vaginitis and the changes in vaginal flora result in an increased risk for UTIs. Treatment with estrogen may reduce the frequency of infection. UTIs have been associated with vaginal spermicides, and alternative contraceptive measures should be considered in women experiencing recurrent UTIs.

Several pharmacologic options are available for women with recurrent cystitis. A single-strength trimethoprim-sulfamethoxazole taken daily for 6 to 12 months reduces the frequency of infection. Postcoital double-strength trimethoprim-sulfamethoxazole or "prn" single-dose treatments at the onset of symptoms are also effective. Nitrofurantoin prophylaxis can be used as an alternative in patients who are pregnant or wishing to conceive. There is a high spontaneous resolution rate in women with recurrent UTIs, and the need for further therapy should be reassessed at 6 to 12 months.

Although prolonged antibiotic courses of 2 weeks are appropriate in pyelonephritis or those at risk for pyelonephritis from a UTI (pregnancy, known tract abnormalities, etc.), treating cystitis episodes longer than 2 weeks has not been shown to decrease the recurrence rate in recurrent cystitis.

Problem 49

All women of childbearing age with abnormal vaginal bleeding should be tested for pregnancy. A complete blood count is helpful

Table 9.22 Etiology of abnormal vaginal bleeding

Causes	Example
Dysfunction uterine bleeding	Immature hypothalamic–pituitary–ovarian axis Perimenopause Obesity Polycystic ovarian syndrome
Pregnancy complications	Threatened, incomplete, or spontaneous abortion Ectopic or molar pregnancy
Infectious causes	Pelvic inflammatory disease Chronic endometritis
Anatomic lesions	Fibroids Endometriosis Polyps Neoplasms Endometrial hyperplasia
Medications	Oral contraceptives Warfarin Aspirin Tricyclic antidepressants Major tranquilizers
Coagulapathies	Leukemia Aplastic anemia Von Willebrand's disease Idiopathic thrombocytopenic purpura Platelet defects Thalassemia major
Systemic illness	Adrenal disorders Thryoid dysfunction Renal insufficiency Hepatic failure Diabetes mellitus
Intrauterine device	
Trauma	

Reproduced with permission from Mick N, Peters J, Silvers S, et al. *Blueprints in Emergency Medicine*. Malden: Blackwell Science; 2002:126.

for ruling out an iron deficiency anemia. Pap smear testing is indicated in a sexually active woman without a recent examination. Thyroid dysfunction may present with menstrual irregularity and obtaining TSH is indicated, particularly in the presence of symptoms suggesting thyroid disease.

Abnormal vaginal bleeding is bleeding that occurs less than 21 or more than 36 days after the last period or in excessive amounts. Terms used to describe abnormal bleeding include menorrhagia—excessive bleeding both in amount and in duration at regular intervals; metrorrhagia—bleeding at irregular intervals; menometrorrhagia—frequent, irregular, excessive and prolonged episodes of bleeding; and oligomenorrhea—infrequent, irregular bleeding episodes at intervals of more than 45 days. In a younger woman as described in this case with a normal examination, a functional disturbance of the hypothalamic–pituitary–ovarian axis is usually the cause. Abnormal bleeding that is excessive (greater than 60 to 80 cc) or is prolonged (longer than 7 days) in the absence of an anatomic lesion or systemic illness is often referred to as dysfunctional uterine bleeding. Dysfunctional bleeding is associated with thyroid disorders, diabetes, polycystic ovarian disease, emotional and physical stress, obesity, anorexia, excessive exercise, and iron deficiency. The etiology of abnormal vaginal bleeding is summarized in Table 9.22. Cervical cultures may be helpful if there is a history of multiple partners, vaginal discharge, and cervical motion tenderness or adnexal tenderness. In an 18-year-old female with a normal examination and a history of stress as a possible cause, ordering a pelvic ultrasound is not indicated. Likewise, endometrial sampling in this case is not indicated unless symptoms persist. Endometrial sampling is indicated in older women to exclude endometrial hyperplasia or uterine cancer.

Since the patient desires contraception, an estrogen and progesterone-containing pill can both regulate periods and provide contraception. Depo-medroxyprogesterone acetate, 150 mg every 3 months, provides contraception and may reduce excessive bleeding. Acute bleeding in a stable individual can be stopped with a course of oral progesterone or by using an intramuscular injection of progesterone. However, this patient is not actively bleeding. Clomiphene therapy should be considered in a patient with chronic anovulatory periods who desires pregnancy. Addressing other factors such as emotional stress or anorexia is also an important component of treatment.

NSAIDs may reduce bleeding by as much as 50% and as an additional benefit may provide relief from associated dysmenorrhea. Since this patient exhibits a mild anemia, she is most likely iron deficient and prescribing iron would be helpful. Confirming the diagnosis with serum iron studies, or monitoring her response to iron therapy (e.g., increase in reticulocyte count or hemoglobin), is also indicated.

Problem 50

Some degree of vaginal discharge is normal. However, a change in color, an increase in amount, or a discharge accompanied by an odor characterize an abnormal discharge.

The differential diagnosis of a vaginal discharge includes both infectious and noninfectious causes. Infectious causes include bacterial vaginosis (BV), trichomonal vaginosis, and candidal vulvovaginitis (CVV) and chlamydial or gonococcal cervicitis. Noninfectious causes include atrophic vaginitis, increased physiologic secretions, allergic reactions (e.g., to perfume or deodorant), foreign bodies such as a retained tampon or sponge, physical irritation from spermicides, or frequent douching. Rarely, genital tract neoplasm can also present with a discharge.

Cervicitis is more common in patients with multiple sexual partners. Although patients may be asymptomatic, symptoms of cervicitis include a mucopurulent discharge that may be accompanied by lower abdominal pain, fever, or dysuria. Physical examination may reveal a friable cervix accompanied by a mucopurulent discharge coming from the cervical os. The absence of risk factors for cervicitis and the patient's symptoms suggest a true vaginitis rather than a cervicitis.

Ninety percent of vaginitis is due to BV, CVV, or trichomonas. BV, formerly known as nonspecific vaginitis, is the most common cause of infectious vaginitis. It accounts for about one-third of all cases. BV is believed to represent an alteration of the bacterial flora causing an overgrowth of anaerobes. *Gardnerella vaginalis* is considered to be the key factor in BV, but its role in the pathogenesis of BV is incompletely understood. *Gardnerella* can also be cultured in a healthy asymptomatic person. CVV is the second most common cause.

BV and yeast are not generally considered to be sexually transmitted. Trichomonas, which is the least common cause of infectious vaginitis, is a protozoan usually transmitted by sexual contact.

CVV is caused by the *Candida* species of fungi, usually *Candida albicans*. CVV infections typically cause a vaginal and/or vulvar itching and are often accompanied by a thick, white vaginal discharge. Risk factors for *Candida* vaginitis include recent use of antibiotics, oral contraceptives, the use of systemic steroids, pregnancy, poorly controlled diabetes, and obesity. Noncandidal yeast infections are more common in immunocompromised individuals.

Determining the pH of the vaginal discharge can be useful. Nitrazine paper turns blue if the pH is greater than 4.5. The pH of a normal physiologic discharge or the discharge seen with a yeast vaginitis is usually less than 4.5. A pH greater than 4.5 suggests trichomonas or BV. The patient's symptoms and physical examination strongly suggest yeast vaginitis. Patients with BV more commonly have a thin, grayish, homogeneous discharge accompanied by a fishy odor. The discharge associated with trichomonas is more profuse with a yellow to greenish discoloration.

The clinical evaluation of vaginitis is inexact and most authorities recommend collecting a sample of the discharge for a wet mount, KOH, and, if appropriate, culturing the secretions. The wet mount may identify clue cells, which are epithelial cells that have a granular or glittery appearance due to the adherence of bacteria. Specific organisms such as trichomonas or yeast may also be identified on a wet mount. Although white blood cells can be seen with CVV or BV, numerous white blood cells on wet mount are most commonly seen with trichomonas vaginitis, atrophic vaginitis, or cervicitis. A "whiff test" is performed by checking for a fishy odor when a few drops of 10% of KOH are added to a vaginal discharge. A positive whiff test suggests BV and will most likely be negative in this patient. A KOH prep lyses epithelial cells but not fungal walls, making it easier to identify hyphae and spores. This test is very specific but has only about a 60% sensitivity. A Gram stain is more sensitive but is more difficult to obtain in the office setting. Although conditions such as diabetes mellitus and HIV are associated with yeast infections, testing for these conditions is usually reserved for those patients with risk factors or recurrent yeast infections.

In the case described, the presence of hyphae confirmed the diagnosis of yeast vaginitis. Treatment regimens include a single oral dose of fluconazole (150 mg) and topical imidazoles such as clotrimazole, miconazole, and terconazole. Although ketoconazole can cure yeast vaginitis, it is usually reserved for recalcitrant infections because of its potential toxicity. Metronidazole is indicated for bacterial vaginitis and trichomonas. The treatment of sexual partners is indicated for trichomonas vaginitis but not for bacterial vaginitis. Topical treatment for a partner with recurrent yeast infections is sometimes recommended in patients with recurrent symptoms. However, an iminazole preparation is used rather than metronidazole gel, which is not active against yeast. Treating the sexual partner is indicated for trichomonas.

Index